Medical Coding Certification Exam Preparation

A COMPREHENSIVE GUIDE

Cynthia L. Stewart, CPC, CPC-H, CPMA, CPC-I, CCS-P

Manhattan Area Technical College

Cynthia L. Ward, CPC, CPC-H, CPMA, CEMC, CCC

Medtech College

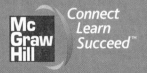

Mc Graw Hill

Connect
Learn
Succeed™

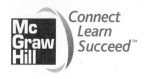

The McGraw-Hill Companies

MEDICAL CODING CERTIFICATION EXAM PREPARATION: A COMPREHENSIVE GUIDE
Published by McGraw-Hill, a business unit of The McGraw-Hill Companies, Inc., 1221 Avenue of the Americas,
New York, NY, 10020. Copyright © 2014 by The McGraw-Hill Companies, Inc. All rights reserved. Printed in
the United States of America. No part of this publication may be reproduced or distributed in any form or
by any means, or stored in a database or retrieval system, without the prior written consent of The McGraw-
Hill Companies, Inc., including, but not limited to, in any network or other electronic storage or transmission,
or broadcast for distance learning.

Some ancillaries, including electronic and print components, may not be available to customers outside the
United States.

This book is printed on acid-free paper.

1 2 3 4 5 6 7 8 9 0 DOW/DOW 1 0 9 8 7 6 5 4 3

ISBN 978-0-07-786205-3
MHID 0-07-786205-8

Senior Vice President,
Products & Markets: *Kurt L. Strand*
Vice President, General Manager,
Products & Markets: *Martin J. Lange*
Vice President, Content Production &
Technology Services: *Kimberly Meriwether David*
Executive Brand Manager: *Natalie J. Ruffatto*
Director of Development: *Rose Koos*
Managing Development Editor:
Michelle L. Flomenhoft
Development Editor: *Raisa Priebe Kreek*
Development Editor: *Jessica Dimitrijevic*
Digital Product Analyst: *Katherine Ward*

Project Manager: *Kathryn D. Wright*
Buyer II: *Debra R. Sylvester*
Senior Designer: *Srdjan Savanovic*
Cover/Interior Designer: *Ellen Pettengell*
Cover Images: lung: *Ingram Publishing;* x-ray: *Fisherss
Artwork/© 2011 KuanZhang;* otoscope: *© Ocean/Corbis;*
acoustic device: *© Tetra Images/Alamy*
Content Licensing Specialist: *Joanne Mennemeier*
Manager, Digital Production: *Janean A. Utley*
Media Project Manager: *Cathy L. Tepper*
Typeface: *10.5/13 Palatino*
Compositor: *Aptara®, Inc.*
Printer: *R. R. Donnelley*

All credits appearing on page or at the end of the book are considered to be an extension of the copyright page.

Library of Congress Cataloging-in-Publication Data

Stewart, Cynthia L. (Cynthia Lorraine), 1963-
  Medical coding certification exam preparation : a comprehensive guide / Cynthia L. Stewart,
Cynthia L. Ward.
     p. ; cm.
  Includes bibliographical references and index.
  ISBN 978-0-07-786205-3 (alk. paper)—ISBN 0-07-786205-8 (alk. paper)
  I. Ward, Cynthia L. (Cynthia Louise), 1949- II. Title.
  [DNLM: 1. Clinical Coding. 2. Problems and Exercises.   WX 18.2]

  616.0076 — dc23

                                     2012050072

All brand or product names are trademarks or registered trademarks of their respective companies.
CPT five-digit codes, nomenclature, and other data are © 2013 American Medical Association. All rights
reserved. No fee schedules, basic units relative values, or related listings are included in CPT. The AMA
assumes no liability for the data contained herein.

CPT codes are based on CPT 2013.
ICD-9-CM codes are based on ICD-9-CM 2013.
ICD-10-CM codes are based on ICD-10-CM 2013.
All names, situations, and anecdotes are fictitious.
They do not represent any person, event, or medical record.
The Internet addresses listed in the text were accurate at the time of publication. The inclusion of a website
does not indicate an endorsement by the authors or McGraw-Hill, and McGraw-Hill does not guarantee the
accuracy of the information presented at these sites.

www.mhhe.com

BRIEF CONTENTS

UNIT FIVE   Coding for Radiology, Pathology/Laboratory, General Medicine, HCPCS Category II and III, and Practice Management   447

● CONTENTS

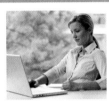
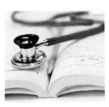
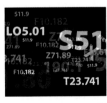
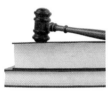
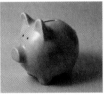

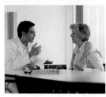
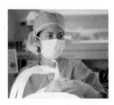
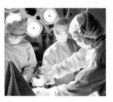
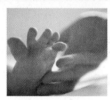
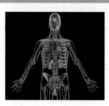

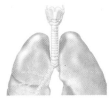

CHAPTER ELEVEN

Surgery Section:
Respiratory System 215

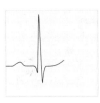

CHAPTER TWELVE

Surgery Section:
Cardiovascular and
Lymphatic Systems 244

UNIT FOUR Coding for Surgical Procedures on Digestive, Urinary, Male and Female Reproductive Systems, Maternity Care, Nervous System, and Eyes, Ears, and Endocrine System 285

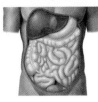

CHAPTER THIRTEEN

Surgery Section:
Digestive System 286

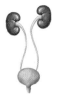

CHAPTER FOURTEEN

Surgery Section: Urinary
System and Male
Reproductive System 323

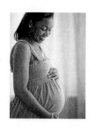
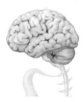
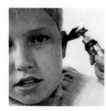
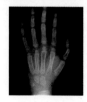

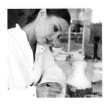
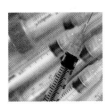
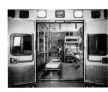
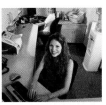
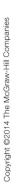

DEDICATION

This book is dedicated to my father, Lee Stewart, who taught me that to learn was only the beginning of a journey—teaching others is the real destination and goal of learning.

—Cynthia Stewart

ABOUT THE AUTHORS

Cynthia L. Stewart, CPC, CPC-H, CPMA, CPC-I, CCS-P

Cynthia has more than 25 years of experience in the medical profession. In the past 16 years she has applied her knowledge and skills in several capacities, providing coding and billing direction as a billing supervisor, practice manager, senior coding specialist, coding and reimbursement consultant, and revenue cycle systems manager of coding and charge entry. As an educator Cynthia was the Director of the Medical Billing and Coding Specialist and Healthcare Management academic programs at Medtech College, Indianapolis campus, and she currently provides direction and instruction at Manhattan Area Technical College. She is an AAPC ICD-10-CM trainer and a workshop presenter, and she has provided instruction through her work as a reviewer, contributing author, and research assistant for various coding and billing texts and periodicals.

Cynthia has been a member of the American Academy of Professional Coders since 1998, serving as the President of the Central Indiana chapter in Indianapolis prior to serving as the 2011–2013 National Advisory Board President. She enjoys spending time with her son Adam, daughter Callie, and grandchildren, Keegan, Mady, and Jaxson. She lives in Fostoria, Kansas, with her boyfriend Shaun, his son Chance, and a small zoo of various pets and farm animals.

Cynthia Ward, CPC, CPC-H, CPMA, CEMC, CCC

Cynthia Ward has 40 years of experience in the healthcare field. She has worked for dermatology, radiology, and cardiology practices in Indianapolis, Indiana. Cynthia held the positions of coding supervisor, billing manager, and coding compliance director during her employment with these practices. For the last 5 years she has provided instruction and direction as Program Director for the Billing and Coding program at Medtech College, Greenwood, Indiana campus. Cynthia has also consulted with practices and taught residents and medical students and has provided instruction through her work as a reviewer for various coding and billing texts.

Cynthia has been a member of the AAPC since 1996 and was a member of the local chapter advisory board for 10 years. Cynthia lives in Indianapolis with her husband, Bob, a retired special education teacher, and her daughter, Emily, who is pursuing a career in coding.

Overview

Medical Coding Certification Exam Preparation is designed to aid in the review for the Certified Professional Coder (CPC) exam. However, much of the information included in this text will also assist the coder in preparation for other coding certification exams. While not intended to be an introduction to medical coding, this text provides an extensive review of the topics students need to know for the CPC exam, including coverage of anatomy, medical terminology, and pathophysiology, as well as the concepts, guidelines, and rules of medical coding. Based on their significant teaching experience and affiliations with AAPC, authors Cynthia Stewart and Cynthia Ward bring a fresh approach to preparing for the exam. The book is organized around the principle that students need the means to learn how to analyze cases and how to then translate services, procedures, and diagnoses from those cases into codes. The importance of understanding and knowing how to locate and use the guidelines inherent to the ICD, CPT, and HCPCS coding manuals is emphasized throughout the book with the use of **Spotlights** and **Mentor Coding Tips.** Each chapter contains questions similar to those found on the CPC exam. In addition, each of the five units of the book ends with a Unit Exam, meant to be a cumulative review. Finally, the book concludes with a comprehensive practice exam on the use of ICD-9-CM codes. (An ICD-10-CM exam is also available to help prepare students for the ICD-10-CM proficiency exam in development by AAPC.) Additional practice is available through *Connect Plus*, McGraw-Hill's online assignment and assessment tool.

A Note from the Authors on Why They Wrote This Book

We began our journey with this text because we felt there was a need to look at preparing coders for the exam and their future career in medical coding in a different way. In our experience as instructors, we found that practicing for the exam by routinely going through numerous cases studies did not benefit the coder in truly understanding why the codes selected were correct or how the codes are supported by the provider's documentation. During our tenure as instructors, we have learned that our students needed the tools to understand how to break the case down and translate services, procedures, and diagnoses into codes. Our purpose in writing this text is to aid the instructor and coder in bringing all of the individually learned pieces together to complete the process of medical coding.

How to Use the Book

As stated in the overview, this book is not designed as, or intended to be used as, an introduction to medical coding. The reader should have an understanding of and foundation in medical coding. Instead, this book is designed to aid in review for the CPC exam.

While preparing for the exam with this text, you will also need:

- Current CPT manual—standard or professional edition (professional edition is author-recommended).
- Current ICD-9-CM manual.
- ICD-10-CM manual (optional).
- Current HCPCS manual.
- A medical dictionary.
- A comprehensive anatomy text.

Throughout this text, instructions identify certain areas, guidelines, or notes within the coding manuals that you should highlight or otherwise flag to remind yourself of the information and to access it quickly when you are taking the exam. To this end, you are encouraged to work through this text with each of the coding manuals open and to use them as additional resources, thus reinforcing the information available to you during the exam.

Organization of *Medical Coding Certification Exam Preparation*

Here is an overview of the five units of the book:

UNIT	COVERAGE
1. Fundamental Coding Guidelines	Discusses coding as a career and the many reasons to become certified. This unit reviews ICD-9-CM and ICD-10-CM coding formats and guidelines. ICD chapter-specific guidelines on conditions such as HIV, septicemia, neoplasms, and diabetes are also found within this unit, along with CPT coding applications.
2. Coding for Evaluation/ Management (E/M), Anesthesia, and Surgery	Provides a review of evaluation and management coding. Specific guidelines along with valuable coding tips for anesthesia procedures and general surgery are included as well.
3. Coding for Surgical Procedures on Integumentary, Musculoskeletal, Respiratory, and Cardiovascular/ Lymphatic Systems	Serves as a comprehensive guide to anatomy, medical terminology, and ICD and CPT coding for the integumentary, musculoskeletal, respiratory, and cardiovascular/lymphatic systems. The use of modifiers with codes for each of these systems is also reviewed.
4. Coding for Surgical Procedures on Digestive, Urinary, Male and Female Reproductive Systems, Maternity Care, Nervous System, and Eyes, Ears, and Endocrine System	Gives an in-depth overview of the urinary, male reproductive, female reproductive, nervous, and endocrine systems' anatomy, ICD and CPT coding, and appropriate use of modifiers with codes for these systems. Coding information is also included for the eyes, ears, and adnexa.
5. Coding for Radiology, Pathology/ Laboratory, General Medicine, HCPCS Category II and III, and Practice Management	Details medical terms, types of procedures, and coding guidelines and their application for radiology, pathology/laboratory, and general medicine services and procedures. Coding foundations for such services as diagnostic imaging, nuclear medicine, drug testing, surgical microscopic exams, immunizations, cardiac procedures, and dialysis are provided. A review of HCPCS coding guidelines, as well as category II and category III code definitions, is found here. This unit also provides a review of practice management issues such as ABNs, compliance, and HIPAA and their effect on coding.

Key Points about the Book

The importance of understanding the guidelines inherent to the ICD, CPT, and HCPCS coding manuals and knowing how to locate and use them is stressed throughout this text by the frequent use of special-feature boxes:

- **Spotlights** within each chapter refer the coder to or provide additional information and direction on specific procedures, conditions, guidelines, and practice management issues.

- **Mentor Coding Tips** are tips and shortcuts the authors have accumulated over the years and learned from other experienced coders in the trenches. These tips aid the coder in breaking down and retaining information necessary for the exam and everyday coding.

While all of the chapters in this text are presented differently from what you might find in other review guides, four chapters in particular should be noted:

- **Chapter Two, Foundations of ICD-9-CM, and Chapter Three, Foundations of ICD-10-CM** These chapters began as a single chapter. However, due to the complications of teaching two similar yet conceptually different coding systems, as well as medical coders' potential need to prepare for the upcoming ICD-10-CM proficiency exam, the authors were prompted to divide these code sets into individual chapters. The intent is for one or the other of these two chapters to be reviewed, depending on the examinee's need. Information about the ICD-10-CM code set is included in Chapters 9 through 20 to help coders gain familiarity with these codes.

- **Chapter Four, ICD Chapter-Specific Guidelines** This chapter includes the four ICD-9-CM coding guidelines that the authors have found to be the most difficult for students and coders to interpret and use: those pertaining to human immunodeficiency virus; septicemia, systemic inflammatory response syndrome (SIRS), sepsis, severe sepsis, and septic shock; neoplasms; and diabetes mellitus. Chapter-specific guidelines pertaining to other ICD chapters are included in the relevant CPT surgery subsection chapters, Chapters 9 through 20.

- **Chapter Eight, Surgery** This chapter begins the Surgery section of CPT. Included is a step-by-step process of documentation analysis. This series of questions maps out many of the thought processes that experienced coders engage in when reviewing operative reports and other documentation. Walking through this process for each case study will help instill this approach in the coder.

It is important to note that *not everything* within the CPT, ICD, and HCPCS coding manuals is addressed in this text. The authors did address concepts and guidelines that in their experience as instructors tended to be difficult for examinees and new coders to master. Taking into account the various learning types, they created and added decision trees for a few of the most difficult coding concepts: pregnancy trimester episode of care, human immunodeficiency, and sepsis, SIRS, and septicemia. Each chapter contains tables that outline the sections of the ICD-9-CM and CPT code sets. Also included in Chapters 9 through 20 are tables comparing ICD-9-CM and ICD-10-CM code sets.

From a pedagogical standpoint, a variety of methods have been included for students to practice applying and developing their skills: review exercises at the end of each chapter section, end-of-chapter reviews and cases studies utilizing the documentation analysis tool where appropriate, and a cumulative unit exam at the end of each unit, designed to prepare students for the final exam at the end of the book (covering ICD-9-CM). The questions in both the unit exams and the final exam are presented in the style of the actual CPC exam questions.

In addition, to help prepare coders for the upcoming ICD-10-CM proficiency exam, the authors have also prepared a final exam covering ICD-10-CM. At the time that this practice exam was developed, very little information regarding the format of the AAPC ICD-10-CM proficiency exam was known. Therefore, the proficiency exam is formatted in a style similar to that of the ICD-9-CM practice exam included in this book.

Key Content Highlights
Pedagogy

- Learning outcomes and key terms are listed at the beginning of each chapter to set the stage for the content to come.
- Major chapter heads are structured to reflect the numbered learning outcomes.
- Key terms are defined in the margins for easy reference, and they are also listed in the Glossary near the end of the book.
- Tips, Spotlights, and Examples help students navigate through the material.
- Chapter summaries, organized by learning outcomes, are presented in a tabular, step-by-step format to help with review of the material.
- End-of-chapter elements are tagged with corresponding learning-outcome numbers.
- The Chapter Review section includes:
  - Using Terminology—matching questions with key terms and definitions.
  - Checking Your Understanding—multiple-choice questions.
  - Applying Your Knowledge—case studies.

Chapter by Chapter

- **Chapter One:** the language and roles of medical coding, benefits of credentialing your knowledge, and CPC exam format and test-taking skills.
- **Chapter Two:** ICD-9-CM manual format, abbreviations, coding conventions, and punctuation; ICD-9-CM chapter, general, section and chapter-specific guidelines; and translation of provider terminology to diagnostic codes.
- **Chapter Three:** ICD-10-CM manual format, abbreviations, coding conventions, and punctuation; ICD-10-CM chapter, general, section and chapter-specific guidelines; and new conventions in ICD-10-CM default codes, extenders, and placeholders.
- **Chapter Four:** ICD chapter-specific general guidelines related to human immunodeficiency virus (HIV) infections; septicemia, systemic inflammatory response syndrome (SIRS), sepsis, severe sepsis, and septic shock; neoplasms; and diabetes mellitus.
- **Chapter Five:** CPT format, conventions, instructional notes, guidelines, and symbols; CPT modifiers; CPT and ICD linkage; and translation of provider documentation to codes.
- **Chapter Six:** Evaluation and management (E/M) guidelines, modifiers, and types of services; and components and levels of an E/M code.

- **Chapter Seven:** anesthesia reimbursement formula and terminology; physical status, qualifying-circumstance modifiers, and HCPCS Level II modifiers; and locating of anesthesia terms in the CPT manual index.
- **Chapter Eight:** general guidelines and format of the Surgery section of the CPT manual; global surgical package and Surgery section modifiers; and use of the index to locate codes for surgical procedures.
- **Chapter Nine:** anatomy of the integumentary system; ICD-9-CM and CPT guidelines for diseases of the skin and subcutaneous tissue; Integumentary subsection modifiers; and common medical and procedural terms used in operative reports.
- **Chapter Ten:** anatomy of the musculoskeletal system; ICD-9-CM and CPT guidelines for diseases of the musculoskeletal system; musculoskeletal system modifiers; and common medical and procedural terms used in operative reports.
- **Chapter Eleven:** anatomy of the respiratory system; ICD-9-CM and CPT guidelines for diseases of the respiratory system; respiratory system modifiers; and common medical and procedural terms used in operative reports.
- **Chapter Twelve:** anatomy of the cardiovascular and lymphatic systems; ICD-9-CM and CPT guidelines for diseases of the cardiovascular system; ICD-9-CM and CPT guidelines for diseases of the lymphatic system; cardiovascular and lymphatic system modifiers; and common medical and procedural terms used in operative reports.
- **Chapter Thirteen:** anatomy of the digestive system; ICD-9-CM and CPT guidelines for diseases of the digestive system; digestive system modifiers; and common medical and procedural terms used in operative reports.
- **Chapter Fourteen:** anatomy of the urinary and male reproductive system; ICD-9-CM and CPT guidelines for diseases of the urinary system; ICD-9-CM and CPT guidelines for diseases of the male reproductive system; urinary and male reproductive system modifiers; and common medical and procedural terms used in operative reports.
- **Chapter Fifteen:** anatomy of the female reproductive system; ICD guidelines and format for complications of pregnancy, childbirth, and the puerperium; CPT guidelines for the female genital system and maternity care and delivery; subsection modifiers; and common medical and procedural terms used in operative reports.
- **Chapter Sixteen:** anatomy of the nervous system; ICD-9-CM and CPT guidelines for diseases of the nervous system; nervous system modifiers; and common medical and procedural terms used in operative reports.
- **Chapter Seventeen:** anatomy of the endocrine system, eye, ocular adnexa, and auditory system; ICD-9-CM guidelines for diseases of the eye, ocular adnexa, and auditory system; CPT guidelines for diseases of the endocrine system, eye, ocular adnexa, and auditory system; endocrine system, eye, ocular adnexa, and auditory system modifiers; and common medical and procedural terms used in operative reports.
- **Chapter Eighteen:** CPT guidelines for the Diagnostic Imaging, Ultrasound, Mammography, and Bone/Joint Studies subsection of the Radiology section; CPT guidelines for the Radiation Oncology and Nuclear Medicine subsections.
- **Chapter Nineteen:** CPT guidelines for pathology/laboratory coding; modifiers most commonly used with codes in the Pathology/Laboratory section of CPT; and common medical and procedural terms used in lab and operative reports.

- **Chapter Twenty:** CPT guidelines for the Medicine section; medical and procedural terms; and modifiers most commonly used with codes in the Medicine section.
- **Chapter Twenty-One:** HCPCS II guidelines and modifiers; common abbreviations and acronyms used in HCPCS Level II; CPT guidelines and format of category II and category III codes.
- **Chapter Twenty-Two:** AAPC professional code of ethics; definitions of providers and payers, including Medicare, Medicaid, TRICARE, and managed care entities; regulations and the parties responsible for maintaining and enforcing the regulations.

Medical Coding Certification Exam Preparation in the Digital World: Supplementary Materials for the Instructor and Student

Instructors, McGraw-Hill knows how much effort it takes to prepare for a new course. Through focus groups, symposia, reviews, and conversations with instructors like you, we have gathered information about what materials you need in order to facilitate successful courses. We are committed to providing you with high-quality, accurate instructor support. Knowing the importance of flexibility and digital learning, McGraw-Hill has created multiple assets to enhance the learning experience no matter what the class format: traditional, online, or hybrid. This product is designed to help instructors and students be successful, with digital solutions proven to drive student success.

A one-stop spot to present, deliver, and assess digital assets available from McGraw-Hill: McGraw-Hill *Connect* Medical Coding Certification Exam Preparation

McGraw-Hill *Connect* Medical Coding Certification Exam Preparation provides online presentation, assignment, and assessment solutions. It connects your students with the tools and resources they'll need to achieve success. With *Connect* you can deliver assignments, quizzes, and tests online. A robust set of questions and activities, including all of the end-of-section and end-of-chapter questions, all of the unit exams, multiple full practice exams (the ICD-9-CM exam from the book plus additional exams, as well as ICD-10-CM exams), interactives, and test bank questions, are presented and aligned with the textbook's learning outcomes. As an instructor, you can edit existing questions and author entirely new problems. *Connect* enables you to track individual student performance—by question, by assignment, or in relation to the class overall—with detailed grade reports. You can integrate grade reports easily with Learning Management Systems (LMSs), such as Blackboard, Desire2Learn, or eCollege—and much more. **Connect Plus Medical Coding Certification Exam Preparation** provides students with all the advantages of *Connect* Medical Coding Certification Exam Preparation *plus* 24/7 online access to an eBook. This media-rich version of the textbook is available through the McGraw-Hill *Connect* platform and allows seamless integration of text, media, and assessments. To learn more, visit **http://connect.mcgraw-hill.com.**

A single sign-on with Connect and your Blackboard course: McGraw-Hill Higher Education and Blackboard

Blackboard, the web-based course management system, has partnered with McGraw-Hill to better allow students and faculty to use online materials and activities to complement face-to-face teaching. Blackboard features exciting social learning and teaching tools that foster active learning opportunities for students. You'll transform your closed-door classroom into communities where students remain connected to their educational experience 24 hours a day. This partnership allows you and your students access to McGraw-Hill's *Connect* and *Create* right from within your Blackboard course—all with a single sign-on. Not only do you get single sign-on with *Connect* and *Create,* but you also get deep integration of McGraw-Hill content and content engines right in Blackboard. Whether you're choosing a book for your course or building *Connect* assignments, all the tools you need are right where you want them—inside Blackboard. Gradebooks are now seamless. When a student completes an integrated *Connect* assignment, the grade for that assignment automatically (and instantly) feeds into your Blackboard grade center. McGraw-Hill and Blackboard can now offer you easy access to industry leading technology and content, whether your campus hosts it or we do. Be sure to ask your local McGraw-Hill representative for details.

Create a textbook organized the way you teach: McGraw-Hill Create

With **McGraw-Hill** *Create,* you can easily rearrange chapters, combine material from other content sources, and quickly upload content you have written, such as your course syllabus or teaching notes. Find the content you need in *Create* by searching through thousands of leading McGraw-Hill textbooks. Arrange your book to fit your teaching style. *Create* even allows you to personalize your book's appearance by selecting the cover and adding your name, school, and course information. Order a *Create* book and you'll receive a complimentary print review copy in 3 to 5 business days or a complimentary electronic review copy (eComp) via e-mail in minutes. Go to **www.mcgrawhillcreate.com** today and register to experience how McGraw-Hill *Create* empowers you to teach *your* students *your* way.

Record and distribute your lectures for multiple viewing: My Lectures—Tegrity

McGraw-Hill Tegrity records and distributes your class lecture with just a click of a button. Students can view it anytime and anywhere via computer, iPod, or mobile device. It indexes as it records your PowerPoint presentations and anything shown on your computer, so students can use keywords to find exactly what they want to study. Tegrity is available as an integrated feature of **McGraw-Hill** *Connect* **Medical Coding Certification Exam Preparation** and as a stand-alone.

Introducing CodeitRightOnline Curriculum!

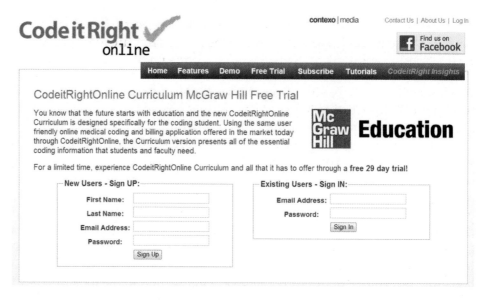

You know that the future starts with education and the new CodeitRightOnline Curriculum is designed specifically for the coding student. Using the same user friendly online medical coding and billing application offered in the market today through CodeitRightOnline, the Curriculum version presents all of the essential coding information that students and faculty need.

CodeitRightOnline Curriculum is offered to students and faculty for up to 12 months, depending on your subscription. You'll get:

- ICD-9-CM: all three volumes, guidelines, and notes
- CPT® codes, modifiers, guidelines, and notes
- HCPCS Level II codes, modifiers, guidelines, and notes
- ICD-10-CM and PCS codes and guidelines, and notes
- Ability to add notes
- E/M Guidelines accessible from the library
- ICD-9-CM official guidelines accessible from the library
- All the searching tools we have in the system
- The ability to make codes a "favorite"
- Anatomy and physiology games
- ICD-10-CM information from Contexo

Curriculum packages include a subscription for 3 months, 6 months, or 12 months. For a limited time, experience CodeitRightOnline Curriculum and all that it has to offer through a free 29-day trial! Simply visit www.codeitrightonline.com/mcgraw-hill to register for a free trial.

Curriculum Pricing:

3 months: $59.95

6 months: $79.95

12 months: $99.95

To learn more about CodeitRightOnline Curriculum, visit http://student.codeitrightonline.com.

CPT® is a registered trademark of the American Medical Association.

Instructor Resources

You can rely on the following materials to help you and your students work through the material in this book. All of these resources are available on the book's website, **www.mhhe.com/stewartcodingprep** (instructors can request a password through their sales representative):

SUPPLEMENT	FEATURES
Instructor's Manual (organized by learning outcomes)	• Lesson plans • Answer keys for all exercises
PowerPoint Presentations (organized by learning outcomes)	• Key terms • Key concepts • Teaching notes
Electronic Test Bank	• EZ Test Online (computerized) • Word version • Questions with tagging for learning outcomes, level of difficulty, level of Bloom's taxonomy, feedback, ABHES, CAAHEP, CAHIIM, and estimated time of completion
Tools to Plan Course	• Correlations of the learning outcomes to accrediting bodies such as ABHES CAAHEP, and CAHIIM • Sample syllabi • Asset Map—a recap of the key instructor resources, as well as information on the content available through *Connect Plus*

Need help? Contact McGraw-Hill's Customer Experience Group (CXG). Visit the CXG website at **www.mhhe.com/support.** Browse our FAQs (frequently asked questions) and product documentation and/or contact a CXG representative. CXG is available Sunday through Friday.

Want to learn more about this product? Attend one of our online webinars. To learn more about the webinars, please contact your McGraw-Hill sales representative. To find your McGraw-Hill representative, go to **www.mhhe.com** and click "Find My Sales Rep."

ACKNOWLEDGMENTS

Suggestions have been received from faculty and students throughout the country. This is vital feedback that is relied on for product development. Each person who has offered comments and suggestions has our thanks. The efforts of many people are needed to develop and improve a product. Among these people are the reviewers and consultants who point out areas of concern, cite areas of strength, and make recommendations for change. In this regard, the following instructors provided feedback that was enormously helpful in preparing the manuscript.

Manuscript Reviews

Many instructors reviewed the manuscript while it was in development, providing valuable feedback that directly impacted the book.

Yvonne Denise Arnold-Jenkins, CMRS, NRCMA, CPC
Remington College

Kathleen Bailey, CPA, MBA, CPC, CPC-I
Everest University

Carolle Battiste, BS, MS
Baker College-Flint

Earl Bills, MAE, CPC
Florida Career College

Suzanne Bitters, RMA, NCICS
Harris School of Business–Wilmington

Tamarra Disco Boggs, CPC, CCP, MCS-P
Bluegrass Community and Technical College

Geraldine Brasin
Premier Education Group

Teresa Buglione, CPC, AHI
Clayton State University

Mary Cantwell, RHIA, CPC, CPC-H, CPC-P, CPC-I
Metro Community College

Michelle Cranney, RHIT, CCS-P, CPC, AHIMA-approved ICD-10-CM/PCS trainer
Everett Community College

Amy Ensign, CMA, RMA
Baker College of Clinton Township

Daniel Figueroa, CBCS, CICS, CPAT
Florida Career College

Amy Files, BS, CPC
Davis College

Madeline Flanagan, MA, CPC
Branford Hall Career Institute

Debi Forcier, CPC
Branford Hall Career Institute

Debbie Gilbert, RHIA, CMA
Dalton State College

Susan Hernandez
San Joaquin Valley College

Amy Jewell, BS, CPC
Baker College–Flint

Patricia King, MA, RHIA, RHIT
Baker College–Flint

Janice Manning, CPC, CMRS
Baker College

Fannie Sue Martin, CPC
YTI Career Institute

Wilsetta McClain, NCICS, NCPT, RMA
Baker College of Auburn Hills

Jeanne McTeigue, CPC
Branford Hall Career Institute

Toni Medina-Allen, CPC
Florida Career College

Susan Miedzianowski, CPC
Baker College

Lane Miller, CHI
Medical Career Institute

Lorraine Papazian-Boyce, CPC, AHIMA-approved ICD-10-CM/PCS trainer
Colorado Technical University Online

Gerry Pape, BA, CPC
Daytona College

Sue Pylant, CCS-P
Sanford-Brown College

Jerri Rowe, CPC
Medvance Institute

Lisa Schaffer, BA, JD, MBA
Newbridge College

Christine Sproles, CMT
Pensacola Christian College

Dr. David Stewart, D.C., FIAMA, DiplAc. IAMA, CPC
Sanford-Brown College–Hazelwood

Wanda Strayhan, CBCS
Florida Career College

Christina Thomas, CPC, CMAA, CCMA, CBCS
Florida Career College

Megan Tober, RHIA
Davenport University

Danielle Ulshafer, NCCT, CPC
Harris School of Business

Susan Ward, CPC, CPC-H, CPC-I, CPCD, CEMC, CPRC
AAPC West Valley Chapter

Market Surveys

Multiple instructors participated in a survey to help guide the early development of the product.

Yvonne Denise Arnold-Jenkins, CMRS, NRCMA, CPC
Remington College

Sheila Batts, CMA (AAMA), MBA
Kaplan Career Institute–Dearborn Campus

Sundy Bellezza
Star Career Institute

Ruth E. Dearborn Berger, MS, RHIA
Chippewa Valley Technical College

Tamarra Disco Boggs, CPC, CCP, MCS-P
Bluegrass Community and Technical College

Mary Cantwell, RHIA, CPC, CPC-H, CPC-P, CPC-I
Metro Community College

Sally Conley, CMPE
American School of Technology

Michelle Cranney, RHIT, CCS-P, CPC, AHIMA-approved ICD-10-CM/PCS trainer
Everett Community College

Ruth Dearborn, CCS, CCS-P
University of Alaska

Barbara Donnally, CPC
University of Rio Grande

Deborah Eid, CBCS, MHA, BA
Carrington College

Madeline Flanagan, MA, CPC
Branford Hall Career Institute

Diana Gardner, CPC, RHIA, CMPE
Florence Darlington Technical College,
Western Governors University

Debbie Gilbert, RHIA, CMA
Dalton State College

Anita Hazelwood, RHIA, FAHIMA
University of Louisiana–Lafayette

Judy Hurtt, MEd
East Central Community College

Carol Johnsons, MBA
Northern Michigan University

Teresa Jolly, MEd
South Georgia Technical College

Fannie Sue Martin, CPC
YTI Career Institute

Laura Michelsen, MS, RHIA, certified ICD-10 trainer
Joliet Junior College

Kris Patterson
Las Positas College

Nehal Rangnekar, MS, CPC-A
Brookhaven College

Darcy Roy, CPC, CMA, RHE
Brevard Community College

Bethany Shirley, CPC, NCICS, AAS
Virginia College–Austin

Christine Sproles, CMT
Pensacola Christian College

Deanna Stephens, AABA, NCICS, CMOA, AABA, RMA, CBCS
Virginia College

Danielle Ulshafer, NCCT, CPC
Harris School of Business

Pamela Webster, CPC
Keiser Career College

Charles Welch, MBA, CPC, CMC, CEC
Everest University

Carole Zeglin, MSEd, BSMT, RMA
Westmoreland County Community College

Technical Editing/Accuracy Panel

A panel of instructors completed a technical edit and review of all the content in the book page proofs to verify its accuracy.

Suzanne Bitters, RMA, NCICS
Harris School of Business–Wilmington

Daniel Figueroa, CBCS, CICS, CPAT
Florida Career College

Debbie Gilbert, RHIA, CMA
Dalton State College

Christina Thomas, CPC, CMAA, CCMA, CBCS
Florida Career College

Acknowledgments from the Authors

We would like to thank all of the students and instructors who have crossed our paths over the years. Their support, encouragement, and enthusiasm contribute to our passion for the coding field. We would also like to thank all of the individuals at McGraw-Hill who have worked with us on this project. Their enthusiasm and backing for the project is appreciated.

Thank you to the textbook exercise contributors: Fannie Sue Martin, Sue Pylant, Lisa Schaffer, Carolle Battiste, Amy Files, Susan Miedzianowski, and Patricia King.

Thank you to the key supplements contributors: Kathleen Bailey, Jerri Rowe, Alyssa Bluhm, and Susan Vana. Thank you to the various reviewers for providing feedback on those supplements.

Thank you to the instructors who helped with the material for *Connect Plus*, including Judy Hurtt, Amy Ensign, Lisa Schaffer, Gerry Pape, Susan Miedzianowski, Lorraine Papazian-Boyce, and Sue Pylant.

A special thank-you to all of our friends and our families for their support and understanding, especially for all the times we said, "I can't right now; I am writing." Our families have made it through many fast-food meals and lost weekends over the past year, and we are grateful for their understanding of what this book means to us.

The authors

Thanks to my parents, Jack and Betty Smith, for their support and the use of their house when I needed a quiet place to write. And thank you Marc for just being there whenever I needed extra encouragement.

Lastly, I would like to thank Cyndi Stewart, with whom I wrote this book. I have learned many new things about coding and myself during this journey with you. There is no one I would have rather shared this experience with, and thanks for being my friend for all of these years.

Cindy Ward

A Commitment to Accuracy

You have a right to expect an accurate textbook, and McGraw-Hill invests considerable time and effort to make sure that we deliver one. Listed below are the many steps we take to make sure this happens.

Our Accuracy Verification Process

First Round—Development Reviews

Step 1: Numerous **health professions instructors review** the draft manuscript and report on any errors that they may find. The **authors** make these corrections in the final manuscript.

Second Round—Page Proofs

Step 2: Once the manuscript has been typeset, the **authors** check the manuscript against the page proofs to ensure that all illustrations, examples, and exercises have been correctly laid out on the pages and that all codes have been updated correctly.

Step 3: An outside panel of **peer instructors** completes a technical edit/review of all content in the page proofs to verify its accuracy. The **authors** add these corrections to the review of the page proofs.

Step 4: A **proofreader** adds a triple layer of accuracy assurance in pages by looking for errors; then a confirming, corrected round of page proofs is produced.

Third Round—Confirming Page Proofs

Step 5: The **authors** review the confirming round of page proofs to make certain that any previous corrections were properly made and to look for any errors that might have been missed on the first round.

Step 6: The **project manager,** who has overseen the book from the beginning, performs **another proofread** to make sure that no new errors have been introduced during the production process.

Final Round—Printer's Proofs

Step 7: The **project manager** performs a **final proofread** of the book during the printing process, providing a final accuracy review.

In concert with the main text, all supplements undergo a proofreading and technical editing stage to ensure their accuracy.

Results

What results is a textbook that is as accurate and error-free as is humanly possible. Our authors and publishing staff are confident that the many layers of quality assurance have produced books that are leaders in the industry for their integrity and correctness. *Please view the Acknowledgments section for more details on the many people involved in this process.*

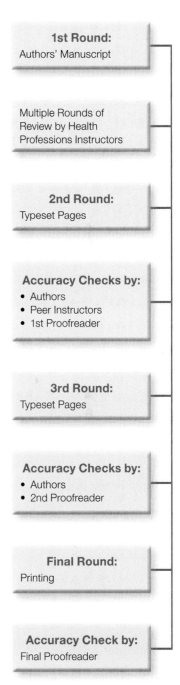

1st Round:
Authors' Manuscript

Multiple Rounds of Review by Health Professions Instructors

2nd Round:
Typeset Pages

Accuracy Checks by:
• Authors
• Peer Instructors
• 1st Proofreader

3rd Round:
Typeset Pages

Accuracy Checks by:
• Authors
• 2nd Proofreader

Final Round:
Printing

Accuracy Check by:
Final Proofreader

Fundamental Coding Guidelines

1

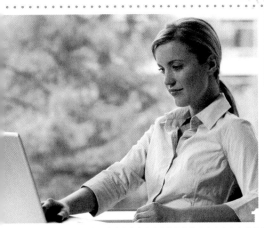

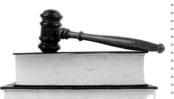

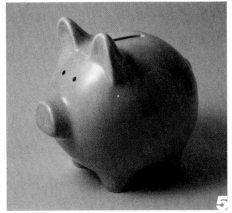

UNIT ONE

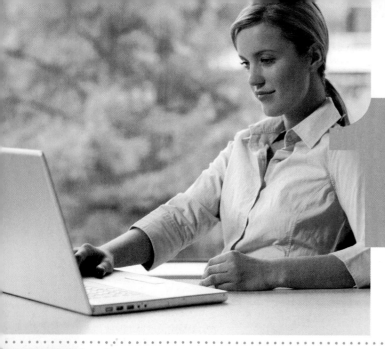

The Certified Professional Coder

Key Terms

Accounts receivable (A/R)

American Academy of Professional Coders (AAPC)

Billing language

Certified Professional Coder (CPC)

Certified Professional Coder (CPC) exam

Clean claim

Compliance language

Medical coding

Medical necessity

Medically managed

Payer language

Provider language

Revenue cycle

Learning Outcomes

After completing this chapter, you will be able to:

1.1 Differentiate between the various languages used in medical coding.

1.2 Determine the many roles a coder plays in the reimbursement and compliance process.

1.3 Recognize the benefits of obtaining medical coding credentials and the importance of AAPC to the medical coder.

1.4 Understand the basic format of the CPC exam.

1.5 Acquire beneficial test-taking skills.

Introduction

Medical coding is the process of translating provider documentation and medical terminology into codes that illustrate the procedures and services performed by medical professionals. A **Certified Professional Coder (CPC)** is an individual who has demonstrated his or her knowledge of medical coding by successfully completing the CPC exam. This exam is designed to test the coder's skill in translating medical information accurately and completely so that the provider is reimbursed correctly and fairly and within compliance guidelines.

1.1 Differentiation of Various Languages in Medical Coding

The process of medical coding requires that the coding professional have an in-depth knowledge of the language and terminology used in medical coding and billing. Coding and billing language is used to assist physician offices, hospitals, patients, third-party administrators, and insurance companies in understanding *why* the patient was seen and *what* services, procedures, or supplies were provided for the patient and in identifying and submitting the claim as codes. These codes used are the Current Procedural Terminology (CPT), Healthcare Common Procedure Coding System (HCPCS), and International Classification of Diseases (ICD) codes.

There are several languages that must be translated in regard to an insurance claim. The identification and application of these languages help determine payment, information stored as data for future healthcare needs of the patient, statistical data for the payer, and financial and medical records for the provider. The list below explains these languages:

- **Provider language** is built on medical terminology, anatomy, and pathophysiology and describes services, procedures, and the medical necessity of those services and procedures.
- **Billing language** includes terms such as *accounts receivable (A/R), clean claims, denials, modifiers,* and *advanced beneficiary notices (ABNs).*
- **Payer language** comprises terms such as *noncovered services, medical necessity, compliance language,* and *unbundling.*
- **Compliance language** brings terms such as *unbundling, fraud, false claim,* and *abuse* into the translation.

The CPT, HCPCS, and ICD codes have been structured to allow for communication of data in a standardized format. This standardized format enables doctors, coders, insurers, and facilities to all use the same language in translating the patient encounter into data that are accurate and consistent and that meet the needs of the individual user of the healthcare data. The ability to interpret the different languages and correctly translate them into data for the CMS-1500 claim form, which becomes the source of the statistical medical data for the practice, payer, and governing bodies, is the foundation of the medical coder's role.

medical coding The process of translating provider documentation and medical terminology into codes that illustrate the procedures and services performed by medical professionals.

Certified Professional Coder (CPC) An individual who has demonstrated his or her knowledge of medical coding by successfully completing the CPC exam.

provider language Language that is built on medical terminology, anatomy, and pathophysiology and describes services, procedures, and their medical necessity.

billing language Language that includes terms such as *accounts receivable (A/R), clean claims, denials, modifiers,* and *advanced beneficiary notices (ABNs).*

payer language Language that comprises terms such as *noncovered services, medical necessity, compliance language,* and *unbundling.*

compliance language Language that brings terms such as *unbundling, fraud, false claim,* and *abuse* into the translation of the medical record.

EXERCISE 1.1

1. Describe the foundation of a coder's role.
2. What are the main languages a coder must be familiar with in order to code accurately?

Also available in Mc Graw Hill **connect** (plus+)

1.2 The CPC's Role in Reimbursement and Compliance

To achieve consistent and accurate communication, providers as well as billing and coding personnel must fully understand coding guidelines and regulations. As guidelines and regulations are frequently updated and may change annually, coders must be diligent in maintaining and updating their knowledge of medical coding and billing policies, requirements, and procedures to be of value to the practices or organizations they work for and the healthcare field in general.

Coder's Impact on the Revenue Cycle

It is helpful to think of the billing process as a cycle of revenue. The health and maintenance of this revenue cycle is the responsibility of everyone within the practice. To meet this responsibility, everyone involved must have the tools needed to submit a clean claim that results in accurate and timely reimbursement for services provided to the patient and the resources used to provide those services. Creating a clean claim requires that all involved in its creation have a good working knowledge of government regulations, payer policies, and the practice/provider-payer contract limitations to remain in compliance with payer regulations.

Confusing government regulations and new and continuing audit programs with costly penalties to providers for errors make it extremely important that all involved in providing patient services understand the role each plays in submitting a clean claim to the insurance carriers.

Medical practices contract with multiple insurance payers. They do this not only to facilitate payment for patients covered by diverse insurance plans but also to maintain or increase the number of patients they serve, since many plans require that patients remain in the plan network. Each practice-payer contract is negotiated separately with various terms. All of the contracts have a specified claim-turnaround time frame, or adjudication period. The adjudication period begins upon receipt of a clean claim.

Coder's Role in Creating Accurate CMS-1500 Claims

The CMS-1500 is the standard billing form used to submit healthcare data from the provider to the payer (see Figure 1.1). A **clean claim** is a CMS-1500 claim that is complete and accurate from the demographic portion to the diagnosis and procedure. If any part of the claim is incomplete or inaccurate, the claim is no longer deemed "clean" and the contractual turnaround, or adjudication, time frame does not have to be met.

The appropriate ICD-9-CM (ninth revision) code for the diagnosis or condition must be linked to the appropriate service or procedure provided. Often, physicians document past conditions that are not being treated or **medically managed** at the present encounter, but these conditions should not be reported on the claim.

ICD-9-CM codes are reported in field 21 of the CMS form, beginning with the first-listed diagnosis followed by any secondary diagnoses that were treated or medically managed. Provider's documentation must support the **medical necessity** reported.

SPOTLIGHT on Terminology

Medically managed A diagnosis which may not receive direct treatment during an encounter but which the provider has to consider when determining treatment for other conditions.

Medical necessity Any diagnosis, condition, procedure, and/or service that is documented in the patient record as having been treated or medically managed.

DRAFT - NOT FOR OFFICIAL USE

HEALTH INSURANCE CLAIM FORM

APPROVED BY NATIONAL UNIFORM CLAIM COMMITTEE (NUCC) 02/12

◀ CARRIER ▶

PICA
PICA

1. MEDICARE ☐ (Medicare#) MEDICAID ☐ (Medicaid#) TRICARE ☐ (ID#/DoD#) CHAMPVA ☐ (Member ID#) GROUP HEALTH PLAN ☐ (ID#) FECA BLK LUNG ☐ (ID#) OTHER ☐ (ID#)
1a. INSURED'S I.D. NUMBER   (For Program in Item 1)

2. PATIENT'S NAME (Last Name, First Name, Middle Initial)
3. PATIENT'S BIRTH DATE MM DD YY   SEX M ☐ F ☐
4. INSURED'S NAME (Last Name, First Name, Middle Initial)

5. PATIENT'S ADDRESS (No., Street)
6. PATIENT RELATIONSHIP TO INSURED Self ☐ Spouse ☐ Child ☐ Other ☐
7. INSURED'S ADDRESS (No., Street)

CITY   STATE
8. RESERVED FOR NUCC USE
CITY   STATE

ZIP CODE   TELEPHONE (Include Area Code) (   )
ZIP CODE   TELEPHONE (Include Area Code) (   )

9. OTHER INSURED'S NAME (Last Name, First Name, Middle Initial)
10. IS PATIENT'S CONDITION RELATED TO:
11. INSURED'S POLICY GROUP OR FECA NUMBER

a. OTHER INSURED'S POLICY OR GROUP NUMBER
a. EMPLOYMENT? (Current or Previous) ☐ YES ☐ NO
a. INSURED'S DATE OF BIRTH MM DD YY   SEX M ☐ F ☐

b. RESERVED FOR NUCC USE
b. AUTO ACCIDENT? ☐ YES ☐ NO   PLACE (State)
b. OTHER CLAIM ID (Designated by NUCC)

c. RESERVED FOR NUCC USE
c. OTHER ACCIDENT? ☐ YES ☐ NO
c. INSURANCE PLAN NAME OR PROGRAM NAME

d. INSURANCE PLAN NAME OR PROGRAM NAME
10d. CLAIM CODES (Designated by NUCC)
d. IS THERE ANOTHER HEALTH BENEFIT PLAN? ☐ YES ☐ NO   *If yes,* complete items 9, 9a, and 9d.

READ BACK OF FORM BEFORE COMPLETING & SIGNING THIS FORM.
12. PATIENT'S OR AUTHORIZED PERSON'S SIGNATURE I authorize the release of any medical or other information necessary to process this claim. I also request payment of government benefits either to myself or to the party who accepts assignment below.
SIGNED _____   DATE _____

13. INSURED'S OR AUTHORIZED PERSON'S SIGNATURE I authorize payment of medical benefits to the undersigned physician or supplier for services described below.
SIGNED _____

◀ PATIENT AND INSURED INFORMATION ▶

14. DATE OF CURRENT ILLNESS, INJURY, or PREGNANCY (LMP) MM DD YY   QUAL.
15. OTHER DATE QUAL.   MM DD YY
16. DATES PATIENT UNABLE TO WORK IN CURRENT OCCUPATION FROM MM DD YY TO MM DD YY

17. NAME OF REFERRING PROVIDER OR OTHER SOURCE
17a.
17b. NPI
18. HOSPITALIZATION DATES RELATED TO CURRENT SERVICES FROM MM DD YY TO MM DD YY

19. ADDITIONAL CLAIM INFORMATION (Designated by NUCC)
20. OUTSIDE LAB? ☐ YES ☐ NO $ CHARGES

21. DIAGNOSIS OR NATURE OF ILLNESS OR INJURY Relate A-L to service line below (24E)   ICD Ind. |
A. |___ B. |___ C. |___ D. |___
E. |___ F. |___ G. |___ H. |___
I. |___ J. |___ K. |___ L. |___

22. RESUBMISSION CODE   ORIGINAL REF. NO.

23. PRIOR AUTHORIZATION NUMBER

24. A. DATE(S) OF SERVICE From MM DD YY To MM DD YY	B. PLACE OF SERVICE	C. EMG	D. PROCEDURES, SERVICES, OR SUPPLIES (Explain Unusual Circumstances) CPT/HCPCS | MODIFIER	E. DIAGNOSIS POINTER	F. $ CHARGES	G. DAYS OR UNITS	H. EPSDT Family Plan	I. ID. QUAL.	J. RENDERING PROVIDER ID. #
1									NPI
2									NPI
3									NPI
4									NPI
5									NPI
6									NPI

25. FEDERAL TAX I.D. NUMBER ☐ SSN ☐ EIN
26. PATIENT'S ACCOUNT NO.
27. ACCEPT ASSIGNMENT? (For govt. claims, see back) ☐ YES ☐ NO
28. TOTAL CHARGE $
29. AMOUNT PAID $
30. Rsvd for NUCC Use

31. SIGNATURE OF PHYSICIAN OR SUPPLIER INCLUDING DEGREES OR CREDENTIALS (I certify that the statements on the reverse apply to this bill and are made a part thereof.)
SIGNED _____   DATE _____
32. SERVICE FACILITY LOCATION INFORMATION
a. NPI   b.
33. BILLING PROVIDER INFO & PH # (   )
a. NPI   b.

◀ PHYSICIAN OR SUPPLIER INFORMATION ▶

NUCC Instruction Manual available at: www.nucc.org   *PLEASE PRINT OR TYPE*   OMB APPROVAL PENDING

Figure 1.1 CMS-1500

1. MEDICARE	MEDICAID	TRICARE	CHAMPVA	GROUP HEALTH PLAN	FECA BLK LUNG	OTHER	1a. INSURED'S I.D. NUMBER	(For Program in Item 1)
X (Medicare#)	☐ (Medicaid#)	☐ (ID#/DoD#)	☐ (Member ID#)	☐ (ID#)	☐ (ID#)	☐ (ID#)	111-22-3333A	

2. PATIENT'S NAME (Last Name, First Name, Middle Initial)	3. PATIENT'S BIRTH DATE			SEX	4. INSURED'S NAME (Last Name, First Name, Middle Initial)
Hutton, Timothy	MM 12	DD 25	YY 1935	M ☐ F X	SAME

5. PATIENT'S ADDRESS (No., Street)	6. PATIENT RELATIONSHIP TO INSURED	7. INSURED'S ADDRESS (No., Street)
281 Green Apple	Self X Spouse ☐ Child ☐ Other ☐	SAME

Figure 1.2 Patient Demographic Portion of CMS-1500

21. DIAGNOSIS OR NATURE OF ILLNESS OR INJURY Relate A-L to service line below (24E)				ICD Ind.	22. RESUMISSION CODE	ORIGINAL REF. NO.
A. 600.00	B.	C.	D.			
E.	F.	G.	H.		23. PRIOR AUTHORIZATION NUMBER	
I.	J.	K.	L.			

24. A.	DATE(S) OF SERVICE						B. PLACE OF SERVICE	C. EMG	D. PROCEDURES, SERVICES, OR SUPPLIES (Explain Unusual Circumstances)		E. DIAGNOSIS POINTER	F. $ CHARGES	G. DAYS OR UNITS	H. EPSDT Family Plan	I. ID. QUAL.	J. RENDERING PROVIDER ID. #
	From MM	DD	YY	To MM	DD	YY			CPT/HCPCS	MODIFIER						
1	03	02	20XX	03	02	20XX	22		55700		A				NPI	

Figure 1.3 Diagnostic Portion of CMS-1500

An inaccurate claim would be one in which the patient demographic information does not support the patient's condition or the nature or type of service performed.

FOR EXAMPLE The patient demographic portion of the claim form (upper portion) identifies the patient as female (see Figure 1.2); the patient's condition is enlarged prostate, and the service performed is a biopsy of the prostate (see Figure 1.3). ▪

Although the patient's condition does support the medical necessity of, or need for, the procedure performed, this condition cannot exist in a female and therefore the claim will be considered inaccurate and not subject to adjudication and payment by the health insurance plan.

Correcting such errors is costly to medical practices, as they result in more days of revenue in the **accounts receivable (A/R)** cycle due to longer adjudication periods and more staff time spent researching, correcting, and resubmitting the claims.

As the patient record may not be altered, errors identified must be corrected so that an auditor can recognize both the error and the correction. All corrections or additions to the medical record (addendums) must be dated and legibly signed or initialed.

accounts receivable (A/R) Revenue that is due to the practice or provider for services or procedures rendered to the patient; may be due from health insurance coverage, workers' compensation, liability coverage, or the patient.

EXERCISE 1.2

1. What are some of the consequences of not submitting a clean claim the first time the claim is submitted to the payer?

2. Give an example of how a service or procedure provided is linked to the medical necessity of that service or procedure.

Also available in 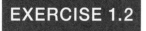 connect plus+

1.3 Medical Coding Credentials and the AAPC

Many practices have found, after doing some internal research, that often they did not need to hire more physicians or office staff, increase patient workload, or take other steps to increase revenue. What they found was that if they were more aware of billing and coding guidelines and if providers and staff worked together, they could increase their revenue considerably. Physicians do not need to know how to code or all of the coding rules. What is important is that they be aware of what is needed in their documentation, whether in a dictated report, a handwritten note in a chart, or a superbill. This documentation is the basis for the decisions made by the billing and coding department in generating a clean claim.

Another important role of coders is compliance. The payers run monthly reports, just as practices do, to identify patterns. Many of the audits being conducted today are determined by these identified patterns. Duplicate claims, incorrect use of modifiers, medical necessity, unbundling, use of invalid codes, and consistent use of the same level of evaluation and management codes are some of the areas being audited. It is important that physicians as well as all office staff understand how to avoid these patterns, and coders play a vital role in relevant education, training, and updating.

Certified coders, on average, earn 20 percent more than noncertified coders and often continue their education, becoming office managers, billing managers, consultants, auditors, and educators.

An additional reason for becoming credentialed is the increased opportunity for employment. According to findings of the Bureau of Labor Statistics, employers prefer to hire credentialed medical coders rather than noncredentialed coders, thereby increasing the chances of employment for CPCs.

The **American Academy of Professional Coders (AAPC)** is a credentialing organization of more than 100,000 members, approximately 80 percent of whom are credentialed as Certified Professional Coders. The AAPC supports its members by providing coding education, identifying job opportunities, and offering networking opportunities.

Credentials validate the knowledge and expertise of the individual who holds them. The AAPC offers members the opportunity to validate their command of medical coding through testing of the medical code sets (ICD, CPT, and HCPCS Level II), the coding rules and regulations, anatomy, physiology, medical terminology, and documentation guidelines.

Upon successful completion of the exam, the student receives the Certified Professional Coder (CPC) credential, which confirms to future employers and others in the medical field his or her knowledge, experience, and abilities as a physician practice–based medical coder.

American Academy of Professional Coders (AAPC) An organization that administers the CPC exam and confers the Certified Professional Coder credential; supports its members by providing coding education, identifying job opportunities, and offering networking opportunities.

1. List three reasons to become a certified coder.
2. Identify some of the impact AAPC has on the coding community.

Also available in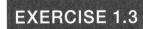

EXERCISE 1.3

1.4 CPC Exam Format

The **Certified Professional Coder (CPC) exam** is a grueling 150-question exam that thoroughly tests the coder's ability within a medical coding subset. As there are multiple versions of this exam, of which any may be administered during examination, the examinee must be prepared to demonstrate her or his knowledge and ability across all code sets: ICD, CPT, and HCPCS Level II codes.

Certified Professional Coder (CPC) exam Exam that tests the coder's skill in translating data from the patient's medical record accurately and completely so that the provider is reimbursed correctly and fairly and within compliance guidelines.

Regardless of the exam version, the time allowed for completing the exam is 5 hours and 40 minutes. The exam tests the coder's ability and understanding of the following:

Anesthesia	Radiology
Medicine	Musculoskeletal system
Endocrine system	Digestive system
Nervous system	Evaluation and management
Urinary system	Respiratory system
Integumentary system	Mediastinum and diaphragm
Pathology	Male/female genital system
Laboratory	Maternity and delivery
Hemic and lymphatic system	Eye and ocular adnexa
ICD-9-CM	HCPCS Level II
Practice management	Coding guidelines
Medical terminology	Anatomy and physiology

The CPC exam is an "open code-book" exam. This means approved current year coding manuals (CPT, HCPCS, and ICD) may be used during the exam. However, some versions of these manuals are not allowed to be used during the exam—a complete and current list of nonapproved manuals can be found at www.aapc.com. It is recommended that this list be reviewed prior to the exam.

EXERCISE 1.4

1. What is the length of the CPC exam, and how many questions are included?
2. List the areas on which a coder is tested on the CPC exam.

Also available in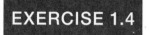

1.5 Test-Taking Skills

Occasionally, coders go into the CPC exam very well versed on the subject matter but fail the exam. One of the more common reasons for this is test anxiety: Some students will begin the exam feeling ready, look at the first question, and forget what they had learned due to panic and fear. Has this ever happened to you?

Here are some tips that will help you improve your test-taking skills:

- Take a mock/practice test a few months before the actual test.
- Use available resources to practice specific areas of weakness identified by the mock/practice test, such as ICD or compliance.
- Form a study group among your peers.
- Know the ICD, CPT, and HCPCS Level II books, and know how to locate codes and use them. Memorization of the guidelines is not required; however, the more you know without having to reference this information during the exam, the better for time management.

MENTOR
Coding Tip

Cramming the night before the test does not help. You know the material by then. Go to bed early, and get a good night's rest.

- Practice exam time management.
- Take a second mock/practice test within a month before the CPC exam.
- Again using available resources, practice any areas of weakness identified by the second mock/practice test.
- Go over the guidelines in both the ICD and the CPT thoroughly during the week of the exam.
- Listen to the proctor carefully, and follow all instructions.
- Leave nothing blank.

We have found the test-taking tips listed above to be beneficial. This list is by no means comprehensive. Don't forget to add your own tips to the list.

MENTOR Coding Tip

Running out of time during the test is a major reason for failing the test. Complete areas or questions about which you are more confident first, as they will take less time. Do not spend considerable time struggling with questions you find difficult. Make your best attempt to answer a question and move on to the next question.

1. What are two of the major factors that can affect a coder's successful completion of the CPC exam?
2. List some test-taking tips from the chapter and some of your own test-taking tips.

EXERCISE 1.5

Also available in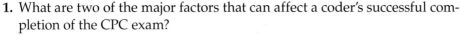

Chapter One Summary

Learning Outcome	Key Concepts/Examples
1.1 Differentiate between the various languages used in medical coding.	Coding is a form of translating billing, compliance, payer, and provider language into standardized billing/reimbursement data.
1.2 Determine the many roles a coder plays in the reimbursement and compliance process.	To achieve consistent and accurate communication, providers as well as billing and coding personnel must fully understand coding guidelines and regulations. As guidelines and regulations are frequently updated and may change annually, coders must be diligent in maintaining and updating their knowledge of medical coding and billing policies, requirements, and procedures to be of value to the practices or organizations they work for and the healthcare field in general.
1.3 Recognize the benefits of obtaining medical coding credentials and the importance of AAPC to the medical coder.	The reasons for becoming certified include increased salary and employment opportunities for the coder and coding and compliance accuracy, as well as increased revenue, for the practice. AAPC is the credentialing organization for professional coders.
1.4 Understand the basic format of the CPC exam.	The CPC exam consists of 150 questions, is 5 hours and 40 minutes in length, and tests the coder's skills in ICD, CPT, HCPCS Level II, anatomy, and medical terminology.
1.5 Acquire beneficial test-taking skills.	Test-taking tips include getting plenty of rest the night before the test, listening closely to instructions, and leaving no answer blank.

Chapter One Review

Using Terminology

Match each key term to the appropriate definition.

_____ 1. [LO1.3] AAPC

_____ 2. [LO1.2] A/R

_____ 3. [LO1.1] CPC

_____ 4. [LO1.2] Billing language

_____ 5. [LO1.2] Clean claim

_____ 6. [LO1.2] Compliance language

_____ 7. [LO1.1] Medical coding

_____ 8. [LO1.2] Medical necessity

_____ 9. [LO1.2] Payer language

_____ 10. [LO1.2] Provider language

A. Certified Professional Coder

B. Diagnoses, conditions, and procedures that are documented in the patient record as being treated or managed

C. American Academy of Professional Coders

D. Includes terms such as *A/R, denials, modifiers,* and *EOB*

E. Includes terms such as *noncovered services, medical necessity,* and *unbundling*

F. Includes term such as *fraud* and *abuse*

G. Language that describes and links services, procedures, and medically necessary diagnoses

H. Revenue that is due to the practice or provider for services or procedures rendered to the patient

I. Form of translating provider documentation and medical terms into codes

J. CMS-1500 form that is complete and accurate

Checking Your Understanding

Choose the most appropriate answer for the following questions.

1. **[LO1. 4]** The CPC exam has _____ questions and is _____ in length.
   - **a.** 50; 3 hours
   - **b.** 150; 5 hours, 40 minutes
   - **c.** 175; 5 hours, 40 minutes
   - **d.** 150; 3 hours

2. **[LO1.1]** The data that are translated by the coder to be submitted to the payer are submitted on which form when billing for the physician?
   - **a.** UB04
   - **b.** HCFA 1500
   - **c.** CMS-1500
   - **d.** The form varies by payer.

3. **[LO1.1]** The "language" that is used by insurance carriers and includes terms such as *noncovered services,* unbundling, and *duplicate claim* is called:
   - **a.** Billing language
   - **b.** Provider language
   - **c.** Compliance language
   - **d.** Payer language

4. **[LO1.2]** To achieve consistent and accurate communication, providers as well as coders must:
   - **a.** Fully understand coding guidelines and regulations
   - **b.** Be willing to communicate with each other on a regular basis
   - **c.** Stay up to date on the guidelines and regulations
   - **d.** All of these

5. **[LO1.3]** Certified coders, on average, earn _____ more than noncertified coders.
   - **a.** 10 percent
   - **b.** 20 percent
   - **c.** 5 percent
   - **d.** They earn approximately the same as noncertified coders.

6. **[LO1.3]** What is used by a coder as the basis for the information required to complete fields 21 and 24 on the CMS-1500?
   - **a.** The superbill
   - **b.** Provider documentation such as a handwritten note
   - **c.** Provider documentation such as a dictated report
   - **d.** Provider documentation, including either handwritten notes and dictated reports

7. **[LO1.2]** A diagnosis may not receive direct treatment during an encounter but the physician still has to consider this diagnosis when determining treatment for other conditions. This is a definition of:
   - **a.** Medical necessity
   - **b.** Medically managed
   - **c.** Medical coding
   - **d.** None of these

8. **[LO1.3]** What is the name of the credentialing organization for the CPC exam?
   - **a.** AHIMA
   - **b.** ABMA
   - **c.** AAMA
   - **d.** AAPC

9. **[LO1.4]** Which books are required for the CPC exam?
   - **a.** HCPCS, current year
   - **b.** ICD-9-CM, current year
   - **c.** CPT, current year
   - **d.** All of these

10. **[LO1.5]** Which of the following would *not* be a good test-taking tip?
    - **a.** Get plenty of rest the night before the test.
    - **b.** Do not leave any questions unanswered.
    - **c.** Study as hard and as long as possible the night before the test.
    - **d.** Follow all instructions given by the proctor on the day of the test.

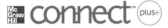 **Enhance your learning by completing these exercises and more at mcgrawhillconnect.com**

Applying Your Knowledge

Use your critical-thinking skills to answer the questions below.

1. **[LO 1.1]** Explain how coding is like translating a language and how realizing this can help a coder pass the CPC exam.

   _____

2. **[LO 1.3]** List other career opportunities for a certified coder.

   _____

3. **[LO 1.5]** Explain which test-taking tips you think will be most beneficial to you in preparing for the CPC exam.

   _____

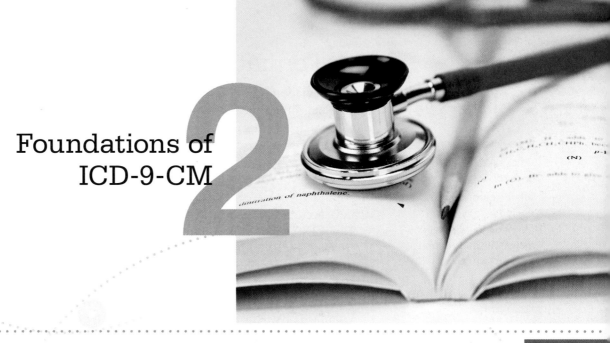

Foundations of ICD-9-CM 2

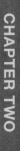

Key Terms

Acute	*Includes*	NOS	Symptom
And	Late effect	Parentheses	Use additional code
Chronic	Main term	Sign	
Code first	Manifestation	Slanted brackets	
Excludes	NEC	Square brackets	

Learning Outcomes

After completing this chapter, you will be able to:

2.1 Understand the format of the ICD-9-CM manual.

2.2 Apply the abbreviations, coding conventions, and punctuation marks used in ICD-9-CM.

2.3 Identify main terms and use the ICD-9-CM index.

2.4 Review ICD-9-CM chapter-specific guidelines.

2.5 Examine ICD-9-CM diagnostic outpatient guidelines.

2.6 Recognize the importance of translating provider terminology into accurate diagnostic codes.

Introduction

The focus of this chapter is a general overview of the ICD-9-CM conventions and guidelines needed to be successful in completing the CPC exam. Later chapters provide more specific detail on the ICD-9-CM codes that are commonly used with specific body systems.

2.1 Format of ICD-9-CM Manual

The abbreviation *ICD-9-CM* stands for "International Classification of Diseases, Ninth Revision, Clinical Modification." The ICD-9-CM manual is the translation dictionary that coders use to translate medical terminology from provider documentation into the codes used to tell a patient's diagnostic story. ICD-9-CM is the "why" for the patient's service or procedure. Understanding the format of the ICD-9-CM manual and being able to implement the guidelines and coding conventions enable coders to not only succeed with the CPC exam but also achieve accuracy and consistency in coding of the medical record.

The ICD-9-CM is published in a two- or three-volume set. The two-volume set is used by providers to identify why the service or procedure was provided. The three-volume set is used exclusively by facilities to identify both why the service or procedure was provided and what service or procedure was provided.

Volume 1, also known as the *tabular portion* of the ICD-9-CM, contains the numerical code section and the full description (nomenclature) of each code. To ease the process of coding for the coder, this volume appears after Volume 2.

Volume 2, also known as the *index* of the ICD-9-CM, contains an alphabetic listing of main terms identifying a patient's condition, injury, sign, or symptom. Subterms follow the main term in a graduated indented format and provide for further clarification of the patient's condition, thus allowing the coder to drill down to a more accurate code before looking up the code in Volume 1.

Volume 3 codes are used by inpatient and outpatient facilities to report procedures and services.

> **MENTOR** Coding Tip
>
> Students have found it very helpful to tab their ICD-9-CM manual. They use self-adhesive tabs or labels to mark the individual tables in the Alphabetic Index (hypertension, neoplasm, table of drugs and chemicals) and the individual chapters in the Tabular List to identify a range of codes. They have found that this saves them considerable time when they are taking the CPC exam since the tabs enable them to quickly locate the code indicated in the index.

EXERCISE 2.1

1. Explain the differences between the three volumes of the ICD-9-CM manual.
2. What is the main function of the ICD-9-CM manual for the coder?

Also available in connect (plus+)

2.2 Abbreviations, Coding Conventions, Guidelines, Instructional Notes, and Punctuation

ICD-9-CM uses several abbreviations, symbols, and punctuation marks within the Tabular List (Volume 1). Many of them are used to save space within the ICD-9-CM manual. The significance of punctuation is reviewed later in this chapter. This section begins with an explanation of two abbreviations that confuse even experienced coders.

Abbreviations

NEC and *NOS* are two coding-convention abbreviations that are important for a coder to differentiate and know how to use. The definitions of each can be found in the Conventions section of the ICD-9-CM manual guidelines.

NEC—not elsewhere classified—means that a more specific code is not provided in the ICD-9-CM manual. In this case, the provider documentation is more specific in its description of the patient's condition than the ICD-9-CM allows for in the code description.

FOR EXAMPLE Hypothyroidism due to autoimmune disorder would be coded as:

secondary hypothyroidism NEC or other specified acquired hypothyroidism (244.8)

This is because the level of detail needed to identify this condition fully is not provided in the description of any of the acquired forms of hypothyroidism listed in the ICD-9-CM manual. ■

NOS—not otherwise specified—is the equivalent of "unspecified." This abbreviation is to be used only when the documentation does not provide enough information to assign a more specific code.

FOR EXAMPLE The diagnostic statement "goiter, nodular nontoxic" would be coded as:

unspecified nontoxic nodular goiter (241.9)

This is because the diagnostic statement does not clarify whether the condition is uninodular or multinodular. ■

MENTOR Coding Tip

Typically, NEC-specified codes are also known as *other-specified* codes and have an 8 as the fourth digit or a 9 as the fifth digit. NOS-specified codes are also known as *unspecified* codes and typically have a 9 as the fourth digit.

Coding Conventions, Guidelines, and Instructional Notes

The official ICD-9-CM coding conventions, as well as the Additional Conventions section, provides detail on the use of the symbols, official footnotes, instructional notes, conventions, and notations found in Volumes 1 and 2 of the ICD-9-CM manual.

Correct use and a comprehensive understanding of these conventions allow for consistency in coding and assist the coder in selecting the most accurate diagnosis code for the disease, condition, or injury as documented by the provider.

Acute and Chronic

One ICD-9-CM guideline addresses the use and sequencing of codes for **acute** and **chronic** conditions. The guideline instructs that when both the acute and chronic forms of a condition are documented, both conditions should be coded. Based on the guidelines, there are two ways these conditions may be coded: together, with a combination code that identifies both the chronic and acute forms of the condition in one code, or separately, with one code for the acute condition and another for the chronic condition.

Both combination codes and distinct codes are recognizable in the Alphabetic Index. After locating the main term of the condition (acute and chronic forms of the same condition are located under the same main term), review both subterms, *acute* and *chronic*. If the subterms *acute* and *chronic* are connected by a *with* statement, ICD-9-CM provides a combination code, or one code to indicate both conditions.

FOR EXAMPLE From the Alphabetic Index:

Bronchitis
   Chronic 491.9
      Obstructive 491.20
         with
            Acute bronchitis 491.22 ■

SPOTLIGHT on Terminology

Acute Conditions with sudden onset, usually without warning, and of brief duration. For example: fractures, intestinal flu, and rhinitis.
Chronic Conditions with slow onset and of long duration, even the lifetime of the patient. For example: diabetes, hypertension, and asthma.

MENTOR Coding Tip

Be sure to review both the *acute* and *chronic* subterms to identify available combination codes, since they are not always found under both terms, as is the case in the previous example.

When a combination code is not available and two distinct codes are needed to fully describe the patient's condition or disease, the ICD-9-CM guidelines instruct the coder to list both the acute and chronic codes with the acute condition listed first, followed by the chronic condition.

And

The ICD-9-CM use of the word **and** is specified in the coding convention and is to be interpreted as meaning "and/or."

FOR EXAMPLE

373.32 Contact and allergic dermatitis of the eyelid

This code is to be used for contact and/or allergic dermatitis of the eyelid. ■

Late Effect

Late effect ICD-9-CM codes are used to describe a residual condition that occurs after the initial illness or injury.

MENTOR Coding Tip

Many coders have trouble with the late-effect residual condition concept. An easy way to distinguish between the two is to remember that the term *late* can be used to describe things or persons of the past (for example, my late husband). Residual refers to the present condition that exists as a result of the past condition or injury.

FOR EXAMPLE

In the following example the past condition is the wound:

906.0   Late effect of open wound of head, neck, and trunk

The residual may be scarring from the now-healed wound. ▪

Excludes

The ICD-9-CM manual provides a list of conditions, diseases, and injuries that are not included in the code being considered in the tabular (Volume 1). The condition, disease, or injury being coded is located elsewhere in the ICD-9-CM manual.

Excludes notes may be found at the beginning of a chapter, section, or category or directly below the code. The placement of an *excludes* note identifies the range of codes to which the note applies.

FOR EXAMPLE

An *excludes* note found at the chapter level, Chapter 3 in this example, is:

endocrine and metabolic disturbances specific to the fetus and newborn (775.0–775.9)

The note placement indicates that these conditions are coded in another chapter of the ICD-9-CM manual. ▪

By contrast, an *excludes* note found at the category level governs only codes within that category (codes beginning with the same three numbers).

FOR EXAMPLE
The *excludes* note found below category 250 provides a list of conditions that are not included in this category but may still be found within the same chapter of ICD-9-CM. ▪

Includes

Includes notes further clarify the code or category being considered by providing definitions or examples of conditions included in the code. Although *includes* notes are not found at the four- and five-digit code levels, inclusion terms may be found at these levels that aid the coder by providing synonyms of the diagnostic statement being coded.

Symptoms and Signs

In addition to listing codes for conditions, diseases, and injuries, the ICD-9-CM manual includes codes to be used by providers when no definitive diagnosis has been established. The Symptoms, Signs, and Ill-Defined Conditions chapter contains a comprehensive list of these codes.

According to the ICD-9-CM Section IV guidelines, providers must use codes for **signs** and **symptoms** instead of codes for diagnosis when a definitive diagnosis has not been made. Review the ICD-9-CM guidelines at Section IV, E and I.

By contrast, signs and symptoms are not coded when they are commonly found with the definitive diagnosis. See the ICD-9-CM coding guideline at Section I, B, 7.

sign An objective condition that can be measured and recorded.

symptom A subjective condition that is relayed to the provider by the patient.

FOR EXAMPLE Pain would be inherent to or normal with appendicitis. ■

SPOTLIGHT on Terminology

Sign A condition that can be measured and recorded. *Sign* is an objective term.

Symptom A condition that is relayed to the provider by the patient. *Symptom* is a subjective term.

Code First and *Use Additional Code*

At times more than one code is needed to clearly define a condition, injury, or disease as documented by the provider. This may occur when the condition is a **manifestation** produced by another condition (etiology) or is a complication of a treatment, disease, or condition.

ICD-9 CM provides the instructional notes **code first** and **use additional code** in the tabular section when additional information is needed to further define the patient's diagnosis. The *use additional code* note differs from the *code also* instruction as *use additional code* implies sequencing of the codes when reported.

manifestation How the condition due to the underlying disease presents itself.

code first and **use additional code** Directional terms that identify required sequencing. The directional "code first" informs the coder that the code being referenced is sequenced second to the primary code. The directional "use additional code" informs the coder that the code being referenced is sequenced as the first listed code in a pairing of codes.

FOR EXAMPLE

acute chest syndrome (517.3) in a patient with Hb-SS sickle-cell disease with crisis (282.62)

For this example, the ICD-9-CM provides guidance within the Tabular List that instructs the coder to code first sickle-cell disease in crisis. The *use additional code* instruction is found below the first-listed code in the tabular section of the ICD-9-CM manual. ■

Regardless of the type of instructional note, the official ICD-9-CM conventions instruct the coder to list the additional code only if the documentation provides the additional information needed to accurately select the code.

Punctuation

Discussed below are some of the more common punctuation marks that a coder needs to be aware of and know how to use effectively. Knowing what information each of these punctuation marks relays and how each impacts the selection of the code will help speed the process of coding as well as increase the accuracy of the codes used. As stated earlier, many of the conventions, abbreviations, and punctuation marks used in the ICD-9-CM manual are means of saving space within the text.

Brackets: Square [ ], Slanted [ ]

ICD-9-CM uses two types of brackets to convey information. **Square brackets**, [ ], are found in the tabular section and are used in two specific ways: to enclose explanatory phrases or to enclose other terms or names of the condition in the nomenclature of the code or inclusion list.

square brackets In ICD-9-CM, punctuation marks used to enclose explanatory phrases or synonyms of the condition and valid fifth digits for the code being reviewed.

FOR EXAMPLE

code 038.2 Pneumococcal septicemia [Streptococcus pneumonia septicemia] ■

Square brackets, [ ], may also be found directly below a code and are used to enclose valid fifth digits for the code being reviewed.

FOR EXAMPLE

678.0-
[0,1,3] ■

By contrast, **slanted brackets, [ ],** are found only in the index and identify mandatory sequencing of etiology/manifestation coding.

slanted brackets In ICD-9-CM, punctuation marks used to identify the mandatory sequencing of etiology/manifestation coding.

FOR EXAMPLE When using the index to find diabetic retinitis, the coder would find:

250.5-, [362.01] ■

SPOTLIGHT on Terminology

Etiology The underlying cause or origin of a condition or disease.

Manifestation How the condition due to the underlying disease presents itself.

parentheses Punctuation marks used to enclose supplemental terms, or nonessential modifiers.

Parentheses ( )

Parentheses, ( ), are found in both the Tabular List and the Alphabetic Index and are used in both to enclose supplemental terms, also known as *nonessential modifiers*. These terms may or may not be included in the provider's documentation, but their noninclusion does not affect the code choice.

FOR EXAMPLE Look up *pneumonia* in the Alphabetic Index (Volume 2). There are multiple words listed in parentheses next to the word *pneumonia*. When any of these words are listed with pneumonia in a diagnostic statement, the appropriate code to use is 486 and not one of the more specific pneumonia codes listed below the main term in the index. ■

EXERCISE 2.2

1. Explain the difference between the abbreviations *NEC* and *NOS*.
2. How do slanted brackets affect the sequencing of codes?
3. What must be present for the coder to report an additional code?

Also available in 📕 **Connect** (plus+)

2.3 Main Terms and the ICD-9-CM Index

One of the main components of correct coding with ICD-9-CM is coding to the highest degree of specificity. This means telling the patient's story to the highest degree of detail allowed by ICD-9-CM. ICD-9-CM has approximately 14,000 codes that can be used to translate the diagnostic story.

The provider's documentation must be reviewed before the coder can translate it into the appropriate ICD-9-CM code(s). The coder must determine whether there is a definitive diagnosis. If none is available, the coder may use the appropriate sign or symptom (as reviewed in Section 2.1).

The coder refers to the index using diagnoses, conditions, signs, symptoms, syndromes, and eponyms. Codes cannot be found in the index under anatomical sites. If a coder looks up a term in the index under an anatomical site, the index will refer the coder to "see condition."

FOR EXAMPLE At the entry "lung" the index states "see condition," meaning that the coder must look under the specific disease, sign, or symptom occurring at this anatomical site. ■

Main Term

The **main term,** as found in the provider's diagnostic statement, identifies, without further descriptive clarifications, the patient's condition, injury, or disease. Determining the main term is the first step in locating a code in the Alphabetic Index (Volume 2) of the ICD-9-CM manual. Main terms are bold-faced, and each is further defined by indented subterms.

FOR EXAMPLE Congestive heart failure:

> Failure
>> Heart
>>> Congestive

MENTOR Coding Tip

When unsure of the main term in a diagnostic statement, ask the question, "What did the patient suffer from?" Nonmain terms should sound out of place as answers to this question.

FOR EXAMPLE The diagnostic statement includes "left ventricular myocardial infarction." Answer the question using each term: The patient suffers from *left*—obvious wrong answer. The patient suffers from *ventricular*—again this answer makes no sense. The same is true of the term *myocardial.* However, the final term resonates as a viable statement: The patient suffers from *infarction.* Therefore, the main term in this statement is *infarction.*

Major Steps in Locating the Appropriate ICD-9-CM Code

After reading the provider documentation thoroughly, the coder should follow these steps:

1. Determine the main term(s) from the documentation.
2. Locate the main term in the Alphabetic Index (Volume 2).
3. Identify and review any subterms listed below the main term in the Alphabetic Index. Then identify in the provider's documentation the subterm that further defines and supports the level of specificity of the condition as documented.
4. Review all notes listed in the Alphabetic Index and Tabular List.
5. Verify the code identified in the Alphabetic Index by checking it in the Tabular List (Volume 1).
6. Determine the code to the highest degree of specificity (use a fourth or fifth digit if required).

Be sure to read all of the instructional notes that exist for the chapter, section, and category of ICD-9-CM code(s) that you are choosing, as these guidelines supersede the chapter-specific guidelines found in the official coding guidelines of the ICD-9-CM manual.

EXERCISE 2.3

Underline the main term in each diagnostic statement below, follow the steps listed above, and determine the appropriate ICD-9-CM code.

1. Capsular congenital cataract.
2. Family history of malignant neoplasm of the bladder.
3. Laceration of the forearm.

Also available in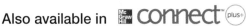

2.4 ICD-9-CM Chapter-Specific Guidelines

In this section we identify various chapter-specific guidelines. Remember: When we refer to chapter guidelines in this section, we are referring to the chapters in the ICD-9-CM manual.

FOR EXAMPLE "Chapter 1" refers to the Infectious and Parasitic Diseases chapter in the ICD-9-CM manual. ■

MENTOR Coding Tip

When preparing for the CPC exam, study the chapter-specific guidelines a few days before taking the exam. This is a good review, and it will remind you during the test that you just "read something about this." This reminder during the exam often takes away the feeling of being overwhelmed.

ICD-9-CM contains 17 chapters plus sections on V and E codes. Table 2.1 presents an overview of some of the guidelines. In this text, we examine these guidelines in detail in the chapters pertaining to particular body systems.

EXERCISE 2.4

1. ICD-9-CM chapter-specific guidelines for Chapter 2 include which type of guidelines?
2. ICD-9-CM chapter-specific guidelines for Chapter 7 include which type of guidelines?
3. ICD-9-CM chapter-specific guidelines for Chapter 17 include which type of guidelines?

Also available in

Table 2.1 Chapter-Specific Guidelines for ICD-9-CM *(Data from ICD-9-CM, Centers for Medicare and Medicaid Services and the National Center for Health Statistics.)*

CHAPTER	GUIDELINES
1. Infectious and Parasitic Diseases	These guidelines are very specific and concern the coding of HIV, septicemia, SIRS, sepsis, and MRSA. The guidelines include selection and sequencing instructions specific to these conditions.
2. Neoplasms	These guidelines pertain to general guidelines for reporting neoplasms and sequencing instructions pertaining to history of malignant neoplasm, administration of chemotherapy, radiotherapy, and complications due to the condition or therapy.
3. Endocrine, Nutritional, and Metabolic Diseases and Immunity Disorders	Included in this chapter are the guidelines for diabetes. The codes in this chapter require fifth digits. There are also multiple-sequencing guidelines, including those on the use of slanted brackets (etiology/manifestation sequencing).
4. Diseases of Blood and Blood-Forming Organs	General and sequencing instructions for anemia are included in these guidelines. Also included are instructions for coding anemia associated with other diseases.
5. Mental Disorders	Currently there are no guidelines for this chapter.
6. Diseases of the Nervous System and Sense Organs	Very specific guidelines for coding pain are included in these guidelines.
7. Diseases of the Circulatory System	Hypertension and hypertensive heart and kidney disease guidelines are located in this chapter, along with guidelines on cerebral infarction, stroke, cerebral vascular accident, late effects, and myocardial infarction.
8. Diseases of the Respiratory System	Instructions and code sequencing for chronic obstructive pulmonary disease (COPD), asthma, bronchitis, and respiratory failure are included in these guidelines.
9. Diseases of the Digestive System	Currently there are no guidelines for this chapter.
10. Diseases of the Genitourinary System	These guidelines include instructions for the coding and sequencing of chronic kidney disease (CKD).
11. Complications of Pregnancy, Childbirth, and the Puerperium	These guidelines include general rules for obstetric care and coding and sequencing instructions for fetal conditions affecting management of pregnancy, HIV infection in pregnancy, normal delivery and postpartum conditions, and abortions.
12. Diseases of the Skin and Subcutaneous Tissue	Guidelines for coding pressure ulcer stages are located in this chapter.
13. Diseases of the Musculoskeletal System and Connective Tissue	Guidelines for the coding of pathologic fractures are included in this chapter.
14. Congenital Anomalies	Currently there are no guidelines for this chapter.
15. Newborn (Perinatal) Guidelines	General perinatal rules and sequencing are included in these guidelines. The use of some V codes is also reviewed here.
16. Symptoms, Signs, and Ill-Defined Conditions	Currently there are no guidelines for this chapter.
17. Injury and Poisoning	Instructions on injuries, fractures, burns, adverse effects, poisoning, and toxic effects are included in these guidelines.
V and E codes:	Guidelines for V and E codes and their sequencing are also included in the chapter-specific guideline section.

2.5 Diagnostic Outpatient Guidelines

The official ICD-9-CM coding guidelines are located in Section IV, I, of the ICD-9-CM manual. These guidelines are used for reporting hospital-based outpatient services and provider-based office visits.

MENTOR Coding Tip

According to ICD-9-CM, "The coding conventions of ICD-9-CM as well as the general and disease specific guidelines take precedence over the outpatient guidelines." When coding, remember that there is a hierarchy to the coding guidelines and conventions. Guidelines or conventions listed at the code level in the Tabular List take precedence over those at the section level. Those listed at the section level take precedence over those at the chapter level. Basically, this means that the closer a guideline or convention is to the code in the Tabular List (Volume 1), the higher it is in the hierarchy of guidelines and thus it supersedes the other guidelines or conventions.

Highlights of Diagnostic Outpatient Guidelines

- **First-listed diagnosis versus principal diagnosis:** The first-listed diagnosis (reason for the visit) is used for provider/outpatient coding. The principal diagnosis (reason for admission after study) is used for facility coding.
- **Signs and symptoms:** Signs and symptoms are acceptable for reporting when a diagnosis has not been confirmed and reported by the provider.
- **Coding to the highest level of specificity:** This guideline refers to the use of fourth and fifth digits when required.
- **Unconfirmed diagnosis term:** Unconfirmed diagnosis terms such as *rule out, probable, access,* and *questionable* may *not* be used in outpatient diagnostic coding. A sign or symptom must be used in place of an unconfirmed diagnosis.
- **Chronic disease:** Chronic conditions may be coded if the chronic condition affects the treatment or management of the presenting condition.

These guidelines are examined in detail in the system-specific chapters of this textbook, as appropriate.

EXERCISE 2.5

1. Explain the difference between a first-listed diagnosis and a principal diagnosis.
2. When is it acceptable to report a sign or symptom?
3. When may a chronic condition be coded?

Also available in McGraw Hill **connect**™ (plus+)

2.6 Translating Provider Documentation to Ensure Medical Necessity

As you work through this text, you will notice that we continue to stress the importance of being able to translate the provider's documentation correctly to ensure that the proper ICD-9-CM code is chosen. One very important aspect of being able to accomplish this translation is the ability to link the medical necessity of the documented encounter to the service provided.

The ability to do this accurately and efficiently and within compliance guidelines is achieved by having a good knowledge of anatomy, medical terminology, physiology, pathophysiology, and basic coding rules and guidelines. The example below demonstrates the importance of this knowledge.

FOR EXAMPLE The provider documents that the patient presents to the provider's office for evaluation of cervical pain and determination of treatment via facet injections. The provider also documents that this patient has diabetes type 2 and benign hypertension. In this example, a coder's knowledge is tested in several ways. First is the term *cervical*. As there are two areas in the female anatomy that may be identified by this main term, the coder needs the additional information provided in the documentation to identify which area is the site of the patient's pain. The proposed treatment of facet injections keys the coder to an anatomical area and provides the additional information necessary to identify the term *cervical* as related to the neck and not the genital/urinary body system.

Next is the understanding of when to code for an additional diagnosis. The ICD-9-CM guidelines for listing additional diagnoses instruct the coder to code for all conditions that affect the patient's care, treatment, or management (Section IV, K). The guidelines further guide the coder in regard to the coding of chronic conditions, such as those in the example, diabetes and hypertension. A chronic condition may be listed if during the encounter the patient receives care or treatment for the condition (Section IV, J). In the example above, there is no documentation to support care or treatment directed at either of the additional chronic conditions listed, and therefore neither would be coded. Finally, the coder's knowledge of pathophysiology is tested to determine whether the conditions that coexist, diabetes and hypertension, with the reason for the encounter, cervical pain, affect either the condition or treatment of the cervical pain. In this example, these chronic conditions do not impact the treatment or management of the condition being treated and therefore would not be coded in addition to the cervical pain. ▪

Throughout this text you will have ample opportunity to test your knowledge of anatomy, medical terminology, physiology, pathophysiology, and basic coding rules and guidelines and to practice translating data in each of these categories into diagnostic codes. The CPC exam will test you on your ability to translate this information.

1. Briefly discuss the importance of translating the medical record into accurate coding data, and explain why it is important to have a thorough knowledge of anatomy, medical terminology, and pathophysiology.

EXERCISE 2.6

Also available in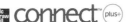

Chapter Two Summary

Learning Outcome	Key Concepts/Examples
2.1 Understand the format of the ICD-9-CM manual.	Volume 1: Tabular List Volume 2: Alphabetic Index Volume 3: Alphabetic Index and Tabular List for Procedures Volumes 1 and 2 are used for hospital-based outpatient services and provider-based office visits.
2.2 Apply the abbreviations, coding conventions, and punctuation marks used in ICD-9-CM.	**Abbreviations** *NEC—not elsewhere classified:* A more specific code is not provided. *NOS—not otherwise specified:* This is the equivalent of unspecified. **Coding conventions/instructional notes** *Acute:* sudden onset, short duration *Chronic:* slow onset, long duration *Excludes:* list of conditions, diagnoses, etc., *not* included in codes in Tabular List *Includes:* further clarifies the definition of terms included in codes in the Tabular List **Punctuation** *Slanted brackets [ ]:* used to identify sequencing of etiology/manifestation *Square brackets [ ]:* used to enclose explanatory phrases or other terms or names of conditions *Parentheses ( ):* used to enclose supplemental terms, which are also known as nonessential modifiers
2.3 Identify main terms and use the ICD-9-CM index.	*Main term:* describes the patient illness or injury (the reason for the present encounter) documented by the provider **Steps in locating the appropriate ICD-9-CM code** After reading the documentation thoroughly: 1. Identify the main term. 2. Locate the main term in the Alphabetic Index. 3. Identify appropriate subterms in the Alphabetic Index. 4. Read all instructional notes. 5. Verify the code in the Tabular List. 6. Code to the highest level of specificity.
2.4 Review ICD-9-CM chapter-specific guidelines.	ICD-9-CM contains 17 chapters and most have specific guidelines. There are also guidelines for V and E codes.
2.5 Examine ICD-9-CM diagnostic outpatient guidelines.	*First-listed diagnosis:* This is the reason for the visit and is used for provider/outpatient coding. *Signs and symptoms:* These may be reported when a diagnosis has not been confirmed. *Code to highest level of specificity:* Use fourth and fifth digits, as appropriate. *Unconfirmed diagnoses:* Do not use unconfirmed terms such as rule out. *Chronic conditions:* A chronic condition may be coded if it affects the treatment or management of the presenting condition.
2.6 Recognize the importance of translating provider terminology into accurate diagnostic codes.	An important aspect is the ability to link the medical necessity of the documented encounter to the service provided.

Chapter Two Review

Using Terminology

Match each key term to the appropriate definition.

_____ 1. [LO2.2] Acute
_____ 2. [LO2.2] And
_____ 3. [LO2.3] Main term
_____ 4. [LO2.2] Brackets
_____ 5. [LO2.2] Slanted brackets
_____ 6. [LO2.2] Late effect
_____ 7. [LO2.2] Includes
_____ 8. [LO2.2] Excludes
_____ 9. [LO2.2] NEC
_____ 10. [LO2.2] Sign
_____ 11. [LO2.2] Symptom
_____ 12. [LO2.2] Chronic
_____ 13. [LO2.2] Manifestation
_____ 14. [LO2.2] Parentheses
_____ 15. [LO2.2] NOS

A. Not elsewhere classified
B. Means "and/or" in ICD-9-CM
C. Describes the patient's illness or injury in the documentation
D. The equivalent of unspecified
E. The way the condition due to the underlying disease presents itself
F. Condition with a slow onset and of long duration
G. A residual condition that occurs after the initial injury or illness
H. Punctuation marks used to enclose supplemental terms, which are also known as nonessential modifiers
I. Condition with a sudden onset and of brief duration
J. Instructional note that provides a list of conditions, diseases, or injuries that are not included in the code listed in Volume 2 (Tabular List)
K. Condition that can be measured and recorded.
L. Condition that is relayed to the provider by the patient
M. Punctuation marks used to enclose explanatory phrases or other appropriate descriptive terms for the code
N. Instructional note that further clarifies the code or category by providing examples of conditions included in the code
O. Punctuation marks that identify mandatory sequencing of etiology/manifestation coding

Checking Your Understanding

Choose the most appropriate answer for each of the following questions.

1. [LO2.2] This abbreviation is next to an ICD-9-CM code when a more appropriate code is not provided elsewhere in the manual:
   a. NOS
   b. NEC
   c. DEF
   d. None of these

2. [LO2.4] Which chapter-specific guidelines include instructions for coding chronic kidney disease?
   a. Chapter 7, Diseases of the Circulatory System
   b. Chapter 10, Diseases of the Genitourinary System
   c. Chapter 16, Symptoms, Signs, and Ill-Defined Conditions
   d. None of these (There are no guidelines for the kidney system.)

3. [LO2.2] Which of the following, when noted in the Alphabetic Index or Tabular List, instructs the coder on the mandatory sequencing of the etiology/manifestation?
   a. Slanted brackets
   b. Brackets
   c. Parentheses
   d. Code first

4. [LO2. 3] Which is *not* an appropriate step in determining an ICD-9-CM code?
   a. Determine the main term from the provider documentation.
   b. Determine any appropriate subterms.
   c. Determine the code directly from the Alphabetic Index.
   d. Code to the highest level of specificity by using appropriate fourth- and fifth-digit codes.

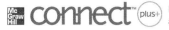

Enhance your learning by completing these exercises and more at mcgrawhillconnect.com

5. **[LO2.5]** According to the diagnostic outpatient guidelines, which of the following best fits the guidelines for the use of signs and symptoms?

   a. They are always to be used.

   b. They are reported only when a diagnosis has not been confirmed and reported by the provider.

   c. There are no specific guidelines as to their use.

   d. They must be documented in the provider records to be used.

6. **[LO2.5]** Coding to the highest level of specificity means:

   a. Coding all the conditions listed in the patient's chart

   b. Coding just the condition for which the patient is being seen

   c. Using a fourth- or fifth-digit when required

   d. None of these

7. **[LO2.6]** Which of the following are important aspects of a coder's being able to translate provider documentation?

   a. Ensuring that the proper ICD-9-CM code is chosen

   b. Being able to stay within compliance guidelines

   c. Linking the medical necessity of the encounter to the service provided

   d. All of these

8. **[LO2.1]** Which volume or volumes of ICD-9-CM are used when taking the CPC exam?

   a. Volume 1   **c.** Volume 3

   b. Volume 2   **d.** Volumes 1 and 2

9. **[LO2.2]** What is the term for a condition due to an underlying disease or condition?

   a. Manifestation   **c.** Sign

   b. Etiology   **d.** Symptom

10. **[LO2.2]** Which term is used to describe a residual condition that occurs after the initial illness or injury?

    a. Sign   **c.** Manifestation

    b. Symptom   **d.** Late effect

Applying Your Knowledge

Use your critical-thinking skills to answer the questions below.

1. **[LO2.3]** Discuss the main steps that a coder needs to follow when translating a provider's documentation and determining the appropriate code using the ICD-9-CM manual.

   _____

2. **[LO2.2]** Explain the differences between *acute* and *chronic,* and list one of the guidelines pertaining to these terms.

   _____

3. **[LO2.2]** Explain the difference between *includes* and *excludes* and the importance each plays in determining the correct ICD-9-CM code.

   _____

4. **[LO2.1–LO2.6]** List five mentor coding tips discussed in this chapter that you considered most helpful.

   _____

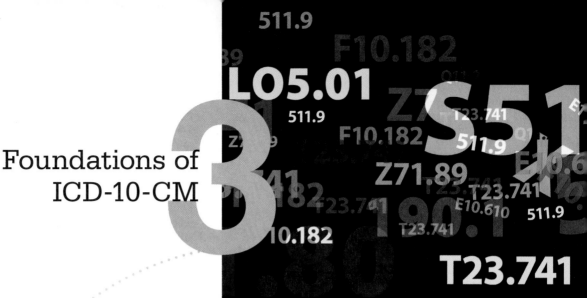

Foundations of ICD-10-CM

3

Key Terms

Acute
And
Chronic
Default code
Excludes 1
Excludes 2

Extenders
Impending condition
Includes
Main term
Manifestation
NEC

NOS
Parentheses
Placeholder characters
Sequela
Sign
Square brackets

Symptom
Threatened condition
With
Without

Learning Outcomes

After completing this chapter, you will be able to:

3.1 Understand the format of ICD-10-CM.

3.2 Explain the abbreviations, coding conventions, and punctuation marks used in ICD-10-CM.

3.3 Identify main terms, default codes, extenders, and placeholders and explain their importance in the use of the ICD-10-CM index.

3.4 Apply ICD-10-CM chapter-specific guidelines.

3.5 Explain ICD-10-CM diagnostic outpatient guidelines.

3.6 Recognize the importance of translating provider terminology into accurate diagnostic codes.

Introduction Upon final implementation, October 1, 2014, ICD-10-CM and ICD-10-PCS (Procedural Coding System) will replace ICD-9-CM for providers as well as outpatient and inpatient facilities. The CPC exam given throughout the year of actual implementation will still be based on the ICD-9-CM manual, and this is the manual coders will use when taking the CPC exam. Beginning January 1 in the year following implementation, the CPC exam will be based on ICD-10-CM. Coders with a current CPC credential will be required to take an ICD-10-CM proficiency exam. An understanding of the ICD-10-CM conventions and guidelines and the differences from the ICD-9-CM manual will be needed for the proficiency exam and CPC exam after the final implementation of ICD-10-CM.

Chapter-specific coding guidelines and details highlighting the changes in diagnostic coding between ICD-9-CM and ICD-10-CM occur in subsequent chapters of this text and encompass the diagnostic codes that are commonly used with specific body systems.

3.1 Format of ICD-10-CM

The abbreviation *ICD-10-CM* stands for "International Classification of Diseases, Tenth Revision, Clinical Modification." The ICD-10-CM manual, like the ICD-9-CM manual, is the translation dictionary that coders use to translate medical terminology from provider documentation into the codes used to tell the patient's diagnostic story. ICD-10-CM is the "why," or the condition, cause, reason for the patient's service or procedure. Understanding the format of the ICD-10-CM manual and being able to implement the guidelines and coding conventions enables coders to not only succeed with the CPC exam but also achieve accuracy and consistency in coding of the medical record.

Unlike the ICD-9-CM, which is published in two and three volume sets, the ICD-10-CM is published in two main parts, or sections, and is used by both providers and facilities to identify why the service or procedure was provided. The ICD-10-CM includes only diagnostic codes. After the final implementation date, facilities will use ICD-10-PCS (Procedural Coding System) to code procedures performed in the facility. The Tabular List of the ICD-10-CM contains the codes and the full description (nomenclature) of each code and is divided into chapters based on body systems or conditions.

The index of the ICD-10-CM contains an alphabetic listing of main terms identifying the patient's condition, injury, sign, or symptom. Subterms follow the main term in a graduated indented format and provide for further clarification of the patient's condition, thus allowing the coder to drill down to a more accurate code before cross-referencing the code in the Tabular List.

> **MENTOR**
> **Coding Tip**
>
> When searching through the index, pay close attention to indentations as you move from one column to the next.

> **MENTOR** Coding Tip
>
> Coding students may find it very helpful to tab the ICD-10-CM manual. They use self-adhesive tabs or labels to mark the individual tables in the Alphabetic Index (hypertension, neoplasm, table of drugs and chemicals) and the individual chapters in the Tabular List to identify a range of codes. They may find that this saves them considerable time when they are taking the CPC exam since the tabs enable them to quickly locate the code indicated in the index.

EXERCISE 3.1

1. What is the function of a subterm?
2. Explain which providers and entities will use ICD-10-CM and/or ICD-10-PCS.

Also available in Mc Graw Hill **connect** (plus+)

3.2 Abbreviations, Coding Conventions, Guidelines, Instructional Notes, and Punctuation

ICD-10-CM uses several abbreviations, symbols, and punctuation marks within the index and tabular listing. Many of these are space-saving devices within the ICD-10-CM manual. The significance of punctuation is reviewed later in this chapter. This section begins with an explanation of two abbreviations that confuse even experienced coders.

Abbreviations

NEC and *NOS* are two coding-convention abbreviations that are important for a coder to differentiate and know how to use. The definitions of each can be found in the Conventions section of the ICD-10-CM manual guidelines.

NEC is an abbreviation that means "not elsewhere classified." It is used when a more specific code is not provided in ICD-10-CM. In this, case the provider documentation is more specific in its description of the patient's condition than the ICD-10-CM allows for in the code description. Such codes are identified with the term *NEC* in the Alphabetic Index of the ICD-10-CM.

NEC Notation meaning "not elsewhere classified"; indicates that a more specific code is not provided in the ICD manual.

> **FOR EXAMPLE** Sepsis due to klebsiella pneumonia in a newborn would be coded as:

other bacterial sepsis of newborn (P36.8)

This is because the level of detail needed to identify this condition fully is not provided in the description of any of the choices listed in the ICD-10-CM for bacterial sepsis of newborns. ■

NOS stands for "not otherwise specified." This is the equivalent of "unspecified." This abbreviation is to be used only when the documentation does not provide enough information to assign a more specific code.

NOS Notation meaning "not otherwise specified"; the equivalent of unspecified.

> **FOR EXAMPLE** A less detailed diagnostic statement of newborn sepsis, bacterial, would be coded as:

bacterial sepsis of newborn, unspecified (P36.9)

This is because the diagnostic statement does not describe the type of bacteria causing the sepsis. ■

Coding Conventions, Guidelines, and Instructional Notes

The official ICD-10-CM coding conventions, as well as the Additional Conventions section, provide detail on the use of the symbols, official footnotes, instructional notes, conventions, and notations found in both the Alphabetic Index and the Tabular List of ICD-10-CM. Correct use and a comprehensive understanding of these conventions allow for consistency in coding and assist the coder in selecting the most accurate diagnosis code for the disease, condition, or injury as documented by the provider.

Acute and Chronic

One ICD-10-CM guideline addresses the use and sequencing of codes for **acute** and **chronic** conditions. The guideline instructs that when both the acute and chronic forms of a condition are documented, both conditions should be coded. Based on the guidelines, there are two ways these conditions may be coded: together, as a combination code that identifies both the chronic and acute forms of the condition in one code, or separately, with one code for the acute condition and another for the chronic condition.

Both combination codes and distinct codes are recognizable in the Alphabetic Index. After locating the main term of the condition (acute and chronic forms of the same condition are located under the same main term), review both subterms, *acute* and *chronic*. If the subterms *acute* and *chronic* are connected by a *with* statement, ICD-10-CM provides a combination code, or one code to indicate both conditions.

FOR EXAMPLE From the Alphabetic Index:

Bronchitis
  Acute or subacute
    with
      Chronic obstructive pulmonary disease J44.0 ■

MENTOR
Coding Tip

Be sure to review both the *acute* and *chronic* subterms to identify available combination codes, since they are not always found under both terms. In the example above, the combination code is found only by reviewing the subterm of *acute*.

SPOTLIGHT on Terminology

Acute Conditions with sudden onset, usually without warning, and of brief duration. For example: fractures, intestinal flu, and rhinitis.

Chronic Conditions with slow onset and of long duration, even the lifetime of the patient. For example: diabetes, hypertension, and asthma.

When a combination code is not available and two distinct codes are needed to fully describe the patient's condition or disease, the ICD-10-CM guidelines instruct the coder to list both the acute and chronic codes with the acute condition listed first, followed by the chronic condition.

And

The ICD-10-CM use of the word **and** is specified in the coding convention and is to be interpreted to mean "and/or."

FOR EXAMPLE

L04.0 Acute lymphadenitis of face, head, and neck

This code may be used for acute lymphadenitis of the face, head, and neck; or of just the face, just the head, or just the neck; or of any combination of these sites. ■

With and Without

In the ICD-10-CM tabular listing there may be codes within the same category or subclassification of a condition that differ only by the presence or absence of an associated complication or comorbidity. The distinction between these codes is identified by the statement of **with** when the condition or complication is present and **without** when the condition or complication is not present.

FOR EXAMPLE

S01.01   Laceration without foreign body of scalp

S01.02   Laceration with foreign body of scalp ▪

Excludes Notes

The ICD-10-CM manual provides a list of conditions, diseases, and injuries that are separate and distinct from the code being considered. There are two types of excludes notes: *Excludes 1* and *Excludes 2*.

Excludes 1 indicates that the condition, disease, or injury being coded is located elsewhere in the ICD-10-CM manual and should never be coded with the code under which the *Excludes 1* note is placed. Conditions identified by this note cannot be present together and therefore are never coded during the same encounter.

FOR EXAMPLE

J37.1   Chronic laryngotracheitis

Excludes 1 chronic tracheitis (J42) ▪

Excludes 2 is used to alert the coder that the condition listed in the *excludes* list is distinct from the code condition and is coded elsewhere in the ICD-10-CM. The condition excluded may occur with the condition represented by the code, and their two codes may be used together during the same encounter.

FOR EXAMPLE

J37.1   Chronic laryngotracheitis

Excludes 2 acute laryngotracheitis (J04.2)

acute tracheitis (J04.1) ▪

Excludes 1 and *Excludes 2* notes may be found at the beginning of a chapter, section, or category or directly below the code. This placement of an *excludes* note identifies the range of codes to which the note applies.

FOR EXAMPLE
An *excludes* note found at the chapter level, Chapter 1 in this example, is:

certain infectious and parasitic diseases (A00–B99)

Excludes 1 certain localized infection and Excludes 2 carrier or suspected carrier of infectious disease

The *Excludes 1* note placement indicates that the conditions listed cannot be coded with other codes from Chapter 1. The *Excludes 2* note indicates that infectious and parasitic diseases specific to the perinatal period are coded in another chapter of the ICD-10-CM manual but may be present with other conditions in Chapter 1. ▪

By contrast an *excludes* note found at the category level governs only codes within that category (codes beginning with the same three characters).

FOR EXAMPLE The *Excludes 1* note found below category A05, "Other bacterial foodborne intoxications, not elsewhere classified," provides a list of conditions that are never coded with the conditions in category A05 but may be found elsewhere in Chapter 1 of ICD-10-CM. ■

Includes

Includes notes further clarify the code or category being considered by providing definitions or examples of conditions included in the code. Although *includes* notes are not found at the fourth- and fifth-digit code levels, inclusion terms may be found at these levels that aid the coder by providing synonyms of the diagnostic statement being coded.

MENTOR Coding Tip

Remember that the inclusion terms are not all-inclusive and other terms may be listed in the index and not included in the tabular list. When this occurs, be sure to double-check the term and code in the index to avoid transposition of code digits before selecting the code.

Symptoms and Signs

In addition to listing codes for conditions, diseases, and injuries, the ICD-10-CM includes codes to be used by providers when no definitive diagnosis has been established. The Symptoms, Signs, and Ill-Defined Conditions chapter contains a comprehensive list of these codes.

SPOTLIGHT on Terminology

Sign An objective condition such as blood pressure reading, heart rate, or measured temperature, which relates to the exam component of an Evaluation and Management service.

Symptom A subjective condition such as cough, chills, pain, or diarrhea, which relates to the history component of an Evaluation and Management service.

According to the ICD-10-CM Section IV guidelines, providers must use codes for **signs** and **symptoms** instead of codes for diagnosis when a definitive diagnosis has not been made. Review the ICD-10-CM guidelines at Section IV, D and H.

By contrast, signs and symptoms are not coded when they are commonly found with the definitive diagnosis. See the ICD-10-CM coding guideline at Section I, B, 4.

MENTOR Coding Tip

If the sign or symptom is inherent to (commonly a part of) the definitive diagnosis, the sign or symptom is not coded in addition to the diagnosis.

FOR EXAMPLE Pain would be inherent to appendicitis. ■

Code First and Use Additional Code

At times more than one code is needed to clearly define the condition, injury, or disease as documented by the provider. This may occur when the condition is a **manifestation** produced by another condition (etiology) or is a complication of a treatment, disease, or condition.

ICD-10-CM provides the instructional notes *code first* and *use additional code* in the tabular section when additional information is needed to further define the patient's diagnosis.

The *use additional code* note differs from the *code also* instruction as *use additional code* implies sequencing of the codes when reported.

FOR EXAMPLE

end stage renal disease (N18.6) due to type 1 diabetes mellitus (E10.22)

For this example, the ICD-10-CM provides guidance within the Tabular List that instructs the coder to code first the underlying disease, type 1 DM with chronic kidney disease (E10.22). In this case the instruction is found directly below the category of N16. The *use additional code* instruction is found below the first-listed code in the tabular section of the ICD-10-CM manual (E10.22). ■

Regardless of the type of instructional note, the official ICD-10-CM conventions instruct the coder to list the additional code only if the documentation provides the additional information needed to accurately select the code.

MENTOR Coding Tip

When searching for additional codes, be aware that unspecified codes may be used for the second-listed code when the provider's documentation is less detailed than needed to select a more accurate code. For example: A41.9 Sepsis, unspecified.

Punctuation

Included in this section are some of the more common punctuation marks that a coder needs to be aware of and know how to use effectively. Knowing what information each of these punctuation marks relays and how each impacts the selection of the code will help speed the process of coding as well as increase the accuracy of the codes used. As stated earlier, many of the conventions, abbreviations, and punctuation marks used in the ICD-10-CM manual are means of saving space within the text.

Brackets

ICD-10-CM uses **square brackets, [ ]**, in the Tabular List to enclose explanatory phrases or other terms or names of the condition in the nomenclature of the code or inclusion list.

FOR EXAMPLE

A30   Leprosy [Hansen's disease] ■

By contrast, in the Alphabetic Index square brackets identify mandatory sequencing of etiology/manifestation coding.

FOR EXAMPLE When reviewing the Alphabetic Index for glaucoma due to amyloidosis, the coder would find:

Glaucoma H40.9

…

In (due to)

    Amyloidosis E85.4 [H42]

According to the ICD-10-CM convention, the first-listed code in the example above would be E85.4—amyloidosis—as the underlying condition (etiology), followed by code H42—glaucoma in diseases classified elsewhere (manifestation).

> **MENTOR** Coding Tip
>
> When the etiology/manifestation coding is identified in the index with the square-bracket convention, the codes must be reported in the sequencing identified by the convention regardless of which condition, etiology or manifestation, is being treated by the provider.

Parentheses

parentheses Punctuation marks used to enclose supplemental terms, or nonessential modifiers.

Parentheses, ( ), are found in both the Tabular List and the Alphabetic Index and are used in both to enclose supplemental terms, also known as *nonessential modifiers.* These terms may or may not be included in the provider's documentation, but their noninclusion does not affect the code choice.

FOR EXAMPLE Look up *pneumonia* in the Alphabetic Index. There are multiple words listed in parentheses following the main term *pneumonia.* When any of these words are listed with pneumonia in a diagnostic statement, the code listed (J18.9) is the appropriate code if no further specificity of the condition is provided in the provider's documentation. ■

EXERCISE 3.2

1. Explain *with* and *without* in ICD-10-CM.
2. Explain *Excludes 1* and *Excludes 2* in ICD-10-CM.

Also available in

3.3 Main Terms, Default Codes, Extenders, Placeholders, and the ICD-10-CM Index

As with ICD-9-CM codes, ICD-10-CM codes are used to translate the patient's story to the highest degree of detail allowed. The provider's documentation must be reviewed before a coder can achieve this translation to the appropriate diagnosis code.

Main Term

The **main term,** as found in the provider's diagnostic statement, identifies, without further descriptive clarifications, the patient's condition, injury, or disease. Determining the main term is the first step in locating a code in the Alphabetic Index of the ICD-10-CM manual. Main terms are bolded, and each is further defined by indented subterms.

FOR EXAMPLE   Congestive heart failure:

Failure
  Heart
    Congestive

MENTOR Coding Tip

When unsure of the main term in a diagnostic statement, ask the question, "What did the patient suffer from?" Nonmain terms should sound out of place as answers to this question.

FOR EXAMPLE   The diagnostic statement includes "left ventricular myocardial infarction." Answer the question using each term: The patient suffers from *left*— obvious wrong answer. The patient suffers from *ventricular*—again this answer makes no sense. The same is true of the term *myocardial.* However, the final term resonates as a viable statement: The patient suffers from *infarction.* Therefore, the main term in this statement is *infarction.*

Default Codes

In ICD-10-CM, a **default code** is a code that either is unspecified or is most often used with a condition. Default codes are located directly after the bold-faced main term and should be used only when the provider's documentation provides no additional detail regarding the patient's condition or disease.

FOR EXAMPLE   From the Alphabetic Index:

Fracture, traumatic T14.8

One of the main components of correct coding with ICD-10-CM is coding to the highest degree of specificity. ICD-10-CM has approximately 69,000 codes that can be used to translate the diagnostic story, with up to seven characters of detail incorporated in each code.

MENTOR Coding Tip

Be sure to review all indented subterms in the Alphabetic Index *and* the code nomenclature in the Tabular List before assigning a code, as a more specific ICD-10-CM code may be available. Also, although the ICD-10-CM index will indicate the need for additional fourth, fifth, and sixth characters by a dash (-) placed after the code, the need for seventh-character extenders is not identified in the Alphabetic Index.

Seventh-Character Extenders

extenders In ICD-10-CM, alphabetic seventh characters used to complete the description of many codes by conveying additional information.

ICD-10-CM makes use of seventh-character **extenders** to complete the description of many codes. This character is alphabetic and conveys information related to the code selected, such as episode of care, type of fracture, late effects, or trimester of pregnancy.

FOR EXAMPLE

S32.012B   Unstable burst fracture of first lumbar vertebra, **initial encounter for open fracture** ■

Placeholder Characters

The structure of ICD-10-CM codes is unique in requiring that the seventh-character extender must always be in the seventh-character position in the code. In ICD-10-CM, complete codes may be three, four, or five characters. ICD-10-CM uses **placeholder characters** to extend these codes to the sixth character. Using placeholder "x" in the fourth-, fifth-, or sixth-character place when needed allows the seventh-character extender to remain in the seventh-character position.

placeholder character In ICD-10-CM, an "x" placed in the fourth-, fifth-, or sixth-character place when needed to enable the seventh-character extender to remain in the seventh-character position.

FOR EXAMPLE

M84.50xA   Pathological fracture in neoplastic disease, unspecified site, initial encounter for fracture ■

Sequela (Late Effect)

sequela The condition produced after the initial injury or condition has healed.

ICD-10-CM **sequela** codes are used to describe a residual condition that occurs after the initial illness or injury. In most cases two codes are needed to describe the patient's condition: one for the residual or current condition and one for the previous injury or illness that led to the current condition.

FOR EXAMPLE

The individual sequela codes related to injuries are identified by the extension "S." ■

FOR EXAMPLE

Scar contracture of a previous nonpenetrating laceration, left anterior chest, would be coded as:

scar conditions and fibrosis of skin (L90.5)

and

laceration without foreign body of left front wall of thorax without penetration into thoracic cavity (S21.112S) ■

At times a combination code is provided by ICD-10-CM that identifies both the residual condition and the sequela.

FOR EXAMPLE

Monoplegia of upper limb following unspecified cerebrovascular disease affecting right dominant side (I69.931) ■

Impending or Threatened Conditions

At times providers may document conditions as **impending** or **threatened conditions**. These terms refer to specific diagnostic conditions and should not be considered synonymous with possible or probable conditions. These specific conditions, although limited, are located in the Alphabetic Index under the term *Impending* or *Threatened.* Their codes are used only when a condition was averted due to medical intervention, such as a myocardial infarction prevented by intervention in the cardiac cath lab.

impending or threatened conditions Specific diagnostic conditions whose codes are used only when the condition was averted due to medical intervention.

> FOR EXAMPLE
>
> **O20.0**   Threatened abortion ▪

If a medical condition did occur, code the condition and do not use the impending- or threatened-condition code. If there is no impending- or threatened-condition code for the patient's condition, code the underlying condition, such as COPD versus impending respiratory failure.

The provider's documentation must be reviewed before the coder can translate it into the appropriate ICD-10-CM code(s). The coder must determined whether there is a definitive diagnosis or impending condition. If neither of these is documented by the provider, the coder may use the appropriate sign or symptom (as reviewed in Section 3.2).

The coder refers to the index using diagnoses, conditions, signs, symptoms, and syndromes. Codes cannot be found in the index under anatomical sites. If a coder looks up a term in the index under an anatomical site, the index will refer the coder to "see condition."

> FOR EXAMPLE

At the entry "lung" the index states "see condition," meaning that the coder must look under the specific disease, sign, or symptom occurring at this anatomical site. ▪

Major Steps in Locating the Appropriate ICD-10-CM Code

After reading the provider documentation thoroughly, the coder should follow these steps:

1. Determine the main term(s) from the documentation.
2. Locate the main term(s) in the Alphabetic Index.

3. Identify and review any subterms listed below the main term in the Alphabetic Index. Then identify in the provider's documentation the subterm that further defines and supports the level of specificity of the condition as documented.

4. Review all notes listed in the Alphabetic Index and Tabular List.

5. Verify the code identified in the Alphabetic Index by checking it in the Tabular List.

6. Determine the code to the highest degree of specificity (use up to seven characters, including placeholder characters, if required).

Be sure to read all of the instructional notes that exist for the chapter, section, and category of ICD-10-CM code(s) you are choosing, as these guidelines supersede the chapter-specific guidelines found in the official coding guidelines of the ICD-10-CM manual.

EXERCISE 3.3

1. Explain default codes and their function in ICD-10-CM coding.
2. Explain extenders and their function in ICD-10-CM coding.
3. Explain placeholders and their function in ICD-10-CM coding.

Also available in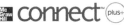

3.4 ICD-10-CM Chapter-Specific Guidelines

In this section we identify various chapter-specific guidelines. When we refer to chapter guidelines in this section, we are referring to the chapters in the ICD-10-CM manual.

FOR EXAMPLE "Chapter 1" refers to the Certain Infectious and Parasitic Diseases chapter in the ICD-10-CM manual.

MENTOR Coding Tip

When preparing for the CPC exam, study the chapter-specific guidelines a few days before taking the exam. This is a good review, and it will remind you during the test that you just "read something about this". This reminder during the exam often takes away the feeling of being overwhelmed.

ICD-10-CM contains 21 chapters. Table 3.1 presents an overview of some of the guidelines. In this text, we examine these guidelines in detail in the chapters pertaining to particular body systems.

Table 3.1 Chapter-Specific Guidelines for ICD-10-CM *(Data from ICD-9-CM and ICD-10-CM, Centers for Medicare and Medicaid Services and the National Center for Health Statistics.)*

CHAPTER	GUIDELINES
1. Certain Infectious and Parasitic Diseases	These guidelines are very specific and concern coding HIV, sepsis, severe sepsis, septic shock, and infections resistant to antibiotics. The guidelines include selection and sequencing. instructions specific to these conditions.
2. Neoplasms	These guidelines include information regarding the sequencing of comorbidities or complications, such as anemia or pathologic fractures, and administration treatment, including surgery, chemotherapy, immunotherapy, and radiation therapy.
3. Diseases of the Blood and Blood-Forming Organs and Certain Disorders Involving the Immune Mechanism	Currently there are no guidelines for this chapter.
4. Endocrine, Nutritional, and Metabolic Diseases	Included in this chapter are the guidelines for diabetes. Most of the codes in this chapter are combination codes. There are also multiple-sequencing guidelines, including those on the long-term use of insulin for both type 2 and secondary diabetes.
5. Mental and Behavioral Disorders	Guidelines for this chapter clarify coding of pain disorders related to psychological factors and to conditions due to a psychoactive substance in remission. They also provide a hierarchy of coding for dependence, use, and abuse of the same substance.
6. Diseases of the Nervous System	Very specific guidelines for coding pain are included in these guidelines.
7. Diseases of the Eye and Adnexa	There are currently no guidelines for this chapter.
8. Diseases of the Ear and Mastoid Process	There are currently no guidelines for this chapter.
9. Diseases of the Circulatory System	Hypertension and hypertensive heart and kidney disease guidelines are located in this chapter. Cerebral infarction, stroke, cerebral vascular accident, late effects, and myocardial infarction guidelines are also discussed.
10. Diseases of the Respiratory System	Instructions and code sequencing for chronic obstructive pulmonary disease (COPD), asthma, bronchitis, and respiratory failure are included in these guidelines.
11. Diseases of the Digestive System	There are currently no guidelines for this chapter.
12. Diseases of the Skin and Subcutaneous Tissue	Guidelines for coding pressure ulcer stages are in this chapter.
13. Diseases of the Musculoskeletal System and Connective Tissue	This chapter contains guidelines for the coding of osteoporosis and pathologic fractures.
14. Diseases of the Genitourinary System	These guidelines include instructions for coding and sequencing chronic kidney disease (CKD).
15. Pregnancy, Childbirth, and the Puerperium	These guidelines include general rules for obstetric care and coding and sequencing instructions for fetal conditions affecting management of pregnancy, fetal extensions, HIV infection in pregnancy, normal delivery and postpartum conditions, and abortions.
16. Certain Conditions Originating in the Perinatal Period	General perinatal rules and sequencing are included in these guidelines.
17. Congenital Malformations, Deformations, and Chromosomal Abnormalities	Guidelines include rules for coding, use of the codes as first-listed or secondary codes, and assignment of additional codes to further define the condition.

(continued)

Table 3.1 Chapter-Specific Guidelines for ICD-10-CM (*concluded*)

CHAPTER	GUIDELINES
18. Symptoms, Signs, and Abnormal Clinical and Laboratory Findings, Not Elsewhere Classified	This chapter includes guidelines on the use of symptom codes with and without definitive diagnosis codes and the use of coma scale codes, as well as rules for sequencing SIRS not due to infection and a description of functional quadriplegia.
19. Injury, Poisoning, and Certain Other Consequences of External Causes	Instructions on coding injuries, fractures, burns, adverse effects, underdosing, poisoning, and toxic effects are included in these guidelines. Also included is a description of seventh-character extenders for this chapter.
20. External Causes of Morbidity	Included in this chapter are guidelines for coding the cause of an injury or condition as related to outside causes. Guidelines contain rules for the use and sequencing of codes for external causes, place of occurrence, abuse, and acts of terrorism.
21. Factors Influencing Health Status and Contact with Health Services	Guidelines cover the coding of reasons other than illness or injury for patient encounters, such as inoculations, vaccinations, contact or suspected exposure to disease, patient status, family or personal history of a medical condition, screening, observation, aftercare or follow-up, and routine and administrative examinations.

EXERCISE 3.4

1. Which guidelines are specific to Chapter 21 in ICD-10-CM?
2. Which guidelines are specific to Chapter 18 in ICD-10-CM?
3. Which guidelines are specific to Chapter 10 in ICD-10-CM?

Also available in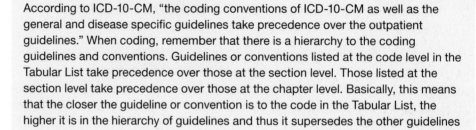

3.5 Diagnostic Outpatient Guidelines

The official ICD-10-CM coding guidelines are located in Section IV, I, of the ICD-10-CM manual. These guidelines are used for reporting hospital-based outpatient services and provider-based office visits.

> **MENTOR** Coding Tip
>
> According to ICD-10-CM, "the coding conventions of ICD-10-CM as well as the general and disease specific guidelines take precedence over the outpatient guidelines." When coding, remember that there is a hierarchy to the coding guidelines and conventions. Guidelines or conventions listed at the code level in the Tabular List take precedence over those at the section level. Those listed at the section level take precedence over those at the chapter level. Basically, this means that the closer the guideline or convention is to the code in the Tabular List, the higher it is in the hierarchy of guidelines and thus it supersedes the other guidelines or conventions.

Highlights of Diagnostic Outpatient Guidelines

- **First-listed diagnosis versus principal diagnosis:** The first-listed diagnosis (reason for the visit) is used for provider/outpatient coding. The principal diagnosis (reason for admission after study) is used for facility coding.

- **Signs and symptoms:** Signs and symptoms are acceptable for reporting when a diagnosis has not been confirmed and reported by the provider.
- **Coding to the highest level of specificity:** This guideline refers to the use of fourth, fifth, and sixth characters and seventh-character extenders when required and placeholder characters if needed.
- **Unconfirmed-diagnosis term:** Unconfirmed-diagnosis terms such as *rule out, probable, access,* and *questionable* may *not* be used in outpatient diagnostic coding. A sign or symptom must be used in place of an unconfirmed diagnosis.
- **Chronic disease:** Chronic conditions may be coded if the chronic condition affects the treatment or management of the presenting condition.

These guidelines are examined in detail in the system-specific chapters of this textbook, as appropriate.

EXERCISE 3.5

1. Explain coding to the highest level of specificity in ICD-10-CM.
2. What is the outpatient guideline concerning an unconfirmed diagnosis?
3. When may a chronic condition be coded?

Also available in **McGraw Hill** **connect** (plus+)

3.6 Translating Provider Documentation to Ensure Medical Necessity

As you read through this text, you will notice that we continue to stress the importance of being able to translate the provider's documentation correctly to ensure that the proper ICD-10-CM code is chosen. A very important aspect of being able to accomplish this translation is the ability to link the medical necessity of the documented encounter to the service provided.

The ability to do this accurately and efficiently and within compliance guidelines is achieved by having a good knowledge of anatomy, medical terminology, pathophysiology, and basic coding rules and guidelines.

FOR EXAMPLE The provider documents that the patient presents to the provider's office for evaluation of cervical pain and determination of treatment via facet injections. The provider also documents that this patient has diabetes type 2 and benign hypertension.

In this example, a coder's knowledge is tested in several ways. First is the term *cervical.* As there are two areas in the female anatomy that may be identified by this term, the coder needs the additional information provided in the documentation to identify which area is the site of the patient's pain. The proposed treatment of facet injections keys the coder to an anatomical area and provides the additional information necessary to identify the term *cervical* as related to the neck and not the genital/urinary body system.

Next is the understanding of when to code for an additional diagnosis. The ICD-10-CM guidelines for listing additional diagnoses instruct the coder to code for all conditions that affect the patient's care, treatment, or management (Section IV, G). The guidelines further guide the coder in regard to the coding of chronic conditions, such as those in the example, diabetes and hypertension. A chronic condition may be listed if during the encounter the patient receives care or treatment for the condition (Section IV, I). In the example above, there is no documentation to support care or treatment directed at either of the additional chronic conditions listed, and therefore neither would be coded.

Finally the coder's knowledge of pathophysiology is tested to determine whether the conditions that coexist, diabetes and hypertension, with the reason for the encounter, cervical pain, affect either the condition or treatment of the cervical pain. In this example, these chronic conditions do not impact the treatment or management of the condition being treated and therefore would not be coded in addition to the cervical pain. ▓

Throughout this text you will have ample opportunity to test your knowledge of anatomy, medical terminology, physiology, pathophysiology, and basic coding rules and guidelines and to practice translating data in each of these categories into diagnostic codes. The CPC exam will test you on your ability to translate this information.

EXERCISE 3.6

1. Briefly discuss the importance of translating the medical record into accurate coding data, and explain why it is important to have a thorough knowledge of anatomy, medical terminology, and pathophysiology.

Also available in ▧ connect™(plus+)

Chapter Three Summary

Learning Outcome	Key Concepts/Examples
3.1 Understand the format of ICD-10-CM.	Volume 1: Tabular List Volume 2: Alphabetic Index ICD-10-PCS (Procedural Coding System): codes for procedures performed in the facility (replaces Volume 3 of ICD-9-CM)
3.2 Explain abbreviations, coding conventions, and punctuation marks used in ICD-10-CM.	**Abbreviations** *NEC—not elsewhere classified:* A more specific code is not provided. *NOS—not otherwise specified:* This is the equivalent of unspecified. **Coding conventions/instructional notes** *Acute:* sudden onset, short duration *Chronic:* slow onset, long duration *Excludes 1:* indicates that the condition, disease, or injury being coded is located elsewhere in the ICD-10-CM manual *Excludes 2:* indicates that the condition listed in the *excludes* list is distinct from the code condition and is coded elsewhere in ICD-10-CM *Includes:* further clarifies the definition of terms included in codes in the Tabular List **Punctuation** *Brackets:* identify mandatory sequencing of etiology/manifestation coding
3.3 Identify main terms, default codes, extenders, and placeholders and explain their importance in the use of the ICD-10-CM index.	*Main term:* describes the patient illness or injury (the reason for the present encounter) documented by the provider **Steps in locating the appropriate ICD-10-CM code** After reading the documentation thoroughly: 1. Identify the main term. 2. Locate the main term in the Alphabetic Index. 3. Identify appropriate subterms and default codes in the Alphabetic Index. 4. Read all instructional notes. 5. Verify the code in the Tabular List. 6. Code to the highest level of specificity.
3.4 Apply ICD-10-CM chapter-specific guidelines.	ICD-10-CM contains 21 chapters and most have specific guidelines.
3.5 Explain ICD-10-CM diagnostic outpatient guidelines.	*First-listed diagnosis:* This is the reason for visit and is used for provider/outpatient coding. *Signs and symptoms:* These may be reported when a diagnosis has not been confirmed. *Code to highest level of specificity:* Use fourth, fifth, sixth, and seventh characters, as appropriate. *Unconfirmed diagnoses:* Do not use unconfirmed terms such as *rule out.* *Chronic conditions:* A chronic condition may be coded if it affects the treatment or management of the presenting condition.
3.6 Recognize the importance of translating provider terminology into accurate diagnostic codes.	An important aspect is the ability to link the medical necessity of the documented encounter to the service provided.

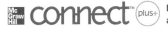 Enhance your learning by completing these exercises and more at mcgrawhillconnect.com

Chapter Three Review

Using Terminology

Match each key term to the appropriate definition.

_____ 1. [LO3.2] Acute

_____ 2. [LO3.2] And

_____ 3. [LO3.3] Main term

_____ 4. [LO3.2] Brackets

_____ 5. [LO3.2] Square brackets

_____ 6. [LO3.2] Late effect

_____ 7. [LO3.2] Includes

_____ 8. [LO3.2] Excludes 1

_____ 9. [LO3.2] NEC

_____ 10. [LO3.2] Sign

_____ 11. [LO3.2] Symptom

_____ 12. [LO3.2] Chronic

_____ 13. [LO3.2] Manifestation

_____ 14. [LO3.2] Parentheses

_____ 15. [LO3.2] NOS

_____ 16. [LO3.3] Default code

_____ 17. [LO3.3] Placeholder

_____ 18. [LO3.2] Excludes 2

_____ 19. [LO3.2] Extender

_____ 20. [LO3.2] Impending or threatened condition

A. Indicates that a more specific code is not provided in the ICD-10-CM manual

B. Means "and/or" in the ICD-10-CM manual

C. Describes the patient's illness or injury in the documentation and is used to locate the code in the Alphabetic Index

D. The equivalent of unspecified

E. The way the condition due to the underlying disease presents itself

F. Condition with a slow onset and of long duration

G. Residual condition that occurs after the initial injury or illness

H. Punctuation marks used to enclose supplemental terms, which are also known as nonessential modifiers

I. Condition with a sudden onset and of brief duration

J. Instructional note indicating that the condition, disease, or injury being coded is located elsewhere in the ICD-10-CM manual.

K. Condition that can be measured and recorded

L. Condition that is relayed to the provider by the patient

M. Punctuation marks used to enclose explanatory phrases or other appropriate descriptive terms for the code.

N. Instructional note that further clarifies the code or category by providing examples of conditions included in the code

O. Punctuation marks that identify mandatory sequencing of etiology/manifestation coding

P. Code that either is unspecified or is most often used with a condition and that should be used only if the documentation provides no additional detail regarding the condition or disease

Q. Character used to extend codes through the sixth character and is represented by an "x," allowing the seventh-character extender to remain in place

R. Instructional note clarifying that the condition listed in the _excludes_ list is distinct from the code condition and is coded elsewhere in the ICD-10-CM manual

S. Character used to complete the description of many codes

T. Terms used only when the condition was averted due to medical intervention

Checking Your Understanding

Choose the most appropriate answer for each of the following questions.

1. [LO3.2] This abbreviation is next to an ICD-10-CM code when a more appropriate code is not provided elsewhere in the manual:

   a. NOS

   b. NEC

   c. DEF

   d. None of these

46

2. **[LO3.4]** Which chapter-specific guidelines include instructions for coding chronic kidney disease?

   a. Chapter 9, Diseases of the Circulatory System

   b. Chapter 14, Diseases of the Genitourinary System

   c. Chapter 18, Symptoms, Signs, and Abnormal Clinical and Laboratory Findings

   d. None of these (There are no guidelines for the kidney system.)

3. **[LO3.2]** Which of the following, when noted in the Alphabetic Index or Tabular List, instructs the coder on the mandatory sequencing of the etiology/manifestation?

   a. Slanted brackets   **c.** Parentheses

   b. Brackets   **d.** Square brackets

4. **[LO3.3]** Which is *not* an appropriate step in determining an ICD-10-CM code?

   a. Determine the main term from the provider documentation

   b. Determine any appropriate subterms and default codes

   c. Determine the code directly from the Alphabetic Index

   d. Code to the highest level of specificity by using appropriate sixth and seventh characters when required.

5. **[LO3.5]** According to the diagnostic outpatient guidelines, which of the following best fits the guidelines for the use of signs and symptoms?

   a. They are always to be used.

   b. They are reported only when a diagnosis has not been confirmed and reported by the provider.

   c. There are no specific guidelines as to their use.

   d. They must be documented in the provider records to be used.

6. **[LO3.5]** Coding to the highest level of specificity means:

   a. Coding all the conditions listed in the patient's chart

   b. Coding just the condition for which the patient is being seen

   c. Using a fourth, fifth, sixth, or seventh digit when required

   d. None of these

7. **[LO3.6]** Which of the following are important aspects of a coder's being able to translate provider documentation?

   a. Ensuring that the proper ICD-10-CM code is chosen

   b. Being able to stay within compliance guidelines

   c. Linking the medical necessity of the encounter to the service provided

   d. All of these

8. **[LO3.2]** According to the ICD-10-CM conventions, if the documentation is unclear or does not state that the complication or comorbidity listed in the code description is present with the condition, the default is:

   a. With   **c.** With or without

   b. Without   **d.** None of these

9. **[LO3.2]** The way the condition due to the underlying disease or condition presents itself is:

   a. Manifestation   **c.** Sign

   b. Etiology   **d.** Symptom

10. **[LO3.2]** Which term is used to describe a residual condition that occurs after the initial illness or injury?

   a. Sign   **c.** Manifestation

   b. Symptom   **d.** Sequela

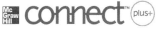 **Enhance your learning** by completing these exercises and more at mcgrawhillconnect.com

Applying Your Knowledge

Use your critical-thinking skills to answer the questions below.

1. **[LO3.3]** Discuss the main steps that a coder needs to follow when translating a provider's documentation and determining the appropriate code using the ICD-10-CM manual.

   _____

2. **[LO3.2]** Explain the differences between *acute* and *chronic,* and list one of the guidelines pertaining to these terms.

   _____

3. **[LO3.3.]** Explain the difference between *includes* and *Excludes 1* and *Excludes 2* and the importance each plays in determining the correct ICD-10-CM code.

   _____

4. **[LO3.1–3.5]** List five mentor coding tips discussed in this chapter that you considered most helpful.

   _____

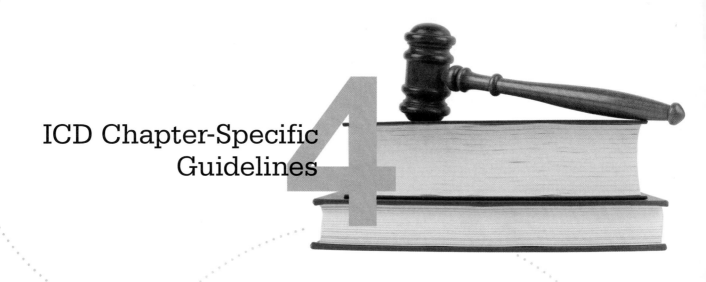

ICD Chapter-Specific Guidelines

CHAPTER FOUR

Key Terms

Benign
Carcinoma in situ
Malignant
methicillin resistant
  *Staphylococcus
  aureus* (MRSA)

Opportunistic infections
  (OIs)
Primary neoplasm
Secondary diabetes
  mellitus

Secondary neoplasm
Sepsis
Septic shock
Septicemia
Severe sepsis

Systemic inflammatory
  response syndrome
  (SIRS)

Learning Outcomes

After completing this chapter, you will be able to:

4.1 Review ICD chapter-specific general guidelines.

4.2 Understand the chapter-specific guidelines on human immunodeficiency virus (HIV) infections.

4.3 Apply the chapter-specific guidelines for septicemia, systemic inflammatory response syndrome (SIRS), sepsis, severe sepsis, and septic shock.

4.4 Recognize the chapter-specific guidelines for coding neoplasms.

4.5 Identify the chapter-specific guidelines for diabetes mellitus.

Introduction

Section I of ICD includes chapter-specific guidelines to help provide clarification and direction for coding the conditions incorporated within the chapter. Although all chapters of the ICD are included in the chapter-specific guidelines, not all chapters have guidelines for coding conditions located within the chapter. Guidelines for some of these chapters have not yet been developed, and the space is being maintained for future use.

Although the chapter-specific guidelines are included to provide instruction and interpretation for the coder, many coders still find many of these guidelines confusing and difficult to interpret. In this chapter of the textbook, we provide explanations that will help clarify the more difficult coding concepts.

4.1 Chapter-Specific General Guidelines

A complete listing of the chapter-specific coding guidelines is located in the ICD-9-CM *Official Guidelines for Coding and Reporting,* Section I, C, Chapter-Specific Guidelines.

The chapter-specific guidelines are more specific and detailed than the general coding guidelines. However, the guidelines and directions provided in the Tabular List at the chapter, section, and code levels supersede the chapter-specific guidelines.

> **MENTOR** Coding Tip
>
> Although coding guidelines listed at the code level (in the tabular list) supersede those listed in the chapter-specific guidelines, many times the tabular guidelines mimic the chapter-specific guidelines by providing a step-by-step process to correct coding, as demonstrated when coding for severe sepsis.

Table 4.1 lists the chapters, locations, and specific guidelines of the coding concepts that are the most difficult to interpret and accurately apply.

EXERCISE 4.1

1. What supersedes the chapter-specific guidelines?

Also available in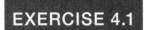

Table 4.1 Difficult Coding Concepts *(Data from ICD-9-CM and ICD-10-CM, Centers for Medicare and Medicaid Services and the National Center for Health Statistics.)*

ICD-9-CM			ICD-10-CM		
CHAPTER	LOCATION (SECTION, SUBSECTIONS)	SPECIFIC GUIDELINE	CHAPTER	LOCATION (SECTION, SUBSECTIONS)	SPECIFIC GUIDELINE
1. Infectious and Parasitic Diseases [4.3]	I, C, 1, a	Human immunodeficiency virus (HIV) infections	1. Certain Infectious and Parasitic Diseases	I, C, 1, a	Human immunodeficiency virus (HIV) infections
	I, C, 1, b	Septicemia, systemic inflammatory response syndrome (SIRS), sepsis, severe sepsis, and septic shock		I, C, 1, d	Sepsis, severe sepsis, and septic shock

Table 4.1 Difficult Coding Concepts (*concluded*)

ICD-9-CM			ICD-10-CM		
CHAPTER	LOCATION (SECTION, SUBSECTIONS)	SPECIFIC GUIDELINE	CHAPTER	LOCATION (SECTION, SUBSECTIONS)	SPECIFIC GUIDELINE
2. Neoplasms	I, C, 2, a	Treatment directed at the malignancy	2. Neoplasms	I, C, 2, a	Treatment directed at the malignancy
	I, C, 2, b	Treatment of secondary site		I, C, 2, b	Treatment of secondary site
	I, C, 2, c	Coding and sequencing of complications		I, C, 2, c	Coding and sequencing of complications
	I, C, 2, d	Primary malignancy previously excised		I, C, 2, d	Primary malignancy previously excised
	I, C, 2, e	Admission/encounter for therapy		I, C, 2, e	Admission/encounter for therapy
	I, C, 2, f	Determining extent of malignancy		I, C, 2, f	Determining extent of malignancy
	I, C, 2, g	Symptoms, signs, and ill-defined conditions associated with neoplasms		I, C, 2, g	Symptoms, signs, and ill-defined conditions associated with neoplasms
	I, C, 2, h	Admission/encounter for pain management		I, C, 2, h	Admission/encounter for pain management
	I, C, 2, i	Malignant neoplasm associated with transplanted organ		I, C, 2, i	Malignant neoplasm associated with transplanted organ
				I, C, 2, l	Sequencing of neoplasm codes
				I, C, 2, m	Current malignancy versus personal history of malignancy
				I, C, 2, n	Leukemia in remission versus personal history of leukemia
				I, C, 2, t	Malignant neoplasm associated with transplanted organ
3. Endocrine, Nutritional, and Metabolic Diseases and Immunity Disorders [4.5]	I, C, 3, a	Diabetes Mellitus	4. Endocrine, Nutritional, and Metabolic Diseases	I, C, 4, a	Diabetes Mellitus

4.2 Human Immunodeficiency Virus Infections—Chapter-Specific Guidelines

When coding for human immunodeficiency virus (HIV) and HIV-related conditions, the coder must understand the current state of the patient in relation to the condition of HIV.

FOR EXAMPLE Was the patient exposed to HIV and seeking testing or counseling, or has the patient been diagnosed as HIV-positive? If the latter, does the patient have an HIV-related condition? ■

Only if the condition is confirmed, *as stated in the provider's documentation,* can a coder assign a code from category V08, "Asymptomatic HIV status," or 042 HIV, "Symptomatic" (also known as *acquired immune deficiency syndrome (AIDS).* As coders are not permitted to interpret lab or pathology findings, the provider's statement is sufficient and a positive test result is not needed to code the patient's condition (Section I, C, 1, a, 1).

opportunistic infections (OIs) HIV-related illness. When documented in conjunction with HIV-positive status, convert the patient's diagnosis from HIV-positive status V08 to AIDS (042).

MENTOR Coding Tip

HIV-related illnesses, or **opportunistic infections (OIs),** when documented in conjunction with HIV-positive status, convert the patient's diagnosis from HIV-positive status V08 to AIDS (042).

As the presence of OIs identify a progression of the HIV disease, once the patient has been diagnosed with AIDS (042) this code remains the correct HIV code for all future encounters regardless of the absence of OIs in future encounters.

SPOTLIGHT on Condition

HIV-related opportunistic infections include:

Bacterial diarrhea (shigellosis, salmonellosis)	Cryptosporidiosis
	Peripheral neuropathy
Bacterial pneumonia *(P. carnii)*	Lymphomas
Pneumocystis pneumonia (PCP)	Kaposi's sarcoma
Mycobacterium avium complex	Cytomegalovirus (CMV)
Mycobacterium kansasii	Herpes simplex or zoster virus
Tuberculosis	Molluscum contagiosum
Syphilis	Progressive multifocal
Candidiasis (thrush or yeast infection)	leukoencephalopathy
Aspergillosis	Isosporiasis
Coccidioidomycosis	Microsporidiosis
Histoplasmosis	Toxoplasmosis
Cryptococcal meningitis	

Sequencing of code V08 and 042 is dependent on the reason for the encounter. However, regardless of the reason for the encounter, a minimum of two codes—one to identify the condition being treated and one or more additional codes to identify the associated conditions—are required.

The examples below and Figure 4.1 illustrate chapter-specific guidelines regarding the selection and sequencing of HIV codes (Section I, 1, a, 2).

When a patient presents for treatment of an HIV-related infection, code first the HIV (AIDS), followed by the infection.

FOR EXAMPLE An HIV-positive patient is seen for Kaposi's sarcoma. Code first the HIV (042), followed by the OI, Kaposi's sarcoma (176.-). ■

When a patient presents for an unrelated condition, first sequence the reason for the encounter—the unrelated condition—followed by the appropriate HIV code (V08 or 042).

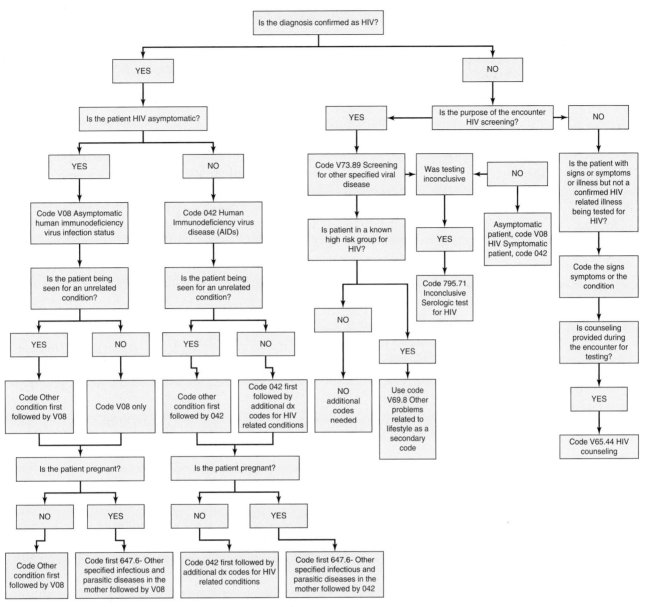

Figure 4.1 HIV Code Selection Flowchart

FOR EXAMPLE An HIV-positive patient is treated for femur fracture. Code first the fracture, followed by the appropriate HIV code. ◼

MENTOR Coding Tip

More than two codes are needed to code for an encounter unrelated to HIV when the appropriate HIV code is 042. Additional codes identifying the OIs are needed to report all HIV-related conditions.

ICD provides several distinct codes to identify various circumstances that may result in a patient presenting for HIV testing. If a patient without signs or symptoms presents for testing, assign V73.89, "Screening for other specified viral disease." An additional code may be used to identify the need for testing, such as high-risk lifestyle (V69.8), or other problems related to lifestyle or behaviors, such as drug use/abuse (304.-) or accidental exposure, which may have occurred while providing medical care to an HIV-positive patient.

At times, HIV testing may result in an inconclusive test result. If a patient is seen in follow-up or to discuss inconclusive test results, the service is identified by code 795.71, "Inconclusive serologic test for human immunodeficiency virus."

ICD code V65.44 is used to identify an encounter in which counseling is provided to an asymptomatic patient or a patient with an HIV-negative or inconclusive test result, either during testing or when the patient returns for test results. Encounters with symptomatic patients presenting for counseling are identified with codes for the signs and symptoms or the condition (HIV) first, followed by the counseling code.

ICD provides specific codes for identifying encounters for HIV-positive pregnant patients. Code 647.6-, "Other specified infectious and parasitic diseases in the mother classifiable elsewhere, but complicating the pregnancy, childbirth or the puerperium," is used to identify the presence of infection or disease in the mother; however, an additional code is needed to identify the status of the HIV (V08 or 042). Sequencing of this code set (647.6-, V08 or 042) when other conditions are present is dependent on the reason for the encounter and follows the sequencing guidelines for nonpregnant patients.

The decision tree in Figure 4.1 depicts the coding process for HIV-related services. Table 4.2 lists the ICD-9-CM codes for HIV and their counterparts in ICD-10-CM.

Table 4.2 HIV ICD-9-CM/ICD-10-CM comparison *(Data from ICD-9-CM and ICD-10-CM, Centers for Medicare and Medicaid Services and the National Center for Health Statistics.)*

ICD-10-CM Guideline Tip: HIV

There are no changes in the coding guidelines for HIV in ICD-10-CM. This table compares the legacy ICD-9-CM codes and the new ICD-10-CM codes identifying HIV and related conditions/encounters.

ICD-9-CM		ICD-10-CM	
042	Human immunodeficiency virus [HIV] disease	B20	Human immunodeficiency virus [HIV] disease
V08	Asymptomatic human immunodeficiency virus [HIV] infection status	Z21	Asymptomatic human immunodeficiency virus [HIV] infection status
795.71	Nonspecific serologic evidence of human immunodeficiency virus [HIV]	R75	Inconclusive laboratory evidence of human immunodeficiency virus [HIV]
647.6-	Other viral diseases complicating pregnancy, childbirth, or the puerperium	O98.7-	Human immunodeficiency virus [HIV] disease complicating pregnancy, childbirth, and the puerperium
V73.89	Special screening examination for other specified viral diseases	Z11.4	Encounter for screening for human immunodeficiency virus [HIV]
V65.44	Human immunodeficiency virus [HIV] counseling	Z71.7	Human immunodeficiency virus [HIV] counseling

Code the following diagnostic statements:

1. An HIV-positive patient presents to the orthopedist for distal shaft fracture of the left radius.

2. The patient presents for severe fever, abdominal pain, and diarrhea; lab test confirmed shigellosis dysenteriae in this HIV-positive patient.

3. Nurse Jaci is seen by the occupational health provider for testing after exposure to an HIV-positive patient by accidental needle stick.

Also available in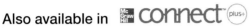

EXERCISE 4.2

4.3 Septicemia, Systemic Inflammatory Response Syndrome, Sepsis, Severe Sepsis, and Septic Shock—Chapter-Specific Guidelines

Septicemia is a progressive condition that may or may not begin with an infectious process but may result in organ failure and loss of life. Several terms are used to describe this condition, and many coders find them confusing:

Septicemia: the presence of toxins or disease in the blood, such as bacteria or a fungus.

Systemic inflammatory response syndrome (SIRS): the body's response to septicemia, trauma, or, in some cases, cancer.

Sepsis: a response specifically to infection.

Severe sepsis: sepsis with organ failure.

Septic shock: a form of organ failure of the vascular system.

> **septicemia** Presence of toxins or disease in the blood, such as bacteria or a fungus.
>
> **systemic inflammatory response syndrome (SIRS)** Body's response to septicemia, trauma, or, in some cases, cancer.
>
> **sepsis** Response specifically to infection.
>
> **severe sepsis** Sepsis with organ failure.
>
> **septic shock** A form of organ failure of the vascular system.

MENTOR Coding Tip

As septic shock is organ failure due to sepsis, documentation of septic shock alone indicates the presence of severe sepsis, and coding this condition requires three codes.

Coding of sepsis requires a minimum of two ICD codes. When the condition is related to an infectious process, the first-listed code identifies the underlying cause of the sepsis, typically a 038 category code, "Septicemia," and the second code identifies the progression of the condition as sepsis or severe sepsis. When the condition is related to or the result of a trauma or another condition such as pancreatitis, the underlying condition or injury is coded first. If severe sepsis or SIRS with organ dysfunction or failure is documented, an additional code (or codes) to identify the failing organs is also needed and is listed after the code for severe sepsis (995.92) or SIRS with organ failure (995.94). Figure 4.2 illustrates the coding process for sepsis, severe sepsis, and SIRS.

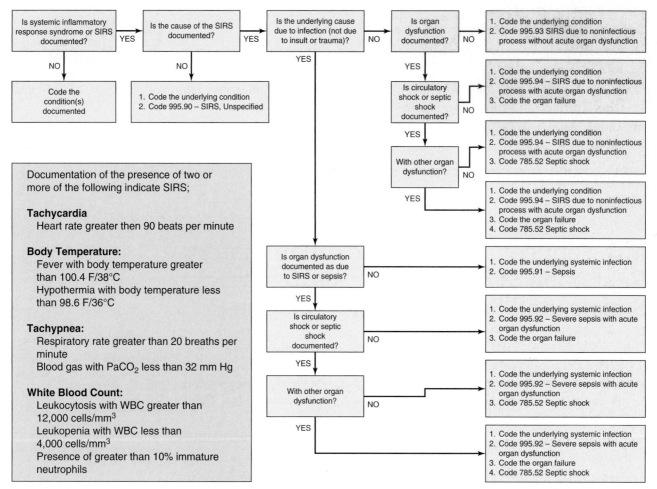

Documentation of the presence of two or more of the following indicate SIRS;

Tachycardia
Heart rate greater then 90 beats per minute

Body Temperature:
Fever with body temperature greater than 100.4 F/38°C
Hypothermia with body temperature less than 98.6 F/36°C

Tachypnea:
Respiratory rate greater than 20 breaths per minute
Blood gas with $PaCO_2$ less than 32 mm Hg

White Blood Count:
Leukocytosis with WBC greater than 12,000 cells/mm³
Leukopenia with WBC less than 4,000 cells/mm³
Presence of greater than 10% immature neutrophils

Figure 4.2 Coding of Sepsis, Severe Sepsis, and SIRS

MENTOR Coding Tip

In coding this condition, the only difference between sepsis and severe sepsis is the presence of organ dysfunction or failure due to the infection, as documented by the physician. Identifying this detail, in review of the documentation, helps to simplify coding this condition.

SPOTLIGHT on a Guideline

To code severe sepsis or SIRS due to a noninfectious process with organ failure, the documentation must clearly reflect that the organ dysfunction/failure is due to sepsis or SIRS in the presence of other comorbidities.

Simply defined, the term *SIRS* is used as the base condition, which ICD further defines by four characteristics: due to infectious (sepsis) or noninfectious (trauma) process and with or without organ dysfunction.

ICD differentiates SIRS related to infection by the term *sepsis* and further defines the progression of SIRS related to infection by the terms *sepsis* or *severe sepsis.* Therefore, a simple statement of "SIRS due to **MRSA** with respiratory failure" would be coded as:

038.12 **(Methicillin resistant *Staphylococcus aureus* septicemia)**

995.92 (severe sepsis)

518.81 (acute respiratory failure)

> **MENTOR** Coding Tip
>
> ICD provides the sequencing directions *code first* and *use additional code* at the code level for each step needed to correctly code this condition and its progression. Using this directional information will guide the coder in coding this condition correctly and completely.

ICD chapter-specific guidelines provide additional sequencing directions when coding for this condition with or due to other conditions:

- **Sepsis due to postprocedural infection:** Code first the complication code, which identifies the type of procedure, followed by the code for septicemia or codes for sepsis or severe sepsis, and use additional codes to identify organ dysfunction or failure if present.
- **Abortion and pregnancy complicated by sepsis:** As with all conditions related to or present with pregnancy, a code from Chapter 11, Complications of Pregnancy, Childbirth, and the Puerperium, is listed first (see categories 647 and 670), followed by the codes to identify sepsis or severe sepsis and, if present, organ dysfunction or failure.
- **Sepsis in newborns:** This condition in newborns requires a combination code from subcategory 771.8- to identify the type of sepsis and the causal organism. If organ dysfunction or failure is present, use an additional code to identify severe sepsis (995.92) and a code (or codes) to identify the organ dysfunction or failure.
- **SIRS due to a noninfectious process:** If SIRS is documented as due to trauma or some other insult to the body and no associated infection is documented, the code for the cause of the SIRS is listed first, followed by either 995.93, "SIRS due to noninfectious process without acute organ dysfunction," or 995.94, "SIRS due to noninfectious process with acute organ dysfunction." If code 995.94 is listed, one or more additional codes for the acute organ dysfunction is needed to identify the organs affected.

Table 4.3 highlights the coding changes in ICD-10-CM for sepsis, severe sepsis, and septic shock.

Code the following:

1. Sepsis with acute renal failure due to *E. coli* following gastric bypass.
2. A 20-day-old infant is admitted in respiratory failure due to sepsis; labs are pending.
3. The patient was admitted to the hospital for streptococcal pneumonia. On day 2 of admission, patient symptoms include tachycardia and labs confirm leukocytosis. Physician is queried and confirms sepsis.

EXERCISE 4.3

Also available in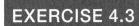

Table 4.3 Sepsis, severe sepsis, and septic shock: ICD-9-CM/ICD-10-CM Comparison *(Data from ICD-9-CM and ICD-10-CM, Centers for Medicare and Medicaid Services and the National Center for Health Statistics.)*

ICD-10-CM Guideline Tip: Sepsis, Severe Sepsis, Septic Shock

ICD-10-CM guidelines and the addition of combination codes require a number of changes in the coding of sepsis, severe sepsis, and septic shock:

- Sepsis without acute organ failure requires only one code, the code for the underlying systemic infection (A40.0–A41.9)
- Severe sepsis requires a minimum of two codes:
  1. Sepsis, A40.0–A41.9, or a code to identify the underlying condition, such as postprocedural infection, trauma, or burn.
  2. The first code is followed by a code to indicate the extent to which the septic condition has progressed: severe sepsis with or without septic shock.
- Combination codes were created for severe sepsis with and without septic shock: (R65.20) (R65.21)
- Additional codes to identify organ dysfunction are still needed in coding for severe sepsis with or without septic shock.

The sequencing rules on codes needed to fully describe the condition of severe sepsis do not change in the ICD-10-CM code set.

ICD-9-CM	ICD-10-CM
038.0 Streptococcal septicemia	A40.0 Sepsis due to streptococcus, group A
	A40.1 Sepsis due to streptococcus, group B
No code	A40.8 Other streptococcal sepsis
No code	A40.9 Streptococcal sepsis, unspecified
038.10 Staphylococcal septicemia, unspecified	A41.2 Sepsis due to unspecified staphylococcus
038.11 Methicillin susceptible *Staphylococcus aureus* septicemia, (includes *Staphylococcus aureus* septicemia NOS)	A41.0 Sepsis due to *Staphylococcus aureus*
038.12 Methicillin resistant *Staphylococcus aureus* septicemia	A41.1 Sepsis due to other specified staphylococcus
038.19 Other staphylococcal septicemia	A41.1 Sepsis due to other specified staphylococcus
038.2 *Streptococcus pneumoniae*	A40.3 Sepsis due to *Streptococcus pneumoniae*
038.3 Septicemia due to anaerobes	A41.4 Sepsis due to anaerobes
038.40 Septicemia due to gram-negative organism, unspecified (includes gram-negative septicemia NOS)	A41.50 Gram-negative sepsis, unspecified
038.41 Septicemia due to *Hemophilus* influenza	A41.3 Sepsis due to *Hemophilus* influenza
038.42 Septicemia due to *Escherichia coli*	A41.51 Sepsis due to *Escherichia coli*
038.43 Septicemia due to pseudomonas	A41.52 Sepsis due to pseudomonas
038.44 Septicemia due to serratia	A41.53 Sepsis due to serratia
038.49 Septicemia due to other gram-negative organisms	A41.59 Other gram-negative sepsis
No code	A41.81 Sepsis due to Enterococcus
038.8 Other specified septicemias	A41.89 Other specified sepsis
038.9 Unspecified septicemia	A41.9 Sepsis, unspecified
995.90 SIRS unspecified	No code
995.91 SIRS due to infectious process without acute organ dysfunction	No code
995.92 SIRS due to infectious process with acute organ dysfunction	R65.20 Severe sepsis without septic shock
995.92 SIRS due to infectious process with acute organ dysfunction	R65.21 Severe sepsis with septic shock
995.93 SIRS due to noninfectious process without acute organ dysfunction	R65.10 SIRS of noninfectious origin without acute organ dysfunction
995.94 SIRS due to noninfectious process with acute organ dysfunction	R65.11 SIRS of noninfectious origin with acute organ dysfunction

4.4 Neoplasms—Chapter-Specific Guidelines

Chapter 2, Neoplasms, contains most, but not all, codes for benign and malignant neoplasms. Some neoplasm codes are located in the chapters that are specific to neoplasms' anatomical sites.

MENTOR Coding Tip

Many coders begin searching for a neoplasm code in the Table of Neoplasms. This is incorrect and typically takes more time or leads to inaccurate coding.

Always begin the selection of neoplasm codes by indexing the histologic term first, such as *lymphoma* or *glioblastoma,* or, if documented as a malignancy of or carcinoma of a particular anatomical site, by indexing the term *carcinoma.* Next, review the subterms for the condition documented. If the condition documented is not listed in the subterms, return to the main term. Most main terms have a *see also* direction that refers the coder to the neoplasm table and identifies whether the neoplasm is benign or malignant.

MENTOR Coding Tip

The morphology codes listed in the Alphabetic Index can aid the coder in determining the correct column of the neoplasm table from which to select a code. The last digit following the forward slash of the morphology code (M code) identifies the neoplasm as follows:

/0 Benign

/1 Uncertain behavior or borderline malignancy

/2 Carcinoma in situ

/3 Malignant, primary

/6 Malignant, secondary

/9 Malignant, uncertain whether primary or secondary

Placing these digits above the corresponding columns of the neoplasm table will aid the coder in quickly selecting the appropriate code in the table.

SPOTLIGHT on Terminology

The neoplasm table is divided into four columns: malignant, benign, unspecified behavior, and uncertain behavior. The malignant column is subdivided by primary, secondary and **carcinoma in situ.**

benign Noninvasive tumor that remains localized.

malignant Invasive tumor that spreads beyond the tumor site.

primary neoplasm Site of origin of the malignancy.

secondary neoplasm Spread or metastases of the malignancy.

carcinoma in situ A neoplasm whose cells are localized in the epithelium and do not invade or metastasize into surrounding tissue.

When sequencing primary and secondary sites of carcinomas, the coder must first determine the site being treated and sequence the code for this site first. A code for the other site, primary or secondary, at which no treatment is directed during the encounter is listed after the code for the site being treated.

FOR EXAMPLE A patient with lung cancer with metastases to the brain is seen for treatment. If the patient is receiving treatment for the brain tumor only, the coding sequence would be carcinoma of the brain (198.3), followed by carcinoma of the lung (162.9). ■

MENTOR Coding Tip

A clear understanding of primary and secondary cancer sites is important when selecting the code for these conditions. As physicians typically do not document using the terms *primary* and *secondary*, the coder must be able to translate terms such as *malignant* (the primary site) and *metastatic* (the secondary site) and phrases such as *with metastases to the* or *metastatic from.*

FOR EXAMPLE

carcinoma of the brain metastatic from the lung
In this example, the lung cancer is the primary site, and the brain tumor is the secondary site. ■

By identifying both the primary and secondary sites, the coder completes the full diagnostic picture of the patient's condition. Thinking of the primary site as an underlying cause, although not a true etiology/manifestation relationship, may help you remember to fully code such cases. Think: "The patient has cancer at this site because . . . "

If the primary site, due to surgical excision or therapy, no longer exists and the patient is receiving treatment for a secondary site, the primary site is coded with a "personal history of" code (V10-) listed in addition to the code for the secondary site. A code (V10-) may also be used as a first-listed code when the patient is being seen in follow-up and no further treatment is needed or provided.

When coding and sequencing a complication due to cancer or the treatment of cancer, such as anemia, dehydration, vomiting, or surgical complications, and the patient is being seen and/or treated for the complication, list the code for the complication first, followed by the code for the site(s) of the cancer.

MENTOR Coding Tip

To help determine sequencing of the codes for a patient with both cancer and a complication of the condition or treatment, ask yourself, "What is the reason for the encounter?" and then, "Why is this complication present?"

Sequencing of admission or encounters for therapy requires that the reason for the encounter be the first-listed code (chemotherapy V58.11, immunotherapy V58.12, or radiation therapy V58.0), followed by the code for the reason the patient is receiving the therapy (carcinoma). Should a complication (e.g., nausea, vomiting) arise during therapy and receive treatment at that time, a code for the complication should also be listed.

FOR EXAMPLE The patient presented for chemotherapy for metastatic carcinoma of the liver. While receiving therapy, the patient became increasingly nauseous and began vomiting, and 1ml of Zofran was administered to relieve nausea.

V58.11 Chemotherapy

197.7 Metastatic liver cancer

787.01 Nausea and vomiting ■

SPOTLIGHT on a Guideline

ICD clarifies at the code level (V58.0) that encounters that involve implantation of a radioactive device should be coded to the condition treated. Do not use the radiotherapy code for these encounters.

However, there may be times when the encounter is for other care or services, such as testing to determine the extent of malignancy, and therapy is also provided. When this occurs, the code to identify the reason for the testing—the malignancy or secondary site—is the first-listed code, followed by the code for the encounter for therapy.

Coding of a malignant neoplasm in a transplanted organ is coded first as "Complication of the transplant (996.8-)" followed by "199.2 Malignancy associated with organ transplant." As neither of these first two codes identifies the organ or site of the malignancy, a third code is needed to indicate the site of the cancer and its status as primary or secondary.

FOR EXAMPLE

Documentation: malignancy of the left lower lobe of lung, left lung transplant 4 years ago.

996.84 Complication of transplanted organ

199.2 Malignant neoplasm associated with transplanted organ

162.5 Malignant neoplasm of lower lobe, bronchus, or lung ■

Table 4.4 summarizes the coding changes in ICD-10-CM for neoplasms.

Code the following:

EXERCISE 4.4

1. Biopsy of a suspicious mass of the lower outer quadrant of the right breast in a 42-year-old female with a maternal history of malignant breast cancer.

2. The patient presents to the operating suite for removal of a malignant neoplasm of the thyroid, metastatic from a previously removed squamous cell carcinoma of the right forearm.

3. Radiation therapy for an occipital lobe lesion is provided for astocytic glioma of unknown origin.

Also available in **McGraw Hill connect** plus+

Table 4.4 Neoplasm: ICD-9-CM/ICD-10-CM Comparison *(Data from ICD-9-CM and ICD-10-CM, Centers for Medicare and Medicaid Services and the National Center for Health Statistics.)*

ICD-10-CM Guideline Tip: Neoplasms

The coding and sequencing guidelines for neoplasms in ICD-10-CM are very similar to those in ICD-9-CM. Changes to and new guidelines are:

- Sequencing of anemia and neoplasms is dependent on the underlying cause of the anemia:

  1. If the anemia is the result of treatment of the neoplasm, such as radiotherapy or chemotherapy, and the primary reason for the encounter is treatment of the anemia, sequence the code for the anemia first, followed by the code for the neoplasm and adverse effect of treatment of the neoplasm (T45.1x5).

  2. If the anemia is due to the neoplasm (e.g., colon cancer causing anemia) and treatment is provided for the anemia, sequence the code for the neoplasm before the appropriate code for the type of anemia, such as "D63.0 anemia in neoplastic disease."

- For advanced metastatic disease in which no primary or secondary site can be determined, ICD-10-CM provides this code:"Disseminated malignant neoplasm, unspecified C80.0"

The lists below compare the legacy ICD-9-CM codes and the new ICD-10-CM codes identifying neoplasms and related conditions and treatment.

ICD-9-CM		ICD-10-CM	
140–239	Neoplasms	C00–D49	Neoplasms
V58.0	Encounter for radiation therapy	Z51.0	Encounter for antineoplastic radiation therapy
V58.11	Encounter for antineoplastic chemotherapy	Z51.11	Encounter for antineoplastic chemotherapy
V58.12	Encounter for antineoplastic immunotherapy	Z51.12	Encounter for antineoplastic immunotherapy
V10	Personal history of malignant neoplasm	Z85	Personal history of primary and secondary malignant neoplasm
V16	Family history of malignant neoplasm	Z80	Family history of primary malignant neoplasm

4.5 Diabetes Mellitus—Chapter-Specific Guidelines

secondary diabetes Diabetes due to an underlying condition or cause.

ICD divides diabetes mellitus into two categories: **secondary diabetes mellitus**—diabetes due to an underlying condition or cause (249)—and diabetes mellitus (250). Many of the guidelines on the use of codes within these two categories are the same. We'll discuss the exception at the end of this section.

Category 250 is subdivided first by the presence or absence of diabetic manifestations, identified by the fourth digit, and then by the type of diabetes and the status of control of the condition. ICD guidelines state that if the type of diabetes is not documented, the condition is coded as type 2; ICD provides a default code (250.00 or 249.00) for use when the documentation does not identify the type or status of control of the condition.

Although all type 1 diabetics must rely on the daily use of insulin, type 2 diabetes may be controlled through diet and exercise, use of oral medications, and/or the use of insulin. When type 2 diabetes is managed long-term by insulin, an additional code is needed to identify the current long-term use of insulin (V58.67).

MENTOR Coding Tip

Consider the description of code V58.67 as meaning that the patient uses insulin in his or her daily management of diabetes mellitus.

Most of the codes listed in each of these categories are combination codes that identify the type of diabetes and an associated manifestation or complication. For diabetes-related complications associated with an organ system (i.e., diabetes with neurologic manifestations), an additional code is needed to identify the condition affecting the organ system (manifestation) due to the underlying cause, diabetes (etiology).

FOR EXAMPLE Documentation: proliferative diabetic retinopathy in a well-controlled type 1 patient.

250.51 Diabetes with ophthalmic manifestations, type 1, not stated as uncontrolled

362.02 Proliferative diabetic retinopathy ▪

In some cases, diabetes is treated by means of an implanted insulin pump. As insulin pumps may malfunction, supplying too little or too much insulin to the patient, ICD has provided guidelines for coding each of these complications:

• When insulin pump malfunction leads to underdosing (too little insulin), code first the mechanical complication due to the insulin pump, 996.57. Follow this with the code for the reason for the pump's presence, the appropriate diabetes code for the patient's diabetic condition. Then list additional codes for any conditions arising from the underdosing, such as ketoacidosis or coma.

• When insulin pump malfunction leads to overdosing (too much insulin), the coding is similar to that for underdosing but involves one additional code. As in underdosing, code first the mechanical complication due to the insulin pump, 996.57, followed by 962.3, poisoning by insulin. Next, code the reason for the presence of the pump, diabetes, followed by any condition resulting from the insulin poisoning.

Correct sequencing of secondary diabetes depends on the underlying cause of the diabetes and the reason for, or focus of, the encounter:

• If the reason for the encounter is treatment of the underlying condition, the cause of the diabetic condition, code the underlying condition first, followed by the secondary diabetes code.

• If the reason for the encounter is treatment of the secondary diabetes or a manifestation of the diabetes, first code the diabetes (249.--) and then list the underlying condition as an additional code.

An exception to this rule occurs when the secondary diabetes is the result of removal of the pancreas. In such cases, a code identifying the reason for the diabetes, such as "Postsurgical hypoinsulinemia, 251.3," must be listed first followed by the appropriate secondary diabetes code, 249, and code V88.1, "Acquired absence of pancreas." Any manifestations of the secondary diabetes should also be coded.

Table 4.5 summarizes the coding changes in ICD-10-CM for diabetes mellitus.

Table 4.5 Diabetes: ICD-9-CM/ICD-10-CM Comparison *(Data from ICD-9-CM and ICD-10-CM, Centers for Medicare and Medicaid Services and the National Center for Health Statistics.)*

ICD-10-CM Guideline Tip: Diabetes Mellitus

The coding and sequencing guidelines for diabetes mellitus in ICD-10-CM are very similar to those in ICD-9-CM. However, in ICD-10-CM diabetes mellitus codes are combination codes identifying the specific type of diabetes by the etiology, the body system impacted, and the specific manifestation. Changes to and new guidelines are:

- Assign Z79.4, "Long-term (current) use of insulin," in addition to the appropriate diabetes mellitus code when the patient uses insulin to manage diabetes on a day-to-day basis. Do not assign Z79.4 with category E10, "Type 1 diabetes mellitus."
- For sequencing of insulin overdosing and underdosing due to insulin pump failure:
  1. List the code identifying the mechanical complication of the insulin pump (T85.6-).
  2. Next, list the code for the overdosing (T38.3x1-, poisoning) or underdosing (T38.3x6-).
  3. Code the type of diabetes mellitus and associated complications due to underdosing.

ICD-9-CM		ICD-10-CM	
249	Secondary diabetes mellitus	E08	Diabetes mellitus due to underlying condition
		E09	Drug- or chemical-induced diabetes mellitus
250.-0	Type 1 diabetes mellitus	E10	Type 1 diabetes mellitus
250.-1	Type 2 diabetes mellitus	E11	Type 2 diabetes mellitus
V58.67	Long-term (current) use of insulin	Z79.4	Long-term (current) use of insulin

---

EXERCISE 4.5

Assign the appropriate ICD-9-CM code(s) for the following:

1. A poorly controlled type 1 DM patient is seen and has elevated ketone levels. The physician query confirms a diagnosis of ketoacidosis.

2. The patient is admitted for diabetic gastroparalysis. The patient history notes total pancreatectomy 6 years ago.

3. The endocrinologist provides a 3-month recheck for a DM patient. The patient had managed DM with diet; however, for the past 4 months the patient has required insulin for adequate control.

Also available in Mc Graw Hill **connect**™ (plus+)

Chapter Four Summary

Learning Outcome	Key Concepts/Examples
4.1 Review ICD chapter-specific general guidelines.	The chapter-specific guidelines are more specific and detailed than the general coding guidelines. However, the guidelines and directions provided in the Tabular List at the chapter, section, and code levels supersede the chapter-specific guidelines.
4.2 Understand the chapter-specific guidelines on human immunodeficiency virus (HIV) infections.	When coding for HIV and HIV-related conditions, the coder must understand the current state of the patient in relation to the condition of HIV. A patient who was exposed to HIV may be seeking testing or counseling, whereas a patient who has been diagnosed as HIV-positive may have HIV-related conditions. When HIV-related illnesses, or opportunistic infections (OIs), are documented in conjunction with HIV-positive status, convert the patient's diagnosis from HIV-positive status V08 to (AIDS) 042.
4.3 Apply the chapter-specific guidelines for septicemia, systemic inflammatory response syndrome (SIRS), sepsis, severe sepsis, and septic shock.	Septicemia is a progressive condition that may or may not begin with an infectious process but may result in organ failure and loss of life. Several terms are used to describe this condition, and many coders find them confusing: *Septicemia:* the presence of toxins or disease in the blood, such as bacteria or a fungus *Systemic inflammatory response syndrome (SIRS):* the body's response to septicemia, trauma, or, in some cases, cancer *Sepsis:* a response specifically to infection *Severe sepsis:* sepsis with organ failure *Septic shock:* a form of organ failure of the vascular system Coding of this condition requires a minimum of two ICD codes.
4.4 Recognize the chapter-specific guidelines for coding neoplasms.	Chapter 2, Neoplasms, contains most, but not all, codes for benign and malignant neoplasms. Some neoplasm codes are located in the chapters that are specific to neoplasms' anatomical sites. Always begin selection of neoplasm codes by indexing the histologic term first. Next, review the subterms for the condition documented.
4.5 Identify the chapter specific guidelines for diabetes mellitus.	ICD divides diabetes mellitus into two categories: secondary diabetes mellitus—diabetes due to an underlying condition or cause (249)—and diabetes mellitus (250). Most of the codes listed in each of these categories are combination codes that identify the type of diabetes and an associated manifestation or complication.

CHAPTER FOUR REVIEW

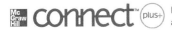
Enhance your learning by completing these exercises and more at mcgrawhillconnect.com

Chapter Four Review

Using Terminology

Match each key term with the appropriate definition.

_____ 1. **[LO4.3]** MRSA

_____ 2. **[LO4.2]** Opportunistic infections (OIs)

_____ 3. **[LO4.4]** Metastases

_____ 4. **[LO4.4]** Primary neoplasm

_____ 5. **[LO4.5]** Secondary diabetes mellitus

_____ 6. **[LO4.3]** Septicemia

_____ 7. **[LO4.3]** Sepsis

_____ 8. **[LO4.3]** Systemic inflammatory response syndrome (SIRS)

_____ 9. **[LO4.3]** Severe sepsis

_____ 10. **[LO4.3]** Septic shock

A. Diabetes due to an underlying condition or cause

B. Methicillin resistant *Staphylococcus aureus* septicemia

C. Sepsis with organ failure

D. A form of organ failure of the vascular system

E. An HIV-related condition

F. Presence of toxins or disease in the blood, such as bacteria or a fungus

G. Site of origin

H. Response specifically to infection

I. Secondary site

J. Body's response to septicemia, trauma, or, in some cases, cancer

Checking Your Understanding

Choose the answer that lists the correct ICD-9-CM code(s) for each of the following questions.

1. **[LO4.5]** The medical record states diabetic proliferative retinopathy in a patient with controlled type 1 diabetes. This is coded as:

   a. 362.02, 249.5

   b. 250.51, 362.02

   c. 250.53, 362.02

   d. 250.11

2. **[LO4.4]** A 49-year-old female patient has been diagnosed with invasive lobular breast cancer in the right breast at 8:00 with spread to the axillary sentinel lymph node. The codes for this are:

   a. 174.5, 196.3

   b. 174.9, 196.3

   c. 196.3, 174.9

   d. 174.5, 198.89

3. **[LO4.2]** A patient who is 32 weeks' pregnant is admitted because of an HIV related illness. The patient spent 3 days in the hospital and was sent home in stable condition. The baby was not delivered during this hospital stay. The codes for this are:

   a. 042, 647.60

   b. 042, 647.63

   c. 647.83, 042

   d. 647.63, 042

4. **[LO4.5]** A 53-year-old obese female was diagnosed with chronic kidney disease, stage III, resulting from malignant hypertension and type 2 diabetes mellitus. Which codes would be reported in this case?

   a. 403.90, 250.41, 585.9

   b. 403.00, 250.40

   c. 403.00, 250.40, 585.3

   d. 403.90, 401.0, 250.40, 585.3

5. **[LO4.4]** A 70-year-old male is brought to the operating room for a biopsy of the pancreas. A wedge biopsy is performed and the specimen sent to pathology. The report comes back immediately indicating that malignant cells are present in the specimen. The code for this case is:

   a. 197.8

   b. 157.8

   c. 157.9

   d. 157.0

6. **[LO4.4]** A 16-year-old patient who is suffering from osteosarcoma located above the right knee begins chemotherapy treatments. Which codes should be reported?

   a. 170.7, V58.1

   b. 171.3, V58.0

   c. V58.1, 170.7

   d. V58.11, 171.9

7. **[LO4.5]** Which of the following is *not* considered a type of diabetes?

   a. Type 1 diabetes mellitus

   b. Non-insulin-dependent diabetes mellitus

   c. Hypertensive diabetes

   d. Gestational diabetes

8. **[LO4.2]** You cannot code HIV if:

   a. The patient is asymptomatic.

   b. There are positive test results but no physician documentation.

   c. The patient has AIDS.

   d. No test results are available.

9. **[LO4.2]** The patient is being admitted for a sprained coccyx due to a fall off a roof. The patient also has been diagnosed with AIDS. This is coded as:

   a. 847.4, 042

   b. 847.4, V08

   c. 042, 847.4

   d. 847.4

10. **[LO4.3]** Septicemia due to pseudomonas with septic shock is coded as:

    a. 785.52, 038.41, 995.92

    b. 038.43, 995.92, 785.52

    c. 038.43, 995.92

    d. 038.42, 785.52

Applying Your Knowledge

[LO 4.4] Case Study

Clinical information Patient has a history of breast cancer with left lumpectomy and radiation 4 years ago. Chest CT shows multiple pulmonary nodules.

Specimen submitted Left lower-lobe lung mass.

Gross description Received, labeled with the patient's name and "lung Bx," are seven white to gray needle biopsy cylinders measuring 1.5 × 1.0 × 0.1 cm in aggregate.

Microscopic and final diagnosis Lung, left lower lobe, needle biopsy: Adenocarcinoma, consistent with breast primary.

Answer the following question.

1. Which is (are) the correct code(s) for this case?

   a. 174.9, 197.0

   b. 197.0, 174.9

   c. 197.0, V10.3

   d. 162.5, 174.9

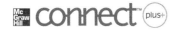

Enhance your learning by completing these exercises and more at mcgrawhillconnect.com

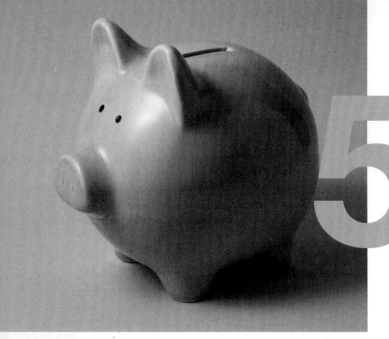

5 Foundations of CPT

Key Terms

Bullet

Bull's-eye

Eponym

Facing triangles

Linkage

Moderate sedation

Modifier

Null zero

Parenthetical notes

Plus sign

Semicolon

Separate procedure

Triangle

Learning Outcomes

After completing this chapter, you will be able to:

5.1 Recognize the importance of linking the CPT and ICD codes.

5.2 Understand the format of CPT.

5.3 Apply the coding conventions, instructional notes, guidelines, and symbols used in CPT.

5.4 Identify main terms and use the CPT index.

5.5 Apply HCPCS Level I CPT modifiers.

5.6 Evaluate the process of accurately translating provider documentation into accurate codes.

Introduction Current Procedural Terminology (CPT) codes are used to translate the services and procedures provided to the patient (what was done to treat the patient's condition). As with diagnosis coding, the translation of these services and procedures begins with the provider's documentation within the medical record. The CPT manual (fourth edition) and the ICD manual are the final destinations for translating written documentation into numeric data that is then submitted to the payers for reimbursement.

Knowledge and understanding of the format and guidelines of the CPT manual are key factors in the correct application of CPT codes, thus leading to the coder's successful completion of the CPC exam and accurate utilization of coding skills in the professional workplace.

5.1 Linking CPT and ICD to Support Medical Services and Procedures

The CPT manual is used to complete the story of the patient's encounter or visit. While the ICD manual tells *why* the visit occurred, the CPT manual tells *what* was provided to the patient during the encounter. Medical necessity requires that the diagnosis, or the *why*, support the service or procedure provided, or the *what*.

Backing up the necessity of the CPT code with the condition documented as the medical reason for the service or procedure is known as *supporting the medical necessity* of the service. Supporting the medical necessity of the CPT code with the ICD code(s) is also referred to as **linkage** on the claim form submitted to payers.

linkage The process of supporting the medical necessity of the CPT code(s) with the ICD code(s).

FOR EXAMPLE Consider a visit for management of benign hypertension and removal of six skin tags. To support the medical necessity of each of these services, a different distinct diagnosis code would need to be linked to each. An example of medical necessity linkage on the CMS-1500 is provided in Figure 5.1. ▪

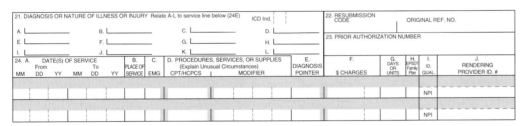

Figure 5.1 CMS-1500 Medical Necessity Linkage

1. Explain linkage in reference to CPT and ICD coding.
2. Explain medical necessity and its importance to CPT coding.

Also available in McGraw Hill **connect**™ (plus+)

EXERCISE 5.1

5.2 CPT Format

CPT is Level I of the Healthcare Common Procedure Coding System (HCPCS). The CPT manual contains six main sections, category II codes, category III codes, and multiple appendices. CPT codes consist of five digits that assist in providing a uniform language to describe medical, surgical, and diagnostic services provided to the patient.

The American Medical Association (AMA) is responsible for annual updates of the CPT manual. Each update occurs in the third quarter of each year for use beginning January 1 of the year immediately following the update.

SPOTLIGHT on a Guideline

Healthcare Common Procedure Coding System (HCPCS)

Level I—CPT codes: five numeric digits except for category II and category III codes.

Level II—national codes: five alphabetic and numeric characters. Codes within this level are not included in Level I.

MENTOR Coding Tip

It is imperative that a coder use the current CPT manual both for the exam and in the workplace.

Table 5.1 lists the sections of the CPT manual, along with the appropriate range of codes in each. Each section is divided into subsections by anatomical site, procedure, condition, eponymn, or descriptive headings based on the type of service being coded to the section.

FOR EXAMPLE The Surgery section is divided into subsections such as Musculoskeletal and Digestive. The Radiology section is divided into subsections such as Diagnostic Ultrasound and Nuclear Medicine. ■

MENTOR Coding Tip

Being familiar with the sections and their code ranges contributes to success on the CPC exam. For example: A CPC exam scenario may depict a surgical procedure with description of the work provided by both the anesthesiologist and the surgeon. The question instructs the coder to code for the surgeon only. One or more of the multiple-choice answers contains a code that begins with 00xxx. By knowing the CPT code ranges, the coder can identify 00xxx codes as anesthesiologist services and thus not a correct answer for this scenario. Therefore, the coder could eliminate one or more choices of the available answers very quickly. Since the CPC exam is a timed test, this type of elimination is important to the coder's timely completion of the exam.

EXERCISE 5.2

1. List the six main sections of the CPT manual.
2. Explain the two levels of HCPCS
3. Who is responsible for the annual CPT updates?

Also available in Mc Graw Hill **connect** (plus+)

Table 5.1 CPT Manual: Sections and subsections *(Data from CPT 2013. © 2013 American Medical Association. All rights reserved.)*

SECTION	CODE RANGE OR DESCRIPTION
Evaluation and Management	99201–99499
Anesthesia	00100–01999
Surgery	**10021–69990**
Integumentary	10021–19499
Musculoskeletal	20005–29999
Respiratory	30000–32999
Cardiovascular	33010–37799
Hemic and Lymphatic	38100–38999
Mediastinum and Diaphragm	39000–39599
Digestive	40490–49999
Urinary System	50010–53899
Male Genital	54000–55899
Reproductive and Intersex surgery	55920–55980
Female Genital	56405–58999
Maternity Care and Delivery	59000–59899
Endocrine	60000–60300
Parathyroid, Thymus, Adrenal Glands, Pancreas, and Carotid Body	60500–60699
Nervous System	61000–64999
Radiology	**70010–79999**
Pathology and Laboratory	80048–89356
Medicine	90281–99607
Category II	0001F–7025F
Category III	0019T–0259T
Appendix A	Modifiers (full description of CPT Level I modifiers)
Appendix B	Summary of Additions, Deletions, and Revisions
Appendix C	Clinical Examples of Evaluation and Management Services
Appendix D	Summary of CPT Add-On Codes
Appendix E	Summary of CPT Codes Exempt from Modifier 51
Appendix F	Summary of CPT Codes Exempt from Modifier 63
Appendix G	Summary of CPT Codes That Include Moderate (Conscious) Sedation
Appendix H	Alphabetic Clinical Topics Listing
Appendix I	Genetic Testing Code Modifiers
Appendix J	Electrodiagnostic Medicine Listing of Sensory, Motor, and Mixed Nerves
Appendix K	Products Pending FDA Approval
Appendix L	Vascular Families
Appendix M	Deleted CPT Codes
Appendix N	Summary of Resequenced CPT Codes
Alphabetic Index	Includes instructions on the use of the CPT index

5.3 Coding Conventions, Guidelines, Instructional Notes, and Symbols

As with the ICD manuals, CPT uses instructional notes, coding conventions, symbols, and guidelines in the alphabetic index and within the specific sections.

Guidelines and Parenthetical Notes

Guidelines are located at the beginning of each major section of the CPT manual. There are also guidelines within many of the subsections, each of which is specific to the subsection in which it appears.

FOR EXAMPLE Surgery guidelines appear before the Surgery section, and more specific guidelines occur within the Musculoskeletal section to instruct coders how and when to code for casting and strapping. ■

The CPT section-specific coding guidelines are reviewed within each body system chapter of this textbook.

> **MENTOR** Coding Tip
>
> As mentioned in earlier chapters, it is a good idea to identify where the guidelines are located and to understand and review their implementation shortly before taking the CPC exam. As with the ICD manuals, students have found it beneficial to tab the different sections and guidelines of the CPT manual.

parenthetical notes In CPT, notes that provide additional information regarding a code or code range; enclosed in parentheses directly below the code or code range to which the note applies; and may inform the coder that the service or procedure described by the code or codes being reviewed are a part of or included in the work of the code for the service or procedure code listed in the parenthetical note.

Parenthetical notes (coding notes enclosed in parentheses) are located directly below the code or code range to which the note applies. Parenthetical notes provide additional information regarding the code being reviewed by the coder. These notes may inform the coder that the service or procedure described by the code or codes being reviewed is a part of or included in the code for the service or procedure listed in the parenthetical note. Such notes also indicate when an additional code or codes may be needed to describe additional work not included in the code being reviewed.

FOR EXAMPLE

20552   Injection(s); single or multiple trigger point(s), 3 or more muscle(s).

(If imaging guidance is performed, see 76942, 77002, 77021) ■

> **MENTOR** Coding Tip
>
> Coders have found it helpful to highlight certain "trigger" words within parenthetical notes. In the example above, a coder might highlight in the CPT book the terms *single, multiple, 3 or more,* and *imaging guidance.* This helps during the timed CPC exam to remind the coder that there are several important notes to this code. Highlighting is a really good approach for sections in which a coder is having particular difficulty determining the right code.

CPT Symbols

Like the ICD manual, CPT uses symbols to more efficiently convey additional information about a code or guideline. The information conveyed does not add to or change the description of the code or the service or procedure described by the code.

The symbols and their definitions are located in the introduction of the CPT manual as well as at the bottom of each page of the manual. Table 5.2 explains the symbols.

MENTOR Coding Tip

Knowing the meaning of each of the symbols at a glance increases the speed at which accurate codes are selected.

Coding Conventions

Semicolon (;)

As a means of saving space within the manual, CPT uses an indented dependent format in the nomenclature or description of many codes. Basically, this means that for its full description, the dependent code must refer to the stand-alone code for a portion of its description. CPT identifies the dependent code by indenting the description of the code.

To determine the full description of the dependent code, the coder must first locate the stand-alone, or parent, code positioned above the dependent code. Stand-alone codes are not indented, and the first word of the description begins with an uppercase, or capital, letter. The stand-alone code shares the verbiage preceding the **semicolon** with all dependent codes that follow it, and in this way a full description of the service or procedure is completed for each dependent code.

semicolon In CPT, the punctuation mark indicating that the verbiage preceding it in a stand-alone code is shared with all dependent codes that follow it, thus providing a full description for each dependent code.

moderate sedation A level of consciousness in which the patient can still respond to verbal commands.

bullet In CPT, the symbol that designates a new code for the current edition of the manual.

triangle In CPT, the symbol designating that a code has been revised.

facing triangles In CPT, the symbols that designate which portion of the text describing a guideline or note has been revised for the current edition of the manual.

bull's-eye In CPT, the symbol designating that the use of moderate sedation is included in the code description and is not to be reported separately.

null zero In CPT, the symbol designating that modifier 51 is not to be used with the code.

plus sign In CPT, the symbol designating that a code is an additional code to be used with the primary procedure and never to be used alone.

Table 5.2 CPT Symbols *(Data from CPT 2013. © 2013 American Medical Association. All rights reserved.)*

SYMBOL	DESCRIPTION
Bullet •	Designates a new CPT code for the current edition of the manual.
Triangle ▲	Designates a CPT code that has been revised for the current edition of the manual.
Facing triangles ►◄	Designate which portion of the text describing a CPT guideline or note has been revised for the current edition of the manual.
Bull's-eye ⊙	Designates that the use of **moderate sedation** is included in the code. description and is *not* to be reported separately.
Null zero θ	Designates that modifier 51 is not to be used with the code.
Plus sign +	Designates that the code is an additional code to be used with the primary procedure. A code with a plus sign may never be used alone.

77761 Intracavitary radiation source application; simple

77762 intermediate

Read code 77762 as "Intracavitary radiation source application; intermediate." ∎

MENTOR Coding Tip

The function of the semicolon is a critical concept for coders to understand. This understanding of the full definition of the indented code is often troublesome for coders and leads to the assignment of the wrong CPT code. To overcome this difficulty, some coders highlight in the CPT the part of the code located before the semicolon and then the indented definition. The highlighting acts as a "trigger" for them to remember this particular coding convention.

Separate Procedure

CPT includes a number of codes for services or procedures that, although they may be performed alone, when performed with a more extensive procedure or service of the same site, are considered a part of the more extensive procedure or service and are therefore not separately reportable. These codes are desig nated **separate procedures,** and each is identified by the term *separate procedure* within the description of the code.

separate procedure In CPT, the term used in a code description to indicate that when the service/procedure is performed with a more extensive service/procedure at the same site, the code is not to be reported along with the extensive procedure. includes a number of codes for services or procedures which, though they may be performed alone, when performed with a more extensive procedure or service of the same site are considered a part of the more extensive procedure or service and are therefore not separately reportable

FOR EXAMPLE Both of the procedures listed below are performed during the encounter:

69210 Removal of impacted cerumen (separate procedure), 1 or both ears

69200 Removal foreign body from external auditory canal; without general anesthesia

In this example, the foreign-body removal (69200) is the only code reportable because the cerumen removal (69210) is designated as a separate procedure and therefore is considered an integral part of the more extensive procedure, the foreign-body removal. ∎

MENTOR Coding Tip

Separate procedures performed in addition to other procedures *not* of the same anatomical or surgical site are reportable in addition to a more extensive procedure. When considering a code designated as a separate procedure, review the documentation to determine the anatomical site or surgical site of the more extensive procedure or procedures.

EXERCISE 5.3

1. Explain the concept of separate procedure.
2. Explain the function of the semicolon in CPT coding.
3. Explain the function of a parenthetical note in CPT coding.

Also available in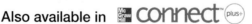

5.4 Main Terms and the CPT Index

Just as with selecting the diagnosis code, the provider's documentation must be reviewed before a coder can translate services or procedures into the appropriate CPT code(s).

Accurate translation of the provider's documentation into CPT codes requires one of two things from the coder: an in-depth understanding of the procedure performed or the ability to target in on key terms, beginning with the main term, as identified in each code description. As developing an in-depth understanding of all procedures takes experience across all specialties and years of hands-on training, it is beyond the scope of this text.

However, developing the ability to target in on key terms takes relatively little time and the tools needed to do so are used each time a coder begins the search for a CPT code.

> **MENTOR** Coding Tip
>
> CPT coding is not memorizing all the terms, guidelines, and so on. Coding is being able to use the CPT manual to translate the medical story in an accurate and compliant manner by utilizing the information that is located throughout the manual. When coding, students are often asked, "Why did you choose that code?" and the response is "because the documentation led me to that code."

Main terms are referenced in the CPT index. Unlike main terms in the ICD manual index, which may be a condition, disease, or injury, main terms in the index of CPT may be a service, procedure, condition, anatomical site, or **eponym.** Procedural terms may be common procedures such as excision, removal, resection, or amputation. They may also be less common, like reimplantation, harvesting, or absence.

eponym The proper name of the person who first identified the condition or disease, the physician who first developed the treatment or procedure for the condition, or the first patient diagnosed with the condition.

> **SPOTLIGHT** on Terminology
>
> An **eponym** may be the proper name of:
>
> The person who first identified the condition or disease.
>
> The physician who first developed the treatment or procedure for the condition.
>
> The first patient diagnosed with the condition.

Major Steps in Locating the Appropriate CPT Code

The coder should begin by reading the provider documentation thoroughly to determine the service or procedure provided to the patient. Then the coder should follow these steps:

1. Determine the main term(s) and subterm(s) from the documentation.
2. Locate the main term and subterm in the alphabetic index.
3. Determine any modifying circumstances that require the use of a modifier.
4. Verify the code identified in the alphabetic index by checking it in the appropriate section of CPT.

5. Review all section-specific instructional notes and guidelines.

6. Determine the CPT code that represents the service or procedure provided to the patient, along with appropriate modifiers.

Be sure to read all of the instructional notes that exist for the main sections and subsections of CPT.

MENTOR Coding Tip

As with ICD, one of the tricks used by successful coding students when checking the main sections or subsections of CPT is to look at the five codes above and five codes below the code identified in the index just to make sure that there is not a more accurate code and that they are not missing subsection guidelines or information found in parenthetical notes.

EXERCISE 5.4

1. List the major steps in locating an appropriate CPT code.
2. How are main terms indexed in the CPT manual.

Also available in **connect** (plus+)

5.5 Modifiers

modifier In CPT, an addition to the code that is used to show that the service or procedure performed was altered in some way.

There are several types of **modifiers** that need to be used in order to translate completely the service or procedure provided to the patient. The purpose of a modifier is to continue to tell the patient's story by showing that the service or procedure performed was altered in some way. The CPT code does not change; only the telling of the story changes.

Table 5.3 lists HCPCS Level I CPT modifiers and their descriptions. Their specific functions within each section and subsection of CPT are explained in later chapters of this textbook. The examples included in Table 5.3 are not all-inclusive and are intended to provide a snapshot of the use of each modifier and facilitate discussion.

HCPCS Level II modifiers and modifiers used within the Anesthesia section are further clarified in subsequent chapters of this text.

EXERCISE 5.5

1. Explain the purpose of a modifier.

2. A screening mammogram is performed on the left breast. CPT code 77057 is reported. Does a modifier need to be attached to this code? If so, which one and why?

3. A 54-year-old patient presents to the office for an annual visit. The patient has no complaints. During the exam, the physician determines that the patient's blood pressure has continued to remain elevated over the past three months and the provider prescribes medication. The coder reports 99396 for the preventive medicine visit. Is it appropriate to also code for the office visit? If so, is a modifier needed, and which one would be appropriate?

Also available in **connect** (plus+)

Table 5.3 HCPCS Level I CPT modifiers *(Data from CPT 2013. © 2013 American Medical Association. All rights reserved.)*

MODIFIER	DESCRIPTION	EXAMPLE
22	Unusual procedural service	Morbidly obese patient requires additional time, resources, and anterior instruments to perform surgery on the posterior spine.
23	Unusual anesthesia	Because of unusual circumstances, a procedure that usually requires either no anesthesia or local anesthesia must be done under general anesthesia.
24	Unrelated E&M service by the same physician during postoperative period	Patient returns to her physician for flu symptoms during the postoperative period for removal of a benign neoplasm.
25	Significant separately identifiable E&M service by the same physician on the same day of a procedure	Patient presents to the office with poison ivy and while there has a wart on the plantar surface of the foot removed.
26	Professional component	Provider interprets and reports on x-ray findings of films taken by the facility.
32	Mandated services	Workers' compensation carrier requests an encounter to determine the extent or course of a patient's injury.
47	Anesthesia by surgeon	Surgeon performs a neuroplasty procedure and administers a nerve block. The modifier is reported with the neuroplasty code.
50	Bilateral procedure	Same procedure identified by the same CPT code is performed on the left and right during the same operative session.
51	Multiple procedures	Multiple lacerations of different anatomical sites: Modifier is appended to the less resource-intense codes, allowing for reimbursement at 100% fee schedule of the primary procedure and multiple-procedure reduction of each additional procedure. Modifier 51 is never to be used with an add-on code.
52	Reduced service	Bilateral service is performed unilaterally (i.e., eye exam) on a patient with absent left eye.
53	Discontinued service	After the start of a surgical procedure, the surgeon stops the procedure due to the patient's condition (i.e., blood pressure drops below safe levels).
54	Surgical care only	Patient, while away from home, fractures the bimalleolar, which is repaired surgically. Surgeon will not be following patient postoperatively.
55	Postoperative care only	Local orthopedist follows up on patient after return home.
56	Preoperative care only	Physician sees patient in the office and by ordering lab work and diagnostic tests determines the patient needs a surgical procedure. The physician is located in a rural area where the procedure is not available and transfers the care of the patient to a surgeon, who then provides the surgery and postoperative care.
57	Decision for surgery	Patient is diagnosed with acute appendicitis, and major surgery is performed the next day. Use of modifier 57 notifies payers that the service performed prior to surgery but within the global period is separately payable.
58	Staged or related procedure or service by the same physician during postoperative period	After an open biopsy of a breast mass, the patient returns in the postoperative period for a total lumpectomy.

(continued)

Table 5.3 HCPCS Level I CPT modifiers (*concluded*)

MODIFIER	DESCRIPTION	EXAMPLE
59	Distinct procedural service	During the same encounter, a patient has a biopsy of a suspicious lesion on the forearm and an excision of a mole on the chest. In this case, use of modifier 59 clarifies to the payer that the biopsy and excision are not of the same lesion.
62	Two surgeons	During an anterior thoracic spine procedure, the neurosurgeon requests that a thoracic surgeon create the approach to the spine (i.e., open and retract vital organs). Both surgeons will report the same code with modifier 62 as both are performing vital parts of the same procedure.
66	Surgical team	Patient is receiving an organ transplant. One surgical team prepares the patient to receive the organ, and another team harvests and prepares the organ for transplant.
76	Repeat procedure by same physician	Within the postoperative period of a hernia repair, the patient reherniates after moving furniture within his home. Patient returns to the same physician for the same procedure (i.e., same CPT code).
77	Repeat procedure by another physician	Again within the poçstoperative period, the patient reherniates and is seen by a new surgeon who surgically repairs the hernia using the same method as the previous surgeon used (same CPT code).
78	Return to operating room for a related procedure during postoperative period	Within the postoperative period of the hernia repair, the patient returns to the surgeon for follow-up, and the surgeon determines that the surgical site is infected, requiring a return to the operative suite for cleaning and debridement. **Mentor Coding Tip:** When in doubt regarding use of modifier 78 versus 79, ask this question: Would the patient have the condition now requiring surgery if not for the previous procedure? If the answer is no, the correct modifier is 78.
79	Unrelated procedure or service by the same physician during postoperative period	While in the postoperative period of a tonsillectomy, the patient falls from a slide and fractures the left ulna, requiring surgical repair.
80	Assistant surgeon	During coronary artery bypass, the cardiothoracic surgeon gains access to the site while the assisting surgeon harvests the saphenous vein and provides additional assistance as needed throughout the entire procedure.
81	Minimum assistant surgeon	In the example above, the minimum assistant would leave upon completion of the vein harvesting, thus only assisting the surgeon for a portion of the procedure.
82	Assistant surgeon, when a qualified resident is unavailable	A neurosurgeon requests the assistance of a nonresident surgeon for a difficult and extensive procedure for which no available residents are qualified to assist. Modifier 82 is used only in teaching facilities. As residents services are not reportable or payable, the reportable service (surgeon assistant) must be identified to the payer.
90	Reference outside laboratory	Provider sends the patient to a lab outside the clinic for testing. The lab has an agreement with the clinic to provide the service and will receive payment from the clinic. The provider will bill the payer for the test and identify the agreement by appending modifier 90 to this service.
91	Repeat clinical diagnostic laboratory test	Patient presents with symptoms of hypoglycemia and is sent to the lab for a fasting blood glucose and then is sent back to the lab later on the same day to check on levels after treatment.
99	Multiple modifiers	The use of this modifier is driven by payer requirements or space limitations in field 24D of the CMS-1500 claim form (allows four modifiers).

5.6 Translating Provider Documentation to Ensure Accurate CPT Code Selection

As explained in Chapters 2 and 3, being able to translate the provider's documentation to select the procedural and diagnostic codes is vital to ensuring accurate and complete coding of services rendered to the patient during each encounter.

Inaccurate or incomplete capture and coding of the services or procedures provided and lack of supporting medical necessity for the provided services are the most common errors, leading to reduced or lost revenue within the medical practice.

Several codes in CPT need very specific information from the medical record in order to tell the most specific and accurate story of the service or procedure provided.

FOR EXAMPLE Some radiology codes are specific on the number of views or whether contrast was administered. The reimbursement for a code with a definition of one view versus a code for three views is different, but if the radiologist's documentation does not specify that a three-view x-ray was taken, the code for one view must be used. Several surgical codes are specific on whether the procedure was partial or complete.

The approach used is important. Likewise, whether a procedure is performed as an open procedure or endoscopic procedure makes a difference in the code used and in the reimbursement the provider receives. ▪

The accurate translation of the medical record into codes is important to the provider as well as the patient. This story decides reimbursement, creates an insurance profile for the patient, and gathers statistical and research data.

---

1. Why is accurate translation of the patient encounter important to both the provider and the patient?
2. Give some examples of situations in which the documentation determines the accurate code selection for radiology.

EXERCISE 5.6

Also available in ꜱꜱ CONNECT (plus+)

Chapter Five Summary

Learning Outcome	Key Concepts/Examples
5.1 Recognize the importance of linking the CPT and ICD codes.	Medical necessity requires that the diagnosis, or the *why*, supports the service or procedure provided, or the *what*. *Linkage* is a term used to show this support on the claim form submitted to the payer.

5.2 Understand the format of CPT.	CPT consists of:
	• Six main sections:
	  1. Evaluation and Management
	  2. Anesthesia
	  3. Surgery
	  4. Radiology
	  5. Pathology and Laboratory
	  6. Medicine
	• Category II and III codes
	• Appendices

5.3 Apply the coding conventions, instructional notes, guidelines, and symbols used in CPT.	**Coding Conventions** *Semicolon:* A stand-alone code shares the first portion of the verbiage to the left of the semicolon with all dependent codes that follow it. *Separate procedure:* This is a procedure that may be performed alone, but when it is performed with a more extensive procedure at the same site, it is considered a part of the more extensive procedure . **Symbols** *Bullet:* designates a new CPT code *Triangle:* designates a CPT code that has been revised *Facing triangles:* designate the portion of the guideline or note that has been revised *Bull's-eye:* designates that the use of moderate sedation is included in the description of the code *Null Zero:* designates that modifier 51 is not to be used with the code *Plus sign:* designates that the code is an add-on code to be used with the primary procedure
5.4 Identify main terms and use the CPT index.	*Main terms* are identified in CPT by service, procedure, condition, eponym, or anatomical site. **Steps in locating the appropriate CPT code** After reading the documentation thoroughly: 1. Determine the main term(s) and subterm(s) from the documentation. 2. Locate the main term and subterm in the alphabetic index. 3. Determine any modifying circumstances from the documentation that require the use of a modifier. 4. Verify the code identified in the alphabetic index by checking it in the appropriate section of the CPT manual. 5. Review all section-specific guidelines and instructional notes. 6. Select the appropriate CPT code, along with appropriate modifiers.
5.5 Apply HCPCS Level I CPT modifiers.	The purpose of a modifier is to show that the service or procedure was altered in some way. The CPT code does not change; only the telling of the patient's story changes.

Learning Outcome	Key Concepts/Examples
5.6 Evaluate the process of accurately translating provider documentation into accurate codes.	Several codes in CPT need very specific information from the medical record in order to tell the most specific and accurate story of the service or procedure provided.

Chapter Five Review

Using Terminology

Match each key term to the appropriate definition.

_____ 1. [LO5.3] Bullet

_____ 2. [LO5.3] Bull's-eye

_____ 3. [LO5.3] Eponym

_____ 4. [LO5.3] Facing triangles

_____ 5. [LO5.3] Parenthetical notes

_____ 6. [LO5.1] Linkage

_____ 7. [LO5.3] Moderate sedation

_____ 8. [LO5.5] Modifier

_____ 9. [LO5.3] Null zero

_____ 10. [LO5.3] Plus sign

_____ 11. [LO5.3] Semicolon

_____ 12. [LO5.3] Separate procedure

_____ 13. [LO5.3] Triangle

A. Term used when the proper name of the person who first identified the condition as a disease is used as a main term in the CPT alphabetic index

B. Symbol indicating an additional code to be used with the primary procedure

C. Indicates that the reporting of the service or procedure was altered and does not change the definition of the CPT code

D. Symbol designating that a new code has been added to the current edition of CPT

E. Term that refers to supporting the CPT code with the medically necessary diagnosis code on the claim form

F. Located directly below the code or code range and provide additional information regarding the code being reviewed.

G. Anesthesia that results in a level of consciousness in which the patient can still respond to verbal commands

H. Symbol designating that the use of moderate sedation is included in the CPT code and is not to be reported separately

I. Coding-convention punctuation mark that is used to help identify the full description of an indented CPT code

J. Symbol indicating that modifier 51 is never to be used with the selected CPT code; located in front of the CPT code

K. Symbol identifying the part of the text of the CPT guideline or note that has been revised

L. Symbol designating that a CPT code has been revised in the current CPT edition

M. Term used within a CPT code description to indicate that when the procedure is performed with a more extensive procedure at the same site, the code is not to be reported along with the extensive procedure.

Checking Your Understanding

Identify the main term in each diagnostic statement and the main section and subsection of the CPT in which the code would appear.

1. [LO5.4] CT scan of the abdomen:

    Main term = _____

    Section = _____

    Subsection = _____

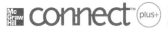
Enhance your learning by completing these exercises and more at mcgrawhillconnect.com

2. **[LO5.4]** Basic metabolic panel:

   Main term = _____

   Section = _____

   Subsection = _____

3. **[LO5.4]** Excision of tendon sheath of the palm:

   Main term = _____

   Section = _____

   Subsection = _____

4. **[LO5.4]** Destruction by laser surgery of a malignant lesion of the arm:

   Main term = _____

   Section = _____

   Subsection = _____

5. **[LO5.4]** Patient is seen in the office for a 2-week follow-up visit for hypertension:

   Main term = _____

   Section = _____

   Subsection = _____

Choose the most appropriate answer for each of the following questions.

6. **[LO5.5]** A patient presented to the ED with a possible fractured femur. A two-view x-ray of the femur was performed, and the radiologist confirmed a fracture of the femur. The patient was sent to the orthopedic department, and the fracture was treated. A few hours later the patient was sent back to radiology for a one-view x-ray of the femur.

   Attach the appropriate modifier to the second x-ray of the femur. The modifier is:

   a. Modifier 51   **c.** Modifier 78

   b. Modifier 52   **d.** Modifier 59

7. **[LO5.1]** A patient is sent to the radiology department with an indication of abdominal pain. A KUB is ordered. The coder inputs data that is then transferred to line 21 of the CMS-1500 form, showing ICD-10-CM 789.01 (abdominal pain RUQ) or CM R10.11, and line 24 field C, showing CPT 74000. The coder has demonstrated which of the following:

   a. Medical necessity   **c.** Medical necessity and linkage

   b. Linkage   **d.** None of these

8. **[LO5.3]** When a code has a bullet symbol, ● before it in the current edition of the CPT, this indicates to the coder that the code is:

   a. New to this edition   **c.** Modifier 51–exempt

   b. Revised for this edition   **d.** An add-on code

9. **[LO5.4]** Identify the appendix to be consulted for examples of levels of office visits:

   a. Appendix D

   b. Appendix H

   c. Appendix N

   d. Appendix C

10. **[LO5.5]** A patient underwent emergency cholecystectomy 6 days after having a lung biopsy. The same surgeon performed both procedures. Assign the correct CPT modifier to tell this patient's story.

    a. Modifier 78   **c.** Modifier 79

    b. Modifier 51   **d.** Modifier 58

11. **[LO5.2]** Which statement is *not* true about HCPCS Level II codes?

    a. Level II HCPCS codes are also referred to as national codes.

    b. Level II HCPCS codes are 5-digit numeric codes.

    c. Level II HCPCS codes are 5-character alphabetic and numeric codes.

    d. Level II HCPCS codes are codes that are not included in CPT.

12. **[LO5.2]** Which entity is responsible for updating CPT, and in which month is the update implemented?

    a. WHO, October   **c.** WHO, January

    b. AMA, October   **d.** AMA, January

13. **[LO5.3]** Determine the full description of code CPT 33244:

    a. Removal of single- or dual-chamber pacing cardioverter-defibrillator electrode(s) by thoracotomy

    b. Removal of single- or dual-chamber pacing cardioverter-defibrillator electrodes(s) by transvenous extraction

    c. By transvenous extraction

    d. Removal of single- or dual-chamber pacing cardioverter-defibrillator electrode(s)

14. **[LO5.3]** CPT code 47011 has a symbol and coding conventions attached to the code. Identify them from the list below:

    a. Moderate sedation is included in this code and is not to be coded separately.

    b. The code is indented, and therefore the full description of the code is the portion of the code above that is to the left of the semicolon along with the description of the indented code.

    c. There are parenthetical notes in parentheses adding additional information.

    d. All of these.

15. **[LO5.2]** In which section of the CPT manual would code 0176T, transluminal dilation of aqueous outflow canal; without retention of device stent, be located?

    a. Radiology   **c.** Category II

    b. Cardiovascular   **d.** Category III

Applying Your Knowledge

Use your critical-thinking skills to answer the questions below.

1. **[LO5.6]** The patient had a pacemaker inserted with atrial and ventricular lead placements. This procedure was coded as 33249 and 33217. Determine whether the codes are correct. If they are incorrect, what code or codes should have been reported and what translation errors were made?

_____

2. **[LO5.3]** In the following scenario, locate the main term and subterms that need to be identified to accurately code for the radiologist. Then choose the appropriate CPT code. The code chosen needs to be supported by a medically necessary diagnosis code.

> A 10-year-old male was seen in the office today, complaining of pain in the right ankle. He had been playing soccer after school and received an injury to the ankle. Mild abrasions and contusions were noticed on the ankle; slight swelling was noted. There was some discomfort when he walked. A two-view x-ray of the ankle was ordered. The x-ray confirmed a mild sprain of the ankle.

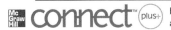
Enhance your learning by completing these exercises and more at mcgrawhillconnect.com

Unit 1 Exam

The questions in this exam cover material in the first five chapters of this book.

Choose the most appropriate answer for each question below.

1. **[LO1.1]** The language that is built on medical terminology, anatomy, and pathophysiology and describes services, procedures, and the medical necessity of those services and procedures is referred to as:
   a. Provider language
   b. Payer language
   c. Billing language
   d. Compliance language

2. **[LO1.2]** The flow of a practice's revenue, which begins when charges for services, procedures, or supplies are incurred and continues until those charges are paid in full or adjusted off the account is known as the:
   a. Claim process
   b. Adjudication
   c. Revenue cycle
   d. Reimbursement cycle

3. **[LO2.2]** The diagnostic statement "goiter, nodular nontoxic" would be coded as an unspecified nontoxic goiter, ICD-9-CM code 241.9 since the diagnosis does not describe the condition as uninodular or multinodular. This is an example of which abbreviation used in ICD?
   a. NEC
   b. NOS
   c. MUE
   d. CCI

4. **[LO2.2]** Identify the true statement or statements concerning acute and chronic conditions and their coding guidelines:
   a. Acute and chronic conditions may be coded as a combination code that identifies both the chronic and acute forms of the condition in one code.
   b. Acute and chronic conditions may be coded separately, with one code for the acute condition and another for the chronic condition.
   c. If the subterms for acute and chronic are connected by a *with* statement, ICD has provided a combination code to indicate both conditions.
   d. All of these statements are true.

5. **[LO2.2]** Identify the true statement or statements concerning signs and symptoms:
   a. Codes for signs and symptoms must be used instead of codes for a diagnosis when a definitive diagnosis has been documented.
   b. A symptom is something that can be measured, such as a blood pressure reading
   c. If the sign or symptom is inherent to or commonly a part of the definitive diagnosis, the sign or symptom is coded in addition to the definitive diagnosis.
   d. Codes for both signs and symptoms must be used instead of codes for a diagnosis when a definitive diagnosis has not been documented; if the sign or symptom is inherent to or commonly a part of the definitive diagnosis, the sign or symptom is not coded in addition to the definitive diagnosis.

6. **[LO2.2]** When a condition is produced as a manifestation of another condition or a complication of a treatment, disease, or condition, more than one code is needed to clearly define the condition, injury, or disease. This is noted by which instructional note or notes in the ICD manual?
   a. Code first
   b. Both code first and use additional code
   c. Use additional code
   d. Excludes

7. **[LO4.4]** A patient who is suffering from osteosarcoma located above the right knee begins chemotherapy treatment at today's encounter. Select the appropriate ICD-9-CM codes to be reported for this encounter:
   a. 170.7, V58.1
   b. 171.3, V58.0
   c. V58.1, 170.7
   d. V58.11, 170.7

8. **[LO4.2]** The patient is admitted to the ER for excessive weight loss and dehydration. The patient has a history of HIV-2 and has been taking nucleoside reverse transcriptase (RT) inhibitors. Assign the appropriate ICD-9-CM codes:

   a. V08, 783.2, 276.51
   b. 042, 079.53, 783.21, 276.51
   c. V08, 042, 783.21, 276.51
   d. V08, 042

9. **[LO4.5]** A 67-year-old female patient with mild chronic kidney disease presents today for dialysis. Choose the appropriate ICD-9-CM codes:

   a. 404.01, V56.8, 585.9
   b. 403.00, V56.0, 585.9
   c. 403.00, V56.0, 585.2
   d. V56.0, 585.2

10. **[LO2.2]** A 32-year-old female was diagnosed with premature menopause that is symptomatic of ovarian failure. Select the correct ICD-9-CM code(s):

    a. 256.39
    b. 256.2, 627.4
    c. 256.31, 627.2
    d. 256.31, V49.81

11. **[LO2.2]** Many conditions and diseases have "late effects," such as a CVA. How much time must elapse between the incident and the acute symptoms for a residual condition to be coded as a late effect?

    a. More than 48 hours
    b. 6 months
    c. No set time
    d. None of these

12. **[LO1.2]** A patient is diagnosed with sickle cell crisis and acute chest syndrome with respiratory failure. Select the correct ICD codes:

    a. 282.60, 518.81
    b. 282.64, 517.3, 289.52
    c. 282.61, 517.3, 518.81
    d. 282.62, 517.3, 518.81

13. **[LO5.3]** Where will a coder locate all the instructions necessary to properly code a procedure in the CPT manual?

    a. Appendix A
    b. Index
    c. Guidelines
    d. Unlisted procedures

14. **[LO5.5]** A physician performed a simple mastectomy on both the left and right breasts—19303 mastectomy, simple, complete. Assign the appropriate modifier to be added to 19303 to indicate that both breasts were removed in the same operative session:

    a. −**50**
    b. −57
    c. −51
    d. −76

15. **[LO5.2]** Why is it necessary for a medical coder to use a current edition of the AMA CPT manual?

    a. This is the law.
    b. Reimbursement will be less.
    c. This ensures accurate coding.
    d. Reimbursement will be more.

16. **[LO5.5]** What is a two-digit modifier used for in CPT coding?

    a. Add-on codes
    b. Code changes
    c. Conscious sedation
    d. Alteration of a procedure or service

17. **[LO5.2]** CPT code range 90281–99607 is located in which section of the CPT manual?

    a. Anesthesia
    b. Radiology
    c. Evaluation and Management
    d. Medicine

18. **[LO2.4]** A nonhealing burn should be coded as which type of burn?

    a. Chronic burn
    b. Acute burn
    c. Late effect
    d. Severe burn

19. **[LO4.5]** The patient has type 2 diabetes mellitus that is controlled with insulin and complicated by proliferative retinopathy, gangrene, and ketonuria. Identify the correct ICD-9-CM codes:

   a. 249.10, 249.70, V58.67, 731.8,
      c. 250.50, 362.02, 250.70, 785.4, 791.6, V58.67

   b. 362.02, 250.30, 785.4, 791.6
      d. V58.67, 250.60, 362.17, 791.6

20. **[LO2.4]** Four people were seen in the ED. Which one will receive a diagnosis of poisoning?

   Patient A: digitalis toxicity

   Patient B: allergic reaction to contrast dye used for a CT exam

   Patient C: syncope after taking antihistamine with alcohol

   Patient D: reaction between two properly administered prescription drugs

   a. Patient A
      c. Patient C

   b. Patient B
      d. Patient D

21. **[LO2.4]** Which is an example of a pathologic fracture?

   a. Greenstick fracture due to fall from bed

   b. Compression fracture after sustaining injury to head

   c. Vertebral fracture with cord injury due to automobile accident

   d. Compression fracture of vertebrae due to metastatic carcinoma

22. **[LO4.3]** The patient is in the intensive care unit with fluid overload with acute renal failure. He has type 2 DM and sepsis. The patient is sedated and on a ventilator because of respiratory failure. Code the diagnoses only:

   a. 782.3, 585.9, 792, 250.40, 039.9, 518.81

   b. 789.59, 584.7, 250.4, 039.9, 518.81

   c. 276.50, 597, 250.00, 038.9, 518.81, 99223

   d. 038.9, 995.91, 584.9, 518.81, 276.6, 250.00

23. **[LO4.4]** The patient is admitted for severe anemia due to chemotherapy treatments for metastatic bone cancer. The primary site is the prostate. What are the correct ICD-9-CM codes?

   a. 185, 198.5, 285.22, E933.1
      c. 285.22, E933.1

   b. 285.22, 198.5, 185, E933.1
      d. E933.1, 285.22

24. **[LO2.4]** An elderly patient was admitted with malnutrition. He had suffered a stroke two years previously that left him with dysphagia. He was treated for the malnutrition with hyperalimentation. He was also diagnosed with hypokalemia. What are the correct codes?

   a. 438.82, 263.9, 787.20
      c. 263.9, 276.8, 438.82

   b. 787.20, 276.8
      d. 263.9, 787.20, 276.8

25. **[LO5.5]** A patient returns to the physician's office with flulike symptoms during the postoperative period for an appendectomy performed 1 month ago. Which modifier would need to be appended to today's office visit?

   a. −24
      c. −55

   b. −25
      d. −58

Coding for Evaluation and Management (E/M), Anesthesia, and Surgery Section

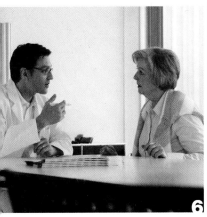
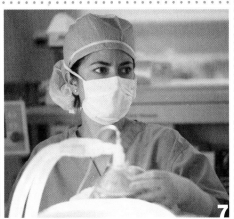
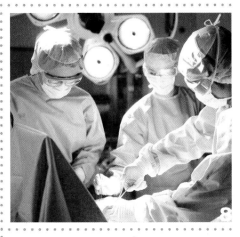

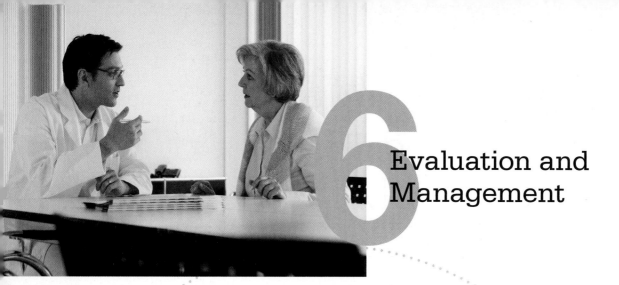

6 Evaluation and Management

CHAPTER SIX

Key Terms

Chief complaint

Consultation

Critical care

Emergency department

Established patient

Face-to-face time

History of present illness (HPI)

Inpatient

Medical decision making (MDM)

New patient

Outpatient

Past, family, and social history (PFSH)

Preventive care

Review of systems (ROS)

Learning Outcomes

After completing this chapter, you will be able to:

6.1 Understand the format and guidelines of the Evaluation and Management (E/M) section of the CPT manual.

6.2 Determine the range of E/M codes required for the service provided.

6.3 Define the components of an E/M code.

6.4 Apply the guidelines for determining the level of service of an E/M code.

6.5 Review the modifiers commonly used with E/M codes.

Introduction

The Evaluation and Management (E/M) section of the CPT manual contains the codes ranging from 99201 to 99499. Some of the categories included in this section are office, hospital, and nursing home services; emergency and critical care services; case management services; and preventive medicine services. This section is used to tell the story of the services provided to the patient in an examination, rather than procedures, which are covered in the remaining sections of the CPT manual.

The E/M section is often the most difficult for coders, physicians, payers, and auditors to understand and use correctly because coding for E/M services is based on applying measurements to the provider's work and interpretation of the patient's condition.

6.1 Format and Guidelines of the E/M Section of the CPT Manual

The Evaluation and Management section of the CPT manual contains ranges of codes that require the coder to abstract information from the documentation. Beyond determining the type of service, place of service, and patient status (new or established), the coder must understand the three key components and identify when time, counseling, and coordination of care are appropriate factors, as well as age of the patient if required. To select the appropriate code from this section and thus tell the complete and accurate story of the patient's encounter, the coder must be able to abstract the necessary information from the provider documentation and translate it into the appropriate code or codes.

Office or Other Outpatient Services (99201–99215)

Codes in this range are used to report services provided to the patient in an office setting or some other outpatient setting such as an ambulatory facility. Such visits require face-to-face time with the patient.

> **SPOTLIGHT on a Guideline**
>
> **Face-to-face time** is the time actually spent by the physician in direct contact with the patient and/or family in the office or outpatient setting. In the hospital the time spent by the physician on the floor or unit that is related to the care given to the patient for that day's encounter is the physician time.

face-to-face time The actual time the provider spends with the patient and or family in the office or outpatient setting.

New Patients: 99201–99205

Codes within this range require that the documentation support the definition of a new patient and that the three key components be met for a level of service.

Established Patients: 99211–99215

Codes within this range require that the documentation support the definition of an established patient and that two of the three key components be met for a level of service.

> **MENTOR Coding Tip**
>
> Code 99211 may not require the presence of a physician. Often this code is referred to as a *nurse visit*. Note that this code has no key-component requirements.

Hospital Observation Services (99217–99220, 99224–99226, 99234–99239)

This code range is appropriate for services provided to a patient in a designated observation status in a hospital setting.

Observation Care Discharge Services: 99217

This code has no key-component or time requirement and is used to report services provided to a patient such as final examination, instructions for post-discharge care, and preparation of discharge forms. Code 99217 is reported only for services provided if the discharge is on a day other than the initial day of observation-status admission. This code is never to be reported with an inpatient initial service (99221–99223).

Initial Observation Care: 99218–99220

This range of codes requires that all three key components be met for the level of service, but it does not require distinction between new and established patients. These codes are for services provided for the initiation of observation status. If the patient is admitted to the hospital after receiving observation care on the same day, an initial hospital care code (99221–99223) would be appropriate in place of the initial observation care code.

If a provider initiates observation care during an encounter at another site, such as the emergency department or the office, all E/M services provided are part of the initial observation care for the same date of service. Codes from the initial-observation care range (99218–99220) would be appropriate, not codes from another section of E/M such as Office and Other Outpatient Services or Emergency Department Services.

Subsequent Observation Care: 99224–99226

This code range requires that two of the three key components be met for the level of service. These codes are appropriate for services provided during observation status after the initial-observation care has occurred.

Observation or Inpatient Care Services (Including Admission and Discharge Services): 99234–99236

This code range is used for observation or inpatient care if the patient is admitted and discharged on the same day. These codes require that all three key components be met for the level of service.

Hospital Discharge Services: 99238–99239

These codes are time-based: 99238 is for 30 minutes or less; 99239 is for more than 30 minutes. They do not have component requirements. These codes are used if the patient is not admitted and discharged on the same day. The time spent on discharge services does not have to be continuous but must be documented.

Hospital Inpatient Services (99221–99223, 99231–99233)

This code range is used to report services provided to inpatients. There is no distinction between new and established patients for this code range.

Initial Hospital Care: 99221–99223

These codes are used for the attending physician's initial (first) encounter with the inpatient. All three key components must be met in determining the level of services for these codes. For the admitting provider the initial hospital care code may be referred to as the *admission versus initial encounter.*

MENTOR Coding Tip

Note that there are only three codes to choose from in this range. To obtain a level 99222 or 99223 code, a comprehensive exam must have been performed and documented. When determining the appropriate level for this code range, coders find it helpful to determine the level of exam first. If a comprehensive exam was not performed and documented, the code choice becomes 99221.

Subsequent Hospital Care: 99231–99233

This code range is used for services provided to an inpatient subsequent to (after) the initial inpatient visit (admit) during the same admission. These codes require that two of the three key components be met for the level of service.

Consultations (99241–99245, 99251–99255)

The **consultation** regarding the patient's condition, treatment options, and/or prognosis must be requested from an appropriate source such as a physician or nonphysician practitioner. The major factor for using this range of codes is the intent of the service: evaluation and the rendering of an opinion (consultation) or the transferring of care for the patient's present illness (referral).

consultation A visit that is requested in writing and that involves the rendering of an opinion and the compilation of a written report.

FOR EXAMPLE

A consultation: The patient presents to the physician office with chest pain, and the physician cannot determine whether the pain is gastric or cardiac in nature and requests in writing that a cardiologist evaluate the patient, render an opinion, and supply a written report stating this opinion.

A transfer of care, or a referral: The patient presents to the physician office with worsening of a known cardiology condition, and the physician feels that she can no longer manage the patient's cardiac care and asks the cardiologist to take over the cardiac portion of the patient's care. ■

MENTOR Coding Tip

Consultation codes are used when the three R's rule can be applied: request, render, and report.

SPOTLIGHT on a Guideline

The three R's can be summarized as follows: The service must be in the form of a written *request* to the consulting physician asking that physician to *render* an opinion and supply a written *report* to the requesting physician.

MENTOR Coding Tip

Some payers, such as Medicare, do not recognize consultation code ranges 99241–99245 and 99251–99255.

Office or Other Outpatient Consultations: 99241–99245

This code range is used to report consultation services provided to patients seen in the office or outpatient settings. There is no distinction between new and established patients for this code range. This code range requires that all three key components be met for the level of service.

Inpatient Consultations: 99251–99255

This code range is used to report consultation services provided to patients seen in the inpatient setting. There is no distinction between new and established patients for this code range. This code range requires that two of the three key components be met for the level of service.

Emergency Department Services (99281–99285)

emergency department Services provided in a 24-hour facility to a unscheduled patient with an immediate concern.

This code range is used to report services provided in an emergency department. CPT defines the **emergency department (ED)** as a hospital-based facility for provision of unscheduled services to patients who present for immediate care. The facility must be open 24 hours a day. If critical care services are provided in the ED, appropriate codes from the critical care range of codes, 99291–99292, would be reported.

There is no distinction between new and established patients for this code range. This code range requires that all three key components be met for the level of service.

Critical Care Services (99291–99292)

These codes are time-based: 99291 is for the first 30 to 74 minutes; 99292 is for each additional 30 minutes. They do not have key-component requirements. For this range of codes to be used appropriately, the provider documentation must state the time spent with the individual patient and must document that the patient is critically ill.

critical care Service that is provided to a patient suffering from an illness or injury that impairs one or more organ systems and has a high potential of life-threatening deterioration.

MENTOR Coding Tip

Remember that 99292 is an add-on code to be used for each additional 30 minutes. Use the grid supplied in some CPT manuals to determine how many times 99292 should be used for the encounter.

If less than 30 minutes is documented as the time spent with the critically ill patient, code 99291 may not be reported and an appropriate E/M code should be chosen.

The total time spent does not have to be continuous, but it must be documented and must show that during this time the provider's full attention was directed toward the individual patient. Time spent on the floor but not directly at the bedside is counted as long as it pertains to the critical condition of the patient. Time spent outside the unit may not be considered in the time documentation.

The CPT manual includes the following services or procedures in the critical care codes:

Interpretation of cardiac output measurements: 93561, 93562

Chest x-ray (CXR): 71010, 71015, 71020

Pulse oximetry: 94760, 94761, 94762

Gastric intubation: 43752, 43753

Temporary transcutaneous pacing: 92953

Ventilatory management: 94002–94004, 94660, 94662

Vascular access procedures: 36000–36410, 36415, 36591, 36600

Nursing Facility Services (99304–99318)

This code range is used to report services provided to patients in a nursing facility, such as a skilled nursing facility (SNF), an intermediate care facility (ICF), or a long-term care facility (LTCF). There is no distinction between new and established patients for this code range, but there is a distinction between initial and subsequent visits.

Initial Nursing Facility Care: 99304–99306

These codes are used for initial services provided to a patient in a nursing facility setting. They require that all three key components be met for the level of service.

If a patient is admitted to a nursing facility from an encounter in the office on the same day, all evaluation and management services provided are part of the initial nursing facility code.

If a patient was discharged from inpatient care on the same day as a nursing facility admit, hospital discharge codes 99238–99239 may be reported separately in order to tell the complete story of the patient encounter. If a patient was discharged from observation status on the same day as a nursing facility admit, code 99217 is reported separately. If a patient was both admitted and discharged from observation status on the same day as the nursing facility admit, a code from range 99234—99236 is reported separately.

Subsequent Nursing Facility Care: 99307–99310

This code range is used for services provided for a patient in a nursing facility setting subsequent to (after) the initial nursing facility visit (admit). These codes require that two of the three key components be met for the level of service.

Nursing Facility Discharge Services: 99315–99316

These codes are time-based: 99315 is for 30 minutes or less; 99316 is for more than 30 minutes. They do not have key-component requirements. The time spent on discharge services does not have to be continuous but must be documented.

Home Services (99341–99350)

This code range is used for services provided for a patient in the patient's home (private residence). These codes are distinguished by whether the patient is a new or established patient.

New Patient: 99341–99345

Services provided to a new patient in a home setting are reported using this code range. These codes require that all three key components be met for the level of service.

Established Patient: 99347–99350

Services provided to an established patient in a home setting are reported using this code range. These codes require that two of the three key components be met for the level of service.

Prolonged Services (99354–99359)

Codes in this range are reported when services are provided that are outside the normal services provided for the condition or injury of the present encounter. According to the CPT guidelines, codes in this range are to be reported along with any level of an appropriate E/M code. Prolonged services of less than 30 minutes duration are not separately reported.

Prolonged Services with Direct Patient Contact: 99354–99357

This range of codes requires direct patient contact (face-to-face) and includes additional non-face-to-face services provided during the same session. These codes are time-based, and the time does not have to be continuous. The codes are also differentiated by place of service—office and other outpatient or inpatient and observation:

+99354   Prolonged service, office or other outpatient setting, first hour

+99355   Prolonged service, office or other outpatient setting, each additional 30 minutes

+99356   Prolonged service, inpatient or observation setting, first hour

+99357   Prolonged service, inpatient or observation setting, each additional 30 minutes

Prolonged Services without Direct Patient Contact: 99358–99359

This range of codes is used to report services provided that are neither face-to-face services in the office or outpatient setting nor additional unit- or floor-time inpatient or nursing facility services. These codes are time-based, and the time does not have to be continuous:

99358   Prolonged E/M services provided before and/or after direct patient care; first hour

+99359   Prolonged E/M services provided before and/or after direct patient care; each additional 30 minutes

MENTOR Coding Tip

Be aware that codes 99354–99357 and 99359 have a plus sign (+) in front of it and therefore can never be used alone or as the first code.

Preventive Services (99381–99397)

This range of codes is for **preventive care** services provided to a patient in order to maintain health and prevent disease. The choice of codes in this range depends on the type of patient, new or established, and the age of the patient.

(New patients 99381–99387 or established patients 99391–99397)

The service provided will include an age- and gender-appropriate history and examination, counseling, risk-factor reduction, and the ordering of lab and diagnostic tests

If a significant new condition or worsening of a preexisting condition is identified during the visit, requiring additional work to support the key components of an appropriate E/M service from the Office or Other Outpatient Services section, this may be reported with the appropriate code from the preventive service range with modifier 25 attached to the office or outpatient code (99201–99215).

FOR EXAMPLE The documentation states that the 45-year-old female was seen today for her annual visit. During the visit, it was determined that her hypertension was worsening and she would need to have a change made in her medication and to return to the office in one week. An expanded problem-focused history and examination was documented, and medical decision making was documented as low. In this case, the appropriate codes to report would be 99213–25 and 99396. The ICD-9-CM codes would be 401.9 linked to 99213 and V70.0 linked to 99396. ∎

MENTOR Coding Tip

The documentation often will not state that the visit is a preventive medicine visit. The coder should look for terms such as *annual visit, yearly checkup, and well-woman check.* The patient will present with no signs or symptoms.

> **preventive care** Service that is provided to a patient in order to maintain health and prevent disease.

Basic Life and/or Disability Evaluation Services (99450)

This code has no key-component, time, or age requirement. It is used for the following services: documentation of height, weight, and blood pressure; medical history; collection of blood sample and urinalysis; and completion of appropriate forms.

Work-Related or Medical Disability Evaluation Services (99355–99356)

This range of codes includes a designation indicating whether the examination is performed by the treating physician or other than the treating physician. These codes are used for the following services: medical history; examination, diagnosis, and assessment of capabilities and impairment; treatment plan; and completion of appropriate forms.

Newborn Services (99460–99465)

This range of codes is for services provided in different settings to newborns (birth to 28 days).

Newborn Care Services: 94460–94463

99460   Initial hospital or birthing center care, per day for E/M of normal newborn infant

99461   Initial care, per day for E/M of normal newborn infant in other than hospital or birthing center

99462   Subsequent hospital or birthing center care, per day for E/M of normal newborn infant

99463   Initial hospital or birthing center care, per day, for E/M of normal newborn infant admitted and discharged on the same date of service

Delivery/Birthing Room Attendance and Resuscitation Services: 99464, 99465

This range of codes is reported when these services are required and may be reported in addition to the normal newborn service codes.

Inpatient Neonatal Intensive Care Services and Pediatric and Neonatal Critical Care Services (99466–99486)

Codes within this range are used to report transportation services for critical care pediatric patients, inpatient neonatal and pediatric critical care, and initial and continuing intensive care services.

Pediatric Critical Care Patient Transport: 99466–99467, 99485–99486

The range of codes 99466–99467 is reported for physician face-to-face contact with critically ill or injured pediatric patients (younger than 24 months of age) during an interfacility transport. Codes 99485 and 99486 are used to report the non-face-to-face or supervision services by the "control physician" as the one directing transport services. The codes in both of these ranges are time based.

MENTOR Coding Tip

If less than 30 minutes of time is recorded, these codes may not be used; instead, an appropriate E/M service code is used. The time reported for these codes is for the physician contact time only; any services provided by others during the transport is not included in the physician time.

Inpatient Neonatal and Pediatric Critical Care: 99468–99476

The definitions for critical care for adults and children apply to neonatal and pediatric critical care codes. The documentation must support that the patient is critically ill or injured and must show the time spent on critical care services.

For neonates or pediatric patients, critical care services in the outpatient setting, such as the ED or office, are reported using the codes for critical care services, 99291–99292. If the patient is seen in both the outpatient and inpatient settings by the provider on the same day, codes from the neonate or pediatric critical care range, 99468–99476, are reported for all critical care services provided that day.

Critical care services provided to pediatric patients 6 years of age and older are reported using code range 99291–99292.

The codes in the 99468–99476 range are designated by initial and subsequent care and by age (28 days through 5 years of age).

Initial and Continuing Intensive Care Services: 99477–99480

This range of codes is for services provided for a patient who is not critically ill or injured but requires intensive care services such as intensive observation and frequent interventions.

Complex Chronic Care Coordination Services (99487–99489)

Per CPT this range of codes is used to report patient-centered management and support services provided to an individual residing at home or in domiciliary, rest home, or assisted living facilities. These services may be provided by physicians, other qualified healthcare professionals, and/or clinical staff. The complexity of the patient's condition requires the coordination of various specialties and services. These codes may be reported only once during a calendar month.

Transitional Care Management Services (99495–99496)

This range of codes is used to report services required for an established patient during transitions in care from inpatient hospital settings, partial hospital, observation status in a hospital, or skilled nursing facility to the patient's community setting (home, domiciliary, rest home, or assisted living). The medical and/or psychosocial condition of the patients require moderate or high complexity medical decision making during this transition.

---

1. Explain the three R's needed to support a consultation code.
2. Define *face-to-face time.*
3. Explain CPT's definition of a critical illness or injury.

Also available in **connect** (plus+)

EXERCISE 6.1

6.2 Determining the Range of E/M Codes Required for the Service Provided

The *first step* in determining a code for an E/M service is to determine the patient's chief complaint. With the exception of preventive medicine visits, documentation of an E/M service must include a chief complaint. The **chief complaint** is the reason, usually expressed in the patient's own words, for the encounter.

> The *second step* is to identify the place of service or setting of the encounter: office, hospital, nursing home.

> The *third step* is to identify the type of service: consultation, admit (or initial).

> The *fourth step* is to identify the status of the patient:

Inpatient: One who has been formally admitted to inpatient status at a healthcare facility.

chief complaint Reason for the present encounter, usually in the patient's own words.

inpatient One who has been formally admitted to a heathcare facility

SPOTLIGHT
on a Guideline

The words *exact* and *subspecialty* were added to the wording of the definition of *new patient* and *established patient* in the 2013 edition of the CPT manual. There is a decision tree in the evaluation and management guidelines that can help with deciding whether a patient is new or established.

Outpatient: One who has not been formally admitted to inpatient status in a healthcare facility.

New patient: One who has *not* received face-to-face services from the physician /qualified healthcare professional or another physician/qualified healthcare professional of the *exact same specialty and subspecialty* in the same group within the past 3 years.

Established patient: One who *has* received face-to-face services from the physician/qualified healthcare professional or another physician/qualified healthcare professional of the *exact same specialty and subspecialty* in the same group within the past 3 years.

The definitions of *new patient* and *established patient* are sometimes different for the clinical setting than they are for coding. For instance, suppose that a patient has not been seen by the practice for 4 years and then returns. Under the coding guidelines, this patient is now a new patient. For the practice, this patient is a returning patient who has a medical record and an account. This is often a difficult concept for physicians, as documentation of the encounter will reflect that the patient is a returning patient. Likewise, if one of the physicians in a group leaves and his or her patients are now being seen by another physician in the group, often the latter physician will consider these patients to be new patients since the physician feels they entail the work of a new visit. However, according to the coding guidelines, they are established patients and would be coded as such.

MENTOR Coding Tip

The concept of same practice, as described in the E/M section guideline defining a new versus established patient, is considered by payers to be all providers providing services under the same tax ID. This means that two providers seeing patients at different physical locations are considered in the same practice if the services are billed under the same tax ID.

In addition to the 3-year period for determining the patient's status, another consideration is the provider's specialty. Patients seen in the same practice by providers of different specialties are considered new patients of the provider of the different specialty.

 A patient returns to his internal medicine physician's office to see the cardiologist in the practice. As the patient has never seen the cardiologist before and the cardiologist's specialty differs from that of the other provider (internal medicine), this patient would be considered a new patient. ▪

Following the four steps outlined above leads the coder to the appropriate range of evaluation and management codes for the patient encounter.

FOR EXAMPLE

Forty-year-old male *returns* to the *office* today with complaints of cough and shortness of breath getting worse. ▪

From this portion of the documentation, it can be determined that the chief complaint is cough and shortness of breath and that the patient was seen in the office and is an established patient. This information indicates that the range of codes needed is 99211–99215, office or other outpatient, established patient.

MENTOR Coding Tip

In the E/M section, the fourth digit identifies the place of service and patient status, as shown in the list below. Knowing this relationship between the fourth digit and the code description helps coders during the CPC exam to quickly eliminate some of the answers included in the E/M section.

99202   The 0 in the fourth place identifies a new patient service in the office.

99212   The 1 in the fourth place identifies an established patient service in the office.

99222   The 2 in the fourth place identifies an initial inpatient service.

99232   The 3 in the fourth place identifies a subsequent inpatient service.

99242   The 4 in the fourth place identifies a consultation service in the office.

99252   The 5 in the fourth place identifies a consultation service in the hospital.

99281   The 8 in the fourth place identifies an emergency service.

99291   The 9 in the fourth place identifies a critical care service.

The fifth digit identifies the level of service.

FOR EXAMPLE   An exam question describes the initial visit by the patient to the office. The coder can quickly scan the answer choices for codes in the range of 99201 to 99205 since the coder knows that the 0 in the fourth place identifies a new patient. ▪

EXERCISE 6.2

1. Define *new patient* and *established patient.*
2. Define *inpatient* and *outpatient.*
3. List the four steps that can lead the coder to the appropriate range of E/M codes for the patient encounter.

Also available in ⬛ connect (plus+)

6.3 Components of an E/M Service

There are seven components of an E/M Service:

History

Examination

Medical decision making

Counseling

Coordination of care

Nature of presenting problem

Time

Three *key* components are used to select the appropriate code for an E/M service:

History

Examination

Medical decision making

Time can be a key factor, for the codes within this section requiring either two or three key components, when 50 percent or more of the visit is spent on counseling and coordination of care.

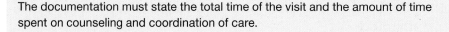

MENTOR Coding Tip

The documentation must state the total time of the visit and the amount of time spent on counseling and coordination of care.

FOR EXAMPLE The documentation states that the patient was seen for 60 minutes and the physician spent 35 minutes of the total time on counseling and coordination of care. If it had stated only that the physician spent 60 minutes with the patient, the documentation would not support using time as the key component. ▪

Some code ranges within this section are time-based only, such as those for critical care (99291–99292), hospital discharge services (99238–99239), nursing facility discharge services (99315–99316), and prolonged services (99354–99359).

The key components are used to determine the appropriate level of service provided. The number of key components that must be used varies by type of service.

FOR EXAMPLE Initial visits require that all three components be met for the level of service, while subsequent visits require only two. ▪

CPT provides the expected key components for each level of service within the E/M code description.

FOR EXAMPLE

99204 Office or other outpatient visit for the evaluation and management of a new patient

This requires these three key components:

A comprehensive history.

A comprehensive examination.

Medical decision making of moderate complexity. ▪

Based on this example, the *expected* components of 99204 are a comprehensive history, a comprehensive exam, and moderate medical decision making. All three key components must be met as required for the initial service.

In contrast to the expected key components are the key components documented by the provider, referred to in this text as the *given* components. For a coder to assign a CPT code to a level of service, the key components given must be equal to or greater than the expected components.

Table 6.1 E/M Level of Service *(Data from CPT 2013. © 2013 American Medical Association. All rights reserved.)*

KEY COMPONENTS	GIVEN COMPONENTS (PROVIDER DOCUMENTATION)	EXPECTED COMPONENTS, CPT 99204
History	Comprehensive	Comprehensive
Exam	Detailed	Comprehensive
Medical decision making	Moderate	Moderate

Table 6.2 E/M Level of Service *(Data from CPT 2013. © 2013 American Medical Association. All rights reserved.)*

KEY COMPONENTS	GIVEN COMPONENTS (PROVIDER DOCUMENTATION)	EXPECTED COMPONENTS, CPT 99203
History	Comprehensive	Detailed
Exam	Detailed	Detailed
Medical decision making	Moderate	Low

FOR EXAMPLE Using 99204 as the expected level of service, compare the given components to the expected components in Table 6.1 and determine whether 99204 is the appropriate code. ▪

In this case, 99204 would not be the appropriate code, since the given components (taken from the documentation) do not meet or exceed the expected components (defined by CPT for the specific level). As shown in Table 6.2, the appropriate code would be 99203, since the given components for this code meet or exceed the expected components.

EXERCISE 6.3

1. When is time a key factor?
2. List the seven components of an E/M service.
3. List the three key components of an E/M service.

Also available in ᴹᶜGraw Hill **connect** (plus+)

6.4 Determining the Level of an E/M Code

As discussed earlier in the chapter, three key components are often used to determine the appropriate level of an E/M code. These key components are history, exam, and medical decision making. Each of these components is then broken down into elements and subelements, which the coder needs to identify from the provider documentation in order to determine and support the level of service reported for the patient encounter. Table 6.3 lists the key components, the elements and their definitions, the subelements with their definitions, and some trigger words to look for in the provider's documentation.

Table 6.3 E/M Key Components, elements, and subelements *(Data from CPT 2013. © 2013 American Medical Association. All rights reserved)*

COMPONENT	ELEMENT	SUBELEMENT AND DESCRIPTIVE TERMS
History	**History of present illness (HPI)** Description of the illness that precipitated the present encounter, from the first sign or symptom to the time of the encounter	• **Location:** Location refers to the anatomical location of present signs and symptoms. • **Duration:** How long have the signs and/or symptoms of the present illness or injury been present? • **Quality:** Quality is the description of present illness, such as *sharp, throbbing,* and *persistent.* • **Severity:** Descriptors such as *mild, moderate,* and *severe* or the use of the pain scale ("Pain is 5/10") are examples of severity. • **Timing:** When do the signs and or symptoms occur? • **Context:** What is happening or happened when the present illness or injury occurred? • **Modifying factors:** What makes the present illness or injury worse or better? • **Associated signs and symptoms:** These are other factors occurring that are related to or affect the present illness or injury.
	Review of systems (ROS) Review of body systems obtained by asking the patient a series of questions that identify any signs, symptoms, or contributing factors related to the present encounter	• Constitutional • Eyes • Ears, nose, mouth, throat • Cardiovascular • Respiratory • Gastrointestinal • Genitourinary • Musculoskeletal • Integumentary • Neurologic • Psychiatric • Endocrine • Hematologic/lymphatic • Allergic/immunologic
	Past, family, and social history (PFSH)	• Past medical and/or surgical history • Family history • Social history
Exam	**Body area**	• **Head, including face:** A descriptive word in documentation is *normocephalic.* • **Neck:** A descriptive word in documentation is *supple.* • **Chest, including breast** • **Abdomen:** Descriptive words in documentation are *soft, tender,* and *nontender.* • **Genitalia, including groin and buttocks** • **Back, including spine** • **Left upper extremity** • **Right upper extremity** • **Left lower extremity** • **Right lower extremity**

Table 6.3 E/M Key Components, elements, and subelements (*concluded*)

COMPONENT	ELEMENT	SUBELEMENT AND DESCRIPTIVE TERMS
	Organ system	• **Constitutional:** Vitals—i.e., blood pressure, weight, height, and pulse (at least three vitals must be recorded)—*or* general appearance. • **Eyes:** Descriptive words in documentation are *conjunctivae* and *PERRLA* (p upils, equal, round, and reactive to light accommodation). • **Ears, nose, mouth, throat:** Descriptive words in documentation are *auditory canal, nasal mucosa, septum, lips, teeth, gums,* and *pharynx.* • **Respiratory:** Descriptive words in documentation are *respiratory effort* and *auscultation of lungs.* • **Cardiovascular:** Descriptive words in documentation are *palpations, S1 sounds,* and *pedal pulses.* • **Gastrointestinal:** Descriptive words in documentation are *bowel sounds* and *organomegaly.* • **Genitourinary:** Descriptive words in documentation are *male or female genitalia examined, urethra,* and *bladder.* • **Musculoskeletal:** Descriptive words in documentation are *gait, range of motion, inspect nails,* and *digits.* • **Skin** Descriptive words in documentation are *rash, bruising,* and *discoloration.* • **Neurologic:** Descriptive words in documentation are *reflexes, focus,* and *sensations.* • **Psychiatric:** Descriptive words in documentation are *mood, alert,* and *oriented times three.* • **Hematologic/lymphatic:** Descriptive word in documentation is *lymphadenopathy.*
Medical decision making (MDM)	Number of diagnoses and management options	• **Self-limiting or minor problem:** e.g., poison ivy • **Established problem:** stable improved • **Established problem:** worsening • **New problem:** no additional workup • **New problem:** additional workup **Mentor Coding Tip:** This is a new problem to the provider, not the patient.
	Amount and complexity of data	• Ordered and reviewed clinical labs (codes from the 80000 series) • Ordered and reviewed radiology (codes from the 70000 series) • Ordered and reviewed test from CPT Medicine section • Discussed test with performing or interpreting physician • Independent visualization and direct view of image or tracing (must be specifically documented) • Decision to obtain old records • Reviewed and summarized old records
	Table of risk	• Presenting problems • Diagnostic procedure • Management options

SPOTLIGHT on a Guideline

The 1995 documentation guidelines are followed for the CPC exam, and the determination of the three key components is based on these guidelines in this textbook.

To determine the appropriate level of code, the coder must determine each component: history, exam, and medical decision making.

Tables 6.4 to 6.6 show each key component (history, exam, and medical decision making), the elements that make up each component (HPI, ROS, PFSH),

history of present illness (HPI) Description of the illness or injury which precipitated the present encounter.

review of systems (ROS) Series of questions presented to the patient which identify any signs and symptoms or contributing factors relevant to the present encounter.

past, family, and social history (PFSH) Listing of patient's past surgeries, allergies, marital status, and family illnesses.(PFSH)

Table 6.4 History component, elements and number of required sub elements for each level of visit *(Data from CPT 2013. © 2013 American Medical Association. All rights reserved.)*

COMPONENT	ELEMENT	NUMBER OF SUBELEMENTS FOR COMPONENT LEVEL
History	**History of present illness (HPI)**	*Brief:* 1–2 subelements documented *Extended:* 4 or more sub elements documented
	Review of systems (ROS)	*Problem pertinent:* 1 subelement documented *Extended:* 2–9 subelements documented *Complete:* 10 or more subelements documented
	Past, family, and social history (PFSH)	*Pertinent:* 1 subelement documented *Complete:* 2 of 3 or 3 of 3 subelements documented *Problem-focused history:* chief complaint and brief HPI *Expanded-focused history:* chief complaint, brief HPI, and pertinent PFSH *Detailed history:* chief complaint, extended HPI, extended ROS, pertinent PFSH *Comprehensive history:* chief complaint, extended HPI, complete ROS, complete PFSH

MENTOR
Coding Tip

Problem-focused, expanded focused, and detailed exams can use documentation supporting examination of a combination of body areas and organ systems. To qualify as a comprehensive exam, the documentation must support a minimum of 8 organ systems examined.

Table 6.5 Exam component, elements and number of required sub elements for each level of visit *(Data from CPT 2013. © 2013 American Medical Association. All rights reserved.)*

COMPONENT	ELEMENT	NUMBER OF SUBELEMENTS FOR COMPONENT LEVEL
Exam	Body area	*Problem-focused exam:* 1 body area or organ system
	Organ system	*Expanded problem-focused exam:* 2–4 body areas and/or organ systems *Detailed exam:* 5–7 body areas and/or organ systems *Comprehensive exam:* 8 or more organ systems

Table 6.6 Medical Decision Making component, elements and number of required sub elements for each level of visit
(Data from CPT 2013. © 2013 American Medical Association. All rights reserved.)

COMPONENT	ELEMENT	NUMBER OF SUBELEMENTS FOR COMPONENT LEVEL
Medical decision making	Number of diagnoses and management options	*Minimal:* 1 self-limiting or minor problem or 1 established problem, stable and improving *Limited:* 2 self-limiting problems; 2 established problems, stable and improved; or 1 established problem, worsening *Multiple:* new problem, no additional workup, or multiple established problems *Extensive:* new problem, additional workup or new problem, no additional workup, and 1 or more established problems
	Amount and complexity of data reviewed	*Minimal:* 1 subelement documented *Limited:* 2 subelements documented; documentation supporting independent visualization of imaging, tracing, etc.; or documentation supporting review and summarization of old records *Moderate:* 3 subelements documented; combination of documentation supporting independent visualization of imaging, tracing, etc.; or review and summarization and 1 order and review subelement (labs, radiology, medicine) *Extensive:* 4 subelements documented; or combination of documentation supporting independent visualization of imaging, tracing, etc.; or review and summarization and physician order and/or review subelements (labs, radiology, medicine)
	Table of risk ***Mentor Coding Tip:*** In this element, the highest level in any one subelement (presenting problem, diagnostic procedure, or management option) determines the overall risk.	**Straightforward** *Presenting problem:* self-limiting or minor problem *Diagnostic:* lab tests, x-rays, EKGs, ultrasound *Management options:* rest, superficial dressings **Low** *Presenting problem:* 2 or more self-limiting, 1 stable chronic, or acute uncomplicated illness or injury *Diagnostic:* noncardiovascular imaging studies with contrast, superficial needle biopsies *Management options:* over-the-counter drugs, minor surgery, physical therapy, IV fluids without additives **Moderate** *Presenting problem:* 1 or more chronic illnesses with mild exacerbation, progression, or side effects of treatment; 2 or more stable chronic illnesses; undiagnosed new problem with uncertain prognosis; or acute illness with systemic symptoms *Diagnostic:* physiologic tests under stress, diagnostic endoscopies, deep needle or incisional biopsy, cardiovascular imaging studies with contrast and no identified risk factors *Management options:* minor surgery with identified risk factor, elective major surgery with no identified risk factor, prescription drug management, therapeutic nuclear medicine, IV fluids with additives, closed treatment of fracture or dislocation without manipulation **High** *Presenting problem:* 1 or more chronic illnesses with severe exacerbation, progression, or side effects of treatment; acute or chronic illnesses or injuries that pose a threat to life or bodily function; or abrupt change in neurologic status *Diagnostic:* cardiovascular imaging studies with contrast, with identified risk factors; cardiac electrophysiologic tests; diagnostic endoscopies with identified risk factors; discography *Management options:* elective major surgery with identified risk factors, emergency major surgery, parenteral control substances, drug therapy requiring intensive monitoring, decision not to resuscitate

(continued)

Table 6.6 Medical Decision Making component, elements and number of required sub elements for each level of visit *(concluded)*

COMPONENT	ELEMENT	NUMBER OF SUBELEMENTS FOR COMPONENT LEVEL
		Straightforward decision making: • Minimal number of diagnoses and management options • Minimal amount of data reviewed • Minimal risk of complication **Low decision making:** • Limited number of diagnoses and management options • Limited amount of data reviewed • Low risk of complication **Moderate decision making:** • Multiple diagnoses and management options • Moderate amount of data reviewed • Moderate risk of complications **High decision making:** • Extensive diagnoses and management options • Extensive amount of data reviewed • High risk of complications ***Mentor Coding Tip:*** In determining the level of the medical decision-making component, only 2 of the 3 subelement requirements must be met or exceeded, regardless of the type of visit or status of patient (new or established office, initial or subsequent hospital care).

medical decision making (MDM) Key component which includes the number of management options or diagnoses, data reviewed, and risk factors the physician encounters during an E/M visit.

the number of subelements needed to determine the specific component level, and the overall level of each key component.

Putting It All Together

The patient presents to the office for an initial visit, complaining of chest pain. The patient states that the pain is a 6 out of 10 on the pain scale, has been occurring for the last 2 days, and is sharp in nature, and he denies any nausea or vomiting. The patient has not had any blurred vision, denies sore throat, has no stomach cramping. He has experienced some shortness of breath and heart palpitations. He has to get up during the night often to urinate. The patient is diabetic. He does not state any symptoms of depression. The patient is in the office today with his wife. His parents are both alive and well. The patient has a history of CABG in 1995.

Let's establish the range of codes, chief complaint, and history component:

Range of codes: 99201–99205, patient is seen in the office for initial visit

Chief complaint: chest pain

History:

- **HPI:** *location*—chest; *duration*—2 days; *severity*—6/10; *quality*—sharp; *associated signs and symptoms*—no nausea or vomiting = 5 subelements
- **ROS:** *eyes*—blurred vision; *ENT*—no sore throat; *gastrointestinal*—no stomach cramping; *respiratory*—shortness of breath; *cardiovascular*—heart palpitations; *genitourinary*—night-type frequent urination; *endocrine*—diabetic; *psychiatric*—not depressed = 8 subelements

- **PFSH:** *past medical history*—CABG 1995; *family history*—parents alive; *social history*—married (patient in office with wife) = 3 subelements

  History level = detailed:
  - Extended HPI (4 or more subelements)
  - Extended ROS (2–9 subelements)
  - Complete PFSH (3 subelements)

Let's take a closer look at the exam component

Physical exam:

Vitals: BP, 140/90; height, 6 ft; weight, 220 lb

Neck: supple

Head: normocephalic

Eyes: pupils equal round reactive to light accommodation (PERRLA)

ENT: nasal mucosa clear

Respiratory: lungs clear

Cardiovascular: some edema of lower extremities, no murmur

Gastrointestinal: normal bowel sounds

Musculoskeletal: normal gait

Neurologic: AOx3

Body areas: neck and head = 2 subelements

Organ systems: constitutional, eyes, ENT, respiratory, cardiovascular, gastrointestinal, musculoskeletal, neurologic (alert and oriented times 3) = 8 subelements

Exam Component: comprehensive, eight organ systems documented

Let's look at the medical decision-making component

Assessment and plan: CBC, CXR, ECG ordered. Records concerning the CABG performed in 1995 will be requested. Patient started on meds and will return in 1 week. Patient is to present to ED if pain increases

Amount of diagnoses and management options:

New problem: chest pain

Established problem: stable diabetes

Extensive = 4 subelements

Data reviewed:

Ordered or reviewed labs: CBC

Ordered or reviewed radiology: CXR

Ordered or reviewed medicine section: ECG

Decision to obtain old records: CABG in 1995

Extensive = 4 or more subelements

Table of risk:

Prescription Management

Moderate

Medical decision making component = high

Now let's put it all together to determine the code:

Final code determination: 99203

Given components:	Expected components—99203:
History: detailed	*History:* detailed
Exam: comprehensive	*Exam:* detailed
Medical decision making: high	*Medical decision making:* low

The documentation does not support level 99204 or 99205, since both codes require a comprehensive history and our history is detailed.

MENTOR Coding Tip

One way that providers dictate is based on the SOAP format. This format correlates with how coders abstract the documentation to support the level of service reported.

SOAP Notes	Component
Subjective	HPI and ROS
Objective	Exam
Assessment	Medical decision making
Plan	Medical decision making

EXERCISE 6.4

1. What year's E/M documentation guidelines are followed for the CPC exam?
2. Define the subelements of the HPI.
3. What determines the overall risk for the table of risk subelement for medical decision making?

Also available in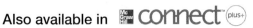

6.5 Modifiers Commonly Used with E/M Codes

As with any other section of CPT, modifiers continue to tell the story for evaluation and management services. These modifiers let the payer know why a patient may have required care for an unrelated service during the postoperative period; that a procedure was performed in the office on the same day the patient was seen for an unrelated E/M service; that the consultation performed was required by the payer; or that the preoperative visit was the visit in which the provider decided surgery was necessary. (See Table 6.7.) When the use of these modifiers is appropriate, their absence does not tell the whole story of the resources used by the provider.

MENTOR Coding Tip

Being familiar with these modifiers and their appropriate use can help when coders are taking the CPC exam. Often, two answer choices can be eliminated by the absence or presence of the correct modifier.

Table 6.7 E/M Code Modifiers *(Data from CPT 2013. © 2013 American Medical Association. All rights reserved.)*

MODIFIER	DEFINITION	EXAMPLE OF USE
24	Unrelated E/M service by the same physician during a postoperative period	Surgeon performs appendectomy, which has a 90-day surgical global period, and the patient returns to office during the 90 days with abdominal pain that is diagnosed as gallstones. The office visit is reported with modifier 24 attached. The ICD code for gallstones also identifies this service as unrelated to the appendectomy.
25	Significant, separately identifiable E/M service by the same physician on the same day of the procedure or other service	Patient presents to the office with a cough and while in the office shows the provider a wart on her foot, and the provider removes the wart. The office visit is reported with modifier 25 attached, and the wart removal is reported with a service code from the Integumentary section. The ICD code for cough is linked to the E/M code, and the ICD code for wart is linked to the wart removal code.
32	Mandated services	Third-party payer requires a second opinion. This modifier is used when the patient asks for a second opinion. The office or hospital consultation code is reported with modifier 32 attached.
57	Decision for surgery	Surgeon is asked to see a patient in the ED for severe abdominal pain. He diagnoses the patient with appendicitis and decides to perform an appendectomy that evening. The CPT code for appendectomy is part of a global surgical package and has a 90-day global period attached. The surgeon reports an outpatient consultation code, 99241–99245 (unless the patient's payer is one that does not recognize consultation codes), with modifier 57 attached. This modifier alerts the payer to the fact that the decision for surgery occurred during this visit. The ICD code for appendicitis is linked to this service. The abdominal pain is not reported since it is considered inherent to the appendicitis.

EXERCISE 6.5

1. Which modifier informs the payer that an unrelated E/M service was provided by the same physician during a postoperative period?

2. A patient presents to the office asking for a second opinion about an upcoming surgery. The patient wants reassurance that the surgery is necessary. Would modifier 32 be appropriate in this case?

3. Which modifier allows for a preoperative visit to be reported separately from the global surgical package?

Also available in connect plus+

Chapter Six Summary

Chapter Outcome	Key Concepts/Example
6.1 Understand the format and guidelines of the Evaluation and Management (E/M) section of the CPT manual.	The Evaluation and Management section of the CPT manual contains ranges of codes that require the coder to abstract information from the provider documentation to determine the appropriate code(s) from this section. The coder must have a full understanding of the distinct requirements for each of the code ranges within this section.
6.2 Determine the range of E/M codes required for the service provided.	Steps followed to determine the range of E/M codes are: 1. Determine the chief complaint. 2. Identify the place of service or setting of the encounter. 3. Identify the kind of service provided. 4. Identify the status of the patient.
6.3 Define the components of an E/M code.	There are seven components of an E/M service, with the three key components being history, exam, and medical decision making. In some instances time can be a deciding factor.
6.4 Apply the guidelines for determining the level of service of an E/M code.	The key components of history, exam, and medical decision making are broken down into elements and subelements that the coder needs to identify from the provider documentation to determine and support the level of service reported for the patient encounter.
6.5 Review the modifiers commonly used with E/M codes.	Modifiers 24, 25, 32, and 57 are the most commonly used modifiers with codes reported from the E/M section of the CPT manual.

Chapter Six Review

Using Terminology

Match each key term to the appropriate definition.

_____ 1. [LO6.2] Chief complaint
_____ 2. [LO6.1] Consultation
_____ 3. [LO6.1] Critical care
_____ 4. [LO6.1] Emergency department
_____ 5. [LO6.2] Established patient
_____ 6. [LO6.1] Face-to-face time
_____ 7. [LO6.4] History of present illness (HPI)
_____ 8. [LO6.2] Inpatient
_____ 9. [LO6.4] Medical decision making (MDM)
_____ 10. [LO6.2] New patient
_____ 11. [LO6.2] Outpatient

A. One who has not been formally admitted to inpatient status
B. Reason for the present encounter, usually in the patient's own words
C. Visit requested in writing, opinion rendered, and written report compiled
D. One who has been formally admitted to a heathcare facility
E. Key component that includes the number of management options or diagnoses, data reviewed, and risk factors the physician encounters during an E/M visit
F. Actual time the provider spends with the patient and/or family in the office or outpatient setting
G. Services provided to a patient suffering from an illness or injury that impairs one or more organ systems and has a high potential of life-threatening deterioration
H. Patient who has not received services from the physician or another physician of the exact same specialty or subspecialty in the same group within the past 3 years
I. Series of questions presented to the patient that identify any signs, symptoms, or contributing factors relevant to the present encounter

_____ 12. **[LO6.4]** Past, family, and social history (PFSH)

_____ 13. **[LO6.1]** Preventive care

_____ 14. **[LO6.4]** Review of systems (ROS)

J. Services provided in a 24-hour facility to an unscheduled patient with an immediate concern

K. Patient who has received services from the physician or another physician of the exact same specialty or subspecialty in the same group within the past 3 years

L. Listing of patient's past surgeries, allergies, marital status, and family illnesses

M. Description of the illness or injury that precipitated the present encounter

N. Services provided to a patient in order to maintain health and prevent disease

Checking Your Understanding

Complete each sentence with the most appropriate term or terms.

1. [LO6.1] It is not the setting but the _____ that defines critical care.

2. [LO6.1] *LTCF* is an abbreviation for _____.

3. [LO6.1] CPT code 99221 is found under the subheading _____ in the E/M section of the CPT manual.

4. [LO6.2] The words _____ and _____ were added to the definitions of new patient and established patient in the 2013 edition of the CPT manual.

5. [LO6.1] A patient presents to the office for an annual visit and has no signs or symptoms. An appropriate code would be chosen from the _____ section.

Choose the most appropriate answer for each of the following questions.

6. [LO6.4] The patient states to the physician that her throat is sore. Which key-component element is this an example of?

a. Review of systems

c. Medical decision making

b. Physical exam

d. History of present illness

7. [LO6.4] The physician observes that the patient's throat is red and swollen. Which key-component element is this an example of?

a. Review of systems

b. Ears, nose, mouth, and throat organ system

c. Medical decision making

d. Physical exam

8. [LO6.3] The number 5 in the CPT code 99252 indicates that the type of service provided to the patient was:

a. Inpatient consultation

b. Established patient in the office or outpatient setting

c. Emergency department service

d. Office consultation

9. [LO6.1] A provider documents spending 35 minutes in the morning and 65 minutes in the afternoon providing critical care for a patient. CPT code(s) _____ would be reported.

a. 99291

c. 99291, 99292 x2

b. 99291, 99292

d. 99292 x3

10. [LO6.1] What are the three R's needed to support the choice of a code from the consultation code ranges 99241–99245 and 99215–99255?

a. Request, render, report

c. Reports, render, request

b. Require, render, report

d. Request, render, retain

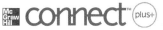

Enhance your learning by completing these exercises and more at mcgrawhillconnect.com

11. [LO6.1] The patient calls the office and asks the cardiologist for a "consultation" regarding his chest pain. The patient is seen, and the physician determines that his chest pain is due to heartburn and sends a report to the patient's family physician. The cardiologist's office reports this visit as a consultation, using codes from range 99241–99245. One of the three R's is missing and therefore the appropriate code range 99201–99205 should be reported. Which "R" is missing?

   a. Request

   b. Render

   c. Report

   d. None of these (Everything is there to support a consultation code.)

12. [LO6.4] The provider documentation states that no abnormal bowel sounds were heard. What element of which one of the key components is this an example of?

   a. Body area; exam

   b. Organ system; exam

   c. Review of systems; history

   d. History of Present Illness:/history

13. [LO6.4] The patient states that her pain occurs upon exertion. Which subelement of the history of present illness (HPI) is this an example of?

   a. Timing

   b. Context

   c. Associated signs and symptoms

   d. Severity

14. [LO6.3] A 45-year-old female patient presents to the office today for her annual visit. During the visit it is discovered that her hypertension needs managing, and the physician changes her medication and orders some lab work. Which modifier needs to be appended to the office visit code for both the preventive medicine visit (annual visit) and the office visit (managing the hypertension) to be reimbursed?

   a. 24

   b. 25

   c. 51

   d. 76

15. [LO6.2] A 30-year-old male patient is seen in the office. He is a returning patient who has not been seen for 4 years by the physician. The patient states that he has been having chronic back pain for several months. The physician performs an expanded, problem-focused history and exam. The physician prescribes medication and asks to see the patient in 3 weeks. The medical decision making is low. What is the appropriate CPT code?

   a. 99202

   b. 99212

   c. 99203

   d. 99242

Applying Your Knowledge

Use your critical-thinking skills to answer the questions below.

1. [LO6.1–6.5] Using the techniques described in this chapter, work through the following case study to determine the appropriate E/M code.

A 17-year-old high school student presents with his mother, complaining of a sore throat which began 3 days ago. He denies any fever or chills but does state that he feels tired and weak. The patient has been seen for frequent bouts of sore throat in the last year.

Physical exam:

   Neck: supple

   General appearance: no acute distress

   Vitals: 98.6, 80, 120/75

   HEENT: pharynx clear; throat mildly red and swollen

   Lungs: normal respiratory effort

Impression: viral URI

Plan: Drink plenty of fluids, Tylenol as needed, rest, and return in a week if no improvement.

Answer the following questions about the above scenario:

Chief complaint = _____

Place of service = _____

Type of service = _____

Status = _____

History component = _____

HPI = _____

ROS = _____

PFSH = _____

Physical exam component = _____

Body areas = _____

Organ systems = _____

Medical Decision-Making Component = _____

Number of diagnoses and management = _____

Options = _____

Amount and complexity of data = _____

Table of risk = _____

Final CPT code = _____

ICD code = _____

2. **[LO 6.1–6.5]** Write a scenario for a new patient seen in the office with a diagnosis of DM and hypertension. The documentation should support a 99203 CPT code. Show the ICD codes.

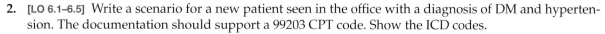

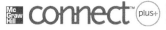

Enhance your learning by completing these exercises
and more at mcgrawhillconnect.com

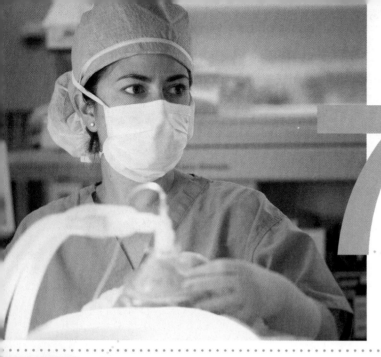

7 Anesthesia

Key Terms

Airway management
Anesthesia
Base unit
Certified Registered Nurse
    Anesthetist (CRNA)

Emergency condition
Extubation
General anesthesia
Intubation
Medical direction

Moderate/Conscious
    Sedation
Monitored anesthesia
    care (MAC)
Physical-status modifiers

Post-anesthesia care unit
    (PACU)
Qualifying circumstances
Time

Learning Outcomes

After completing this chapter, you will be able to:

7.1 Recognize the anesthesia reimbursement formula.

7.2 Apply physical-status and qualifying-circumstance modifiers.

7.3 Define HCPCS Level II modifiers and explain their function in anesthesia billing.

7.4 Identify medical terminology specific to anesthesia billing.

7.5 Examine the types of anesthesia used for specific procedures.

7.6 Explain other procedures or services provided during anesthesia and locate anesthesia terms in the CPT manual index.

Introduction When you break down the word **anesthesia,** you will see that it means "without sensation." This loss of sensation can be partial or complete, and it can be achieved by different types of anesthesia. The type of anesthesia used is determined by the surgical procedure and the condition of the patient. An anesthesiologist administers medication to achieve this loss of sensation. The coding for anesthesiology and the format of its section in the CPT manual is somewhat different from the other codes and sections of the manual. The basis for reimbursement is also different from that in the other sections.

7.1 Reimbursement Formula

The reimbursement formula of time-based general anesthesia services is built on three components: base units (B), total time of anesthesia care (T), and modifying factors (M).

The American Society of Anesthesiologists (ASA), in its Relative Value Guide (RVG), has assigned units of value, known as **base units,** to all CPT codes that qualify as surgical procedures. These units are the first component in assigning a cost-revenue value to anesthesia services. When assigning codes for anesthesia services, the coder assigns only one CPT code for the anesthesia; therefore, only the code with the highest base unit is assigned, regardless of the number of procedures performed.

The next component of the reimbursement formula is time. For anesthesia services, **time** begins when the patient is being prepared for anesthesia by the anesthesiologist and ends when the patient is no longer being attended to by the anesthesiologist. This total time is then converted into units—typically, 15 minutes equal 1 unit according to ASA recommendation—and these units are added to the base units allotted for the surgical procedure. As the time needed to perform multiple surgical procedures is greater than the time needed to perform the base procedure alone, reporting time as well as base units for the primary anesthesia service allows for capture of the additional work provided by the anesthesiologist.

The last component is *modifying factors*. There are two categories of modifying factors and two types of modifiers used to identify these circumstances: physical status and qualifying circumstances. As with the anesthesia procedure code and time units, each of these modifying factors has a unit of value assigned to it based on the increase in risk or difficulty that each circumstance adds to the anesthesia service provided.

Each of these three components is then added together to determine the total number of units. The formula B + T + M is known as the anesthesia reimbursement formula.

> **anesthesia** Anesthesia is without sensation or loss of sensation, partial or complete.

> **base unit** Units of value that are the beginning of the formula for assigning a cost/revenue value to an anesthesia service.

> **time (anesthesia)** Component of the reimbursement formula that begins when the patient is being prepared for anesthesia and ends when the patient is no longer being attended to by the anesthesiologist.

EXERCISE 7.1

1. Define the term *anesthesia*.
2. Define *time* in the context of anesthesia coding.
3. What is the anesthesia reimbursement formula?

Also available in Mc Graw Hill **connect** (plus+)

7.2 Physical-Status Modifiers and Qualifying Circumstances

Physical-status modifiers are used with all anesthesia procedure codes to rank the physical condition of the patient and the level of anesthesia complexity inherent to each ranking.

> **physical-status modifiers** Modifiers that are used with all anesthesia procedure codes to rank the physical condition of the patient and the level of anesthesia complexity inherent to each ranking.

FOR EXAMPLE Consider the complexity of managing anesthesia on a patient with COPD and malignant hypertension versus the complexity of managing anesthesia for a normal healthy patient. ▪

Table 7.1 Physical-Status Modifiers *(Data from CPT 2013. © 2013 American Medical Association. All rights reserved.)*

MODIFIER (ASSIGN ONLY ONE)	DEFINITION	ADDITIONAL UNITS
P1	A normal, healthy patient	0
P2	A patient with mild systemic disease	0
P3	A patient with severe systemic disease	1
P4	A patient with severe systemic disease that is a constant threat to life	2
P5	A moribund patient who is not expected to survive without the operation	3
P6	A declared-brain-dead patient whose organs are being removed for donor purposes	0

Only one physical-status modifier may be assigned to each patient during the anesthesia service. The physical-status modifiers and the units assigned to each are listed in Table 7.1.

At times, anesthesia may be provided under more challenging circumstances such as extreme patient age, condition of patient, conditions under which the surgical procedure is performed, or emergency situations in which the patient's medical history or history of previous anesthesia response is not available before initiation of anesthesia. For reporting such circumstances, CPT provides additional codes called **qualifying-circumstance modifiers.**

qualifying-circumstance modifiers These codes are used to report challenging circumstance in which anesthesia may be provided.

> **MENTOR Coding Tip**
>
> Use as many qualifying-circumstance modifiers as needed to completely identify the patient and/or procedure conditions.

The qualifying-circumstance modifiers and the units assigned to each are listed in Table 7.2.

Table 7.2 Qualifying-Circumstance Modifiers *(Data from CPT 2013. © 2013 American Medical Association. All rights reserved.)*

MODIFIER	DEFINITION	ADDITIONAL UNITS
+99100	Anesthesia for patient of extreme age: younger than 1 year old and older than 70	1
+99116	Anesthesia complicated by utilization of total body hypothermia	5
+99135	Anesthesia complicated by utilization of controlled hypotension	5
+99140	Anesthesia complicated by **emergency conditions**	2

emergency condition Exists when delay in treatment would lead to significant increase in the threat to life or body part.

1. What is the function of a qualifying-circumstance modifier?
2. What is the function of a physical-status modifier?
3. A 72-year-old patient is taken to the operating room for emergency surgery. The patient is known to be diabetic. What physical-status modifier and qualifying-circumstance modifiers, if any, would be appended to this patient's anesthesia code?

Also available in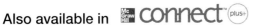

7.3 Modifiers Specific to Anesthesia Billing

At times, anesthesia services may be provided by different levels of providers performing different levels of service, for example, an anesthesiologist providing the services or a **Certified Registered Nurse Anesthetist (CRNA)** may act under the direction of an anesthesiologist or may provide the service without medical direction.

As these providers and the level of service being provided are reimbursed at different rates, several anesthesia-specific modifiers are used to identify these circumstances. Modifiers which identify the provider or level of supervision provided by an anesthesiologist are located in HCPCS Level II and are included in Table 7.3 below.

Certified Registered Nurse Anesthetist (CRNA) Certified Registered Nurse Anesthetist. A provider of anesthesia care.

Table 7.3 Anesthesia-Specific Modifiers: Anesthesiologists *(Data from HCPCS, Centers for Medicare and Medicaid Services and the National Center for Health Statistics.)*

MODIFIER	DEFINITION	FUNCTION
AA	Anesthesia services performed personally by an anesthesiologist	Append this modifier to the anesthesiologist service to identify that the service was provided by an anesthesiologist.
QY	Medical direction of one CRNA by an anesthesiologist	Append this modifier only to the anesthesiologist's (MD's) charges to identify the medical direction of a CRNA. (See medical direction requirements in Section 7.4.)
QK	Medical direction of 2, 3, or 4 concurrent anesthesia procedures involving qualified individuals	Append this modifier only to the anesthesiologist's (MD's) charges when he or she is providing medical direction for up to 4 patients at the same time. (See medical direction requirements in Section 7.4.)
AD	Medical supervision by a physician; more than 4 concurrent anesthesia procedures	Append this modifier only to the anesthesiologist's (MD's) charges when he or she is providing anesthesia supervision for 5 or more patients at a time

Table 7.4 Anesthesia-Specific Modifiers: CRNAs *(Data from HCPCS, Centers for Medicare and Medicaid Services and the National Center for Health Statistics.)*

MODIFIER	DEFINITION	FUNCTION
QX	CRNA service with medical direction by a physician	Use of this modifier requires medical direction by an anesthesiologist. (See medical direction requirements in Section 7.4.)
QZ	CRNA service without medical direction by a physician	Use of this modifier identifies that the service was performed by the CRNA with no medical direction or supervision.

MENTOR Coding Tip

When coding for anesthesia services both during the CPC exam and in the field, coders must first identify the provider of service (MD or CRNA), the level of service provided, and which provider's service is being coded in order to be able to apply the correct anesthesia billing modifier.

FOR EXAMPLE Suppose you encounter this case on a test: An anesthesia service for a closed procedure on the radius (01820) is being provided by a CRNA under the medical direction of an anesthesiologist who is directing three anesthesia services concurrently. The instructions for the question state that you are to code for the services of the anesthesiologist only.

The correct code with modifier for this case is 01820-QK. By knowing which modifiers append to which provider's services, the coder can quickly rule out any answer choices that include the incorrect modifiers. ■

EXERCISE 7.3

1. What is the purpose of the anesthesia-specific modifiers?
2. To select the appropriate anesthesia-specific modifier, what must a coder be able to identify from the documentation?
3. Which anesthesia-specific modifier identifies that the service was performed by the CRNA with no medical direction or supervision?

Also available in **connect** (plus+)

7.4 Medical Terminology Specific to Anesthesia

There are several terms that are specific to anesthesia services. Understanding these terms helps the coder determine what service or procedure is being rendered to the patient. This knowledge also helps the coder understand if any additional services or procedures should be coded separately or if they are a part of the primary service.

Medical direction, as it applies to anesthesia services, is physician involvement with and direction of anesthesia that is carried out by a qualified provider.

SPOTLIGHT on a Guideline

Requirements of Medical Direction

The anesthesiologist must:

- Complete preanesthetic examination and evaluation.
- Set the anesthesia plan.
- Attend to patients during the most demanding procedures of the anesthesia plan.
- Ensure that any procedures that are not personally performed are performed by individuals qualified to do so.
- Monitor the course of anesthesia in frequent intervals.
- Remain physically present and available for emergencies.
- Provide indicated postoperative care.

Another term that coders should key in on when coding for anesthesia services is **airway management.** This information helps the coder distinguish between the types of service provided.

airway management Endotracheal through existing tracheotomy, or via a mask, or nasal cannula are examples of the type of method.

FOR EXAMPLE The documentation reports that the patient was *intubated* or *extubated,* the patient's airway was then managed by endotracheal means, and the type of anesthesia was general. ■

SPOTLIGHT on Terminology

Intubation Placement of a flexible tube into the trachea to maintain an open airway, act as a conduit to administer drugs, or allow for ventilation of the lungs during anesthesia.

Extubation Removal of a previously placed intubation tube.

intubation Placement of a flexible tube into the trachea to maintain an open airway or allow for ventilation of the lungs during anesthesia.

extubation Removal of a flexible tube previously placed in the trachea for airway management.

Upon completion of the surgical procedure, the anesthesiologist will monitor the patient for a period of time postoperatively and then relinquish the patient to the **postanesthesia care unit (PACU),** where the patient will be monitored by a nurse specializing in postsedation care. The transfer of the patient to PACU signals the end of the anesthesia time.

post-anesthesia care unit (PACU) The unit where the patient is monitored by a nurse specializing in postsedation care.

1. Define *intubation.*
2. Define *extubation.*
3. List the requirements of medical direction.

EXERCISE 7.4

Also available in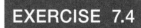

7.5 Procedures and the Type of Anesthesia Used for Specific Procedures

The only two types of anesthesia sedation services reported with an Anesthesia section code (CPT codes beginning with 0) are **general anesthesia** and **monitored anesthesia care (MAC).**

The key to understanding when to report general anesthesia and when to report MAC is knowing whether the patient's airway was managed during the anesthesia service.

When the documentation of the anesthesia service states that the patient managed her airway on her own or when no information is documented indicating that the patient's airway was managed, the anesthesia was monitored anesthesia care. Table 7.5 indicates the modifiers specific to monitored anesthesia care.

General anesthesia, by contrast, requires that the patient's airway is managed by the anesthesiologist or qualified person providing the service. Methods of airway management include endotracheal, through an existing tracheostomy, or via a mask or nasal cannula.

Another form of anesthesia is **conscious sedation,** or **moderate sedation.** This is the lightest form of anesthesia and is typically performed by the surgeon. It is included in the codes of many procedures, indicated by the ⊙ symbol. Conscious, or moderate, sedation codes are located in the Medicine section of CPT .

EXERCISE 7.5

1. The only two types of anesthesia sedation services reported with an Anesthesia section code (CPT codes beginning with 0) are general anesthesia and monitored anesthesia care. What is the key to understanding when to report general anesthesia and when to report MAC?

2. The documentation of the anesthesia service states that the patient managed his airway on his own and there was no documentation indicating that the patient's airway was managed. Which type of anesthesia care is this an example of?

3. List some of the methods of airway management.

Also available in **MᶜGraw Hill** **connect** (plus+)

general anesthesia Type of anesthesia that requires patient airway to be managed by anesthesiologist or qualified providing the service.

monitored anesthesia care (MAC) Patient manages airway on their own or no information is documented that airway was managed, this term is used.

moderate (conscious) sedation A level of consciousness where the patient can still respond to verbal commands.

Table 7.5 MAC-Specific Modifiers *(Data from HCPCS, Centers for Medicare and Medicaid Services and the National Center for Health Statistics.)*

MODIFIER	DESCRIPTION
QS	MAC service
G8	MAC for a deep, complex, complicated, or markedly invasive surgical procedure
G9	MAC for a patient who has a history of a severe cardiopulmonary condition

7.6 Other Procedures and Services Provided during Anesthesia

There are several procedures or services that might be performed and documented by the provider of anesthesia services that, although they may have a distinct CPT code to identify them, are considered part of the work of the anesthesia service and as such are not coded separately. These services include:

- Preoperative and postoperative visits
- General or regional anesthesia and patient care
- Administration of fluids and/or blood
- Usual monitoring services (e.g., ECG, temperature, blood pressure, oximetry, capnography, and mass spectrometry)

Several procedures or services often provided and documented by the anesthesia provider are not considered part of the anesthesia service. They should be billed and coded in addition to the anesthesia service when documented:

- Insertion of central venous catheter (36555–36558, 36568–36569)
- Insertion of an intra-arterial catheter (36620–36625)
- Insertion of Swan-Ganz (93503)
- Transesophageal echocardiography (TEE) (93312–93318)
- Procedures performed for postoperative pain management

Locating Terms in the Index

The main term indexed for anesthesia services is always *anesthesia.* The terms listed after the Anesthesia header are listed by surgical procedure and/or the anatomical site being operated on.

FOR EXAMPLE

Anesthesia
    Bypass Graft
        Leg, Lower 01500 ▪

EXERCISE 7.6

1. List services that are considered part of the work of the anesthesia service and as such are not coded separately.

2. Several procedures or services that are often provided and documented by the anesthesia provider are not considered part of the anesthesia service and thus should be billed and coded in addition to the anesthesia service when documented. List these services.

Also available in Mc Graw Hill **connect**™ (plus+)

Chapter Seven Summary

Learning Outcome	Key Concepts/Examples
7.1 Recognize the anesthesia reimbursement formula.	The reimbursement formula of time-based general anesthesia services consists of three components: base units (B), total time of anesthesia care (T), and modifying factors (M). Therefore, the formula is $B + T + M$
7.2 Apply physical-status and qualifying-circumstance modifiers.	*Physical-status modifiers:* used with all anesthesia procedure codes to rank the physical condition of the patient and the level of anesthesia complexity inherent to each ranking. *Qualifying-circumstances* modifiers: used when anesthesia is provided under circumstances such as extreme patient age, medical condition of patient or surgical procedure, or emergency situations.
7.3 Define HCPCS Level II modifiers and explain their function in anesthesia billing.	Anesthesia-specific modifiers: Anesthesia services may be provided by an anesthesiologist or by a Certified Registered Nurse Anesthetist acting under the direction of an anesthesiologist or acting without medical direction. As these providers and the level of service being provided are reimbursed at different rates, the anesthesia-specific modifiers are used to identify these circumstances.
7.4 Identify medical terminology specific to anesthesia billing.	*Medical direction*: As it applies to anesthesia services, this term refers to physician involvement with and direction of anesthesia that is carried out by a qualified provider. *Airway management:* The documentation reports that the patient was intubated or extubated, the patient's airway was then managed by endotracheal means, and the type of anesthesia is general. *Post-anesthesia care unit (PACU)*: This is where the patient is monitored by a nurse specializing in postsedation care.
7.5 Examine the types of anesthesia used for specific procedures.	The only two types of anesthesia sedation services reported with an Anesthesia section code (CPT codes beginning with 0) are general anesthesia and monitored anesthesia care.
7.6 Explain other procedures or services provided during anesthesia and locate anesthesia terms in the CPT manual index.	Some services are considered part of the work of the anesthesia service and as such are not coded separately. These services include: • Preoperative and postoperative visits • General or regional anesthesia and patient care • Administration of fluids and/or blood • Usual monitoring services (e.g., ECG, temperature, blood pressure, capnography, and mass spectrometry) Several procedures and services often provided and documented by the anesthesia provider are not considered part of the anesthesia service and should be billed and coded in addition to the anesthesia service when documented: • Insertion of central venous catheter (36555–36558, 36568–36569) • Insertion of an intra-arterial catheter (36620–36625) • Insertion of Swan-Ganz (93503) • Transesophageal echocardiography (93312–93318) • Procedures performed for postoperative pain management The main term indexed for anesthesia services is always *anesthesia.* The terms listed after the Anesthesia header are listed by surgical procedure and/or the anatomical site being operated on.

Chapter Seven Review

Using Terminology

Match each key term to the appropriate definition.

_____ 1. [LO7.4] Airway management

_____ 2. [LO7.1] Anesthesia

_____ 3. [LO7.1] Base unit

_____ 4. [LO7.3] CRNA

_____ 5. [LO7.2] Emergency condition

_____ 6. [LO7.4] Extubation

_____ 7. [LO7.5] General anesthesia

_____ 8. [LO7.4] Intubation

_____ 9. [LO7.5] MAC

_____ 10. [LO7.4] Medical direction

_____ 11. [LO7.5] Moderate/conscious sedation

_____ 12. [LO7.4] PACU

_____ 13. [LO7.2] Physical-status modifiers

_____ 14. [LO7.2] Qualifying-circumstance modifiers

_____ 15. [LO7.1] Time

A. The removal of a flexible tube previously placed in the trachea for airway management

B. Units of value that are the first component of the formula for assigning a cost-revenue value to an anesthesia service

C. Without sensation or loss of sensation, partial or complete

D. Component of the reimbursement formula that begins when the patient is being prepared for anesthesia and ends when the patient is no longer being attended by the anesthesiologist

E. Used with all anesthesia procedure codes to rank the physical condition of the patient

F. A provider of anesthesia care other than a physician

G. Refers to physician involvement with and direction of anesthesia that is carried out by a qualified provider

H. Additional codes that are used to report challenging circumstances in which anesthesia may be provided

I. Term used when the documentation states that the patient managed his airway on his own or when no information is documented indicating that the airway was managed

J. Condition that exists when a delay in treatment would lead to a significant increase in the threat to life or a body part

K. The unit where a patient is monitored by a nurse specializing in postsedation care

L. Examples of this method include endotracheal, through an existing tracheotomy, or via a mask or nasal cannula

M. Lightest form of anesthesia, in which the patient can still respond to commands

N. This type of anesthesia requires that the patient airway be managed by the anesthesiologist or qualified practitioner providing the service

O. Placement of a flexible tube into the trachea to maintain an open airway

Checking Your Understanding

Choose the most appropriate answer for each of the following questions.

1. [LO7.4] As it applies to anesthesia services, which of the following terms describes physician involvement with and direction of anesthesia that is carried out by a qualified provider?

   a. Direct supervision

   b. Medical management

   c. Medical direction

   d. General supervision

2. [LO7.5] The correct modifier to report for monitored anesthesia care (MAC) for a patient who has a history of severe cardiopulmonary condition is:

   a. QS

   b. G8

   c. QZ

   d. G9

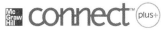

Enhance your learning by completing these exercises and more at mcgrawhillconnect.com

3. **[LO7.1–7.6]** A 72-year-old normal, healthy patient presents to the operating room for a corneal transplant. The anesthesiologist administers general anesthesia. Choose the appropriate codes the anesthesiologist would report:

    a. 00140, P3, 99100

    b. 65710, 00144, P1, 99100

    c. 00144, P1, 99100

    d. 00144, P1

4. **[LO7.1–7.6]** An 8-month-old boy was transported to the ED after being involved in an automobile accident. He required emergency surgery for an injury to the larynx and trachea. The general anesthesia was administered by the anesthesiologist. Choose the appropriate codes:

    a. 00326, P1, 99140

    b. 00350, P1, 99140

    c. 00326, P1, 99100, 99140

    d. 00326

5. **[LO7.1]** Choose the appropriate description of when time begins and ends for anesthesia procedures:

    a. Time begins when the anesthesia is actually administered in the operating room, and it ends when the patient leaves the operating room.

    b. Time begins when the anesthesiologist begins to prepare the patient for the induction of anesthesia, and it ends when the anesthesiologist is no longer in personal attendance.

    c. Time begins when the anesthesiologist begins to prepare the patient for the induction of anesthesia, and it ends when the patient leaves the operating room.

    d. Time begins when the anesthesiologist begins to prepare the patient for the induction of anesthesia, and it does not end until the patient leaves the postoperative room.

Applying Your Knowledge

Note: All anesthesia services in the following cases are performed on the same day by Thames Anesthesiology Group, which provides services at General Medical Hospital.

[LO 7.1–7.7] Case 1

The patient presents for anesthesia for an open appendectomy needed for acute appendicitis (Base Units 6). The patient is 19 and otherwise in good health. Under the medical direction of Dr. Thames, the anesthesiologist, the CRNA begins to prepare the patient for induction of endotracheal anesthesia at 7:45 a.m. The procedure is performed without incident, and the patient is released to PACU at 9:05 a.m.

Answer the following questions.

CPT Coding for Anesthesia Services Only

1. What type of sedation is provided for this service?

2. What is the main term for this service?

3. What is the surgical procedure and/or anatomical site of the procedure (subterm)?

4. What is the correct CPT code for this anesthesia service?

    a. 44950

    b. 00840

    c. 00860

    d. 00800

ICD-9-CM Coding

1. What is the main diagnostic term for this patient's condition?

2. What subterm(s) is (are) indicated in the documentation that would further specify the ICD-9-CM code? What other question(s) might you ask to specify the code even further?

3. Are any additional signs, symptoms, or conditions needed to complete this diagnosis?

4. What is the correct ICD-9-CM code for this anesthesia service?
   a. 540.9   c. 542
   b. 541   d. 540.0

Modifiers

1. What level of provider performed the service?

2. Under what level of service did the provider perform?

3. What is the correct modifier to identify the provider and level of supervision for this service?

4. What is the physical status of this patient?

5. What is the correct physical-status modifier for this service?

6. Were there any unusual circumstances for this patient or procedure?

7. What is the qualifying-circumstance modifier for this service?

Units of Service

1. What is the number of base units assigned to this service?

2. Using the ASA standard of 15 minutes per unit, how many time units are assigned?

3. What is the total number of units listed on the claim for this anesthesia service?

[LO 7.1–7.7] Case 2

Following Dr. Thames' anesthesiologist prescribed plan for a patient with type 2 diabetes mellitus not well controlled, the CRNA intubates the patient at 8:58 a.m. The surgeon performs an excision of a benign tumor on the olecranon process (Base Units 4). At 10:18 a.m. the patient is extubated and sent to the PACU.

Answer the following questions.

CPT Coding for Anesthesia Services Only

1. What type of sedation is provided for this service?

2. What is the main term for this service?

3. What is the surgical procedure and/or anatomical site of the procedure (subterm)?

4. What is the correct CPT code for this anesthesia service?
   a. 01732   c. 01740
   b. 24120   d. 01830

ICD-9-CM Coding

1. What is the main diagnostic term for this patient's condition?

2. What subterm(s) is (are) indicated in the documentation that would further specify the ICD-9-CM code? What other question(s) might you ask to specify the code even further?

3. Are any additional signs, symptoms, or conditions needed to complete this diagnosis?

4. What are the correct ICD-9-CM codes for this anesthesia service?
   a. 170.4, 250.00   c. 250.00, 213.4
   b. 250.02, 170.4   d. 213.4, 250.02

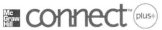

Enhance your learning by completing these exercises
and more at mcgrawhillconnect.com

Modifiers

1. What level of provider performed the service?

2. Under what level of service did the provider perform?

3. What is the correct modifier to identify the provider and level of supervision for this service?

4. What is the physical status of this patient?

5. What is the correct physical-status modifier for this service?

6. Were there any unusual circumstances for this patient or procedure?

7. What is the qualifying-circumstance modifier for this service?

Units of Service

1. What is the number of base units assigned to this service?

2. Using the ASA standard of 15 minutes per unit, how many time units are assigned?

3. What is the total number of units listed on the claim for this anesthesia service?

[LO 7.1–7.7] Case 3

Using the information from Cases 1 and 2 above, provide the coding information needed to bill for Dr. Thames's services.

For Case 1

CPT	_____
ICD-9-CM	_____
Provider-of-service modifier	_____
Physical-status modifier	_____
Qualifying-circumstance modifier	_____
Total number of units	_____

For Case 2

CPT	_____
ICD-9-CM	_____
Provider-of-service modifier	_____
Physical-status modifier	_____
Qualifying-circumstance modifier	_____
Total number of units	_____

[LO 7.1–7.7] Case 4

Arthroplasty right hip

DJD of right hip

After satisfactory anesthesia by Dr. Thames, the surgeon completed the arthroplasty of the right hip of the 72-year-old male. Patient comorbidities include well-controlled type 2 DM and benign hypertension.

Both the head of the femur at the greater trochanter and the acetabulum were replaced during this procedure (Base Units 8). Induction of the patient began at 11:02 a.m., and the patient was extubated and sent to postanesthesia recovery at 1:48 p.m.

Answer the following questions.

CPT Coding for Anesthesia Services Only

1. What type of sedation is provided for this service?

2. What is the main term for this service?

3. What is the surgical procedure and/or anatomical site of the procedure (subterm)?

4. What is (are) the correct CPT code(s) for this anesthesia service?
   a. 01210
   b. 01214
   c. 01210, 27130
   d. 27130

ICD-9-CM Coding

1. What is the main diagnostic term for this patient's condition?

2. What subterm(s) is (are) indicated in the documentation that would further specify the ICD-9-CM code? What other question(s) might you ask to specify the code even further?

3. Are any additional signs, symptoms or conditions needed to complete this diagnosis?

4. What is (are) the correct ICD-9-CM code(s) for this anesthesia service?
   a. 715.95
   b. 250.00, 715.95, 401.0
   c. 715.95, 250.00, 401.1
   d. 715.95, 250.00

Modifiers

1. What level of provider performed the service?

2. Under what level of service did the provider perform?

3. What is the correct modifier to identify the provider and level of supervision for this service?

4. What is the physical status of this patient?

5. What is the correct physical-status modifier for this service?

6. Were there any unusual circumstances for this patient or procedure?

7. What is the qualifying-circumstance modifier for this service?

Units of Service

1. What is the number of base units assigned to this service?

2. Using the ASA standard of 15 minutes per unit, how many time units are assigned?

3. What is the total number of units listed on the claim for this anesthesia service?

[LO 7.1–7.7] Case 5

A 6-year-old boy presents to the OR for closed reduction of a distal ulnar fracture at 3:45. Dr. Thames monitors the patient's vital signs and respirations on room air. The total time of the procedure is 48 minutes. (Base Units 3)

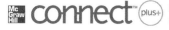

Answer the following questions.

CPT Coding for Anesthesia Services Only

1. What type of sedation is provided for this service?

2. What is the main term for this service?

3. What is the surgical procedure and/or anatomical site of the procedure (subterm)?

4. What is the correct CPT code for this anesthesia service?
   - **a.** 01820
   - **b.** 01820-RT
   - **c.** 01830
   - **d.** 01830-RT

ICD-9-CM Coding

1. What is the main diagnostic term for this patient's condition?

2. What subterm(s) is (are) indicated in the documentation that would further specify the ICD-9-CM code? What other question(s) might you ask to specify the code even further?

3. Are any additional signs, symptoms, or conditions needed to complete this diagnosis?

4. What is the correct ICD-9-CM code for this anesthesia service?
   - **a.** 813.53
   - **b.** 813.43
   - **c.** 813.44
   - **d.** 813.54

Modifiers

1. What level of provider performed the service?

2. Under what level of service did the provider perform?

3. What is the correct modifier to identify the provider and level of supervision for this service?

4. What is the physical status of this patient?

5. What is the correct physical-status modifier for this service?

6. Were there any unusual circumstances for this patient or procedure?

7. What is the qualifying-circumstance modifier for this service?

Units of Service

1. What is the number of base units assigned to this service?

2. Using the ASA standard of 15 minutes per unit, how many time units are assigned?

3. What is the total number of units listed on the claim for this anesthesia service?

Surgery Section

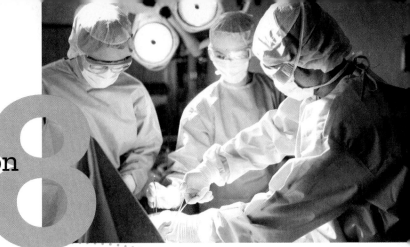

8

Key Terms

Approach

Biopsy

Closed procedure

Destruction

Endoscopy

Excision

Global surgical package

Incision

Laparoscopy

Open procedure

Percutaneous

Repair

Separate procedure

Learning Outcomes

After completing this chapter, you will be able to:

8.1 Recognize and understand the general guidelines and format of the Surgery section of the CPT manual.

8.2. Define *global surgical package.*

8.3 Identify the modifiers most commonly used with codes in the Surgery section.

8.4 Examine the common medical and procedural terms used in operative reports.

8.5 Practice using the index to locate codes for surgical procedures.

Introduction The largest section in the CPT, the Surgery section, includes codes that describe diagnostic as well as therapeutic procedures. Full knowledge of this section in its entirety comes with time and experience. However, with practice and an understanding of the medical terminology used in this section, along with practical knowledge of the Surgery section guidelines, less experienced coders can succeed in correctly coding for the therapeutic and diagnostic procedures listed in the Surgery section.

8.1 General Guidelines and Format of the CPT Surgery Section

The guidelines at the beginning of the Surgery section as well as the beginning of each subsection provide the framework for use of the codes located in this section. Guidelines and instructional notes appear throughout the entire Surgery section. Reviewing these guidelines before deciding on the appropriate code is imperative for correct use of these codes. Coders should be in the practice of consulting the guidelines and notes each time they use this section until they develop an in-depth understanding of these rules.

> **MENTOR** Coding Tip
>
> When deciding on a code, be sure to look at the bottom of each CPT page for the tips that appear there relating to the codes above.

FOR EXAMPLE The + (plus sign) indicates that a code with this designation is an add-on code to be used with the primary procedure code. ■

The Surgery section is divided into six subsections that are based on organ systems or body areas, for example, the integumentary and musculoskeletal subsections. (See Table 8.1.) The Surgery section guidelines contain information

Table 8.1 Surgery Section and Subsection Code Ranges *(Data from CPT 2013. © 2013 American Medical Association. All rights reserved.)*

SECTION	CODE RANGE
Surgery	10021–69990
Subsections:	
General	10021–10022
Integumentary	10040–19499
Musculoskeletal	20005–29999
Respiratory	30000–32999
Cardiovascular	33010–37799
Hemic and Lymphatic	38100–38999
Mediastinum and Diaphragm	39000–39599
Digestive	40490–49999
Urinary System	50010–53899
Reproductive and Intersex Surgery; Male Genital	54000–55899
Female Genital	56405–58999
Maternity Care and Delivery	59000–59899
Endocrine	60000–60300
Parathyroid, Thymus, Adrenal Glands, Pancreas, and Carotid Body	60500–60699
Nervous System	61000–64999
Eye and Ocular Adnexa	65091–68899
Auditory System	69000–69979

and rules that pertain only to the Surgery section, and, as with all other sections, knowing these guidelines and how to use them is one of the keys to correct coding in the Surgery section.

One of the most misunderstood guidelines in the Surgery section is the separate-procedures rule. Codes designated as **separate procedures** are procedures that, when performed with another procedure at the same anatomical site at the same time, are bundled into the other procedure and not coded and reported separately.

FOR EXAMPLE The removal of impacted cerumen (69210) would not be separately reportable when performed at the same time as the removal of a foreign body of the ear canal (69200). There are several examples of the use of separate procedures throughout this chapter. ■

At times, providers may perform and document a service or procedure for which there is no specific Level I CPT code. CPT has provided two means of coding for services or procedures when this occurs: category III codes and unlisted codes.

Category III codes are temporary codes for services, procedures, or emerging technology for which there is no CPT code available. These codes allow for data tracking, and the service or procedure indicated by the code may or may not become a CPT code in the future. These codes follow category II codes in the CPT.

SPOTLIGHT on a Guideline

When available, category III codes must be used instead of an unlisted code because category III codes provide more information regarding the service or procedure performed than do the unlisted codes. Unlisted procedure codes are considered the codes of last resort and are used only when the service or procedure provided is not identified by a distinct CPT or category III code.

MENTOR Coding Tip

With only a few exceptions, unlisted service or procedure codes end in 99. A complete list for each section of the CPT is located in the section guidelines. Category III codes are five-character alphanumeric codes that always end in a "T," which indicates emerging technology.

Several different **approach** methods by which a procedure may be performed are located in the Surgery section of CPT. Regardless of the method of approach, when it is the means by which the provider gains access to the body to complete a service or procedure, it is included in the code for the procedure and not coded separately.

Methods of approach and a brief description of each are provided in Table 8.2.

One guideline that applies throughout the Surgery section pertains to surgical and diagnostic scope procedures that are performed at the same operative session and same anatomical site. CPT clarifies that when this occurs,

Table 8.2 Surgical Approach Methods

APPROACH	DESCRIPTION
Endoscopy	An optic instrument (scope) is inserted into the body for visualization within the body cavity or organ. Typically introduced via a natural opening, the scope may also be inserted through an incision. The type of endoscopic procedure is dependent on the body area or organ being viewed and the intent of the procedure (diagnostic versus surgical). There are several different types of endoscopic procedures: • *Laparoscopy:* The scope is inserted into the abdominal cavity via an incision in the abdomen wall. Procedures or inspection of the outside of the organs contained within the abdominal cavity, such as the colon, intestines, ovaries, fallopian tubes, and uterus, may be completed via this approach. • *Colonoscopy:* The scope is inserted via a natural opening (anus) to examine the inside of the colon, obtain biopsies, or complete procedures within the colon. • *Thoracoscopy:* The scope is inserted into the thoracic cavity via an incision in the skin to view the pleurae, lungs, and mediastinum. Soft tissue from the outside of the lungs or the cavity may be obtained for testing. • *Bronchoscopy:* The scope is inserted via a natural opening (mouth) or a tracheostomy to view the tracheobronchial tree. Examination of the trachea and bronchus is performed. Suctioning, obtaining a biopsy, or removing a foreign body may also be completed. • *Arthroscopy:* The scope is inserted into the joint via an incision in the skin. An arthroscopy may be diagnostic or therapeutic (surgical).
Open (-otomy)	Through an incision in the skin or other membranes, the provider has full view of the organs or structures as needed for the procedure. Example: a laparotomy.
Closed	This type of procedure is completed without incision and is considered noninvasive in nature. Example: a closed reduction of a fracture.
Percutaneous	This type of procedure is completed through the skin; however, the surgical site is not open to view as in a laparotomy. The surgeon views the site indirectly via fluoroscopy or other means and completes the procedure through the skin. Example: placement of pins through the skin to maintain patency of a reduced fracture.

closed procedure Procedures completed without incision and considered noninvasive in nature.

percutaneous Procedures completed through the skin.

open procedure Through an incision in the skin or other membranes the provider has full view of the organs or structures as needed

only the surgical scope procedure is reportable. Since a diagnostic scope procedure is part of all surgical scope procedures, it is bundled into the surgical scope when performed on the same anatomical site during the same operative session.

In addition to the diagnostic-therapeutic scope guideline, there is a scope–open procedure guideline. Since a diagnostic scope is *only* considered part of a surgical scope, it is not bundled with open surgical procedures. This means that if the provider performs an arthroscopy and then, based on the findings, opens the joint to complete the therapeutic procedure, both the diagnostic scope and the therapeutic open procedure would be reported.

MENTOR Coding Tip

In reporting a diagnostic scope with an **open procedure,** a modifier is needed to explain the change. Append modifier 59, distinct procedural service, to the diagnostic scope procedure to identify it as a separate procedure performed during the same operative session.

1. Explain the format of the Surgery section.
2. List some of the approach methods described in the Surgery section.
3. Explain a laparoscopic procedure.
4. Explain the guideline regarding diagnostic and surgical scope procedures performed at the same operative session.

EXERCISE 8.1

Also available in ![McGraw-Hill] **connect**™ (plus+)

8.2 Global Surgical Period and Global Surgical Package

The global surgical period, also known as the *postoperative* or *post-op period*, is a prescribed period of time surrounding the surgical procedure. Each surgical procedure code, except those identified as modifier 51 exempt, is divided into two categories: minor procedures and major procedures. Minor procedures typically have a 0- to 10-day post-op period, and major procedures typically have post-op periods of 90 days or more. Major procedures also include the day prior to surgery, or the pre-op day.

Although the **global surgical package** is defined by each payer, the CPT guidelines include a description of the surgical package. The surgical package specifies what services are bundled with, or a part of, the surgical service. While these services, when not provided during the surgical period, may be coded and reported separately, they are not reportable with the surgical procedure. These services include:

- The anesthesia needed to perform the procedure, such as topical, local, and digital blocks. Forms of anesthesia not included are general, MAC, and moderate sedation when not indicated as included in the procedure.

- Postoperative care including documenting operative notes, writing orders, and providing typical follow-up care. Not included in postoperative care are complications related to the surgery (e.g., infection, post-op bleeding) that require a return to the operating room (OR). (See modifiers 76, 77, and 78 in Section 8.3.) Also not included in the postoperative package are E/M or surgical services for a condition unrelated to the surgery. (See modifier 79 in Section 8.3.)

- History and physical exam on the day of or day prior to the procedure. However, the E/M service on which the need for surgery was determined, regardless of the date on which it was completed, is not included in the global package.

global surgical package Also known as the postoperative or post-op period, is a prescribed period of time surrounding the surgical procedure.

MENTOR Coding Tip

The global surgical period for major surgical procedures includes the day prior to surgery. Thus, if the E/M service that resulted in the decision for surgery was completed the day before or the day of surgery, it must be identified to the payer by appending modifier 57 to the E/M code.

1. Explain the use of modifier 57 in regard to the global surgical package.
2. List some services that are included in the global surgical package and not reported separately.
3. How many postoperative days are typically allocated for minor and major procedures?

Also available in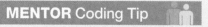

8.3 Modifiers and the Surgery Section

Modifiers tell the rest of the surgical story by adding the details that are not or cannot be expressed in the CPT or ICD code. Modifiers are used to relay unusual circumstances of the procedure itself or those that may have occurred during the procedure. Modifiers relay such information as laterality, services provided that significantly increase or decrease the code description, multiple procedures, discontinued procedures, staged procedures, and reasons for additional services provided during the global surgical period.

When determining the need for modifiers based on the documented procedure, the coder must find the answers to several questions. The answers will identify the need to append modifiers as well as the correct modifier to use. The questions are listed below:

Was the procedure performed as described by the nomenclature of the code?

- Was the procedure more difficult or time-consuming or did it require extra work on the part of the surgeon, as in an unusual anatomy? *If yes,* append modifier 22.
- Did the procedure performed involve less than the procedure described by the code? *If yes,* verify that the code is correct. If it is correct, append modifier 52.
- Was the procedure discontinued after anesthesia but prior to completion? *If yes,* append modifier 53.

Was the procedure performed on an anatomical site that has laterality?

- Was the procedure performed unilaterally? *If yes,* append the RT or LT modifier to identify the site.

> **MENTOR** Coding Tip
>
> If the code describes a bilateral procedure and the procedure is completed unilaterally, append modifier 52 as well as the correct site modifier (RT or LT).

- Was the procedure performed bilaterally? *If yes,* append modifier 50.

> **MENTOR** Coding Tip
>
> Before appending modifier 50, verify that a bilateral code is not available for the procedure performed.

Was the procedure performed in the global period of another procedure?

- Was the procedure the same (same CPT code) as the previous procedure? *If yes:*
  - Was the procedure performed by the same surgeon? *If yes,* append modifier 76.
  - Was the procedure performed by a different surgeon? *If yes,* append modifier 77.
- Was the procedure performed as the result of a complication of the previous procedure? *If yes,* append modifier 78. *If no,* append modifier 79.
- Was the procedure planned or expected or was it more extensive than the original procedure? *If yes,* append modifier 58.

Were additional procedures performed during the operative session?

- Was the additional procedure performed through a separate incision, on a different organ or anatomical site, or on a separate lesion or injury? Would this procedure normally not be reportable with the primary surgical code, but is it appropriate in this circumstance? *If yes,* append modifier 59.
- Was the additional procedure performed one that is normally reportable in addition to the primary procedure? *If yes,* append modifier 51.

Did the surgeon have help from another surgeon or other appropriate person?

- Did each surgeon perform integral parts of the same procedure (i.e., approach and definitive procedure)? *If yes,* append modifier 62.
- Did the assist at surgery remain and assist during the entire procedure? *If yes,* append modifier 80.
- Did the assist at surgery attend and assist for only a portion of the procedure? *If yes,* append modifier 81.

Did the same physician provide the preoperative, postoperative, and intraoperative parts of the procedure? If yes, no modifier is needed. If no, which portion did the surgeon provide?

- Preoperative only: Append modifier 56.
- Postoperative only: Append modifier 55.
- Intraoperative only: Append modifier 54.

Table 8.3 lists modifiers that are used with codes in the Surgery section.

Examples of the use of specific modifiers are given in the specific body system chapters of this textbook.

Table 8.3 Surgery Section Modifiers *(Data from CPT 2013. © 2013 American Medical Association. All rights reserved.)*

MODIFIER	DESCRIPTION
RT	Right side
LT	Left side
22	Increased procedural service
23	Unusual anesthesia
47	Anesthesia by surgeon
50	Bilateral procedure
51	Multiple procedures
52	Reduced services

(continued)

Table 8.3 Surgery Section Modifiers (*concluded*)

MODIFIER	DESCRIPTION
53	Discontinued procedure
54	Surgical care only
55	Postoperative management only
56	Preoperative management only
58	Staged or related procedure or service by the same physician during the postoperative period
59	Distinct procedural service
62	Two surgeons
63	Procedure performed on an infant less than 4 kg
66	Surgical team
76	Repeat procedure or service by same physician or other qualified healthcare professional
77	Repeat procedure or service by another physician or other qualified healthcare professional
78	Unplanned return to the operating room by the same physician or other qualified healthcare professional following the initial procedure for a related procedure during the postoperative period
79	Unrelated procedure or service by the same physician during the postoperative period
80	Assistant surgeon
81	Minimum assistant surgeon

EXERCISE 8.3

1. What questions must a coder answer when determining whether the procedure was performed as described by the nomenclature of the code or requires a modifier to define the variance from the description?

2. What questions must a coder answer when determining whether the procedure was performed in the global period of another procedure and requires a modifier to report why this procedure should be reported separately?

3. What questions must a coder answer from the documentation to determine the appropriate use of modifier 62, 80, or 81?

Also available in **connect** (plus+)

8.4 Common Medical and Procedural Terms Used in Operative Reports

Chapter 1 explained the importance of being able to translate the provider's documentation into a complete story that conveys to the payer, compliance department, or other regulating bodies the patient's diagnosis and treatment at the present encounter. Although the story written by the provider for services rendered to the patient may be in many different formats, the operative report is the documentation primarily used when surgeons tell the story. In addition to using different formats, not all surgeons will use the same language to tell this story.

Some surgeons may use the language used in CPT or ICD to describe services or conditions; however, most do not. This differing language will be among the biggest challenge coders must conquer when coding for services listed in the Surgery section.

MENTOR Coding Tip

A clear understanding of medical terminology, pathophysiology, and anatomy pertaining to the body system affected by the present encounter is critical to accurate coding within the Surgery section.

While the language used may differ, many medical terms used in describing surgical services are common throughout the medical field. Table 8.4 provides a brief introduction to some of these medical terms and lists alternative

biopsy The removal of all or part of a lesion for pathological examination.

destruction Destroying of tissue using heat, cold, or chemicals.

endoscopy Visual examination within a cavity.

excision Removal by cutting all or part. Suffix is -ectomy.

incision Creating an opening by surgically cutting into the skin or other tissue. Suffix is -otomy.

laparoscopy Process of inserting a scope through the skin of the abdomen for examination.

repair Suture, revise or restore are terms which could be used in a documentation to describe this type of procedure.

Table 8.4 Terms for Surgery Section

TERM AND SUFFIX	DEFINITION	DOCUMENTATION KEYS
Biopsy	Removal of all or part of a lesion for pathologic examination	Incisional, excisional, needle aspiration, punch, shave
Destruction	Destroying of tissue by means of heat, cold, or chemicals (*Note*: There is no tissue to send for pathology.)	Cautery, cryo, laser
Endoscopy	Process of using a scope inserted through a natural opening or stoma to examine the *inside* of an organ or system (e.g., respiratory or gastrointestinal)	Orifice, cavity, lumen, pylorus, sphincter, advanced, trachea, bronchus
Excision	Removal by cutting all or part	-ectomy Example: appendectomy
Harvest	Removal of donor organ, tissue, or bone for implantation to another anatomical site or patient (e.g., harvesting of a vein or artery for CABG)	Procurement
Incision	Creation of an opening by surgically cutting into the skin or other tissue	-otomy
Laparoscopy	Process of using a scope inserted through the skin of the abdomen to examine the *outside* of organs or systems (e.g., uterus or intestines)	Insufflation, port, peritoneum, cavity (e.g., abdominopelvic or peritoneal), pleura, stab wound incision
Repair	Restoration of diseased or damaged tissue, organ, bone, etc.	Suture, revise, restore
-ectomy	Surgically removing by cutting	Excision, removal
-plasty	Reshaping or replacing by surgical means	Repair, reconstruction, revision, augmentation
-oscopy	Visually examining through a scope	Advancement, cavity
-ostomy	Surgically creating an artificial opening	Stoma
-otomy	Cutting into or incising	Stab, incision, nick

terms and suffixes that might be in the provider's documentation and that translate to the main term in CPT language, as well as key terms found in the documentation that help the coder identify the procedure, approach, or method of the services documented. Additional terms are discussed in later chapters of this text in terms of their relevance to specific body systems.

8.5 Indexing Surgical Procedures

While language and format of the surgical documentation may differ, the information needed to code the case is still contained within the document. This information is the primary procedure and the condition for which the procedure was performed, as well as any additional services or conditions that were provided and documented during the operative session. It is this information that a coder must learn to target in on when assigning codes.

MENTOR Coding Tip

Keep a medical dictionary handy when coding, as many terms used in the documentation of surgical cases may be new and easily misunderstood.

The key to coding surgical cases is knowing and understanding what to identify during the review of documentation for services provided and conditions supporting the need for those services. Experienced coders have developed a series of questions that are answered as they read through the documentation. The questions build on each other, depending on the type of service or procedure documented. Although it takes practice to develop the skill of using questions, the process of doing so is at the fingertips of every coder and is the main focus of this text.

Coding an operative report is done in three separate processes: procedural (CPT) coding, diagnostic (ICD) coding, and addition of modifiers. Each of these processes is outlined below, with examples.

For the remainder of this section, and for the following chapters in this text, you will need the CPT, ICD, and HCPCS manuals. It is highly recommended that you use these manuals as you work through the processes below. In other words, do *not* just read through the processes; work through them following the examples as a guide when needed.

Using the surgical documentation in Case Study 8.1, you will work through the processes outlined for coding in CPT and ICD and adding modifiers. Do not read the case study yet.

Case Study 8.1

Preoperative diagnosis: DJD left hip

Postoperative diagnosis: DJD left hip

Operation performed: Left hip arthroplasty

Comorbidities: DM type 2 and hyperlipidemia

Under general anesthesia the patient was placed in the left lateral decubitus position. The left hip was prepped and draped in the usual fashion. A 12-inch incision was made, centering over the greater trochanter. The incision was deepened, and small bleeders were cauterized. The short external rotator was divided close to bone, together with the posterior capsule. The hip was dislocated posteriorly. Severe osteoarthritis was noted.

The femoral neck was cut at the appropriate level and angle and acetabulum was exposed. The acetabulum was reamed progressively to 51 mm in diameter. This was under-reamed by 2 mm. A trial with a 53-mm trial acetabular component was done. Fit and alignment were found to be good. The component was removed. The 53-mm porous-coated acetabular component was press-fit into place. Alignment and fixation were found to be excellent. The liner was inserted with the overhang posteriorly and inferiorly. The femoral canal was then prepped by reaming and broaching to 13.5-mm stem size. A trial was made with the neutral neck 31-mm head component. The hip was reduced, and a stable range of movement was noted. An AP view taken showed good position and length.

The hip was re-dislocated, and the trial femoral component was removed. The femoral canal was prepared for cementing by brushing and washing. The canal was plugged with the Universal cement restrictor plug. Using the cement syringe, a 13.5-mm nonporous stem with a 13-mm centralizer was cemented in place. Excellent alignment and fixation were noted. The 4-mm neck, 32-mm head component was tapped onto the femoral stem, and the hip was reduced.

A stable range of movement was noted. Hemostasis was checked.

Closure was done using #1 Vicryl to reattach the short external rotators and the posterior capsule. The fascial layer was closed with #1 Vicryl, the subcutaneous layer with 2-0 and 3-0 Vicryl, and the skin with staples.

The patient tolerated the procedure well and left for the recovery room in stable condition.

Process 1: Procedural Coding

This process involves identifying and translating the services documented.

As you work through development of each question, remember to review the surgical documentation to answer the question and begin targeting in on the code.

1. *Ask yourself, "What is the primary procedure?"* Do *not* read the entire documentation of the case yet; just identify the primary procedure. It should be identified as a single main term, in this case "Arthroplasty."

2. *Locate the main term in the index.* In reviewing the documentation, the next question or set of questions is built on any terms or subterms listed under the main term in the CPT index.

Arthroplasty

...

Hip 27132

    Partial Replacement 27125

       Revision 27134–27138

          Total Replacement 27130

Based on the choices available in the subterms, the next two questions are:

- How much was replaced?
- Was this a revision of a previous arthroplasty of the hip?

> **MENTOR**
> **Coding Tip**
>
> Although the primary procedure is typically documented in the header of the operative report, it is imperative that the coder briefly review the documentation to make sure the procedure listed was actually performed.

3. *Review all the code choices identified in the index to develop additional questions.* Identifying the differences in the code choices available leads to the next question:

 • If this was a partial replacement or partial revision, what portion was replaced?

EXERCISE 8.5a

CPT Coding: With these questions at hand, read the entire report of the surgical case (Case Study 8.1), answering each question below as you read through the case.

1. How much of the hip was replaced?
2. Was this a revision of a previous arthroplasty?
3. If this was a partial replacement or partial revision, what portion was replaced?
4. Based on the answers found in the documentation for this case, identify the correct CPT code for this case.
5. Based on your review of the documentation, were any other procedures performed that should be coded in addition to the primary procedure?

Also available in **connect** (plus+)

MENTOR Coding Tip

Many coders find it helpful to highlight or circle the answer to each of these questions before coding the report. Care should be taken not to highlight the entire report, as this makes it impossible to pick out the target information. To avoid the coloring-book effect, highlight only after all necessary questions have been developed.

Process 2: Diagnostic Coding

This is the process of identifying and translating the condition(s) documented. As in process 1, you will need to develop and answer several questions as the foundation for drilling down to the correct diagnostic code or codes as documented in the operative report. Although you now need to read the operative (op) report in its entirety, begin by reading only enough to identify the primary reason for the procedure. You may *start* this process by reviewing the pre- and postoperative diagnoses. Please note that this is only a starting point, as the pre-op and post-op diagnostic statements documented may be incomplete or incorrect. Reading the entire op report before coding the condition is needed to verify that the information contained in the header is correct and complete.

EXERCISE 8.5b

ICD Coding: Read the entire report of the surgical case (Case Study 8.1), answering each question below as you read through the case.

1. Based on the operative report header, what is the preoperative diagnosis?
2. Is the postoperative diagnosis the same as or different from the preoperative diagnosis? If the post-op diagnosis is different, review the documentation and verify that the post-op diagnosis is supported by the documentation.

Also available in **connect** (plus+)

3. Review the documentation and determine whether the post-op diagnosis is supported in the body of the report. Was the post-op diagnosis supported?

4. Locate the main term in the Alphabetic Index. Just as in process 1, the next question or set of questions for reviewing the documentation is built on the subterms listed below the main term:

Degeneration, degenerative

joint disease (see also Osteoarthrosis) 751.9✓

multiple sites 715.09

spine (see also……

Or:

Osteoarthrosis (degenerative) (hypertrophic) (rheumatoid) 715.9✓

……

……

5 pelvic region and thigh

……

……

generalized 715.09

juvenilis (Kohler's) 732.5

localized 715.3✓

idiopathic 715.1✓

primary 715.1✓

secondary 715.2✓

multiple sites, not specified as generalized 715.89

polyarticular 715.09

……

Based on the subterm choices, you can develop the next questions for this condition:

- What was the anatomical site for the condition?
- Was the condition localized or generalized?
- Was a specific form of the condition documented?

5. Read through the documentation, answering the questions you developed. As you do so, also identify any additional conditions that are documented. Based on the answers from the documentation, what is the primary ICD-9-CM code for the procedure in Case Study 8.1?

MENTOR Coding Tip

As you read through the op report, circle or highlight any additional conditions; these conditions are considered working diagnoses. Many of the working diagnoses will become nonessential once you have applied the ICD-9-CM coding guidelines regarding additional diagnosis codes.

---

6. Determine whether additional conditions are documented and should or should not be coded by comparing each working diagnosis to the questions below, which are based on the ICD-9-CM coding guidelines:
   - Is the condition, sign, or symptom an integral part of the primary (or other) condition coded? *If it is,* it is a nonessential diagnosis. Do not code.
   - *If it is not:* Does the condition require or affect patient care treatment or management? *If no,* the condition is a nonessential diagnosis. Do not code.
   - Has any working diagnosis been determined as being essential. *If yes,* code it in addition to the primary diagnosis.

   Applying step 6 to this case indicates that there are two additional conditions, diabetes mellitus type 2 and hyperlipidemia, for which no signs and symptoms are identified. Ask these questions:
   - Is the condition, sign, or symptom an integral part of the primary (or other) condition coded?
   - Does the condition require or affect patient care treatment or management?

EXERCISE 8.5c

ICD-10-CM Coding: Read the entire report of the surgical case (Case Study 8.1), answering each question as you read through the case.

1. Based on the operative report header, what is the preoperative diagnosis?
2. Is the postoperative diagnosis the same as or different from the preoperative diagnosis? If the post-op diagnosis is different, review the documentation and verify that the post-op diagnosis is supported by the documentation.
3. Review the documentation, and determine whether the post-op diagnosis is supported in the body of the report. Is the post-op diagnosis supported?
4. Locate the main term in the Alphabetic Index. Following the direction "see osteoarthritis," develop the next question or set of questions for reviewing the documentation on the basis of the subterms listed below the main term:

   Osteoarthritis M19.90-

   .....

   Hip M16.1-
       Bilateral M16.0
       Due to hip dysplasia (unilateral) M16.3-

Bilateral M16.2

…..

Post-traumatic

…..

Hip M16.5-
Bilateral M16.4

…..

Primary

…..

Hip 16.1-
Bilateral M16.0

Secondary

…..

Hip M16.7
Bilateral M16.6

Based on the subterm choices, you can develop the next questions for this condition:

- What was the anatomical site for the condition?
- Was the condition primary, secondary, or post-traumatic?
- Was the condition unilateral or bilateral?

5. Locate the code in the Tabular List, and determine whether additional questions are needed to further specify the diagnosis. Based on the information in the Tabular List, is additional information needed to determine the appropriate diagnosis code?

6. Read through the documentation, answering the questions you developed. As you do so, also identify any additional conditions that are documented. Based on the answers from the documentation, what is the primary ICD-10-CM code for the procedure in Case Study 8.1?

7. Determine whether additional conditions are documented and should or should not be coded by comparing each working diagnosis to the questions below, which are based on the ICD-10-CM coding guidelines:

- Is the condition, sign, or symptom an integral part of the primary (or other) condition coded? *If it is,* it is a nonessential diagnosis. Do not code.
- *If it is not:* Does the condition require or affect patient care treatment or management? *If no,* the condition is a nonessential diagnosis. Do not code.
- Has any working diagnosis been determined as being essential? *If yes,* code it in addition to the primary diagnosis.

Applying step 6 to Case Study 8.1 indicates that there are two additional conditions, diabetes mellitus type 2 and hyperlipidemia, for which no signs and symptoms are identified. Ask these questions:

- Is the condition, sign, or symptom an integral part of the primary (or other) condition coded?
- Does the condition require or affect patient care treatment or management?

Also available in

Process 3: Adding Modifiers

The last process in coding surgical cases is identifying the need for modifiers, thereby completing the story. This process involves only a series of questions that can be answered by reviewing either the operative report or the patient's medical record.

EXERCISE 8.5d

Modifiers: Read the entire report of the surgical case (Case Study 8.1), answering each question below as you read through the case.

1. Was the procedure performed different from that described by the nomenclature of the code?

2. Was the procedure performed on an anatomical site that has laterality?

3. Was the procedure performed in the global period of another procedure?

4. Were additional procedures performed during the operative session, and does the documentation support them?

5. Did the surgeon have help from another surgeon or another appropriate person?

6. Did a physician different from the surgeon perform the preoperative or postoperative portion of the procedure.

Based on the answers to the questions above, append modifier LT to the CPT code to identify that this procedure was performed on the left side of a bilateral site.

Also available in Mc Graw Hill **connect**™ (plus+)

Chapter Eight Summary

Learning Outcome	Key Concepts/Examples
8.1 Recognize and understand the general guidelines and format of the Surgery section of the CPT manual.	The guidelines at the beginning of the Surgery section as well as the beginning of each subsection provide the framework for the use of the codes located in this section. The Surgery section is divided into six subsections that are based on organ systems or body areas. Codes designated as separate procedures are procedures that, when performed with another procedure at the same anatomical site at the same time, are bundled into the other procedure and not coded and reported separately. When reporting services for which there is no specific CPT Level I code, CPT provides two means of coding: category III codes and unlisted codes.
8.2 Define *global surgical package.*	This package specifies what services are bundled with, or a part of, the surgical service. While these services, when not provided during the surgical period, may be coded and reported separately, they are not reportable with the surgical procedure. These services include: • The anesthesia needed to perform the procedure, such as topical, local, and digital blocks. Forms of anesthesia not included are general, MAC, and moderate sedation when not indicated as included in the procedure. • Postoperative care including documenting operative notes, writing orders, and providing typical follow-up care. Not included in postoperative care are complications related to the surgery (e.g., infection, post-op bleeding) that require a return to the operating room (OR). (See modifiers 76, 77, and 78 in Section 8.3.) Also not included in the postoperative package are E/M or surgical services for a condition unrelated to the surgery. (See modifier 79 in Section 8.3.) • History and physical exam on the day of or day prior to the procedure. However, the E/M service on which the need for surgery was determined, regardless of the date on which it was completed, is not included in the global package.
8.3 Identify the modifiers most commonly used with codes in the Surgery section.	Modifiers relay information such as laterality, services provided that significantly increase or decrease the code description, multiple procedures, discontinued procedures, staged procedures, and reasons for additional services provided during the global surgical period
8.4 Examine the common medical and procedural terms used in operative reports.	*Biopsy:* removal of all or part of a lesion for pathologic examination *Destruction:* destroying of tissue by means of heat, cold, or chemicals. (*Note:* There is no tissue to send for pathology.) *Excision:* removal by cutting all or part (suffix: *-ectomy*) *Harvest:* removal of a donor organ, tissue, or bone for implantation to another anatomical site or patient (e.g., harvesting of a vein or artery for CABG) *Incision:* creation of an opening by surgically cutting into the skin or other tissue (suffix: *-otomy*) *Repair:* restoration of diseased or damaged tissue, organ, bone, etc.
8.5 Practice using the index to locate codes for surgical procedures.	The language and format of surgical documentation may vary, but the information needed to code the case is still contained within the document. This information is the primary procedure and the condition for which the procedure was performed, as well as any additional services or conditions that were provided and documented during the operative session.

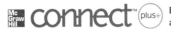

Chapter Eight Review

Using Terminology

Match each key term to the appropriate definition.

_____ 1. [LO8.1] Approach

_____ 2. [LO8.4] Biopsy

_____ 3. [LO8.1] Closed procedures

_____ 4. [LO8.4] Destruction

_____ 5. [LO8.4] Endoscopy

_____ 6. [LO8.4] Excision

_____ 7. [LO8.2] Global surgical package

_____ 8. [LO8.4] Incision

_____ 9. [LO8.4] Laparoscopy

_____ 10. [LO8.1] Open procedures

_____ 11. [LO8.1] Percutaneous

_____ 12. [LO8.4] Repair

_____ 13. [LO8.1] Separate procedures

_____ 14. [LO8.4] -oscopy

_____ 15. [LO8.4] -ostomy

_____ 16. [LO8.4] -plasty

A. Removal of all or part of a lesion for pathologic examination

B. Removal by cutting all or part

C. The means by which the provider gains access to the body to complete a service or procedure

D. Procedures that, when performed with another procedure at the same anatomical site at the same time, are bundled into the other procedure and not coded separately

E. Procedures that are completed without incision and are considered noninvasive in nature

F. Creation of an opening by surgically cutting into the skin or other tissue

G. Suffix meaning "to reshape or replace by surgical means"

H. A prescribed period of time surrounding the surgical procedure; also known as the postoperative or post-op period

I. Destroying of tissue by means of heat, cold, or chemicals

J. A type of procedure that could be documented with the term suture, *revise*, or *restore*

K. Visual examination within a cavity

L. Suffix meaning "surgically creating an artificial opening"

M. Process of inserting a scope through the skin of the abdomen for examination

N. Suffix meaning "visual examination through a scope"

O. Procedure in which, through an incision in the skin or other membranes, the provider has full view of the organs or structures as needed

P. Procedures completed through the skin

Checking Your Understanding

Choose the most appropriate answer for each of the following questions.

1. [LO8.1] The Surgery section of CPT is divided into _____ subsections based on _____.
   a. four; organ systems
   b. six; organ systems or body areas
   c. seven; body areas
   d. eight; diagnoses

2. [LO8.1] When a provider documents a service or procedure for which there is no specific HCPCS Level I code, the following (if a code exists) should be used first to report the service or procedure:
   a. A category III code
   b. A category II code
   c. An unlisted code
   d. The CPT code with the closest description to the procedure performed

3. [LO8.3] Which of the following modifiers would be appropriate to use if each surgeon performed integral parts of the same procedure?
   a. 81
   b. 80
   c. 62
   d. 59

4. [LO8.2] CPT coding for breast procedures is categorized in which section of the CPT manual?
   a. Female Reproductive
   b. Integumentary
   c. Endocrine
   d. Surgery

5. **[LO8.4]** The process of using a scope inserted through a natural opening or stoma to examine the inside of an organ or system (e.g., respiratory or gastrointestinal) is referred to as:

a. Laparoscopy
b. Endoscopy
c. Colonoscopy
d. Arthroscopy

Applying Your Knowledge

Case Study

Preoperative diagnosis: Possible torn medial meniscus

Postoperative diagnosis: Torn medial meniscus

Operation: Diagnostic arthroscopy

The patient was brought to the operating room and placed on the operating table in the supine position. The left lower extremity was prepped in usual sterile fashion. The knee was inflated with normal saline; a 2-centimeter incision was made anteriolaterally. The arthroscope was inserted.

One additional 1-centimeter incision was made anteriomedially. The medial compartment was first visualized; very minimal erosion of the medial femoral condyle and medial plateau was found. A tear was noted at the posterior horn of the medial meniscus. Basket forceps were used, and this area was repaired. Meniscal shaving was completed as well. The remainder of the medial compartment was grossly normal.

The scope was then moved to the intracondylar notch region. The anterior cruciate ligament was found to be intact.

The knee was then flexed to approximately 60 degrees, and the lateral compartment was visualized. The lateral femoral condyle, lateral meniscus, and lateral tibial plateau were patent. As were the popliteus idis and tendon. No loose bodies noted.

The scope was then moved into the suprapatellar pouch with the knee extended. The patellofemoral joint was inspected, with no erosion of the patellar surface noted.

At this point, the instruments were withdrawn and the wounds closed with 4-0 nylon sutures and compression dressing. Pneumatic pressure cuff was released, with good return of capillary refill to the toes. The patient was moved to the recovery room in good condition.

Process 1: Procedural Coding (CPT)

To identify and translate the services documented, answer the following questions.

1. What is the primary procedure?

2. Locate the main term in the index. What additional questions or set of questions can be determined based on any terms or subterms listed under the main term?

3. Upon review of all the code choices identified in the index, what additional questions can be determined?

4. Based on the documentation, what is (are) the correct code(s) for this case?

a. 29880
b. 29881
c. 29877, 29881
d. 29877

Process 2: Diagnostic Coding (ICD)

To identify and translate the condition(s) documented, answer the following questions.

ICD-9-CM Coding

1. Based on the operative report header, what is the preoperative diagnosis?

2. Is the postoperative diagnosis the same as or different from the preoperative diagnosis?

3. Is the post-op diagnosis supported?

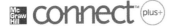

Enhance your learning by completing these exercises and more at mcgrawhillconnect.com

4. What is the main term for this condition?

5. Based on the subterm choices, what question can be developed for this condition?

6. Is any sign, symptom, or additional condition documented?

7. Is the additional condition, sign, or symptom an integral part of the primary (or other) condition coded?

8. Does the condition require or affect patient care, treatment, or management?

9. Based on the documentation, what is (are) the correct ICD-9-CM code(s) for this case?
   a. 836.0
   b. 836.1
   c. 836.0, 733.99
   d. 717.0

ICD-10-CM Coding

1. Based on the operative report header, what is the preoperative diagnosis?

2. Is the postoperative diagnosis the same as or different from the preoperative diagnosis?

3. Is the post-op diagnosis supported?

4. What is the main term for this condition?

5. Based on the subterm choices, what question can be developed for this condition?

6. Based on the information in the Tabular List, is additional information needed to determine the appropriate diagnosis code?

7. Is any sign, symptom, or additional condition documented?

8. Is the additional condition, sign, or symptom an integral part of the primary (or other) condition coded?

9. Does the additional condition require or affect patient care, treatment, or management?

10. Based on the documentation, what is the correct ICD-10-CM code for this case?
    a. S83.211A
    b. S83.222A
    c. S83.212A
    d. S83.252A

Process 3: Adding Modifiers

To identify the components needed to complete the story, answer the following questions.

1. Was the procedure performed different from that described by the nomenclature of the code?

2. Was the procedure performed on an anatomical site that has laterality?

3. Was the procedure performed in the global period of another procedure?

4. Were additional procedures performed during the operative session, and does the documentation support them?

5. Did the surgeon have help from another surgeon or another appropriate person?

6. Did a physician different from the surgeon perform the preoperative or postoperative part of the procedure?

7. Which modifier should be appended to the CPT code for this case?
   a. 57
   b. LT
   c. 25
   d. 22

Unit 2 Exam

The questions in this exam cover material in Chapters 6 through 8 of this book.

Choose the most appropriate answer for each question below.

1. **[LO6.3]** A physician who is part of a medical group practice saw a patient today who had not been treated by the practice for 7 years. The patient presented with a persistent cough and some congestion. The physician performed a comprehensive history and detailed exam. The patient is diabetic, which is controlled with diet and medication. The physician ordered lab work and a CXR. The physician prescribed medication for the cough and congestion and gave the patient a new prescription for his diabetic medication. The patient was asked to return in 1 week. Choose the appropriate evaluation and management code for today's encounter:

    a. 99204   **c.** 99203

    b. 99214   **d.** 99213

2. **[LO6.2]** A patient was admitted into the observation unit of the hospital at 8 a.m. after presenting with pain in the lower back. After reviewing the test results of the lab work and discussing the ultrasound results with the radiologist, the physician diagnosed kidney stones. The physician performed a comprehensive history and comprehensive examination of the patient. The physician approved a plan of treatment and discharged the patient at 1:30 p.m. the same day. Choose the appropriate CPT code(s):

    a. 99221   **c.** 99218, 99217

    b. 99235   **d.** 99236

3. **[LO6.2]** A 92-year-old woman is confined to a wheelchair and cannot live by herself. She resides in a residential facility for the elderly. Once every month, the facility has a physician come to the facility to examine and monitor the health of the residents. The physician makes recommendations to the facility and/or family members on the course of care to be given to the woman each month to maintain her health. At today's encounter the physician performs a problem-focused examination and interval history. The decision making is straightforward. Choose the appropriate CPT code:

    a. 99324   **c.** 99328

    b. 99335   **d.** 99334

4. **[LO6.2]** Choose the appropriate CPT code for a care-plan oversight service performed by a physician for 45 minutes:

    a. 99358   **c.** 99375

    b. 99326   **d.** 99380

5. **[LO6.3]** Which of the following is *not* an element of a history component for evaluation and management coding?

    a. Number of diagnoses and management options   **c.** Chief complaint

    b. Review of systems   **d.** Social history

6. **[LO6.3]** Mary Somner was admitted to the hospital with congestive heart failure by her primary care physician, and cardiology was consulted on the day of admission. On the second day, the cardiologist made hospital rounds and stopped by to see Mary. An expanded problem-focused interval history was obtained, and an expanded problem-focused examination was performed. Mary is showing some improvement with IV therapy. Select the appropriate code for Mary's encounter with the cardiologist today:

    a. 99232   **c.** 99213

    b. 99253   **d.** 99233

7. **[LO6.4]** Jonathan Snyder is a 12-year-old whose mother took him to his pediatrician for his annual exam. While examining him, his pediatrician discovered that he had an inguinal hernia and performed

a problem-focused history, a problem-focused exam, and straightforward medical decision making. The pediatrician is referring Jonathan to a surgeon for the hernia repair, and Jonathan is to return to his pediatrician in 1 year. Choose the appropriate code(s) for Jonathan's visit:

a. 99394

b. 99212

c. 99394, 99212-25

d. 99384, 99212-25

8. **[LO6.4]** The patient presented today with swelling and pain in the right knee. The patient suffers from osteoarthritis. Following an expanded problem-focused history and expanded problem-focused examination, the physician aspirated the joint and gave the patient an injection of steroid medication. Select the appropriate codes for today's visit:

a. 99213, 20610, 716.9

b. 99213-25, 20610, 715.96

c. 99213-25, 20610, 716.9

d. 99213, 20610, 715.96

9. **[LO6.3]** A 19-year-old male was jumping off the roof of his home onto a trampoline. After several successful jumps, he was careless and misjudged the distance on his next jump. He missed the trampoline and landed on the ground, injuring his right foot. The next day the teen was taken to his physician's office. The physician ordered a three-view x-ray of the right foot. The physician performed a detailed history and a detailed examination, and the medical decision making was of moderate complexity. After determining that the teen has suffered a fracture of one of the bones in his right foot, the physician refers the teen to an orthopedic surgeon. Select the appropriate code(s) for the family physician:

a. 99214, 825.20

b. 99204, 852.20

c. 99215, 825.22

d. 99205, 825.25

10. **[LO6.3]** Which of the following statements best describes when time becomes a factor in determining the appropriate evaluation and management code?

a. Time is always one of the key components in determining the level of the code.

b. The physician needs to dictate only that he or she spent extra time with the patient.

c. Time is a factor only when counseling and/or coordination of care represents more than 50 percent of the patient-provider encounter and is documented in the medical record.

d. Time is never a factor in determining the appropriate code.

11. **[LO7.2]** What anesthesia codes would be assigned for harvesting organ(s) from a brain dead person?

a. 00580, P6

b. 01999

c. 01990, P6

d. 01990

12. **[LO7.2]** Peter Dixon was found to have an esophageal stricture, so he consented to esophageal dilation under general anesthesia to reduce this stricture. Select the appropriate anesthesia code(s):

a. 00100

b. 00500, 99140

c. 00500, P1

d. 00500, P4

13. **[LO7.3]** Code the appropriate anesthesia service for Fowler-Stephens orchiopexy. The patient is a normal, healthy 30-year-old male.

a. 00926

b. 00930, P1

c. 00924

d. 00928

14. **[LO7.2]** P1 and P6 are examples of which of the following?

a. Anesthesia qualifying circumstances

b. Anesthesia time-reporting format

c. Anesthesia physical-status modifiers

d. Indications of multiple procedures

15. **[LO7.4]** A donor was brought to the operating room and placed under general anesthesia for harvesting of bone marrow. Select the correct code(s) to report the anesthesia services:

a. 01112, P1, V59.02

b. 01120, P1, V59.3

c. 01120, P1, V59.02

d. 01112, P1, V59.3

16. **[LO7.4]** The patient is a weight lifter who was training with heavy weights. While doing bicep curls, the patient experienced pain in the left forearm. A hematoma occurred, and he sought immediate medical treatment. He was diagnosed with a ruptured vein in his forearm. General anesthesia was administered in order to suture the vein. Which of the following codes is the appropriate code for reporting this service?

   a. 01840   **c.** 01842

   b. 01852   **d.** 01850

17. **[LO7.1]** Which of the following is a type of medication used to relieve pain?

   a. Corticosteroid   **c.** Analgesic

   b. Muscle relaxant   **d.** NSAID

18. **[LO7.1]** Which of the following is the type of anesthesia that makes a large portion of the body numb?

   a. Moderate sedation   **c.** General anesthesia

   b. Local anesthesia   **d.** Regional anesthesia

19. **[LO8.3]** Which modifier would be assigned to an anterior packing of both nares for a nose bleed?

   a. Modifier 51   **c.** Modifier 50

   b. Modifier 22   **d.** Modifier 59

20. **[LO8.1]** An examination of joints using a scope is an:

   a. Arthrography   **c.** Arthroplasty

   b. Arthroscopy   **d.** Arthrodesis

21. **[LO8.1]** CPT codes that contain a set of temporary codes used for emerging technology, services, and procedures can be found in which of the following sections of the CPT manual?

   a. Category II   **c.** Category III

   b. Appendix B   **d.** Appendix D

22. **[LO8.1]** Which one of the following procedures is completed without incision and is considered noninvasive in nature?

   a. Open procedure   **c.** Percutaneous procedure

   b. Endoscopic procedure   **d.** Closed procedure

23. **[LO8.2]** Dr. G was asked to provide a cardiology consultation in the emergency department for a patient who was experiencing atrial fibrillation. Dr. G determined that the patient needed to have a dual-chamber pacemaker inserted, and he scheduled the patient to have this procedure on the following morning. To correctly code the outpatient consultation visit in the ED, which of the following modifiers needs to be appended?

   a. Modifier 51   **c.** Modifier 24

   b. Modifier 57   **d.** Modifier 58

24. **[LO8.3]** A screening mammogram is performed unilaterally. Choose the appropriate code for this service:

   a. 77057   **c.** 77057-52

   b. 77055   **d.** 77057 with the charge reduced

25. **[LO8.2]** A perineoplasty, nonobstetrical, was performed on a 37-year-old female patient. Which range of CPT codes is appropriate for this procedure?

   a. 50010–53899   **c.** 59000–55980

   b. 59000–59899   **d.** 56405–58999

Coding for Surgical Procedures on Integumentary, Musculoskeletal, Respiratory, and Cardiovascular/ Lymphatic Systems

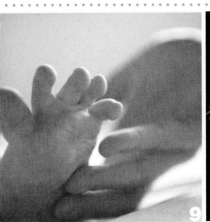
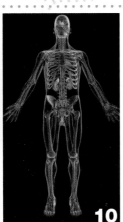
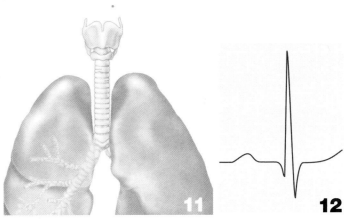

9   10   11   12

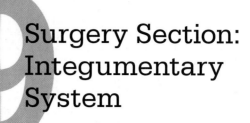

9 Surgery Section: Integumentary System

CHAPTER NINE

Key Terms

Adjacent tissue transfer
Allograft
Autograft
Benign
Complex repair
Debridement

Destruction
Escharotomy
Fissure
Incision and drainage
Infection
Inflammation

Intermediate repair
Laceration
Lesion
Malignant
Mohs surgery
Paring

Shaving
Simple repair
Total body surface area
 (TBSA)
Xenograft

Learning Outcomes

After completing this chapter, you will be able to:

9.1 Recognize the anatomy of the integumentary system.

9.2 Review ICD-9-CM guidelines for diseases of the skin and subcutaneous tissue.

9.3. Understand the general guidelines and format of the Integumentary System subsection of the CPT Surgery section.

9.4 Apply the CPT subheading guidelines for the Integumentary System subsection.

9.5 Identify the modifiers most commonly used with codes in the Integumentary System subsection.

9.6 Examine the common medical and procedural terms used in operative reports.

Introduction The word *integumentary* actually translates from a Latin word that means "to cover." The integumentary system, or skin, is the largest organ of the body. In coding, we translate *integumentary* to the organ system *skin.* The Integumentary subsection is used to code procedures or services provided to a patient with a diagnosis concerning the components of the integumentary system, which are the skin, glands, hair, and nails.

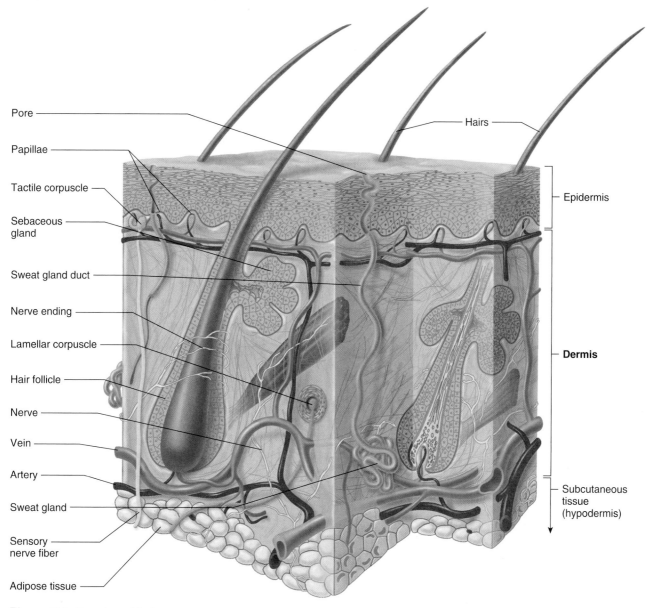

Pore
Papillae
Tactile corpuscle
Sebaceous gland
Sweat gland duct
Nerve ending
Lamellar corpuscle
Hair follicle
Nerve
Vein
Artery
Sweat gland
Sensory nerve fiber
Adipose tissue

Hairs

Epidermis

Dermis

Subcutaneous tissue (hypodermis)

Figure 9.1 Dermis and Its Layers

9.1 Anatomy of the Integumentary System

Each of the skin's layers encompasses the structures needed for each to complete its function within and around the body. (See Figure 9.1 and Table 9.1.)

Nails serve to protect the distal ends of the phalanges and consist of five parts. (See Figure 9.2 and Table 9.2.)

MENTOR Coding Tip

Many coders find it helpful to refer to the diagrams supplied in the CPT manual to help identify the layers of the skin when coding for integumentary procedures.

Table 9.1 Structures of the Integumentary System

STRUCTURE	DEFINITION AND FUNCTIONS

Skin layers:
Epidermis
	• Is the outer layer of the skin.
	• Forms a protective covering for the other layers of the integumentary system.
	• Contains no blood vessels, receiving nutrients from the dermis below.
	• Is the thinnest layer of the three stratums.
	• Consists of two layers:
	   Outermost layer: consists of cells devoid of nuclei and filled with keratin, a hard fibrous protein.
	   Basal layer: the deepest layer of the epidermis, made up of living cells that continue to divide and work their way to the surface, becoming keratin during the process.
	• Contains melanocytes, which give the skin its pigment and protect the skin's DNA from the sun's ultraviolet light. It is in the melanocytes that melanoma, a malignant neoplasm of the skin, begins its formation.
	• Contains cholesterol, which is converted by sunlight into vitamin D, which is stored in the integumentary's subcutaneous layer.

Dermis	• Is the middle layer of the skin, directly below the epidermis.
	• Is made up of elastin and collagen fibers. • Contains arteries and veins, which supply nutrients and remove waste. Blood vessels in this layer also help regulate body temperature by dilating, bringing more blood to the surface of the body and thereby allowing heat to radiate through the epidermis and out of the body.
	• Contains nerves, which provide sensory reception of pain, temperature, and pressure to the skin. • Contains hair follicles, sebaceous glands, and sweat glands.
Subcutaneous	• Is the deepest layer of the integumentary system, located below and attached to the dermis but not extending beyond the fascia, which covers the muscle. • Consists mainly of adipose tissue; contains lipocytes, or fat cells, which store energy for the body. • Serves as insulation for the body, conserving internal body heat, and provides cushioning for the bony structures and internal organs of the body.
Glands	• Sweat glands, or sudoriferous glands, produce sweat, which travels to the surface of the body and exits through pores located in the epidermis. • Sweat is made up of water, sodium, and, in slight amounts, urea, creatinine, and ammonia. • The sweat glands' primary function is cooling the body through evaporation of sweat on the skin's surface. • Diaphoresis is a secondary condition that causes profuse sweating. Conditions that lead to this manifestation include hyperthyroidism, myocardial infarction, and drug withdrawal.

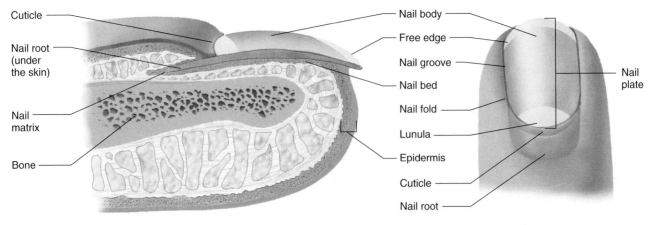

Figure 9.2 Diagram of the Nail

Table 9.2 Parts of the Nail

PART	DESCRIPTION
Plate	Composed of hard keratin Protects toes and fingers
Cuticle	Acts as a seal between the nail plate and the skin Prevents microorganisms from entering the area of the matrix
Bed	Contains nerves and blood vessels
Luna	Moon-shaped whitish area located beneath the proximal end of the nail Tip of the nail root
Matrix	Located beneath the skin of the finger at the proximal end of the nail Produces keratin cells that form the nail plate

1. In which layer of the skin are the sweat pores located?
2. Describe the two layers of the epidermis.
3. What is the function of melanocytes, and in which layer are they located?

EXERCISE 9.1

Also available in **McGraw Hill connect** (plus+)

9.2 ICD-9-CM Guidelines for Diseases of the Skin and Subcutaneous Tissue

Some of the more common conditions of the skin and subcutaneous tissue are cellulitis, pilonidal cyst, dermatitis, psoriasis, corns and callosities, dermatoses such as seborrheic keratosis, and pressure ulcers. When coding these conditions, coders must thoroughly review the provider documentation as well as the guidelines and instructional notes.

ICD-9-CM: Diseases of the Skin and Subcutaneous Tissue is Chapter 12 in the ICD-9-CM manual, with the code range 680–709.

ICD-10-CM: Diseases of the Skin and Subcutaneous Tissue is Chapter 12 in the ICD-10-CM manual, with the code range L00–L99.

Table 9.3 lists the Chapter 12 subheadings and their code ranges.

Infections of Skin and Subcutaneous Tissue (680–686), ICD-9-CM

Infections of Skin and Subcutaneous Tissue (L00–L08), ICD-10-CM

These sections identify conditions due to infections and include:

- **Carbuncles and furuncles:** These are coded by anatomical site of the infection and are category 680 (L02, ICD-10-CM).
- **Cellulitis and abscess:** These are also coded by anatomical site, with a separate category to identify the finger or toe. Cellulitis and abscess are coded to categories 681 and 682 (L03.-, ICD-10-CM).

SPOTLIGHT on Diagnosis

Carbuncle A group or cluster of furuncles most often caused by staphylococcal infection.

Furuncle A localized skin infection originating in a gland or hair follicle. Also called a boil.

Cellulitis A bacterial infection of the dermis and subcutaneous tissues of the skin.

Abscess A collection of pus that forms at the site of tissue which has become infected.

infection Invasion of the body by a pathogenic organism.

inflammation A localized response to an injury or destruction of tissue.

Table 9.3 ICD Skin and Subcutaneous Tissue Subheadings *(Data from ICD-9-CM and ICD-10-CM, Centers for Medicare and Medicaid Services and the National Center for Health Statistics.)*

ICD-9-CM		ICD-10-CM	
SUBHEADING	**CODE RANGE**	**SUBHEADING**	**CODE RANGE**
Infections of Skin and Subcutaneous Tissue	680–686	Infections of Skin and Subcutaneous Tissue	L00–L08
Other Inflammatory Conditions of Skin and Subcutaneous Tissue	690–698	Bullous Disorders	L10–L14
		Dermatitis and Eczema	L20–L30
		Papulosquamous disorders	L40-L45
		Urticaria and Erythema	L49–L54
		Radiation-Related Disorders of the Skin and Subcutaneous Tissue	L55–L59
Other Diseases of Skin and Subcutaneous Tissue	700–709	Disorders of Skin Appendages	L60–L75
		Intraoperative and Postprocedural Complications of Skin and Subcutaneous Tissue	L76
		Other Disorders of the Skin and Subcutaneous Tissue	L80–L99

- **Pilonidal cyst:** The codes in this category are further defined by the presence of an abscess at the site of the cyst.

SPOTLIGHT on Condition

A pilonidal cyst (ICD-9-CM 685.0–685.1 or ICD-10-CM L05.01–L05.91) forms at the bottom of the coccyx (tailbone) and may cause pain, erythema, and swelling at the site just above the crack of the buttocks. If left untreated, the cyst may become infected, becoming an abscess.

Other Inflammatory Conditions of Skin and Subcutaneous Tissue (690–698), ICD-9-CM
Bullous Disorders (L10–L14), ICD-10-CM
Dermatitis and Eczema (L20–L30), ICD-10-CM
Urticaria and Erythema (L49–L54), ICD-10-CM
Radiation-Related Disorders of the Skin and Subcutaneous Tissue (L55–L59), ICD-10-CM

Included in these sections are various types of dermatitis, erythema, and psoriasis:

- **Erythematosquamous dermatosis:** In category 690 (L21, ICD-10-CM), this is an inflammatory condition of the skin that causes the skin, usually of the scalp and face, to become scaly. The category is first divided by seborrheic conditions and other erythematosquamous dermatosis and further divided based on the type of seborrheic dermatitis.
- **Contact dermatitis:** This may be due to ingestion of or direct contact of the skin with detergents, solvents, food, medicine, or other chemicals, resulting

in a rash. Contact dermatitis is coded to categories 692 and 693 (L23.-through L27.-, ICD-10-CM). These categories are further divided by the method of contact and then by the agent, irritant, or allergen causing the rash.

Other Diseases of Skin and Subcutaneous Tissue (700–709), ICD-9-CM
Disorders of Skin Appendages (L60–L75), ICD-10-CM
Other Disorders of the Skin and Subcutaneous Tissue (L76), ICD-10-CM

Some common conditions listed in these sections include:

- **Corns and callosities:** category 700 (L84, ICD-10-CM).
- **Hypertrophic and atrophic conditions:** category 701 (L91.0, ICD-10-CM); includes scleroderma, keloid scar, and skin tags.

SPOTLIGHT on Condition

Skin tags, also known as *cutaneous papilloma,* are a benign outward growth of skin usually occurring on the neck, axillary, and chest of older persons. The ICD-9-CM code for this type of skin tag, regardless of site, is 701.9.

Also included in these sections are chronic ulcers of the skin. Category 707 (L89.-, ICD-10-CM) is divided into two groupings of codes used to identify the site of the ulcer (707.0- and 707.1-) and the stage of the ulcer (707.2-). ICD-9-CM provides chapter-specific guidelines regarding the use and reporting of these codes, summarized as follows:

- To completely code the condition, two codes are needed: one to identify the site and one to identify the stage.
- For pressure ulcers whose stage cannot be determined, assign code 707.25, "Pressure ulcer, unstageable," in addition to the code for the site of the ulcer.
- Only one ICD-9-CM code is needed to identify bilateral pressure ulcers at the same anatomical site and at the same stage.
- For pressure ulcers of different stages at the same bilateral site (e.g., hip) assign one code for the site and a separate code for each stage documented.
- Assign codes for each anatomical site and stage when multiple ulcers and sites are documented.
- Pressure ulcers documented as healing should be assigned both a code for the site and a code for the stage of the ulcer documented. If the documentation does not provide the stage of a healing ulcer, assign code 707.20, "Pressure ulcer, stage unspecified."
- As the stage of a pressure ulcer may continue to evolve until healing begins, code the stage to the highest stage reported.

In addition to listing conditions of the skin, this section includes conditions related to the hair and hair follicles, such as alopecia, hirsutism, and conditions that may affect treatment of nails, including injury, onychomycosis, paronychia, and improper growth such as ingrown nails, which may result from injury to the nail matrix.

Onychomycosis Fungal infection of the nail root that deforms and discolors the nails of the fingers or toes. The nail becomes misshaped, thickened, and raised from the nail bed.

Paronychia Bacterial infection of the cuticle that causes inflammation, tenderness, erythema, and swelling at the site of abscess.

EXERCISE 9.2

1. Explain the difference between inflammation and infection.
2. Explain the possible causes of contact dermatitis, and identify the factors a coder must know before assigning the appropriate ICD-9-CM code.
3. Discuss the guidelines concerning the coding of pressure ulcers.

Also available in

9.3 General Guidelines and Format of the Integumentary Subsection of CPT

The Integumentary System subsection of CPT contains the code range 10040–19499. The codes are defined by the subsections listed in Table 9.4.

Table 9.4 CPT Integumentary System Subsections *(Data from CPT 2013. © 2013 American Medical Association. All rights reserved.)*

SUBSECTION	CODE RANGE
Skin, Subcutaneous, and Accessory Structures	**10040–11646**
Incision and Drainage	10040–10180
Debridement	11000–11047
Paring or Cutting	11055–11057
Biopsy	11100–11101
Removal of Skin Tags	11200–11201
Shaving of Epidermal or Dermal Lesions	11300–11313
Excision—Benign Lesions	11400–11471
Excision—Malignant Lesions	11600-11646
Nails	**11719–11765**
Pilonidal Cyst	**11770–11772**
Introduction	**11900–11983**
Repair (Closure)	**12001–16036**
Simple Repair	12001–12021
Intermediate Repair	12031–12057
Complex Repair	13100–13160

Table 9.4 CPT Integumentary System Subsections (*concluded*)

SUBSECTION	CODE RANGE
Adjacent Tissue Transfer or Rearrangement	14000–14350
Skin Replacement Surgery	15002–15278
Surgical Preparation	15002–15005
Autografts/Tissue Cultured Autograft	15040–15261
Skin Substitute Grafts	15271–15278
Flaps (Skin and/or Deep Tissue)	15570–15738
Other Flaps and Grafts	15740–15777
Other Procedures	15780–15879
Pressure Ulcers (Decubitus Ulcers)	15920–15999
Burns, Local Treatment	16000–16036
Destruction	**17000–17999**
Destruction, Benign or Premalignant Lesions	17000–17250
Destruction, Malignant Lesions, Any Method	17260–17286
Mohs Micrographic Surgery	17311–17315
Other Procedures	17340–17999
Breast	**19000–19499**
Incision	19000–19030
Excision	19100–19272
Introduction	19290–19298
Mastectomy Procedures	19300–19307
Repair and/or Reconstruction	19316–19396
Other Procedures	19499

The Integumentary subsection of the Surgery section has several specific guidelines and trouble areas for coders. Converting inches to centimeters is just one of these trouble areas. Coders must know that 1 inch (in.) equals 2.54 centimeters (cm) to be able to convert inches to centimeters, as needed for CPT codes. When calculating square centimeters (sq cm), as needed for many grafting procedures, coders must know that the equation to do so is length times width, or $L \times W$.

MENTOR
Coding Tip

Many coders find it helpful to write these two equations in the guidelines of the Integumentary subsection:
1 inch = 2.54 cm
and $L \times W$ = sq cm.

FOR EXAMPLE 4 cm × 6 cm = 24 sq cm ■

1. The physician dictates the size of the lesion as 2 inches × 3 inches. Convert the inches to centimeters.

2. The physician dictates the size of a malignant lesion as 3 cm × 5 cm. Calculate the square centimeters.

3. For coding a Z-plasty, which is an adjacent tissue transfer procedure, what is the appropriate range of codes?

EXERCISE 9.3

Also available in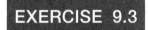

9.4. CPT Subheading Guidelines for the Integumentary System SubSection

Incision and Drainage (10040–10180)

Three main questions need to be answered from the medical record before selecting the appropriate codes for incision and drainage procedures:

- **Site:** Is it integumentary or some other body area?
- **Condition:** Is the condition part of the CPT description?
- **Complexity:** Is this a simple or complex I&D?

incision and drainage (I&D) Procedure completed with either a needle or scalpel which is used to open or access and then drain the area or site.

Incision and drainage (I&D) may be completed with either a needle or a scalpel, which is used to open or access and then drain the area or site. Incision and drainage may be performed in many areas of the body, including organs such as the lungs or colon, so it is necessary when coding for this procedure to first identify the site of the I&D. I&D of the integumentary is considered a minor procedure with postoperative periods of 0 to 10 days.

CPT: Codes for I&D are divided based on the condition and complexity of the procedure. The incision and drainage CPT codes are very specific as to what is being incised and drained, such as pilonidal cyst, foreign body, hematoma, and complex postoperative wound infections.

Simple procedures involve opening and draining the pus or cyst and leaving the site open to heal on its own. Complex procedures require work such as placement of drains and packing in addition to the work done in simple I&Ds.

ICD: I&Ds may be performed for some of the following conditions: abscess, cyst, furuncle, carbuncle, foreign body, hematoma, and postoperative wound infection.

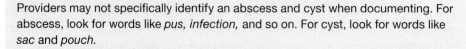

MENTOR Coding Tip

Providers may not specifically identify an abscess and cyst when documenting. For abscess, look for words like *pus*, *infection*, and so on. For cyst, look for words like *sac* and *pouch*.

FOR EXAMPLE Using a scalpel, the physician entered the site located on the posterior of the left shoulder and purulent material was expressed from the wound. The wound was packed with sterile gauze, allowing approximately 3 cm of gauze to remain outside the wound to act as a wick and aid in continued drainage. ▪

CPT code: 10061 I&D of abscess, complicated. As a drain a gauze wick was left, this is considered a complex I&D of an abscess.

ICD-9-CM code: 682.3 Abscess of upper arm and forearm. Pus (purulent material) was drained from the site, making this an abscess.

ICD-10-CM code: L02.414 Cutaneous abscess of left upper limb.

debridement Removal of foreign object, damaged tissue, either by excision or non excision, such as brushing or irrigating.

Debridement (11000–11047)

Debridement is the removal of necrotic or devitalized tissue to reduce the risk of infection and aid in healing or in preparation of grafting. It may be accomplished surgically, using sharp instruments; chemically, using topical drugs; or mechanically, using wet to dry dressings.

MENTOR Coding Tip

Debridement may also be described as *excisional*, which involves surgical removal or cutting away of tissue, or *nonexcisional*, which involves nonsurgical brushing, irrigating, scrubbing, or washing of tissue.

CPT: Codes for debridement are divided based on the condition and the depth, site, and surface area debrided. Several of these codes have add-on codes for additional percentage or centimeters of debrided area. When coding for multiple debridement sites of the same depth and condition, add the surface areas together and select the code or codes to report the service. Do not code these sites separately by listing a primary code for each. These services may be performed for injuries, infections, wounds, and ulcers.

FOR EXAMPLE Using sharp dissection, the provider debrided necrotic subcutaneous tissue from nonhealing wounds: 2 × 4 cm from right shoulder, 2 × 2 cm from right forearm, and 3 × 4 sq cm from right upper arm. ∎

CPT codes: 11042 and 11045. Total surface area is 24 sq cm. Only one primary code, 11042, is used to identify the first 20 sq cm of multiple body sites. The add-on code 11045 is used to report the addition 4 sq cm.

$$2 \times 4 = 8 \text{ sq cm}$$
$$2 \times 2 = 4 \text{ sq cm}$$
$$3 \times 4 = \underline{12 \text{ sq cm}}$$
$$\text{Sum for total: } 24 \text{ sq cm}$$

ICD-9-CM codes: 884.1 complicated wound of multiple sites of shoulder and upper arm, and 881.10 complicated wound of forearm. These wounds are considered complicated as they are infected.

ICD-10-CM codes: S41.001A Unspecified open wound of right shoulder, S41.101A Unspecified open wound of right upper arm, S51.801 Unspecified open wound of right forearm. The seventh character "A" identifies these services as initial encounters since the patient is still receiving active treatment for these wounds.

MENTOR Coding Tip

The index of the ICD includes a text box below the main term "Wound, Open" that identifies complicated wounds as those with delayed healing, delayed treatment, a foreign body, or infection.

Paring or Cutting (11055–11057)

Paring or cutting is the removal of cornified (hyperkeratotic) epithelial layers by skinning or trimming back the overgrowth. The provider removes enough to relieve pressure but not enough to draw blood, as occurs when shaving procedures are performed. The procedure is performed for conditions such as a corn or callus that may cause pain as they continue to grow and exert pressure on the tissue beneath.

CPT codes are divided based on the number of lesions pared.

paring Paring is the removal by skinning or trimming back overgrowth of cornified epithelial layers

Biopsy (11100–11101)

A biopsy is performed to obtain tissue for pathologic examination. Like I&D procedures, a biopsy may be performed in various body areas; therefore, before selecting the CPT code, coders must identify the site of the biopsy as skin and not deeper structures, which may be the case in breast biopsy procedures,.

Biopsy codes 11100 and 11101 are used to identify the work of the provider obtaining a tissue sample from a lesion but not excising the entire lesion. When simple closure is performed, it is included in the biopsy code; however, intermediate and complex closures should be reported in addition to the biopsy code.

Removal of Skin Tags (11200–11201)

Skin tag removal may be completed by cutting with scissors or scalpel, by destruction with cautery or chemicals, or by strangulation with ligature.

CPT: There are only two CPT codes to identify the removal of skin tags, regardless of the method of removal: 11200 and 11201. These codes are divided based on the number of tags removed and include cauterization, electrical or chemical, of the wound and local anesthesia when used.

Code 11200 is used to report removal of up to the first 15 tags and 11201 to report removal of each additional, or any part thereof, 10 or fewer tags.

FOR EXAMPLE removal of 19 skin tags from the neck using electrocautery on 11 and placement of ligature on the remaining 8 tags

CPT code: 11200 for first 15 and 11201 for additional 4 tags.
ICD-9-CM code: 701.9 Unspecified hypertrophic and atrophic conditions of skin.
ICD-10-CM code: L91.8 Other hypertrophic disorder of the skin, unspecified. ■

Shaving of Epidermal or Dermal Lesions (11300–11313)

CPT defines **shaving** as "sharp removal by transverse incision or horizontal slicing." In essence the provider lays the blade next to the skin and shaves off the lesion much like shaving hair from the body. As the wound is not sutured closed, bleeding is controlled by cauterization, either electrical or chemical. The codes include cauterization and local anesthesia.

The CPT codes are divided based on size of the lesion and body area. Each lesion removed is coded separately.

shaving Shaving is a sharp removal by transverse incision or horizontal slicing.

11300   Shaving of epidermal or dermal lesion, single lesion, trunk, arms or legs; lesion diameter 0.5 cm or less

11301   lesion diameter 0.6 to 1.0

11302   lesion diameter 1.1 to 2.0 cm ▦

ICD: Shaving can be performed for a variety of conditions, such as nevus (216.0–216.9), seborrheic keratosis (702.11–702.19), and neurodermatitis (690–698).

Excision of Benign and Malignant Lesions (11400–11646)

Before selecting the appropriate codes for excision procedures, coders need to find answers in the medical record to these questions:

- **Pathology:** Benign or malignant?

  Benign lesions are noninvasive tumors that remain localized.

  Malignant lesions are invasive tumors that spread beyond the tumor site.

- **Site:** Where is the lesion located anatomically?
- **Size:** What is the largest diameter of lesion plus the narrowest margin × 2?
- **Closure:** Was more than simple closure necessary to repair the wound site?

Lesions are classified as abnormal or pathologic changes in tissues due to disease or injury.

Often the term *neoplasm* is used interchangeably with *lesion* in the documentation of lesion removal since a neoplasm is a lesion. However, neoplasms may be benign, such as moles or seborrheic keratoses, or malignant, such as a melanoma or basal cell carcinoma.

CPT first divides lesion excision codes based on the pathology of the lesion: benign lesions (11400–11471) and malignant lesions (11600–11646). For this reason, the coder must refer to the pathology of the excised lesion before coding for this service. In the absence of confirmed pathology, the provider's documented statement of benign or malignant is used for determining the lesion excision category.

The next division of these codes is based on the anatomical site of the lesion. As with the codes for shaving of epidermal lesions, coders find it helpful to highlight the anatomical site and bracket each anatomical grouping of the lesion excision codes.

The last division of these codes is based on the size of the lesion and of its excised margin. Specifically, the size is the largest diameter of the lesion plus the narrowest margin times 2 (once for each side, but only two sides).

benign: Benign lesions are noninvasive tumors that remain localized

malignant Invasive tumor that spreads beyond the tumor site.

lesion Abnormal or pathologic changes in tissues due to disease or injury

If the dimensions of the lesion are documented as 4 cm × 2.5 cm × 1 cm and of the margins are documented as 0.3 cm and 0.5 cm, use 4 cm as the size of the lesion and use the narrowest margin, 0.3 cm × 2, for a total of 0.6 cm for the margin. Adding the lesion and margin figures results in a total excised lesion of 4.6 cm. ▦

Included in the excision procedure are simple repairs needed to close the wound site; therefore, simple closure should not be reported in addition to the excision code. However, intermediate or complex closures, when performed to close the wound site, are separately reportable.

Conversely, excision of lesions, whether benign or malignant, is included in adjacent tissue transfers and not separately reportable when the transfer is performed to cover the defect of the lesion removal.

Correct ICD coding of neoplasms, as with CPT coding, requires a pathology report or the physician's interpretation of the lesion as malignant or benign or of uncertain behavior. If the pathology is unknown or not stated by the physician at the time of reporting, the lesion should be coded as unspecified.

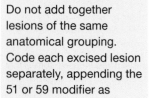

Nails (11719–11765)

CPT services or procedures involving the nail plate include trimming, debridement, removal (avulsion), or evacuation of subungual hematomas.

Ingrown or deformed nails may be treated by removing the nail temporarily, by removing only the nail plate (avulsion, 11730–11732), or permanently by removing all or part of the matrix with the nail plate (11750–11752). A wedge excision of the skin around the deformed nail may also be completed to relieve pain and pressure due to ingrown toenails (11765).

Pilonidal Cyst (11770–11772)

Treatment of a pilonidal cyst involves removal of the cyst, and CPT coding for this procedure is divided by the nature of the cyst and complexity of the procedure required:

Simple (11770): This includes I&D of the cyst or sinus, with a simple closure of the wound.

Extensive (11771): The cyst is more complex, branching into the subcutaneous layer, and intermediate closure is required.

Complicated (11772): The cyst is complex, and either complex closure or grafting is required to close the site or the wound may be left open to heal.

Repair (Closure) (12001–16036)

Before selecting the appropriate codes for repairs, coders need to find answers in the medical record to these questions:

- Type of closure?
  - Simple: single layer
  - Intermediate: in layers or grossly contaminated
  - Complex: required retention sutures; scar or wound revision
- Anatomical site? (grouping)
- Wound size? (prior to closure, in centimeters)
- Multiple wounds of same grouping? (sum for total length of repair)

Repairs of wounds may be accomplished using different methods depending upon the type and depth of the wound however, repair codes include only repairs completed by suturing, stapling, or tissue glue.

MENTOR Coding Tip

Closures using only adhesive strips or butterflies are not coded as repairs. Such work is captured in the E/M code reported for the encounter.

Included in all repair codes is the simple examination and ligation of blood vessels and exploration of any nerves or tendons exposed by the injury.
CPT first divides repairs into three categories:

Simple repairs (12001–12021), also known as *single-layer closure,* involve closing the wound in one layer regardless of wound depth.

Intermediate repairs (12031–12057), are reported for wounds closed in layers, as in suturing the subcutaneous in one layer followed by the dermis in a second layer. Intermediate repairs may also be reported for wounds that are contaminated to the point that they require extensive cleaning to prepare them for closure, even if that closure is completed in a single layer.

Complex repairs (13100–13160) are those that require additional work beyond that of an intermediate repair, such as retention sutures, debridement, or placement of stents or drains.

Each of these categories is then subdivided into anatomical groupings. For each of these anatomical groupings, only a single code may be reported—multiple repairs of the same complexity of the same grouping are added together and reported with one code.

FOR EXAMPLE The provider performed an intermediate repair of three separate lacerations of the forearm. Only one code from the 12031–12037 grouping would be reported. ▪

To determine the correct code in the example above, the documented sizes of all three wounds, prior to closure, would be added together to determine the total length of the repair.

FOR EXAMPLE

3-cm, 8-cm and 1.2-cm open wounds of the right forearm, all requiring layered closure

simple repair A simple layer closure involving closing of the wound in one layer regardless of wound depth.

intermediate repair Repairs for wounds closed in layers, such as suturing the subcutaneous in one layer followed by the dermis in a second layer.

MENTOR Coding Tip

Don't confuse the type of repair with the type of wound.

complex repair Repairs that require additional repair work such as retention suturing, debridement, or placement of stents or drains.

As all are of the same anatomic grouping and of the same complexity of repair, intermediate, the lengths of all three wounds are added together and one repair code is reported:

CPT: 12034 Repair, intermediate, wound of scalp, axillae, trunk and/or extremities; 7.6 to 12.5 cm (total length, 3 cm + 8 cm + 1.2 cm = 12.2 cm).

ICD-9-CM: 881.00 Open wound, forearm.

ICD-10-CM: S51.801A Unspecified open wound of right forearm. ■

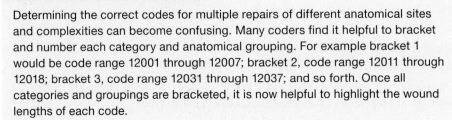

MENTOR Coding Tip

Determining the correct codes for multiple repairs of different anatomical sites and complexities can become confusing. Many coders find it helpful to bracket and number each category and anatomical grouping. For example bracket 1 would be code range 12001 through 12007; bracket 2, code range 12011 through 12018; bracket 3, code range 12031 through 12037; and so forth. Once all categories and groupings are bracketed, it is now helpful to highlight the wound lengths of each code.

12001	Simple repair of superficial wounds of scalp, neck, axillae, external genitalia, trunk and/or extremities; 2.5 cm or less
12002	2.6 cm to 7.5 cm
12004	7.6 cm to 12.5 cm
12005	12.6 cm to 20.0 cm
12006	20.1 cm to 30.0 cm
12007	over 30.0 cm

Using the bracket and number system, the coder can categorize each repair, sum the lengths of those that are in the same bracket, and correctly report the repair services.

FOR EXAMPLE The patient presents with multiple lacerations; right thigh had a 12.2-cm laceration that was closed in layered fashion and a 2.4-cm wound that required closure of the dermis only. A 2.1-cm laceration of the right cheek was closed in a single layer, and a superficial wound of the forehead was closed with sterile adhesive strips. Two lacerations of the right arm: A 3.4 cm laceration was closed in a single layer, and a 5.4-cm deep wound required closure of both the subcutaneous and the dermis.

Bracket 1: Right thigh 2.4 cm

    Right arm 3.4 cm

        5.8 cm = code 12002

Bracket 2: Right cheek 2.1 cm = code 12011

Bracket 3: Right thigh 12.2 cm

    Right arm 5.4 cm

        17.6 cm = code 12035 ■

MENTOR
Coding Tip

When coding for cellulitis, rely on the physician documentation. When the condition is documented with an injury or burn, report one code for injury and one code for cellulitis. Sequencing depends on circumstances of admission.

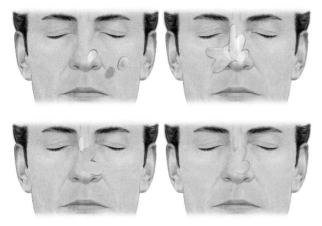

Figure 9.3 A Flap Graft

Adjacent Tissue Transfers and Flaps (14000–14350, 15570–15738)

Before selecting the appropriate codes for adjacent tissue transfers and flaps, coders need to find answers in the medical record to these questions:

- Did the tissue remain in its original location?
- What is the anatomical site of the defect?
- What is the total size of the defect? (primary + secondary defect = total)

Unlike tissue grafts, in which the donor tissue is completely lifted and moved from its origin, **adjacent tissue transfers** remain attached to the original anatomical location either permanently or temporarily(15570–15738).

Tissue transfers, which may be documented as a flap by some surgeons, are designed, cut, and placed by the surgeon in a manner that allows tissue of the flap to cover both its original site and the defect being repaired. (See Figure 9.3.)

CPT divides codes for adjacent tissue transfers (14000–14350) first by anatomical site and then by size, in square centimeters, of the total defect, that is, the total of both the primary and secondary defects.

- The primary defect is the site that is being repaired or covered, such as a pressure ulcer or excised lesion site.
- The secondary defect is the flap that is created to complete the repair.

adjacent tissue transfer
During this type of tissue transfer the tissue remains attached to its original anatomic location.

> **FOR EXAMPLE** The primary defect created by the removal of a 3.1-cm by 2.0-cm excised lesion would be 6.2 sq cm (3.1 cm × 2.0 cm = 6.2 sq cm). The secondary defect created by the surgeon for the flap is 2.1 cm by 6.0 cm, totaling 12.6 sq cm. By summing the size of both the primary and secondary defects, the size of the adjacent tissue transfer is 18.8 sq cm. ■

> **MENTOR Coding Tip**
>
> The surgeon's work to remove a lesion or otherwise prepare the primary defect site is included in the code with the adjacent tissue transfer and is not separately reported.

As with an adjacent tissue transfer, a flap remains attached at some point to its original anatomical site. The other portion is surgically attached to the recipient site prior to transfer of the donor tissue (15570–15576). The flap is left attached to its donor site until vascularity has been established at the recipient site. Once that is established, the flap is surgically released from its site of origin (15650–15731). Any donor tissue that is still attached to its original site and not used to cover the defect is then surgically reattached to its original site (15600–15630).

Flaps may be full-thickness—all layers of skin and subcutaneous tissue—or may be deeper structures such as muscle or both myocutaneous or fasciocutaneous flaps (15732–15738).

If the donor site requires skin grafting or an adjacent tissue transfer to close the site, these services are reported in addition to the flap procedure.

Grafts and Skin Replacement Procedures (15002–15278)

Before selecting the appropriate codes for grafts and skin replacement procedures, coders need to find answers in the medical record to these questions:

- Was the site surgically prepared to receive the graft?
  - What is the anatomical site of the defect?
  - What is the age of the patient?
  - What is the size or percentage of the area prepared?
- What is the source of the graft used?
- What type of graft was used?
- What is the anatomical location of the recipient site?
- Did the donor site require repair?

Grafts may be performed for a variety of conditions, such as scar contracture due to a previous injury or trauma resulting in injuries such as burns or avulsions that require donor tissue or skin substitutes to close the defect.

Not all graft recipient sites require preparation of the site to receive the graft. For example, a clean bleeding wound site may need little or no preparation to receive a graft, and in such cases surgical preparation codes should not be reported.

When surgical preparation is performed to prepare the wound bed or create the recipient site, such as cutting away scar or removing devitalized or necrotic tissue, surgical preparation codes (15002–15005) should be reported in addition to graft placement codes.

The CPT codes for surgical preparation are divided and grouped first anatomically, by the recipient site, and then by the size or percentage of area being prepared. The determination of size, in square centimeters, versus percentage is based on the patient's age at the time of the procedure. Percentage is used only for patients younger than 10 years of age.

Only one code from each anatomical grouping should be reported. When surgical preparation of multiple sites of the same anatomical grouping is performed, sum the size or percentage of each and select the code based on the total size or percentage.

There are many different sources and types of skin grafts. Sources include **autografts,** from the patient's body, which may be harvested for immediate use or be harvested and cultured or grown detached from the body for later

autograft A graft harvested from a patient's own body.

use, as in code 15040. Skin substitute grafts include nonautologous grafts, or **allografts** (from another human donor), **xenografts** (from a nonhuman donor, as with porcine grafts), and biological product grafts.

Types of grafts include:

- **Dermal grafts:** dermis only. (The epidermal layer remains at the donor site.)
- **Epidermal grafts:** epidermal layer only.
- **Split-thickness grafts:** the epidermis and part of the dermis.
- **Full-thickness grafts:** all layers through the subcutaneous.

CPT divides the graft codes based first on the source of the graft: autografts/tissue cultured autografts (15040–15261) and skin substitute grafts (15271–15278). The next division of the codes is based on the type of graft and the recipient site, grouped anatomically. Add-on codes are provided to capture additional square centimeters or percentages of the recipient site beyond that of the initial code. As with the surgical preparation codes, multiple sites of the same anatomical grouping should be added together before selecting the code or codes to report the procedure.

MENTOR Coding Tip

Read the descriptions of each add-on code carefully. Most are reported for any additional size or percentage beyond that included in the initial code. However, some do not, follow this convention, for example 15156 and 15157. Lack of attention to the information contained in these codes can lead to incorrect code reporting.

Should the donor site require repair, either by skin graft, flap, transfer, or closure, report these services in addition to the graft procedure.

Burns, Local Treatment (16000–16036)

Burns may be from thermal, electrical, or chemical sources. Burns are classified by degrees, which identify the depth and extent of tissue damage. (See Figure 9.4.) Medically there are six degrees of burns, and the method of treatment differs for each:

First: limited to the epidermis and top layer of the dermis. Local topical treatment to cool and sooth the burn is usually provided at home. However, a provider in the office or emergency department may render treatment.

Second: extending beyond the epidermis and deeper into the dermis. Results in blistering and significant pain for the patient. Depending on the size and location of the burn, treatment may be similar to that of a first-degree burn or may require dressing and limited debridement of the burn.

Third: extends through all layers of the skin and into the subcutaneous tissue and results in destruction of the nerves as well. Treatment involves surgical removal of all destroyed tissue and dressing of the adjacent burns of lesser degrees. The patient may be placed in a hyperbaric chamber to prevent infection and aid in healing. Grafts may be needed to replace the destroyed tissue.

Fourth: extends beyond the subcutaneous tissue, involving the underlying structures of muscle, tendon, and ligament but not the bone. Treatment is

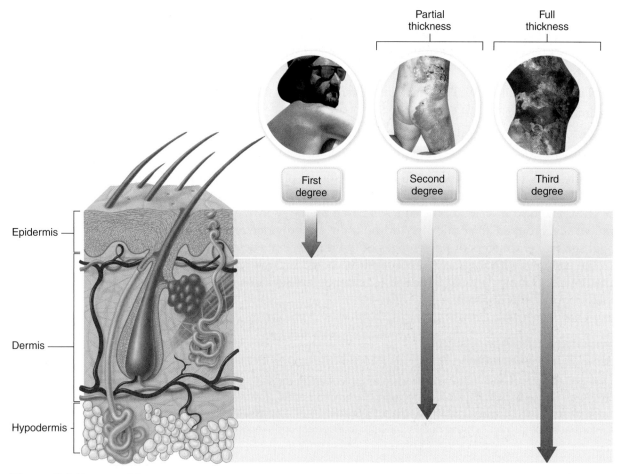

Figure 9.4 Degrees of Burn

> **MENTOR**
> Coding Tip
>
> The rule of nines is located in the guidelines and in the Tabular List of burn codes in many editions of the ICD manual.

total body surface area (TBSA) Total body surface area is based on the rule of nines, which divides the patient's body into segments of 9 percent.

similar to that of a third-degree burn; however, amputation may also be medically warranted.

Fifth and Sixth: extend into the bone and beyond to the underlying organs, typically resulting in the demise of the patient.

CPT codes in the Integumentary subsection are for nonsurgical treatment of burns regardless of the type or source of the burn. These codes are divided based on the degree and size of the burn. Partial-thickness burns, as described in codes 16020–16025, may be second- or third-degree burns.

Total body surface area (TBSA) is based on the rule of nines, which divides the patient's body into segments of 9 percent. However, the percentages assigned to infants and children differ from those of adults, due to their proportionally larger heads.

> **MENTOR** Coding Tip
>
> The rule of nines is a general guideline of body surface area. As patients are proportioned differently based on body type or condition, the percentage of any given body area may differ from that assigned by the rule. For example, the anterior portion of a morbidly obese patient's trunk may be considered 20 percent of TBSA versus the 18 percent assigned by the rule. Provider's documentation of TBSA will dictate the percentage of TBSA in these cases.

Third- and fourth-degree burns also result in scarring that may contract over time, requiring additional treatment to release the scar. **Escharotomy** is the release of scar from underlying tissue by means of incising or cutting (CPT 16035–16036).

Diagnostic coding of burns requires that the coder know the anatomical location of the burn, depth or degree of the burn, and extent of body area burned. Although clinically there are six degrees of burns, for ICD-9-CM coding purposes there are only three categories of burns, identified by the fourth digit of the burn diagnosis codes:

First degree: erythema (fourth digit: 1).

Second degree: blistering or epidermal loss (fourth digit: 2).

Third degree: full-thickness skin loss and beyond (fourth digit: 3).

ICD codes for deep third-degree burns are further divided based on destruction and loss of underlying tissue with or without loss of a body part (fourth digit: 4 or 5).

Multiple burns of different anatomical sites are coded separately. Burns of the same anatomical site, as identified by the category code (first three digits of the ICD code), but of different degrees are coded once to the highest degree of the burn.

ICD category 948 identifies the TBSA involved and what percentage of the TBSA is a third-degree burn.

FOR EXAMPLE The patient has a second-degree burn of the thighs involving 10 percent of TBSA and second- and third-degree burns of full thickness of the abdomen involving 12 percent of TBSA. Three codes are reported:

942.33 third-degree burn, abdomen

945.26 second degree burn, thigh

948.21 Burn 20–29% of body surface, 10–19% at 3rd degree ▪

Destruction of Benign, Premalignant, and Malignant Lesions (17000–17999)

Before selecting the appropriate codes for destruction procedures, coders need to find answers in the medical record to these questions:

- What is the nature of the lesion?
- How many lesions are being destroyed?
- What is the size of the lesion(s)?
- What is the anatomical site of the lesion(s)?

Destruction is the ablation or eradication of tissue by any method, including laser or chemical treatment, cryosurgery, or electrosurgery. The lesion destroyed may be benign, premalignant, or malignant.

Unlike the excision of lesions, destruction procedures destroy the entire lesion, leaving no remaining tissue for pathologic analysis. Therefore, the type of lesion is determined based on the clinical judgment of the provider.

CPT divides destruction of lesions first by type: premalignant (17000–17004), cutaneous vascular proliferative (17106–17108), benign (17110–17111), and malignant (17260–17286).

escharotomy Release of scar from underlying tissue. This is often accomplished by making an incision into scar or necrotic tissue resulting from a severe burn when needed to prevent edema from causing interstitial pressure impairing blood flow to surrounding tissue.

MENTOR
Coding Tip

Nonhealing burns are acute burns. Necrosis is a nonhealing burn and, therefore, an acute burn.

destruction Destroying of tissue using heat, cold, or chemicals.

Table 9.5 Skin Lesions *(Data from CPT 2013. © 2013 American Medical Association. All rights reserved.)*

LESION	NATURE	CPT CODE RANGE
Actinic keratosis	Premalignant	17000–17004
Seborrheic keratosis	Benign	17110–17111
Pyogenic granuloma	Benign	17110–17111
Melanoma	Malignant	17260–17286
Basal cell	Malignant	17260–17286
Squamous cell	Malignant	17260–17286

These codes are further divided based on the number of lesions destroyed or the size of the lesion to be destroyed. The malignant lesion destruction codes are also divided based on the anatomical site of the lesion.

Although there are many different types of skin lesions, each with its own pathologic nature, there are several that most coders are familiar with as they are the most commonly documented by providers. (See Table 9.5.)

MENTOR Coding Tip

Many resources are available to the coder to determine the nature of the lesion and therefore the correct destruction category. During the CPC exam, you may refer to your ICD-9-CM manual for this information, and the category of the condition many times includes the nature of the lesion as benign or malignant or of uncertain behavior (premalignant).

Mohs Micrographic Surgery: 17311–17315

Mohs surgery The physician acts as both the surgeon and pathologist during this procedure.

Mohs is a procedure performed in a manner that allows the physician to excise 100 percent, including margins, of a premalignant or malignant lesion. The physician acts as both the surgeon and the pathologist, excising, mounting, staining, and examining each block of the specimen as it is removed. The physician continues this process, removing one stage at a time, until all malignant tissue has been excised.

CPT divides the codes for this procedure anatomically and by the number of stages and blocks. A stage is a transverse slice of the lesion. The surgeon cuts the stage or slice into individual blocks of tissue to be examined. Codes 17311 and 17313 indicate the first stage or slice of a lesion based on its anatomical site. Add-on codes 17312 and 17314 indicate each additional stage or slice of the lesion for each of the anatomical sites, respectively.

Codes 17311 to 17314 describe a division of each stage into up to five blocks for examination. If a stage is divided into more than five blocks, add-on code 17315 is reported for each additional block for any stage.

Conditions for which this procedure is most commonly performed include squamous and basal cell lesions.

MENTOR Coding Tip

Although Mohs terminology seems complex, it can easily be applied to an everyday item. Using a loaf of bread slices stacked vertically to represent the tumor, remove the top slice from the loaf, cut it into five pieces, and place it in a bowl. The contents of this bowl, the slice with its pieces, represent your first stage and blocks (up to five) or CPT codes 17311 or 17313. Now remove the next slice and cut it into seven pieces. Place five of these pieces into the next bowl. The contents of this bowl, the five pieces of the second slice, represent your second stage and up to five blocks, codes 17312 or 17314. The remaining pieces represent additional blocks after the first five (any stage) and are coded as 17315 for each block.

Breast (19000–19499)

Services and procedures included under the Breast subheading are both diagnostic and therapeutic in nature and may be through-the-skin, percutaneous, or open surgical procedures. Although several of these procedures are similar in description to those found earlier in the Integumentary subsection, such as needle biopsy or excision of lesions, the procedures under the Breast subheading are for deeper structures found below the integument or skin.

Incision: 19000–19030

The codes located under this subheading include drainage of a cyst or abscess lying below the subcutaneous layer in the deeper tissue of the breast (19000–19020). The distinction between these codes is the condition being treated and the method of treatment. In codes 19000 and 19001 the provider, using a needle, punctures and aspirates a cyst. Code 19020 requires an incision into the breast to locate and drain an abscess. Depending on the size of the abscess, the wound site of the abscess may be packed with gauze to allow for continued drainage.

Excision: 19100–19272

This subheading includes codes for biopsies of the breast (19100–19103). The approach used in this code rage is percutaneous, and the codes are further divided by the surgical tools used to complete the procedure. Also included in this subheading is excisional removal of benign or malignant lesions (19120–19272). The codes are further divided by the location or depth of the lesion and the preprocedure placement of a radiological marker.

Introduction: 19290–19298

These codes identify the placement of localization or treatment devices into the breast. Codes 19290 to 19295 indicate preoperative placement of markers to aid in lesion identification during the excisional procedure.

If the physician placing the marker uses imaging to place the marker (ultrasound, stereotactic, or mammography), this service is reported separately in addition to the code for placement of the marker.

MENTOR
Coding Tip

As procedures performed involve the breast structure and not the skin, it is appropriate and correct to append laterality modifiers to services performed on the breast (50, LT, or RT).

MENTOR
Coding Tip

CPT provides guidance throughout regarding additional services that are separately reportable when provided by the *same* physician as the one providing the primary procedure or service. Many coders find it helpful to highlight these parenthetical notes.

The remaining codes in this subheading are used for the placement of radiotherapy devices. The codes are divided based on the timing of the procedure, at the time of or following partial mastectomy (19296–19297), and the type of device, expandable (balloon) or brachytherapy catheters (19298).

Mastectomy Procedures: 19300–19307

The mastectomy procedure codes are divided based on the amount of tissue removed with the tumor.

Codes 19301 and 19302 identify a partial mastectomy that includes excision of both the tumor and a margin of healthy tissue surrounding the tumor. Code 19302 includes a lymphadenectomy of the axillary lymph nodes, which may be completed through a separate incision.

A simple complete mastectomy (19303) is the removal of the entire breast including the subcutaneous tissue and skin, with or without the nipple.

In contrast to the simple complete mastectomy, a subcutaneous mastectomy (19304) allows the patient to retain the skin, and only the breast tissue below the subcutaneous tissue to the fascia is removed.

The remainder of the mastectomy procedures (19305–19307) are radical mastectomies and are divided based on the muscle removed with the tumor.

MENTOR Coding Tip

Radical procedures, such as described in CPT codes 19305 and 19306, are more invasive and include the excision of the tumor, tissue surrounding the tumor, and all lymph nodes in the area of the excised tumor.

Repair and/or Reconstruction: 19316–19396

The codes included in this subheading may be cosmetic or reconstructive, depending on the intent of the procedure. For example, in both a mastopexy and a reduction mammaplasty healthy breast tissue is excised to change the appearance of the breast. However, the intent of the mastopexy procedure (19316) is to lift the breast to create a more youthful look, while the reduction mammaplasty (19318) is performed to reduce the size and weight of the breast to reduce back, neck, and shoulder pain and grooving caused by the breast.

MENTOR Coding Tip

The surgical approaches and descriptions of both of these procedures are the same, with the exception of the amount of tissue removed. Correct coding requires that the coder understand the surgeon's intent.

Breast reconstruction procedures (19340–19369) may be immediate, occurring during the mastectomy, or delayed, occurring after the mastectomy (or mastopexy, as in code 19340) at a different surgical session. These procedures differ, and the codes are divided based on the method or device used to complete the reconstruction and the timing of the procedure.

The devices used may be prostheses (19340–19342), which are prefilled implants or tissue expanders that allow for gradual expansion of the breast and skin tissue as the expander is filled over time via saline injections.

Another method of breast reconstruction is completed using muscle flaps (19367–19369). These codes are divided based on the muscle used to complete the flap. In code 19361 the surgeon utilizes a muscle from the midback, latissimus dorsi, while code 19367 (TRAM) identifies utilization of the abdominal muscle, rectus abdominis.

MENTOR Coding Tip

Another clue that helps the coder distinguish between these codes is the incision site of the flap. The incision site of the latissimus dorsi flap is on the back, and for the TRAM the incision site is the low abdomen.

Codes 19370 and 19371 describe periprosthetic capsulotomy (19370) and capsulectomy (19371), which are performed when scar tissue forms and contracts around the previously implanted prosthetic device, causing pain. Code 19370 is the incisional release of scar tissue around the prosthesis without its removal, and 19371 is the removal of scar tissue and the prosthesis.

This complication is identified by ICD-9-CM code 996.79, "Other complications of prosthetic device, implant, and graft," or ICD-10-CM code T85.44xxA, "Capsular contracture of breast implant, initial encounter."

MENTOR Coding Tip

For all breast reconstruction procedures, it is important that the coder identify the timing of the procedures to properly append modifiers.

---

1. Explain the difference between a simple incision and drainage and a complex I&D.
2. List the different ways that debridement can be accomplished.
3. Describe the difference between excisional and nonexcisional debridement.
4. Define *simple*, *intermediate*, and *complex repair.*
5. List and define the six degrees of burns.

EXERCISE 9.4

Also available in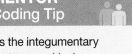

MENTOR
Coding Tip

As the integumentary system, or skin, is considered one organ, there are no bilateral sites. Therefore, if procedures are performed on the skin at separate sites, such as right arm and left arm, it would be incorrect to use the bilateral modifier, 50. Instead, use the 59 or 51 modifier, as appropriate.

9.5 Modifiers Most Commonly Used with Codes in the Integumentary Subsection

Modifiers tell the rest of the surgical story by adding the details that are not or cannot be expressed in the CPT or ICD-9-CM code. While any appropriate surgical modifier may be used with integumentary procedure codes when needed to provide additional information, there are three that are used more commonly than others: modifiers 51, 58, and 59 (see Table 9.6).

Table 9.6 Integumentary Subsection Modifiers *(Data from CPT 2013. © 2013 American Medical Association. All rights reserved.)*

MODIFIER	DEFINITION	EXAMPLE
51	Multiple procedures	Multiple related surgical procedures are performed on the same day, in the same session.
58	Staged or related procedure or service by the same physician during the postoperative period	Reexcision of a malignant lesion is performed during the postoperative period of the primary excision procedure.
59	Distinct procedural service	A nonroutine histochemical stain on frozen tissue is utilized during Mohs surgery (report 88314 with modifier 59).

EXERCISE 9.5

1. Explain the function of a modifier in coding a procedure involving the integumentary system.
2. Explain why modifier 50, bilateral procedure, is not used with codes for the integumentary system.

Also available in Mc Graw Hill **connect** (plus+)

9.6 Common Medical and Procedural Terms Used in Operative Reports

As with all sections of CPT, the Integumentary subsection includes medical terms and procedural terms that are specific to the system involved. Many of the common medical terms have other terms that can be used in provider documentation to describe a condition or procedure. Tables 9.7 and 9.8 list some of the CPT and ICD terms for the integumentary system.

Table 9.7 Terms for Integumentary System

TERM	DEFINITION	DOCUMENTATION KEYS
Adjacent tissue transfer	Rearrangement procedure involving the transfer of healthy skin or tissue to an adjacent wound, scar, etc.	Z-plasty, rotation flap
Allograft	Human skin graft applied from donor to recipient	Homograft
Biopsy	Removal of all or part of a lesion for pathologic examination	Incisional, excisional, needle aspiration, punch, shave
Debridement	Removal of devitalized or necrotic tissue	Removal of foreign object, damaged tissue
Destruction	The destroying of tissue by means of heat, cold, or chemicals. (*Note:* There is no tissue to send for pathology.)	Cautery, cryo, laser
Excision	Removal by cutting all or part	-ectomy,
Harvest	Removal of a donor organ or vein or artery for bypass	Procurement

Table 9.7 Terms for Integumentary System (*concluded*)

TERM	DEFINITION	DOCUMENTATION KEYS
Incision	Creation of an opening by surgically cutting into the skin or other tissue	-otomy
Incision and drainage (I&D)	Incision is made to release pus or pressure under the skin	Expressed material from, Lanced
-plasty	Process of reshaping or replacing by surgical means	Repair, reconstruction, revision, augmentation
Repair	Restoration of diseased or damaged tissue	Suture, revision, restore, closure
Shaving	Removal of epidermal or dermal lesions without full-thickness dermal excision	Transverse incision Tangential excision
Xenograft	Tissue procured from another species	Porcine graft

Table 9.8 Additional Terms for Integumentary System

TERMS	DEFINITION/DOCUMENTATION KEYS
Abrasion	Scrape, contusion, bruise, scratch
Blister	Bulla, pustule, vesicle
Boil	Furuncle, carbuncle
Chickenpox	Herpes zoster, herpes varicella
Dermatitis	Inflammation of skin
Erythema	Redness of skin
Fissure	Groove or crack
Hive	Urticaria
Itching	Pruritis
Laceration	Tear, cut, wound (open)
Lice	Impetigo, pediculosis
Macule	Papule
Scar	Cicatrix, callus
Wart	Verruca

fissure A groove or a crack

laceration A laceration is a tear, cut, or open wound.

List other terms that could be used for the following in a physician dictation:

EXERCISE 9.6

1. Abrasion: _____

2. Laceration: _____

3. Harvesting: _____

4. Adjacent tissue transfer: _____

5. Repair: _____

6. Shaving: _____

7. Blister: _____

8. Scar: _____

9. Boil: _____

10. Hive: _____

Also available in Mc Graw Hill **connect**™ plus+

Chapter Nine Summary

Learning Outcome	Key Concepts/Examples
9.1 Recognize the anatomy of the integumentary system.	The anatomy of the integumentary system includes: • *Epidermis:* the outer layer of the skin, which forms a protective covering for the other layers of the integumentary system. • *Dermis:* the middle layer of the skin, directly below the epidermis. It is made up of elastin and collagen fibers and contains arteries and veins, which supply nutrients and remove waste. • *Subcutaneous:* the deepest layer of the integumentary system, located below and attached to the dermis but not extending beyond the fascia, which covers the muscle. • *Sweat glands,* or *sudoriferous glands:* glands that produce sweat, which travels to the surface of the body and exits through pores located in the epidermis.
9.2 Review ICD-9-CM guidelines for diseases of the skin and subcutaneous tissue.	Some of the more common conditions of the skin and subcutaneous tissue include cellulitis, pilonidal cyst, dermatitis, psoriasis, corns and callosities, dermatoses such as seborrheic keratosis, and pressure ulcers. When coding these conditions, coders must thoroughly review the provider documentation as well as the guidelines and instructional notes. *ICD-9-CM:* Diseases of the Skin and Subcutaneous Tissue is Chapter 12 in the *ICD-9-CM* manual, with the code range 680–709. *ICD-10-CM:* Diseases of the Skin and Subcutaneous Tissue is Chapter 12 in the ICD-10-CM manual, with the code range L00–L99.
9.3 Understand the general guidelines and format of the Integumentary System subsection of the CPT Surgery section.	The Integumentary subsection contains the code range 10040–19499. This subsection has several specific guidelines and trouble areas for coders. Translating inches to centimeters is just one of these trouble areas. Coders must know that 1 inch equals 2.54 centimeters to be able to convert inches to centimeters, as needed for CPT codes. When calculating square centimeters, as needed for many grafting procedures, coders must know that the equation to do so is length times width, or $L \times W$.
9.4 Apply the CPT subheading guidelines for the Integumentary System subsection.	Before selecting the appropriate codes for specific procedures, coders need to find answers in the medical record to questions on the following: • *I&D procedures:* site, condition, and complexity. • *Excision procedures:* pathology, site, size, and type of closure. • *Repairs:* type of closure, anatomical site, wound size, and multiple wounds of same anatomical grouping. • *Adjacent tissue transfers and flaps:* tissue location, anatomical site of the defect, and total size of the defect. • *Destruction procedures:* nature, number, size, and anatomical site of the lesion(s).
9.5 Identify the modifiers most commonly used with codes in the Integumentary System subsection.	Modifiers 51, 58, and 59 are the most commonly used modifiers for this section.
9.6 Examine the common medical and procedural terms used in operative reports.	Many of the common medical terms have other terms that can be used in provider documentation to describe a condition or procedure.

Chapter Nine Review

Using Terminology

Match each key term to the appropriate definition.

_____ 1. [LO9.4] Adjacent tissue transfer

_____ 2. [LO9.4] Complex repair

_____ 3. [LO9.4] Debridement

_____ 4. [LO9.4] Destruction

_____ 5. [LO9.1] Epidermis

_____ 6. [LO9.4] Escharotomy

_____ 7. [LO9.4] Incision and drainage

_____ 8. [LO9.4] Infection

_____ 9. [LO9.4] Inflammation

_____ 10. [LO9.4] Intermediate repair

_____ 11. [LO9.6] Laceration

_____ 12. [LO9.4] Mohs surgery

_____ 13. [LO9.4] Paring

_____ 14. [LO9.4] Shaving

_____ 15. [LO9.4] Simple repair

A. Outer layer of the skin that forms a protective covering for the other layers of the integumentary system

B. Localized response to an injury or destruction of tissues

C. Removal of cornified epithelial layers by skinning or trimming back the overgrowth

D. Invasion of the body by a pathogenic organism

E. Removal of a foreign object or damaged tissue either by excision or nonexcision, such as brushing or irrigating

F. Sharp removal by transverse incision or horizontal slicing

G. Closure that involves closing the wound in one layer regardless of the wound depth

H. Repairs that require additional work, such as retention suturing, debridement, or placement of stents or drains

I. Repairs for wounds closed in layers, such as suturing the subcutaneous in one layer followed by the dermis in a second layer

J. Tissue transfer in which the tissue remains attached to its original anatomical location

K. Ablation or eradication of tissue by any method, including laser or chemical treatment, cryosurgery, or electrosurgery

L. Tear, cut, or open wound

M. Procedure in which the physician acts as both surgeon and pathologist

N. Release of scar from underlying tissue

O. Procedure completed with either a needle or scalpel, which is used to open or access and then drain the area or site

Checking Your Understanding

Choose the most appropriate answer for each of the following questions.

1. [LO9.1] The _____ layer, made up of living cells that continue to divide and work their way to the surface, becoming keratin, is the deepest layer of the epidermis.

   a. outermost layer

   b. basal layer

   c. dermis

   d. subcutaneous

2. [LO9.1] Which layer of the skin consists of mainly adipose tissue and contains lipocytes, or fat cells, which store energy for the body?

   a. Dermis

   b. Epidermis

   c. Subcutaneous

   d. Basal

3. [LO9.5] Which modifier would *not* be used with the codes in the Integumentary subsection?

   a. 58

   b. 59

   c. 51

   d. 50

4. [LO9.2] One inch equals _____ centimeters.

   a. 3

   b. 2.5

   c. 2.54

   d. 1.54

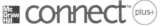

5. **[LO9.4]** The correct CPT and ICD-9-CM codes for a complicated I&D of purulent material from the upper arm are:

   a. 10060, 682.3

   b. 10061, 682.3

   c. 10080, 682.3

   d. 10081, 682.3

6. **[LO9.4]** An area of subcutaneous necrotic tissue from a nonhealing wound was debrided from a patient's forearm. The area debrided was 2 × 4 cm. The appropriate CPT and ICD-9-CM codes are:

   a. 11042, 11045, 884.1

   b. 11042, 881.10

   c. 11042, 884.1

   d. 11043, 881.10

7. **[LO9.4]** The _____ acts as a seal between the nail plate and the skin.

   a. bed

   d. luna

   c. cuticle

   d. matrix

8. **[LO9.4]** The patient presented to the ED with two lacerations on the right arm. The first laceration measured 7 cm, and the second measured 9 cm. Intermediate repair was needed for these lacerations. There was also a 5-cm laceration of the face, and a simple closure was performed. Select the appropriate code(s):

   a. 12036

   b. 12035, 12013

   c. 12035

   d. 12004

9. **[LO9.4]** The patient has an ischial ulcer that is excised, including an ostectomy with a skin flap closure. Select the appropriate code(s):

   a. 15940, 15941

   b. 15945

   c. 15941

   d. 15946

10. **[LO9.4]** Which of the following is true about an adjacent tissue transfer?

   a. One portion remains attached at some point along the flap to its original anatomical site.

   b. Z-plasty and rotation flap are types of adjacent tissue transfer.

   c. The flap is left attached to its donor site until vascularity has been established.

   d. All of these.

11. **[LO9.4]** When coding flaps and tissue transfer, which of the following questions should a coder ask before choosing the appropriate code?

   a. Did the tissue remain in its original location?

   b. What is the anatomical site of the defect?

   c. What is the total size of the defect?

   d. All of these.

12. **[LO9.4]** A porcine graft is a(n):

   a. Xenograft

   b. Homograft

   c. Autograft

   d. Allograft

13. **[LO9.4]** The patient presents with a burn that extends beyond the epidermis and deeper into the dermis. The patient is experiencing pain and blistering. If coders see this type of description in a report, they would code the condition as what degree of burn?

   a. First

   b. Second

   c. Third

   d. Fifth or sixth

Applying Your Knowledge

Answer the following questions and code the following case study. Be sure to follow the process steps as illustrated in chapter 8

Case Study

Preoperative diagnosis: Lacerations of right palm and forearm and left leg

Postoperative diagnosis: Same

An 8-year-old male was brought to the emergency room. While playing basketball with friends, he ran through a sliding glass door. He suffered lacerations on his right hand and arm and on his left leg just above and at the knee.

Procedure: The patient was placed on the table in the supine position. Satisfactory local anesthesia was obtained. All wounds were cleaned and examined, and no sign of glass or other foreign bodies was found. The laceration of the left thigh, right above the patella, was repaired first by layered closure, and the 4.8-cm laceration was carefully sutured.

The lacerations on the hand and arm were attended to next. A 3-cm laceration on the right-hand palm and a 4-cm laceration on the right forearm proximal to the elbow were carefully sutured in a single layer with 4-0 Vicryl, as well.

Process 1: CPT

1. What is the procedure?

2. Locate the main term in the index. What additional questions or set of questions can be determined?

3. Upon review of all the code choices identified in the index, what additional questions can be determined?

4. Based on the documentation, what is (are) the correct code(s) for this case?
   - **a.** 12002 × 2, 12032
   - **b.** 12004
   - **c.** 12032, 12002
   - **d.** 12034

Process 2: ICD

ICD-9-CM

1. Based on the operative report header, what is the preoperative diagnosis?

2. Is the postoperative diagnosis the same as or different from the preoperative diagnosis?

3. Is the postoperative diagnosis supported?

4. What is the main term for this condition?

5. Based on the subterm choices, what question(s) can be developed for this condition?

6. Is any sign, symptom, or additional condition documented?

7. Is the additional condition, sign, or symptom an integral part of the primary (or other) condition coded?

8. Does the additional condition require or affect patient care, treatment, or management?

9. Based on the documentation, what are the correct ICD-9-CM codes for this case?
   - **a.** 890.0, 881.00, 882.0
   - **b.** 890.0, 884.0
   - **c.** 891.0, 884.0
   - **d.** 882.0, 881.10, 890.1

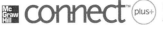 **connect** (plus+) Enhance your learning by completing these exercises and more at mcgrawhillconnect.com

ICD-10-CM

1. Based on the operative report header, what is the preoperative diagnosis?

2. Is the postoperative diagnosis the same as or different from the preoperative diagnosis?

3. Is the postoperative diagnosis supported?

4. What is the main term for this condition?

5. Based on the subterm choices, what question(s) can be developed for this condition?

6. Based on the information in the Tabular List, is additional information needed to determine the appropriate diagnosis code?

7. Is any sign, symptom, or additional condition documented?

8. Is the additional condition, sign, or symptom an integral part of the primary (or other) condition coded?

9. Does the additional condition require or affect patient care, treatment, or management?

10. Based on the documentation, what are the correct ICD-10-CM codes for this case?
    a. S71.102A, S61.401A, S51.801A
    b. S71.112A, S61.411A, S51.811A
    c. S71.111A, S61.411A, S51.812A
    d. S71.112A, S61.412, S51.812A

Process 3: Modifiers

1. Was the procedure performed different from that described by the nomenclature of the code?

2. Was the procedure performed on an anatomical site that has laterality?

3. Was the procedure performed in the global period of another procedure?

4. Were additional procedures performed during the operative session, and does the documentation support them?

5. Did the surgeon have help from another surgeon or another appropriate person?

6. Did a physician different from the surgeon perform the preoperative or postoperative portion of the procedure?

7. Which modifier should be appended to the CPT code for this case?
    a. 50
    b. 51
    c. None
    d. 59

Surgery Section: Musculoskeletal System

10

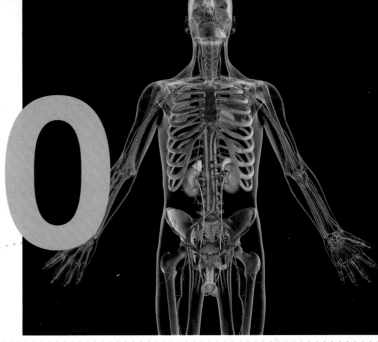

Key Terms

Appendicular skeleton
Axial skeleton
Closed fracture
Diaphysis
Dislocation
Epiphysis
External fixation

Internal fixation
Ligament
Malunion
Manipulation
Nonsegmental
  instrumentation
Nonunion

Open fracture
Osteoarthritis
Osteoporosis
Pathologic fracture
Segmental
  instrumentation

Skeletal traction
Sprain
Tendon

Learning Outcomes

After completing this chapter, you will be able to:

10.1 Review the anatomy of the musculoskeletal system.

10.2 Recognize the general guidelines and format of ICD codes for the musculoskeletal system.

10.3 Understand the general guidelines and format of the Musculoskeletal subsection in the CPT manual.

10.4 Apply the subheading guidelines.

10.5 Identify the modifiers most commonly used with codes in the Musculoskeletal subsection.

10.6 Examine the common medical and procedural terms used in operative reports.

Introduction

The Musculoskeletal System subsection of the CPT manual contains the largest number of codes. This section includes procedures performed on muscles, soft tissues, joints, bursae, cartilage, and bones. The section is formatted by anatomical site, approach or technique, and treatment or condition. A detailed explanation of the formatting of this section and the specific guidelines is presented later in this chapter.

10.1 Anatomy of the Musculoskeletal System

Understanding the anatomy and specific medical terminology pertinent to the musculoskeletal system will aid the coder in selecting the appropriate codes.

Muscular System

Some of the functions of the muscular system are to hold the body erect, make movement possible, generate body heat, and move food through the digestive system. See Figure 10.1 and Table 10.1 for additional information of the muscular system anatomy.

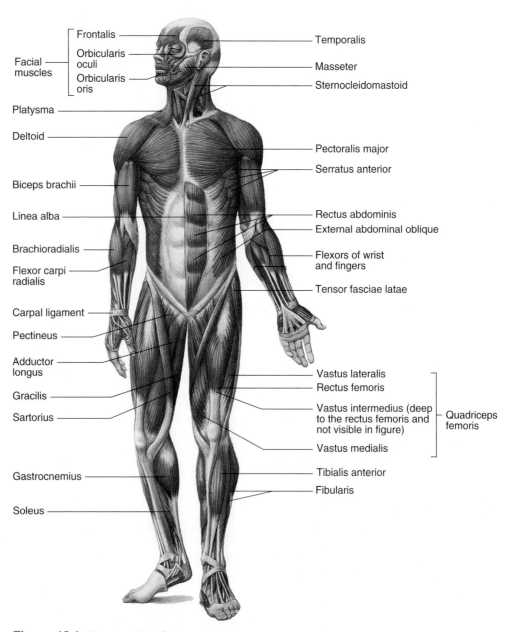

Figure 10.1 Muscles of the Body

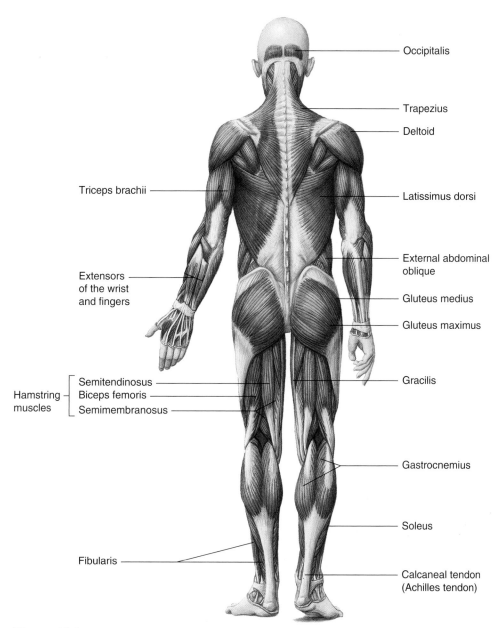

Occipitalis

Trapezius

Deltoid

Triceps brachii

Latissimus dorsi

External abdominal oblique

Extensors of the wrist and fingers

Gluteus medius

Gluteus maximus

Gracilis

Hamstring muscles
- Semitendinosus
- Biceps femoris
- Semimembranosus

Gastrocnemius

Soleus

Fibularis

Calcaneal tendon (Achilles tendon)

Figure 10.1 Muscles of the Body *(concluded)*

Table 10.1 Structures of the Musculoskeletal System

STRUCTURE	DEFINITION/FUNCTION
Soft tissues:	
Muscle fibers	Group of fibers that are held together by connective tissue and enclosed in a fibrous sheath
Fascia	Sheet of fibrous connective tissue that covers, supports, and separates muscles Word root = fasci Myofascial = pertaining to fascia and muscle My/o = muscle; fasci = fascia; al = pertaining to

(continued)

> **MENTOR**
> Coding Tip
>
> Deep fascia lies beneath the second layer of subcutaneous tissue.

Table 10.1 Structures of the Musculoskeletal System (*concluded*)

STRUCTURE	DEFINITION/FUNCTION
Tendon	Narrow band of nonelastic, dense, fibrous connective tissue Attaches muscle to a bone Word root = ten/o, tend/o Tendonitis = inflammation of a tendon Tend/o = tendon; -itis = inflammation (See Figure 10.2)
Ligament	Bands of fibrous tissue that connect two or more bones or cartilage (See Figure 10.3)
Skeletal muscles	Attached to bones of skeleton Make motion such as walking possible Striated muscle Voluntary muscle
Smooth muscles	Located in walls of internal organs Move and control the flow of fluids Unstriated muscles Involuntary muscles Visceral (internal organs) muscles
Myocardial muscles	Cardiac muscles Form muscular wall of the heart Like striated muscle in appearance but similar to smooth muscle in action Myocardial = pertaining to the heart muscle My/o = muscle; cardi/o = heart; -al = pertaining to

tendon Narrow band of non elastic, dense, fibrous connective tissue which attaches muscle to a bone

ligament Bands of fibrous tissue that connect two or more bones or cartilage.

Skeletal System

Some of the functions of the skeletal system are to support and shape the body, protect internal organs, anchor muscles, and make blood cells.

The muscular and skeletal systems work together to support the body and produce movement.

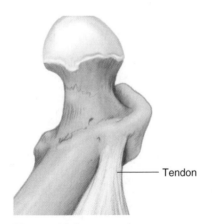

Figure 10.2 Muscle Tendon Attachment to Bone

Tendon

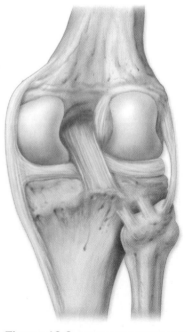

Figure 10.3 Ligament Attachment of bone to bone

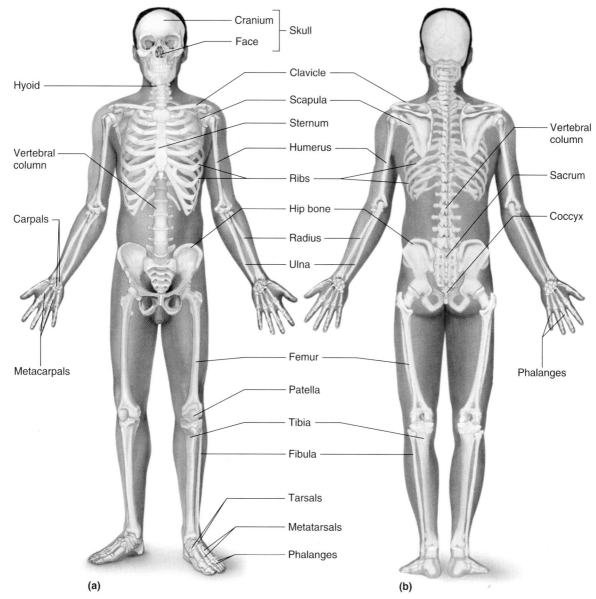

Figure 10.4 Axial and Appendicular Skeletons

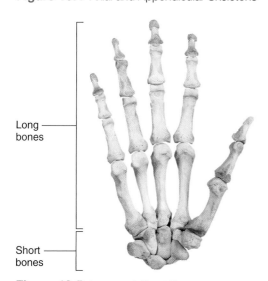

Figure 10.5 Long and Short Bones

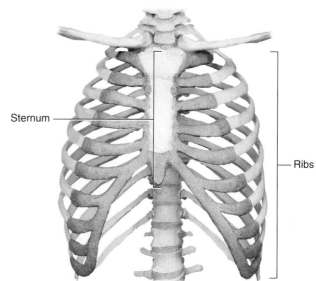

Figure 10.6 Flat Bones

CHAPTER 10 Surgery Section: Musculoskeletal System **189**

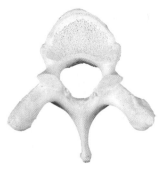

Figure 10.7 Irregular bones

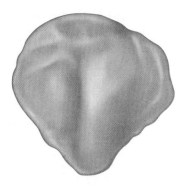

Figure 10.8 Sesamoid bone

Table 10.2 Structures of the Skeletal System

STRUCTURE	DEFINITION/FUNCTION
Bone:	Hardest tissue in the body Word root = oste/o, ost/o Living structure that changes and is capable of healing itself
Tissues of the bone Periosteum	Tough, fibrous tissue Forms outermost covering of bone Peri = surrounding; oste/o = bone
Compact bone	Hard, dense, strong bone Forms outer layer of the bones **Diaphysis:** shaft of a long bone; made up of compact bone
Spongy bone	Found in ends and inner portions of long bones, such as the femur Red bone marrow located here **Epiphyses:** ends of a long bone; made up of spongy bone covered by compact bone
Medullary cavity	Located in the shaft of a long bone Surrounded by compact bone Contains yellow bone marrow Medullary = pertaining to inner section
Cartilage	Smooth, rubbery, blue-white connective tissue Acts as a shock absorber between bones More elastic than bone Makes up the flexible parts of the skeleton, such as the outer ear and the tip of the nose Word root = chondr/o = cartilage
Joints:	Articulation (to join or come together in a manner that allows motion between parts) Places where two or more bones meet Word root = arthr/o = joint Arthroplasty = surgical repair of a joint Arthro = joint; -plasty = surgical repair
Suture joint	Immovable joint Bones join along a jagged line to form a joint that does not move

diaphysis This is the shaft of a long bone.

epiphyses The ends of a long bone.

Table 10.2 Structures of the Skeletal System (*continued*)

STRUCTURE	DEFINITION/FUNCTION
Synovial joint	Movable joint Ball-and-socket joint (hips, shoulders) Hinge joint (knees, elbows)
Axial skeleton:	Consists of the skull, spinal column, ribs, and sternum Protects major organs of the nervous, respiratory, and circulatory systems Axis is an imaginary line running lengthwise through the center of the body Axial = pertaining to an axis Axi = axis; -al = pertaining to (See Figure 10.4)
Bones of the skull	*Frontal:* forehead *Parietal:* roof and upper sides of cranium *Occipital:* posterior floor and walls of cranium *Temporal:* sides and base of cranium *Sphenoid:* part of the base of the skull and floor and sides of the orbit *Ethomoid:* forms part of the nose, orbit, and floor of cranium (See Figure 10.9) These bones are flat bones.
Bones of the face	*Nasal:* upper part of bridge of nose *Zygomatic:* cheekbones *Maxillary:* most of the upper jaw *Palatine:* part of the hard palate of mouth and floor of mouth *Lacrimal:* part of the orbit at the inner angle of eye *Vomer:* base for the nasal septum *Mandible:* lower jawbone These bones are irregular bones. (See Figure 10.9)

Vertebrae	*Cervical:* C1–C7
	  1st set, consists of 7 vertebrae
	  Word root = cervic/o = neck
	Thoracic: T1–T12
	  2nd set, consists of 12 vertebrae
	  Word root = thorac/o = thorax
	Lumbar: L1–L5
	  3rd set, consists of 5 vertebrae
	  Word root = lumb/o = lumbar
	These bones are irregular bones. (See Figure 10.7)
	
	Mentor Coding Tip: One way to remember the number of vertebrae in each section: breakfast at 7, lunch at 12, and dinner at 5.

Appendicular skeleton:	Consists of the upper and lower extremities, which make body movement possible Appendicular = pertaining to an appendage (See Figure 10.4)
Bones of the shoulder	*Clavicle:* collar bone *Scapula:* shoulder blade *Acromion:* extension of the scapula; forms the point of the shoulder These bones are flat bones. (See Figure 10.6)

axial skeleton Consists of the skull, spinal column, ribs, and sternum. It protects major organs of the nervous, respiratory, and circulatory systems.

appendicular skeleton Consists of the upper and lower extremities and makes body movement possible.

(*continued*)

Table 10.2 Structures of the Skeletal System *(concluded)*

STRUCTURE	DEFINITION/FUNCTION
Bones of the arms	*Humerus:* upper arm *Radius:* smaller bone in the forearm *Ulna:* larger bone in the forearm *Olecranon process ("funny bone"):* large projection on the upper end of the ulna that forms the point of the elbow These bones are long bones.
Bones of the wrists, hands, and fingers	*Carpals:* wrists *Metacarpals:* palms of the hands *Phalanges:* fingers The bones of the hands are long bones. The bones of the wrists are short bones. (See Figure 10.5)
Bones of the pelvis and hips	*Ilium:* upper portion of each hip bone *Ischium:* lower and back part of the hip bone *Pubis:* front arch of pelvis These bones are flat bones. **Mentor Coding Tip:** Remember not to confuse *ilium* with *ileum,* which is the small intestine.
Bones of the legs	*Femur:* upper leg bone, thigh bone; largest bone in the body *Knees:* complex joint enabling movement between the upper leg and the lower leg. *Patella:* kneecap *Tibia:* larger, anterior lower leg bone *Fibula:* smaller lateral bone of lower leg These bones are long bones.
Bones of the ankles, feet, and toes	*Tarsals:* ankles; short bones *Metatarsals:* form the part of the foot to which the toes are attached *Phalanges:* toes; long bones *Sesamoid:* bone embedded in the tendon near the first digit of each foot (see Figure 10.8)

EXERCISE 10.1

1. Explain the difference between a tendon and a ligament.
2. Identify the functions of skeletal, smooth, and myocardial muscles.
3. Where is the deep fascia?
4. Describe the bones that make up the axial skeleton.
5. Describe the bones that make up the appendicular skeleton.

Also available in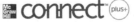

10.2 General Guidelines and Format of ICD Codes for the Musculoskeletal System

Some of the more common conditions of the musculoskeletal system include diseases of the connective tissue, such as systemic lupus erythematosus; poliomyelitis; arthropathy; osteoarthrosis; derangement joint disorders; spondylosis; and disorders of muscles, ligaments, and fascia. When coding these conditions, coders must thoroughly review the provider documentation as well as the guidelines and instructional notes.

ICD-9-CM: Diseases of the musculoskeletal system and connective tissues are located in Chapter 13 in the ICD-9-CM manual, with the code range 710–739.

ICD-10-CM: Diseases of the musculoskeletal system and connective tissues are located in Chapter 13 in the ICD-10-CM manual, with the code range M00–M99.

Table 10.3 lists the Chapter 13 subheadings and their code ranges.

Table 10.3 ICD Musculoskeletal System Subheadings *(Data from ICD-9-CM and ICD-10-CM, Centers for Medicare and Medicaid Services and the National Center for Health Statistics)*

ICD-9-CM		ICD-10-CM	
SUBHEADING	**CODE RANGE**	**SUBHEADING**	**CODE RANGE**
Arthropathies and Related Disorders	710–719	Infectious Arthropathies	M00–M02
		Osteoarthritis	M15–M19
		Other Joint Disorders	M20–M25
		Systemic Connective Tissue Disorders	M30–M36
Dorsopathies	720–724	Deforming Dorsopathies	M40–M43
		Spondylopathies	M45–M49
		Other Dorsopathies	M50–M54
Rheumatism, Excluding the Back	725–729	Inflammatory Polyarthropathies	M05–M14
		Disorders of Muscles	M60–M63
		Disorders of Synovium and Tendon	M65–M67
		Other Soft Tissue Disorders	M70–M79
Osteopathies, Chondropathies, and Acquired Deformities	730–739	Disorders of Bone Density and Structure	M80–M85
		Other Osteopathies	M86–M90
		Chondropathies	M91–M94
		Dentofacial Anomalies and Other Disorders of Jaw	M26–M27
		Other Disorders of the Musculoskeletal System and Connective Tissue	M95
		Intraoperative and Postprocedural Complications and Disorders of Musculoskeletal System, Not Elsewhere Classified	M96
		Biomechanical Lesions, Not Elsewhere Classified	M99

Arthropathies and Related Disorders (710–719), ICD-9-CM
Infectious Arthropathies (M00–M02), ICD-10-CM
Osteoarthritis (M15–M19), ICD-10-CM
Other Joint Disorders (M20–M25), ICD-10-CM
Systemic Connective Tissue Disorders (M30–M36), ICD-10-CM

These code ranges do not include disorders of the spine. Conditions of the spine are reported using codes from range 720–724 (ICD-9-CM) or M40–M54 (ICD-10-CM).

Disorders of the connective tissue, such as systemic lupus erythematosus (SLE); systemic sclerosis; and poliomyelitis are codes found within these ranges.

SPOTLIGHT on Condition

Systemic lupus erythematosus (ICD-9-CM 710.0 and ICD-10-CM M32.9) is a chronic inflammatory disease that affects many organ systems. Signs and symptoms include fever, rash, redness, and muscle and joint pain.

MENTOR
Coding Tip

Category 711 includes codes describing infections of joints of the bones, whereas infections of the bone are reported using codes from category 730.

Codes within these ranges may need an additional code to identify manifestations of the condition or an E code to identify drugs, if the condition is drug-induced.

Arthropathies associated with infections are reported with codes from category 711.

The codes within this category require fifth digits that identify the anatomical site.

FOR EXAMPLE Pyogenic arthritis of the upper arm is reported with code 711.02 (ICD-9-CM) or M00.81- (ICD-10-CM). ■

Many codes within these ranges also require that the underlying disease be coded first.

FOR EXAMPLE Arthropathy associated with mycoses of the lower leg is reported with ICD-9-CM code 711.66, with a code from range 110.0–118 reported first to identify the underlying disease. ■

Category 714 (ICD-9-CM) or M06 (ICD-10-CM) is used to report rheumatoid arthritis and other inflammatory polyarthropathies. There is an instructional note with this category excluding rheumatic fever and rheumatoid arthritis of the spine from this category.

Category 715 (ICD-9-CM) or M15–M19 (ICD-10-CM) is used to report osteoarthritis (OA). There is an instructional note that directs the coder to use this category for the diagnosis of degenerative joint disease (DJD).

SPOTLIGHT
on a Guideline

This range of codes has several *excludes* notes that coders must refer to before selecting the appropriate code.

The fourth digit in this category of codes defines whether the condition is generalized or localized and whether it is primary or secondary.

The fifth digit in this category of codes defines the anatomical site.

FOR EXAMPLE Osteoarthrosis of the hand that is generalized and primary would be assigned code 715.04 (ICD-9-CM) or M15.0 (ICD-10-CM). ■

Category 717 is used to report internal derangements of the knee, such as an old bucket handle tear of the medial meniscus, ICD-9-CM code 717.0 (ICD-10-CM M23.20–).

Dorsopathies (720–724), ICD-9-CM
Deforming Dorsopathies (M40–M43), ICD-10-CM
Spondylopathies (M45–M49), ICD-10-CM
Other Dorsopathies (M50–M54), ICD-10-CM

Conditions reported with codes from these code ranges include conditions related to the spine and intervertebral discs, such as ankylosing spondylitis, spondylosis, displacement of intervertebral discs, spinal stenosis, and lumbago.

FOR EXAMPLE Cervical spondylosis with myelopathy is reported with ICD-9-CM code 721.1 or ICD-10-CM code M47.12. ■

Rheumatism (725–729), ICD-9-CM
Inflammatory Polyarthropathies (M05–M14), ICD-10-CM
Disorders of Muscles (M60–M63), ICD-10-CM
Disorders of Synovium and Tendon (M65–M67), ICD-10-CM
Other Soft Tissue Disorders (M70–M79), ICD-10-CM

These code ranges include disorders of muscles and tendons and their attachments. Some disorders of the rotator cuff, such as a partial tear, are included in these code ranges. Bursitis is included, but the ranges exclude "frozen shoulder" (capsulitis), which is reported using ICD-9-CM code 726.0. or ICD-10-CM M75.0–.

Osteopathies, Chondropathies, and Acquired Musculoskeletal
Deformities (730–739), ICD-9-CM
Disorders of Bone Density and Structure (M80–M85), ICD-10-CM
Other Osteopathies (M86–M90), ICD-10-CM
Chondropathies (M91–M94), ICD-10-CM

Osteomyelitis is a condition defined within these code ranges. It is further defined as acute, chronic, or unspecified by the fourth-digit assignment, and its anatomical site is identified by the fifth-digit assignment.

FOR EXAMPLE Unspecified osteomyelitis of the ankle is reported with ICD-9-CM code 730.27 or ICD-10-CM M86.9. ■

Traumatic fractures and dislocations are reported with codes located in the Injury and Poisoning chapters of ICD, along with sprains and strains. Other conditions associated with the musculoskeletal system are located in the Congenital Anomalies; Symptoms, Signs, and Ill-defined Conditions; Neoplasms; and Diseases of the Nervous System chapters of the ICD manual.

EXERCISE 10.2

1. List some of the more common conditions associated with the musculoskeletal system that would be reported using codes from this chapter of ICD.

2. List some of the other chapters of ICD containing codes that could be used to report conditions associated with the musculoskeletal system.

3. In reporting osteoarthritis (OA), what elements of the condition are defined by the fourth and fifth digits?

Also available in **McGraw Hill connect** (plus+)

10.3 General Format of the Musculoskeletal Subsection of CPT

The Musculoskeletal subsection of CPT is arranged in anatomical order from the head down (see Table 10.4). Each anatomical site is then divided based on the approach or technique and describes the type of treatment or condition.

There are several questions a coder needs to ask when reading an operative report and coding a procedure from this subsection. The following questions will help the coder, when reading through the report, to understand what actually was done and how the procedure should be coded:

- Was the procedure performed on muscle, soft tissue, or bone?
- Was the treatment for a traumatic injury (acute) or a medical condition (chronic)?
- What approach or technique was used (open, scope, or percutaneous)?
- What is the most specific anatomical site (e.g., cervical, thoracic, or lumbar)?
- Does the code description include grafting, reduction, or fixation?
- Does the code describe a procedure done at a single site or at multiple sites?

Several of the anatomical sections have very specific guidelines and notes unique to the section that the coder must read before assigning the appropriate code. The following anatomical headings have these specific notes: Head, Spine, Shoulder, Humerus and Elbow, Forearm and Wrist, Pelvis and Hip Joint, and Femur and Knee Joint.

The Application of Casts and Strapping and Endoscopy/Arthroscopy headings also have unique notes.

Each anatomical heading is then divided into the following subheadings consisting of approach, technique, treatment, or condition:

- Incision
- Excision
- Introduction or Removal

Table 10.4 Musculoskeletal Subsection Code Ranges *(Data from CPT 2013. © 2013 American Medical Association. All rights reserved.)*

HEADING	CODE RANGE
General	20005–20999
Head	21010–21499
Neck (Soft Tissues) and Thorax	21501–21899
Back and Flank	21920–21936
Spine (Vertebral Column)	22010–22899
Abdomen	22900–22999
Shoulder	23000–23929
Humerus (Upper Arm) and Elbow	23930–24999
Forearm and Wrist	25000–25999
Hands and Fingers	26010–26989
Pelvis and Hip Joint	26990–27299
Femur (Thigh Region) and Knee Joint	27301–27599
Leg (Tibia and Fibula) and Ankle Joint	27600–27899
Foot and Toes	28001–28899
Application of Casts and Strapping	29000–29799
Endoscopy/Arthroscopy	29800–29999

- Repair, Revision, and/or Reconstruction
- Fracture and/or Dislocation
- Manipulation
- Arthrodesis
- Amputation
- Other Procedures

MENTOR Coding Tip

- When complication defines the code, this can refer to infection or treatment delay.
- Intermediate repair in this section is an integral part of the surgery and is not reported separately.
- Surgical arthroscopies always include diagnostic arthroscopies.
- Superficial injuries occurring at the site of a more serious injury are not coded; examples: contusions and abrasions at the site of dislocation or fracture.
- When a fracture is not described as closed or open, the coder defaults to closed.

1. List terms found in provider documentation that would lead the coder to assign the ICD code in which "complicated" appears in the code description.

EXERCISE 10.3

2. List some of the subheadings that contain specific instructional notes.

3. CPT codes for procedures of the upper arm are located in which range of codes?

4. CPT codes for procedures of the thigh region are located in which range of codes?

Also available in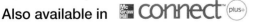

10.4 Subheading Format and Guidelines of the Musculoskeletal Subsection of CPT

General (20005–20999)

The first subheading in this section contains guidelines for general procedures that are not listed elsewhere within the subsection.

Incision: 20005

This code is used to report an incision and drainage of a soft tissue abscess at a site that is not listed elsewhere in the subsection or other surgery subsections. The code is further defined as subfascial, or below the fascia. If the report describes the site as cutaneous or subcutaneous, codes from the Integumentary subsection would be reported.

This code is to be used with an ICD code describing an abscess.

Wound Exploration—Trauma: 20100–20103

These codes are used to report wound exploration due to trauma, such as a gunshot or stab wound, which penetrates through the skin and into the soft tissue. These codes include surgical exploration, enlargement of the wound, extended dissection in order to determine wound penetration, debridement, and removal of foreign bodies. If it is necessary to perform a thoracotomy or laparotomy, codes from the appropriate surgery subsection should be reported instead of the codes in this range.

The ICD code linked with these code ranges needs to indicate that there was a penetrating wound.

Excision: 20150–20251

This range of codes includes biopsies performed on muscle or bone.

Some of the notes in this area ask the coder to determine whether imaging guidance was performed or whether the specimen was obtained by excision or percutaneously (through the skin) by the use of a needle.

Introduction or Removal: 20500–20697

This range of codes includes therapeutic injections of a sinus tract, a tendon sheath, and trigger points. There is an instructional note in this section that instructs the coder to reference the anatomical area if the injection procedure is for arthrography.

Arthrocentesis, aspiration, and/or injection of a joint or bursa, codes 20600–20610, are included in this subheading. These codes are divided by the size of the joint or bursa: A small joint or bursa is a finger or toe, an intermediate joint or bursa is a wrist, elbow, or ankle, and a large joint or bursa is a hip, shoulder, or knee.

Also included in this subheading is the application of cranial tongs, stereotactic frame, halo, and uniplane and multiplane external fixation systems. Codes for the removal of these appliances are also located under this subheading.

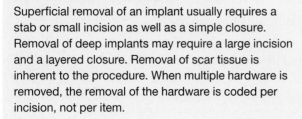

Replantation: 20802–20838

Procedures included in this subheading are used to report replantation of extremities and digits. When reporting a replantation of an incomplete amputation, coders are instructed to see specific codes for repair of bone, ligaments, tendons, nerves, or blood vessels with the use of modifier 52 (reduced service).

MENTOR Coding Tip

Remember that an allograft is also a homograft.

Grafts (or Implants): 20900–20938

Bone, cartilage, and tendon grafts are included in this range.

The remainder of this subsection is divided into anatomical subheadings with further division by approach, technique, treatment, or condition and with specific guidelines and instructional notations for the anatomical site.

Incision and Excision Subheadings

These subheadings are listed in Table 10.5.

MENTOR Coding Tip

Being familiar with the subheadings and the divisions of each speeds the location and selection of the code, aiding the coder when taking the CPC exam.

Table 10.5 Subheadings with Incision and/or Excision Code Ranges *(Data from CPT 2013. © 2013 American Medical Association. All rights reserved.)*

SUBHEADING	CODE RANGE
Head (skull, facial bones, and temporomandibular joint)	21010 Incision 21011–21070 Excision
Neck (soft tissues) and Thorax	21501–21510 Incision 21550–21632 Excision
Back and Flank	21920–21936 Excision
Spine (vertebral column)	22010–22015 Incision 22100–22116 Excision 22206–22226 Osteotomy
Abdomen	22900–22905 Excision
Shoulder	23000–23044 Incision 23065–23220 Excision
Humerus (upper arm) and Elbow	23930–24006 Incision 24065–24155 Excision
Forearm and Wrist	25000–25040 Incision 25065–25240 Excision
Hand and Fingers	26010–26080 Incision 26100– 26262 Excision
Pelvis and Hip Joints	26990– 27036 Incision 27040 –27080 Excision
Femur (thigh region) and Knee Joint	27301–27310 Incision 27323–27365 Excision
Leg (tibia and fibula) and Ankle Joint	27600–27612 Incision 27613–27647 Excision
Foot and Toes	28001–28035 Incision 28039–28175 Excision

Excision of cysts—benign and malignant tumors of subcutaneous soft tissue and bone of the specific anatomical site—are reported with the codes under this subheading. Code selection in the Excision subheading is based on the location of the tumor and the size of the tumor. The size of the tumor is determined by measuring the greatest diameter of the tumor plus the margin required for complete excision of the tumor.

FOR EXAMPLE The surgeon excises a 3.8-cm lipoma of the back. The tumor was located to the right of the spine, just below the fascia covering the latissimus dorsi and superficially descending into the muscle below the fascia. The narrowest excised margin of healthy tissue was 0.2 cm.

CPT: 21932 Excision, tumor, soft tissue of back or flank, subfascial; less than 5 cm

ICD-9-CM: 214.8 Lipoma, Other specified site

ICD-10-CM: D17.7 Benign lipomatous neoplasm of other sites ∎

Specific coding guidelines at the beginning of the Musculoskeletal subsection of the CPT manual address excision of subcutaneous and fascial or subfascial soft tissue tumors.

Excision of subcutaneous soft tissue tumors involves tumors located below the skin but above the deep fascia.

Excision of fascial or subfascial soft tissue tumors involves tumors confined to the tissue within or below the deep fascia.

Radical resection of soft tissue or bone tumors requires excision of surrounding soft tissue. Excision of this tissue is included in the tumor excision and is not coded separately.

Fracture and/or Dislocation Subheadings

These subheadings and their code ranges are listed in Table 10.6.

Bones of the skull and face are shown in Figure 10.9. Knowledge of this anatomy will aid coders in determining the correct code for procedure of this anatomic site.

Coders must be able to determine from the medical documentation the anatomical site of the fracture, the type of the fracture (ICD code), the type of

Table 10.6 Subheadings for Fractures and/or Dislocations *(Data from CPT 2013. © 2013 American Medical Association. All rights reserved.)*

SUBHEADING	CODE RANGE
Head (skull, facial bones, and temporomandibular joint)	21310–21497
Neck (soft tissues) and Thorax	21800–21825
Spine (vertebral column)	22305–22328
Shoulder	23500–23680
Humerus (upper arm) and Elbow	24500–24685
Forearm and Wrist	25500–25695
Hand and Fingers	26600–26785
Pelvis and Hip Joints	27193–27269
Femur (thigh region) and Knee Joint	27500–27566
Leg (tibia and fibula) and Ankle Joint	27750–27848
Foot and Toes	28400–28675

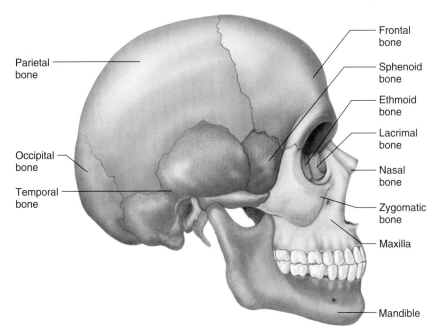

Figure 10.9 Lateral View of Skull

fracture treatment, and the method of reduction and immobilization (CPT code) in order to tell the complete story of the patient encounter.

MENTOR Coding Tip

There can be open treatment of a closed fracture. Therefore, it is important that the coder understand and differentiate between the type of fracture and the type of treatment.

Closed treatment of a fracture occurs when the fracture is not surgically opened and directly visualized. This type of treatment may be performed with or without manipulation, with or without traction, and with casting or splinting.

Open treatment of a fracture occurs when the skin is surgically opened and the fracture is visualized or when the fracture site is opened remotely in order to insert intramedullary nails across the fracture site.

Percutaneous skeletal fixation treatment is neither open nor closed. The fixation of the fracture site is accomplished by other methods, such as a pin placed through the skin and across the fracture site. X-ray imaging is often used to aid in the placement of the fixation device.

internal fixation Wires, pins, or screws are placed through or into the fractured bone to stabilize the fracture.

external fixation Pins attached to an external device are inserted through the skin and into bone near the fracture site. May also be the application of a cast or splint.

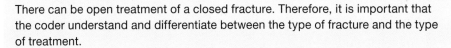

SPOTLIGHT on a Guideline

Internal fixation involves the use of wires, pins, screws, and the like, which are placed through or within the fracture site in order to stabilize the fracture.

External fixation involves skeletal pins attached to an external mechanism.

Traction

Skeletal traction is the application of force to a limb through a wire, pin, screw, or clamp that is attached to a bone.

Skin traction is the application of force to a limb through felt or strapping applied directly to the skin only.

Manipulation is the attempted reduction or restoration of a fracture or joint dislocation to its normal anatomical alignment by the application of manually applied force.

SPOTLIGHT on a Guideline

The definitions of *fixation*, *traction*, and *manipulation* are located in the general guidelines at the beginning of the Musculoskeletal subsection of the CPT manual.

Repair, Reconstruction, and Revision

Before selecting the appropriate codes for repair, reconstruction, and revision, coders need to find answers in the medical record to these questions:

- What is the anatomical site?
- What is the nature of the procedure, such as augmentation, reduction, graft, or arthroplasty?
- What is the nature of the condition: acute or chronic?
- What is the approach used to perform the procedure: open or arthroscopic?

MENTOR
Coding Tip

An instructional note below these codes refers the coder to a different code if the procedure is performed arthroscopically.

FOR EXAMPLE

23410 Repair of ruptured musculotendinous cuff (e.g., rotator cuff), open; acute

23412 Repair of ruptured musculotendinous cuff (e.g., rotator cuff) open; chronic ■

Subheadings of the Musculoskeletal subsection

Codes in these subheadings often include bone grafts, and the code specifically includes the harvesting of the graft, which would not be coded separately.

Table 10.7 Repair, Reconstruction, and Revision *(Data from CPT 2013. © 2013 American Medical Association. All rights reserved.)*

SUBHEADING	CODE RANGE
Head (skull, facial bones, and temporomandibular joint)	21120–21296
Neck (soft tissues) and Thorax	21685–21750
Shoulder	23395–23491
Humerus (upper arm) and Elbow	24300–24498
Forearm and Wrist	25260–25492
Hand and Fingers	26340–26596
Pelvis and Hip Joints	27097–27187
Femur (thigh region) and Knee Joint	27380–27499
Leg (tibia and fibula) and Ankle Joint	27650–27745
Foot and Toes	28200–28360

21151 Reconstruction midface, LeFort II; any direction, requiring bone grafts (including obtaining autografts) ▪

CPT code selection for repair, revision, and reconstruction of tendons and/or muscles depends on the anatomical site, such as the hand; the specific muscle or tendon, such as flexor or extensor; and the type of procedure, such as repair, transfer, lengthening, or shortening. To select the appropriate code to tell the complete story, the coder may also need to know whether the repair was primary or secondary and whether the code selected includes obtaining a graft.

Arthrodesis Subheadings

Arthrodesis, or fusion, may be performed to strengthen an area, such as the spine, after other surgical procedures or to eliminate pain upon flexion and extension at the site of a joint. This procedure may be performed alone as the therapeutic treatment or in conjunction with other procedures such as spinal fixation or complex fracture repairs.

Harvesting of a bone graft for an arthrodesis procedure in which the bone is harvested through a separate skin and or fascial incision is reported only when the primary code does not include harvest of the graft.

Bone obtained through the same surgical incision as the primary procedure, regardless of the type of bone graft (e.g., structural, morselized) is reported with code 20936. As this code has no reimbursement value, it is used internally for tracking and trending purposes.

The codes for arthrodesis of the spine are divided based on the surgeon's approach to the spine and include minimal removal of the intraspinal disc when needed to promote fusion of the vertebral bodies. However, when a discectomy is performed for decompression of the spinal cord or nerve roots, it is reported in addition to the arthrodesis procedure.

Spinal arthrodesis codes are reported according to interspace or vertebral segment. An interspace is the space between the vertebral bodies (bones of

Table 10.8 Subheadings for Arthrodesis *(Data from CPT 2013. © 2013 American Medical Association. All rights reserved.)*

SUBHEADING	CODE RANGE
Spine:	
Lateral Extracavitary Approach Technique	22532–22534
Anterior or Anterolateral Approach Technique	22548–22586
Posterior, Posterolateral, or Lateral Transverse Process Technique	22590–22634
Spine Deformity (scoliosis, kyphosis)	22800–22819
Shoulder	23800–23802
Humerus and Elbow	24800–24802
Forearm and Wrist	25800–25830
Hand and Fingers	26820–26863
Pelvis and Hip Joint	27280–27286
Femur and Knee Joint	27580
Leg (tibia and fibula) and Ankle Joint	27870–27871
Foot and Toes	28705–28760

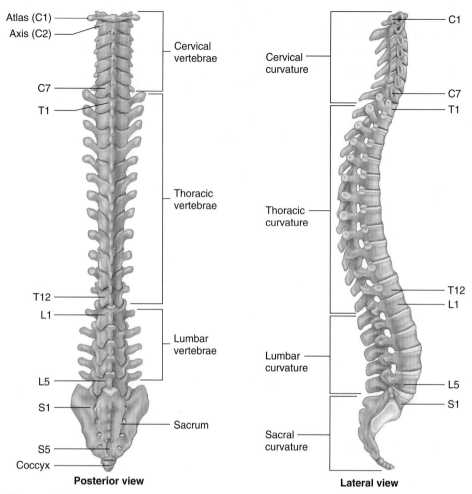

Atlas (C1)
Axis (C2)
Cervical vertebrae
C7
T1
Thoracic vertebrae
T12
L1
Lumbar vertebrae
L5
S1
Sacrum
S5
Coccyx

Posterior view

Cervical curvature
C1
C7
T1
Thoracic curvature
T12
L1
Lumbar curvature
L5
S1
Sacral curvature

Lateral view

Figure 10.10 Spinal Column

the spine), where the intervertebral disc is located, and it includes the disc. A vertebral segment is the vertebral body including the articulating processes (joints of the spine, aka facet joints). (See Figure 10.10.)

> **MENTOR** Coding Tip
>
> When reviewing the documentation for spine procedures, the coder must first determine whether the procedure was performed on the bony structures (segments) or the disc (interspace). A simple means of determining this is the description of the procedure's location. Bony structures are listed by each individual site, for example, T1, T2, T3. Interspaces are identified by the two bony structures above and below the interspace, for example, T1–T2, T2–T3. This description also allows for quick determination of the number of interspaces: Just count the dashes between each identified bony structure.

Spinal Instrumentation (22840–22851)

There are three main types of spinal instrumentation: posterior, anterior, and intervertebral. Spinal instrumentation is performed to provide stability to the spine after therapeutic spinal procedures are performed that may destabilize the vertebral column.

The codes for posterior instrumentation (22841–22844) are divided based on the type of instrumentation, segmental versus nonsegmental, and the number of vertebral segments the device spans. A **nonsegmental instrumentation** is one in which the device (rod) is attached by hooks or screws to the spine *only* at each end of the device. **Segmental instrumentation** is likewise attached to the spine at each end *and* at least one other point of the spine along the device.

Anterior instrumentation codes (22845–22847) are divided based on the number of vertebral segments the instrumentation spans. These codes may be used alone or with other spinal instrumentation codes, and they are often used in conjunction with intervertebral instrumentation codes.

There currently is only one intervertebral instrumentation code. CPT 22851 is used to indicate the placement of biomechanical devices, such as cages, between vertebral segments of the spinal column (anterior bony portion of the spine). These devices may be placed anteriorly or posteriorly. The code is reported once per interspace regardless of the number of cages used at each interspace.

Application of Cast and Strapping Subheading

There are very specific guidelines for use of codes located in the Application of Cast and Strapping subheading (see Table 10.9). According to CPT (2013), the procedures in this subheading "apply when the cast application or strapping is a replacement procedure used during or after the period of follow up care or when the cast application or strapping is an initial service performed without a restorative treatment or procedure(s) to stabilize or protect a fracture, injury, or **dislocation** (displacement of a bone from its original location) and/or to afford comfort to a patient. Restorative treatment or procedure(s) rendered by another physician following the application of the initial cast/splint/strap may be reported with a treatment of fracture and/or dislocation code."

CPT further instructs: "An individual who applies the initial cast, strap or splint and also assumes all of the subsequent fracture, dislocation or injury care cannot use the application of casts and strapping codes as an initial service, since the first cast/splint or strap application is included in the treatment of fracture and/or dislocation codes. If cast application or strapping is provided as an initial service (casting of a sprained ankle or knee) in which no other procedure or treatment (surgical repair, reduction of a fracture, or joint dislocation) is performed or is expected to be performed by a

nonsegmental instrumentation A device (rod) is attached by hooks or screws to the spine only at each end of the device.

segmental instrumentation A device (rod) is attached by hooks or screws to the spine at each end of the device and to at least one other point of the spine along the device.

dislocation Displacement of a bone from its normal location.

Table 10.9 Casts, Splints, and Strapping *(Data from CPT 2013. © 2013 American Medical Association. All rights reserved.)*

SUBHEADING	CODE RANGE
Body and Upper Extremity:	
Casts	29000–29086
Splints	29105–29131
Strapping	29200–29280
Lower Extremity:	
Casts	29305–29450
Splints	29505–29515
Strapping	29520–29584
Removal or Repair	29700–29750

physician rendering the initial care only, use the casting, strapping, and/or supply code 99070 in addition to an evaluation and management code."

The removal and repair codes are reported only if the casts are applied by another physician.

Endoscopy/Arthroscopy Subheading (29800–29999)

The word *endoscopy* means to visualize within a cavity. Arthroscopy is the visualization of a joint through a scope. When a diagnostic arthroscopic procedure is done and then surgical treatment is performed through the scope during the same operative session on the same anatomical site, only the surgical arthroscopic procedure is reported.

EXERCISE 10.4

1. How would a coder report a replantation of an incomplete amputation of an extremity or digit?
2. Code selection in the excision subheading is based on the location of the tumor and the size of the tumor. How is the size of the tumor determined?
3. Explain the guidelines for coding excision of subcutaneous and fascial or subfascial soft tissue tumors.
4. Explain the difference between skeletal traction and skin traction.
5. Explain why an arthrodesis or fusion procedure would be performed.
6. Explain when codes within the Application of Cast and Strapping subheading may be reported.

Also available in **connect** (plus+)

10.5 Modifiers Most Commonly Used with Codes in the Musculoskeletal Subsection

As with all sections of the CPT manual, modifiers are used in the Musculoskeletal subsection to continue or modify the story of the patient's encounter. In the Musculoskeletal subsection, modifiers are most commonly used to indicate bilateral procedures, reduced services, multiple procedures, and/or two surgeons performing distinct parts of a single procedure. (See Table 10.10.)

Table 10.10 Musculoskeletal Subsection Modifiers *(Data from CPT 2013. © 2013 American Medical Association. All rights reserved.)*

MODIFIER	DEFINITION	EXAMPLE
50	Bilateral procedure	*Code 21060:* meniscectomy, partial or complete, temporomandibular joint. For a bilateral procedure, report 21060-50.
51	Multiple procedures	• Arthroscopy performed at the same time as an arthrotomy. • When arthrodesis is performed in addition to another procedure, the arthrodesis is reported in addition to the original procedure with -51. *Note:* Bone grafts and instrumentation are never performed without arthrodesis. **Example from CPT:** Treatment of a burst fracture of L2 by *corpectomy (original procedure)* followed by *arthrodesis* of L1–L3, utilizing *anterior instrumentation* L1–L3 and structural *allograft.* *Codes:* 63090, 22558-51, 22585, 22845, and 20931. Do *not* append modifier 62.
52	Reduced service	• Replantation of incomplete amputation.
62	Two surgeons	• When two surgeons work together as primary surgeons performing distinct parts of a single reportable procedure, each surgeon should report his or her distinct operative work by appending modifier 62. **Example from CPT:** Male with history of post-traumatic degenerative disc disease at L3–L4 and L4–L5 underwent surgical repair. Surgeon A performed an anterior exposure of the spine with mobilization of the great vessels. Surgeon B performed anterior discectomy and fusion at L3–L4 and L4–L5 using anterior interbody technique. Report surgeon A: 22558-62 22585-62 Report surgeon B: 22558-62 22585-62 20931 Do *not* append modifier 62 to spinal instrumenation codes or bone grafts.

---

1. For what type of procedures within the Musculoskeletal subsection would it not be appropriate to append modifier 62?

2. Arthrodesis may be performed in the absence of other procedures, but when it is performed with another procedure, such as a corpectomy, it would be appropriate to code using modifier 51 to report multiple procedures. Would it also be appropriate to use a modifier with a code such as 22614 when reporting arthrodesis of each vertebral segment?

EXERCISE 10.5

Also available in **Mc Graw Hill connect**™ (plus+)

10.6 Common Medical and Procedural Terms Used in Operative Reports

There are many procedural and diagnostic terms that are specific to the musculoskeletal system or are shared with other organ systems. Coders need to be aware of when the terms used in the medical documentation define the procedure and/or service and diagnosis of the system they are coding. Tables 10.11 and 10.12 list some of the CPT and ICD terms for the musculoskeletal system.

Table 10.11 Terms for Musculoskeletal System

TERM	DEFINITION	DOCUMENTATION KEYS
Biopsy	Removal of all or part of a lesion for pathologic examination	Incisional, excisional, needle aspiration, punch, shave
Destruction	Destroying tissue by means of heat, cold, or chemicals (*Note:* There is no tissue to send for pathology.)	Cautery, cryo, laser
Excision	Removal by cutting all or part	-ectomy
Fascioplasty	Fasci/o = fascia plasty = surgical repair Surgical repair of fascia	Plastic repair of a fascia
Incision	Creation of an opening by surgically cutting into the skin or other tissue	-otomy
-plasty	Reshaping or replacing by surgical means	Repair, reconstruction, revision, augmentation
Repair	Restoration of diseased or damaged tissue	Suture, revision, restore

Table 10.12 Additional Terms for Musculoskeletal System

TERM	DEFINITION	DOCUMENTATION KEYS
Atrophy	Weakness or wearing away of body tissues and structures	Degeneration, decline of tissue, organs, wasting
Closed fracture	Fracture closed to the environment; does not protrude outside the skin	Greenstick
Contracture	Tightening of fascia, muscles, tendons, ligaments, or skin	Scarring
Cramp	Localized muscle spasm named for its cause	Heat cramp, writer's cramp
Impingement syndrome	Condition of inflamed and swollen tendons caught in the narrow space between the bones within the shoulder joint	Rotator cuff injury
Malunion	Incorrectly healing fracture	Faulty union, incomplete union
Myalgia	Muscle tenderness or pain	Fibromyalgia (muscle and connective tissue pain)
Myolysis	Degeneration of muscle tissue	Breaking down of tissue
Nonunion	Nonhealing fracture	Failed to heal
Open fracture	Fracture open to the environment; protrudes outside the skin	Compound, missile
Osteoarthritis	Inflammation of the bone and joint; occurs when protective cartilage on the ends of the bones wear down	Wear-and-tear arthritis
Osteoporosis	Thinning of bone tissue and loss of bone density over time, causing bones to become weak and brittle	Porous bones
Pathologic fracture	Fracture caused by disease, not trauma	Fracture due to: neoplasm, osteoporosis, or other non-traumatic condition
Sprain	Injury to the ligament of a joint, ankle, wrist, or knee	stretched or torn ligament overuse injuries; stretched or torn muscle or tendon attachment
Strain	Injury to the body of the muscle or the attachment of a tendon	
Shin splint	Painful condition caused by muscle tearing away from the tibia	repeated stress to the lower leg
Hamstring injury	Strain or tear on any of the three hamstring muscles that straighten the hip and bend the knee	sudden and severe pain in the back of the thigh

closed fracture A fracture which is closed to the environment or does not protrude through the skin. An example is a greenstick fracture.

malunion An incorrect (faulty, incomplete) healing fracture.

nonunion A nonhealing fracture

open fracture Fracture is open to the environment and does protrude outside of the skin. Examples of an open fracture are compound and missile fractures.

osteoarthritis A condition in which there is inflammation of the bone and joint. Also called wear and tear arthritis

osteoporosis A condition of thinning of bone tissue and loss of bone density and the bones become brittle and weak.

pathologic fracture A pathologic fracture is caused by disease and not trauma.

sprain A sprain is an injury to a joint and usually involves a stretched or torn ligament.

---

1. Explain the difference between a sprain and a strain.

2. Explain the difference between osteoarthritis and osteoporosis.

3. If the word *cautery, cryo,* or *laser* is part of the description of the procedure performed, what main term could be used to describe all of these words?

EXERCISE 10.6

Also available in ⊞ **connect** (plus+)

Chapter Ten Summary

Learning Outcome	Key Concepts/Examples
10.1 Review the anatomy of the musculoskeletal system.	Recognizing the anatomy and specific medical terminology pertinent to the musculoskeletal system will aid the coder in selecting the appropriate codes.
	Some of the functions of the muscular system are to hold the body erect, make movement possible, generate body heat, and move food through the digestive system.
	Some of the functions of the skeletal system are to support and shape the body, protect internal organs, anchor muscles, and make blood cells.
10.2 Recognize the general guidelines and format of ICD codes for the musculoskeletal system.	Some of the more common conditions of the musculoskeletal system include diseases of the connective tissue, such as systemic lupus erythematosus; poliomyelitis; arthropathy; osteoarthrosis; derangement joint disorders; spondylosis; and disorders of muscles, ligaments, and fascia. When coding these conditions, coders must thoroughly review the provider documentation as well as the guidelines and instructional notes.
	ICD-9-CM: Diseases of the musculoskeletal system and connective tissues are located in Chapter 13 in the ICD-9-CM manual, with the code range 710–739.
	ICD-10-CM: Diseases of the musculoskeletal system and connective tissues are located in Chapter 13 in the ICD-10-CM manual, with the code range M00–M99.
10.3 Understand the general guidelines and format of the Musculoskeletal subsection in the CPT manual.	The Musculoskeletal subsection of CPT is arranged in anatomical order from the head down. Each anatomical site is then divided based on the approach or technique and on the type of treatment or condition.
10.4 Apply the subheading guidelines.	Each anatomical heading is divided into the following subheadings consisting of approach, technique, treatment, or condition:
	Incision
	Excision
	Introduction or Removal
	Repair, Revision, and/or Reconstruction
	Fracture and/or Dislocation
	Manipulation
	Arthrodesis
	Amputation
10.5 Identify the modifiers most commonly used with codes in the Musculoskeletal subsection.	In the Musculoskeletal subsection modifiers are most commonly used to indicate bilateral procedures, reduced services, multiple procedures, and/or two surgeons performing distinct parts of a single procedure.
10.6 Examine the common medical and procedural terms used in operative reports.	There are many procedural and diagnostic terms that are specific to the musculoskeletal system or are shared with other organ systems. Coders need to be aware of when the terms used in the medical documentation define the procedure and/or service and diagnosis of the system they are coding.

Chapter Ten Review

Understanding Terminology

Match each key term to the appropriate definition.

_____ 1. [LO10.1] Axial skeleton

_____ 2. [LO10.1] Appendicular skeleton

_____ 3. [LO10.1] Closed fracture

_____ 4. [LO10.1] Diaphysis

_____ 5. [LO10.1] Dislocation

_____ 6. [LO10.1] Epiphyses

_____ 7. [LO10.4] External fixation

_____ 8. [LO10.4] Internal fixation

_____ 9. [LO10.1] Ligament

_____ 10. [LO10.6] Malunion

_____ 11. [LO10.4] Manipulation

_____ 12. [LO10.4] Nonunion

_____ 13. [LO10.4] Open fracture

_____ 14. [LO10.6] Osteoarthritis

_____ 15. [LO10.6] Osteoporosis

_____ 16. [LO10.6] Pathologic fracture

_____ 17. [LO10.1] Tendon

A. Fracture caused by disease, not trauma

B. Connects muscle to a bone

C. Displacement of a bone from its normal location

D. Attempted reduction of a fracture by application of manually applied force

E. Nonhealing fracture

F. Fracture that protrudes outside the skin; also identified as *compound* or *puncture*

G. Fracture that does not protrude outside the skin; also identified as *comminuted, greenstick, spiral,* or *simple*

H. Shaft of a long bone

I. The part of the skeleton that consists of the skull, spinal column, ribs, and sternum

J. Connects two or more bones or cartilage

K. Ends of a long bone

L. The part of the skeleton that makes body movement possible and consists of the upper and lower extremities

M. Treatment that involves the use of wires, pins, or screws that are placed through or within the fracture site

N. Incorrect healing of a fracture

O. Treatment that involves skeletal pins attached to an external mechanism

P. Inflammation of the bone and joint

Q. Thinning of the bone tissue and loss of bone density

Checking Your Understanding

Complete each of the following statements with the most appropriate answer or code.

1. [LO10.1] The correct procedure code for subcutaneous foreign body removal from the elbow is _____.

2. [LO10.1] When a fracture is not described as open or closed in the medical documentation, the coder defaults to using _____.

3. [LO10.1] Some examples of irregular bones are _____, _____, and _____.

4. [LO10.3] The Musculoskeletal subsection of CPT is arranged by anatomical order, and each anatomical site is then divided based on the approach or technique and also on the _____.

5. [LO10.3] Some trigger words to look for in an operative report to support using the wound exploration codes are _____, _____, and _____.

Choose the most appropriate answer for each of the following questions.

1. [LO10.1] This lies beneath the layer of subcutaneous tissue of the integumentary system, lines extremities, and holds together groups of muscles:

   a. Visceral fascia

   b. Superficial fascia

   c. Deep fascia

   d. All of these

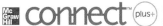

Enhance your learning by completing these exercises and more at mcgrawhillconnect.com

2. **[LO10.1]** Skeletal muscles make motion such as walking possible and are:

   a. Striated muscles

   b. Voluntary muscles

   c. Smooth muscles

   d. Both striated muscles and voluntary muscles

3. **[LO10.4]** What is the correct code for an open repair of an acute ruptured rotator cuff?

   a. 23410

   b. 23405

   c. 23412

   d. 23420

4. **[LO10.4]** Report the appropriate code(s) for the following procedures:
   Diagnostic knee arthroscopy of the right knee, followed by surgical arthroscopy with synovectomy in both medial and lateral components of the right knee.

   a. 29870

   b. 29874, 29870-51

   c. 29876

   d. 29876, 29870-51

5. **[LO10.1]** This type of joint is movable and also called a ball-and-socket joint:

   a. Suture joint

   b. Synovial joint

   c. Hinge joint

   d. Synovial and hinge joint

6. **[LO10.3]** When the description of a code includes the term complicated, it can refer to:

   a. Infection

   b. Delayed healing

   c. Infection and delayed healing

   d. Increased physician time

7. **[LO10.3]** What is the appropriate code for arthrocentesis of the shoulder?

   a. 20605

   b. 20610

   c. 20600

   d. 20612

8. **[LO10.4]** _____ is the attempted reduction or restoration of a fracture or joint dislocation to its normal alignment by the application of manually applied force.

   a. Traction

   b. Manipulation

   c. Internal fixation

   d. External fixation

9. **[LO10.4]** When an arthroscopy is performed at the same time as an arthrotomy, which modifier would be appended?

   a. 58

   b. 59

   c. 51

   d. 76

10. **[LO10.1]** A muscle that is like a striated muscle in appearance but similar to a smooth muscle in action is a:

    a. Skeletal muscle

    b. Myocardial muscle

    c. Smooth muscle

    d. None of these

Applying Your Knowledge

Answer the following questions and code the following case study. Be sure to follow the process steps as illustrated in Chapter 8

Case Study

Preoperative diagnosis: Cervical spondylosis, central stenosis C5–C6

Postoperative diagnosis: Cervical spondylosis, central stenosis C5–C6

Procedure: Anterior cervical arthrodesis anterior body C5–C6 using PEEK cages and DynaTran 18-mm Stryker plate, autologous local bone, and putty

Anesthesia: General anesthesia

The patient was placed in a supine position on the operating table with an interscapular roll. The anterior aspect of the neck was prepped and draped in a sterile fashion. Interoperative fluoroscopy was used to center our incision over the C5 through C6 interspace. A transverse incision was made across the sternocleidomastoid on the right side, and the incision was carried down through the subcutaneous tissues, controlling bleeding with unipolar cautery. Initially, retraction was done using a small Weitlaner, and the anterior border of the sternocleidomastoid was identified. I followed a plane medial to this and medial to the carotid artery but lateral to the esophagus and trachea. I followed this plane until the prevertebral space was identified and the longus colli muscles were divided in the midline. The self-retaining blades of the Trimline retractor were placed underneath this muscle, and then we placed a marker at the C4–C5 level, which was the most inferior, still visible identifiable disc space.

From here I counted down to the C4–C5 level and proceeded with a minimal anterior cervical discectomy and decompression at C5–C6. The ventral osteophytes were removed using a Leksell rongeur, and then the disc was incised using a 15-blade knife in the interspace distracted using the Caspar distraction system. The discectomy was performed; the disk was quite collapsed using a combination of curettes and Midas Rex drill. The discectomy and bony removal was followed posteriorly until the posterior longitudinal ligament was identified. This was opened and removed, and then working carefully over the dura, bilateral foraminotomies were performed.

After verifying that the spinal cord was well decompressed in the midline, the roots out laterally, the area was irrigated with an antibiotic saline solution. I then selected a 6-mm in height PEEK cage, which was filled with some local bone that had been harvested as part of our bony removal combined with autologous bone putty. The cage was then tapped into position and distraction was released.

I then selected an 18 mm in length DynaTran translational plate, and this was secured with two variable-angle screws into C5 and two into C6. Once the screws were partially in position, the translational stops were removed and the screws were secured beyond the backup stops for all screws. The muscles were reapproximated with 2-0 Vicryl, a 2-0 Vicryl subcutaneous closure including the platysma, and a running 4-0 Vicryl subcuticular stitch in the skin.

Process 1: CPT

1. What is the procedure?

2. Locate the main term in the index. What additional questions or set of questions can be determined?

3. Upon review of all the code choices identified in the index, what additional questions can be determined?

4. Based on the documentation, what are the correct codes for this case?
    a. 22551, 22851
    b. 22845, 22851×2
    c. 22551, 22845, 22851
    d. 22551, 22845-51, 22851-51

Process 2: ICD
ICD-9-CM

1. Based on the operative report header, what is the preoperative diagnosis?

2. Is the postoperative diagnosis the same as or different from the preoperative diagnosis?

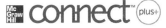 plus+ Enhance your learning by completing these exercises and more at mcgrawhillconnect.com

3. Is the postoperative diagnosis supported?

4. What is the main term for this condition?

5. Based on the subterm choices, what question(s) can be developed for this condition?

6. Is any sign, symptom, or additional condition documented?

7. Is the additional condition, sign, or symptom an integral part of the primary (or other) condition coded?

8. Does the additional condition require or affect patient care, treatment, or management?

9. Based on the documentation, what are the correct ICD-9-CM codes for this case?
   a. 721.1, 723.0
   b. 721.1, 724.00
   c. 721.0, 723.0
   d. 721.0, 724.00

ICD-10-CM

1. Based on the operative report header, what is the preoperative diagnosis?

2. Is the postoperative diagnosis the same as or different from the preoperative diagnosis?

3. Is the postoperative diagnosis supported?

4. What is the main term for this condition?

5. Based on the subterm choices, what question(s) can be developed for this condition?

6. Based on the information in the Tabular List, is additional information needed to determine the appropriate diagnosis code?

7. Is any sign, symptom, or additional condition documented?

8. Is the additional condition, sign, or symptom an integral part of the primary (or other) condition coded?

9. Does the additional condition require or affect patient care, treatment, or management?

10. Based on the documentation, what are the correct ICD-10-CM codes for this case?
    a. M47.12, M99.71
    b. M48.02, M99.71, M47.12
    c. M47.812, M48.02
    d. M47.12, M48.02

Process 3: Modifiers

1. Was the procedure performed different from that described by the nomenclature of the code?

2. Was the procedure performed on an anatomical site that has laterality?

3. Was the procedure performed in the global period of another procedure?

4. Were additional procedures performed during the operative session, and does the documentation support them?

5. Did the surgeon have help from another surgeon or another appropriate person?

6. Did a physician different from the surgeon provide the preoperative or postoperative portion of the procedure?

7. Which modifier should be appended to the CPT code for this case?
   a. 51
   b. 50
   c. 78
   d. None

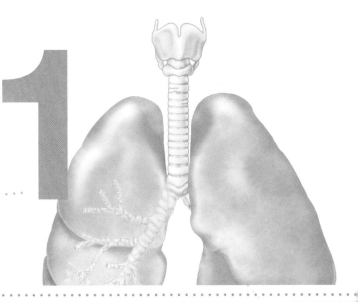

Surgery Section: Respiratory System

11

Key Terms

Alveoli
Anterior nasal
 hemorrhage control
Bronchi
Diaphragm
Direct laryngoscopy

Epiglottis
Ethmoid sinus
Expiration/exhalation
External approach
Indirect laryngoscopy
Inspiration/inhalation

Internal approach
Larynx
Maxillary sinus
Nasal hemorrhage
Pharynx
Pleura

Posterior nasal
 hemorrhage control
Sphenoid sinus
Trachea

Learning Outcomes

After completing this chapter, you will be able to:

11.1 Review the anatomy of the respiratory system.

11.2 Understand the chapter-specific ICD guidelines and format for the respiratory system.

11.3 Identify the guidelines and format of the Respiratory subsection of CPT.

11.4 Apply the modifiers most commonly used with codes in the Respiratory subsection.

11.5 Examine the common medical and procedural terms used in operative reports.

Introduction The respiratory system's primary function is to supply oxygen to the blood, which then delivers it to all parts of the body. The respiratory system accomplishes this during the process of breathing. Oxygen is inhaled, and carbon dioxide is exhaled. The exchange of gases occurs at the **alveoli**. The alveoli disperse the inhaled oxygen into the arterial blood. The veins discharge carbon dioxide into the alveoli, from which it is exhaled out of the lungs.

11.1 Anatomy of the Respiratory System

The respiratory system is divided into the upper and lower respiratory tracts. The upper respiratory tract includes the nose, sinuses, pharynx, and larynx, and the lower respiratory system includes the trachea (windpipe), bronchial tubes, and lungs. (See Figure 11.1.)

Flow of Air through the Respiratory System

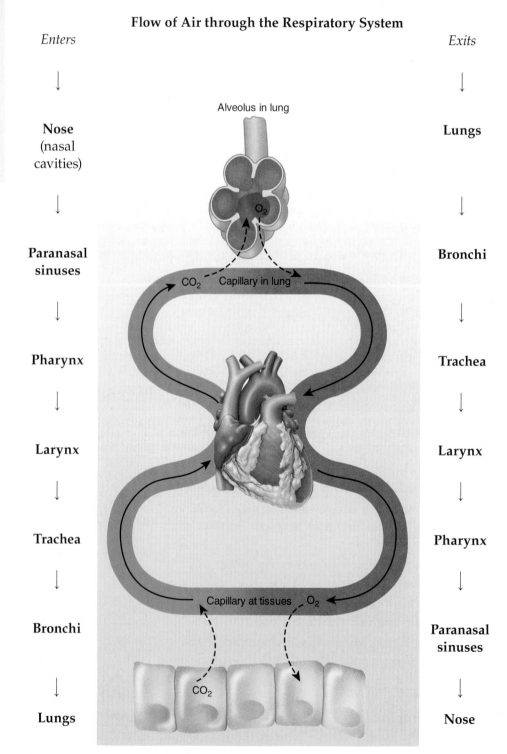

Enters		Exits
↓		↓
Nose (nasal cavities)		**Lungs**
↓		↓
Paranasal sinuses		**Bronchi**
↓		↓
Pharynx		**Trachea**
↓		↓
Larynx		**Larynx**
↓		↓
Trachea		**Pharynx**
↓		↓
Bronchi		**Paranasal sinuses**
↓		↓
Lungs		**Nose**

Alveolus in lung

O_2

CO_2 Capillary in lung

Capillary at tissues O_2

CO_2

Figure 11.1 Gas Exchange of Respiratory System

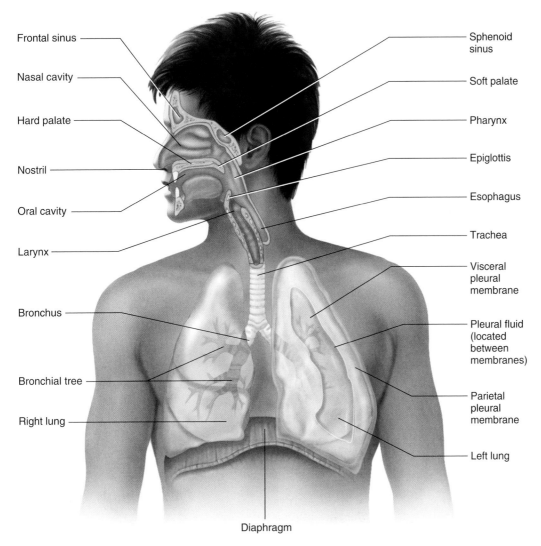

Figure 11.2 Anatomy of the Respiratory System

Figure 11.2 and Table 11.1 refer to the anatomy and definition of the structures of the respiratory system which will aid coders in understanding and reviewing operative reports when assigning codes from the respiratory system.

Table 11.1 Structures of the Respiratory System

STRUCTURE	DEFINITION/FUNCTION
Nose: Nares/nostril	Olfaction (smelling) Assists in producing sound Warms and humidifies the air
Nasal cavities	Contains the turbinates (inferior, middle, and superior), which warm the air as it passes through to the lungs
Nasal septum	Partition of cartilage that divides the left and right nasal cavities

(continued)

MENTOR
Coding Tip

There are instructional notes in CPT regarding procedures performed on the middle and superior turbinates.

Table 11.1 Structures of the Respiratory System (concluded)

STRUCTURE	DEFINITION/FUNCTION
Paranasal sinuses	Cavities in the skull that open into the nasal cavity: *Frontal:* superior to the eye ***Ethmoid:*** between the nose and the eyes ***Sphenoid:*** center of the skull base *Maxillary:* largest sinus cavity; under the eyes, within the maxillary bone
Pharynx	Also referred to as *throat* Connects the nose and the mouth to the larynx Divided into three parts: *Nasopharynx:* upper section *Oropharynx:* middle section *Laryngopharynx:* lower section Is a passage through which both air and food pass The **epiglottis,** a small flap of cartilage that closes over the trachea, prevents food from entering the larynx and thus the lungs
Larynx	Also referred to as *voice box* Vocal cords located here *Glottis:* space between the vocal cords Sound produced as air passes through the spaces between the cords Protects the trachea from foreign objects and particles
Trachea	Also referred to as *windpipe* Made up of muscular tissue Kept open by C-shaped cartilage rings Branches into the bronchi
Bronchi	Tubular structures Branch into smaller tubes called *bronchioles* Bronchioles end in small air sacs called *alveoli,* through which oxygen and carbon dioxide pass: oxygen into the alveoli and on to the bloodstream and the rest of the body; carbon dioxide into the alveoli to be expelled during exhalation
Lungs	Organ Bronchi, bronchioles, alveoli located here Made up of lobes: *Right lung:* three lobes *Left lung:* two lobes *Apex:* upper part of lung *Base:* lower part of lung ***Pleura:*** membrane surrounding the lung; consists of two layers, one covering the lung and the other lining the chest cavity; space between the two layers is the pleural space
Diaphragm	Separates the thoracic and abdominal cavities. Contracts as air is drawn into the lungs—inspiration/inhalation. Relaxes as air is pushed out of the lungs—expiration/exhalation.

ethmoid sinus Cavity in the skull which opens into the nasal cavity located between the nose and eyes.

sphenoid sinus Cavity in the skull which opens into the nasal cavity located in the center of the skull base.

pharynx Also referred to as throat and connects the nose and the mouth to the larynx

epiglottis A small flap of cartilage that closes over the trachea preventing food from entering the larynx and thus the lungs.

larynx Also referred to as the voice box. The vocal cords are located here.

trachea Also referred to as the windpipe. It branches into the bronchi.

bronchi Tubular structures which branch off the trachea.

pleura Membrane surrounding the lung. It contains two layers, one covers the lungs and the other lines the chest cavity.

diaphragm Separates the thoracic and abdominal cavities.

inspiration/inhalation Diaphragm and intercostal muscles contract. Air is drawn into the lungs.

expiration/exhalation Opposite of inspiration, as the diaphragm and intercostals muscles relax, air is pushed out of the lungs.

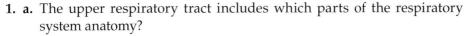
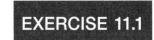

11.2 ICD Chapter-Specific Guidelines and Format of the Respiratory System Subsection

Some common diseases coded to the Respiratory subsection of ICD are asthma, bronchitis, chronic obstructive pulmonary disease (COPD), emphysema, influenza, pneumonia, respiratory failure, and tuberculosis (TB). When coding these conditions, coders must thoroughly review the provider documentation as well as the guidelines and instructional notes.

ICD-9-CM: The Respiratory section is Chapter 8 in the ICD-9-CM manual, with the code range 460–519.

ICD-10-CM: The Respiratory section is Chapter 10 within the ICD-10-CM manual, with the code range J00–J99.

Table 11.2 lists the Respiratory section subheadings and their code ranges.

Table 11.2 ICD Respiratory System Subheadings *(Data from ICD-9-CM and ICD-10-CM, Centers for Medicare and Medicaid Services and the National Center for Health Statistics.)*

ICD-9-CM		ICD-10-CM	
SUBHEADING	CODE RANGE	SUBHEADING	CODE RANGE
Acute Respiratory Infections	460–466	Acute Upper Respiratory Infections	J00–J06
		Other Acute Lower Respiratory Infections	J20–J22
Other Diseases of the Upper Respiratory Tract	470–478	Other Diseases of the Upper Respiratory Tract	J30–J39
Pneumonia and Influenza	480–488	Influenza and Pneumonia	J09–J18
Chronic Obstructive Pulmonary Disease and Allied Conditions	490–496	Chronic Lower Respiratory Diseases	J40–J47
Pneumoconioses and Other Lung Diseases due to External Agents	500–508	Lung Disease due to External Agents	J60–J70

(continued)

Table 11.2 ICD Respiratory System Subheadings (*concluded*)

ICD-9-CM		ICD-10-CM	
SUBHEADING	**CODE RANGE**	**SUBHEADING**	**CODE RANGE**
Other Diseases of the Respiratory System	510–519	Other Respiratory Diseases Principally Affecting the Interstitium	J80–J84
		Suppurative and Necrotic Conditions of the Lower Respiratory Tract	J85–J86
		Other Diseases of the Pleura	J90–J94
		Other Diseases of the Respiratory System	J96–J99
		Intraoperative and Postprocedural Complications and Disorders of Respiratory System, Not Elsewhere Classified	J95

Acute Respiratory Infections (460–466), ICD-9-CM
Acute Upper Respiratory Infections (J00–J06), ICD-10-CM
Other Acute Respiratory Infections (J20–J22), ICD-10-CM

Acute bronchitis An inflammation, due to an infectious organism or irritant, of the bronchus, the main branch of the bronchial tube.

Acute bronchiolitis An inflammation, due to an infectious organism or irritant, of the smaller branches of the bronchial tree.

In ICD-10-CM sub-category acute bronchitis and bronchiolitis is now included in the category "Other acute lower respiratory infections" (J20–J22).

These sections include codes used to identify respiratory infections that are severe in nature and sudden in onset, that is, infections known as *acute*. Although pneumonia and influenza are not coded to this code range, these sections do contain the codes to be reported for conditions such as the following:

- Acute nasopharyngitis, also known as "the common cold," is category 460 (J00, ICD-10-CM).
- Acute sinusitis is category 461 (J01, ICD-10-CM), which is further divided based on the sinus cavity and includes infections, inflammation, and empyema of the sinuses.
- Acute pharyngitis may also be documented as *sore throat*. Both viral and bacterial forms of pharyngitis are coded to 462 (J02.-, ICD-10-CM). An additional code should be assigned if the infectious agent is known.
- Acute tonsillitis is category 463 (J03.-, ICD-10-CM).
- Acute laryngitis and tracheitis—a severe inflammation of either the larynx, trachea, or epiglottis due to an infection—is coded to category 464 (J04.- and J05.-, ICD-10-CM). The condition is further defined by the anatomical site and the presence of obstruction of the site.
- Acute upper respiratory infection of multiple or unspecified sites is category 465 (J06.-, ICD-10-CM).
- Acute bronchitis and bronchiolitis are coded to category 466 (J20.- and J21.-, ICD-10-CM). The category is further defined by the condition, bronchitis or bronchiolitis, and the infectious organism.

Be careful to watch for *excludes* notes in these categories of codes. Often during the CPC exam, since time is a factor, coders will choose what they think is the appropriate code and move on without checking the instructional notes.

Other Diseases of the Upper Respiratory Tract (470–478), ICD-9-CM

Other Diseases of the Upper Respiratory Tract (J30–J39), ICD-10-CM

The upper respiratory tract includes all the respiratory system structures at or above the larynx. These structures are lined with mucous membrane and begin at the nasal cavity and includes the sinus cavities, middle ear, and eustachian tube. These sections contain codes to be reported for conditions such as the following:

- Deviated septum is coded to category 470 (J34.2, ICD-10-CM).
- Nasal polyps are coded to category 471 (J33.-, ICD-10-CM) and are further defined by the site of the polyp(s).
- Chronic pharyngitis and nasopharyngitis are persistent inflammations of the pharynx and/or nasopharynx and are coded to category 472 (J31.-, ICD-10-CM).
- Chronic sinusitis is a persistent inflammatory condition of the sinuses and, like acute sinusitis, is coded to the anatomical site of the condition. See category 473 (J32.-, ICD-10-CM).

  The sinus cavities and their locations are shown in Figure 11.3.

- Chronic diseases of tonsils and adenoids are coded to category 474 (J35.-, ICD-10-CM). The codes are further defined by the anatomical structure and conditions such as inflammation or hypertrophy.
- Peritonsillar abscess is tonsillitis that has extended beyond the tonsils to the soft palate and/or structures around the tonsils. It is coded to category 475 (J36, ICD-10-CM).

ICD-10-CM requires the identification of the organism causing sinusitis or tonsillitis. ICD-10-CM has a new subcategory to report acute recurrent sinusitis.

maxillary sinus Cavity in the skull which opens into the nasal cavity located under the eyes within the maxillary bone.

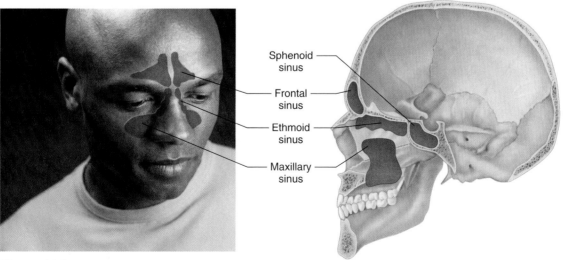

Sphenoid sinus
Frontal sinus
Ethmoid sinus
Maxillary sinus

Figure 11.3 Sinus Cavities

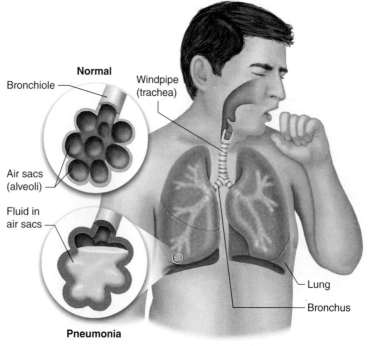

- Chronic laryngitis and laryngotracheitis are coded to category 476 (J37.-, ICD-10-CM) and are further defined by the structures involved.
- Allergic rhinitis may also be documented as hay fever or chronic rhinitis and is coded to category 477 (J30.1- through J30.9, ICD-10-CM). The codes are further defined by the cause of the condition.
- "Other diseases of upper respiratory tract," category 478, includes a variety of respiratory conditions such as paralysis of the vocal cords, stenosis of the larynx, and cellulitis.

Pneumonia and Influenza (480–488), ICD-9-CM
Influenza and Pneumonia (J09–J18), ICD-10-CM

Pneumonia is an inflammatory condition of the lungs affecting the alveoli by filling the air space with fluid (see Figure 11.4). There are numerous causes of pneumonia, and ICD classifies this condition according to its underlying cause. Categories of pneumonia included in these sections are:

- Viral pneumonia, 480 (J12, ICD-10-CM)
- Pneumococcal pneumonia, 481 (J13, ICD-10-CM)
- Other bacterial pneumonia, 482 (J14, ICD-10-CM)
- Pneumonia due to other specified organism, 483 (J16, ICD-10-CM)
- Pneumonia in infectious diseases classified elsewhere, 484 (J16–J17, ICD-10-CM)
- Bronchopneumonia, organism unspecified, 485 (J18, ICD-10-CM)
- Pneumonia, organism unspecified, 486 (J18.9, ICD-10-CM)

Excludes some types of pneumonia such as allergic, aspiration, and rheumatic.

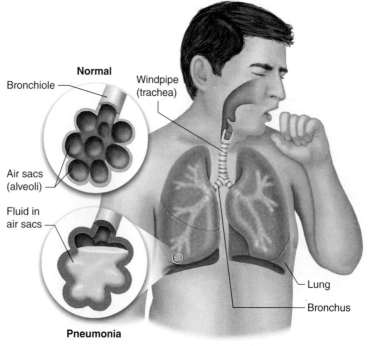

Normal
Bronchiole
Windpipe (trachea)

Air sacs (alveoli)

Fluid in air sacs

Lung

Bronchus

Pneumonia

Figure 11.4 Pneumonia

Also included in these sections is influenza. An acute respiratory infection, influenza is caused by orthomyxoviruses. The condition may present as a mild upper respiratory "cold" or may progress to pneumonia. ICD categorizes influenza as:

- Influenza, 487 (J11, ICD-10-CM)
- Influenza due to certain identified influenza viruses, 488 (J09, ICD-10-CM)

Influenza Chapter-Specific Guidelines

The ICD-9-CM guidelines state: "Code only confirmed cases of avian influenza (488.01–488.02, 488.09), or novel H1N1 influenza virus (H1N1 or swine flu, 488.11–488.12, 488.19)."

The confirmation can be based on a provider documentation statement that the patient has avian or novel H1N1 (H1N1 or swine flu) influenza. Suspected or probable documentation of these conditions would take the coder to category 487 ("Influenza") versus the more specific category 488 ("Influenza due to identified avian influenza virus").

Chronic Obstructive Pulmonary Disease and Allied Conditions (490–496), ICD-9-CM
Chronic Lower Respiratory Diseases (J40–J47), ICD-10-CM

Chronic obstructive pulmonary disease, or COPD, is a group of conditions, each of which causes persistent difficulty in exhaling air from the lungs.

These sections contain codes to be reported for each of these conditions, such as:

- Bronchitis, not specified as acute or chronic, 490 (J40, ICD-10-CM)
- Chronic bronchitis, 491 (J41–J42, ICD-10-CM)
- Emphysema, 492 (J43, ICD-10-CM)
- Asthma, 493 (J45, ICD-10-CM)
- Bronchiectasis, 494 (J47, ICD-10-CM)
- Extrinsic allergic alveolitis, 495
- Chronic airway obstruction, not elsewhere classified, 496 (J44.9, ICD-10-CM)

COPD and Asthma Chapter-Specific Guidelines

According to the ICD-9-CM guidelines, chronic obstructive pulmonary disease comprises obstructive chronic bronchitis and emphysema. Code 496 (chronic airway obstruction) should be reported only when the specific type of COPD being treated is *not* provided in the documentation. In ICD-9-CM, asthma is reported using category 493. There are many overlapping conditions pertaining to asthma and COPD. Both ICD-9-CM and ICD-10-CM distinguish between uncomplicated cases of asthma and those with acute exacerbations.

> **FOR EXAMPLE** Chronic asthma with acute exacerbation of COPD is reported as 493.22 (ICD-9-CM) or J44.1 (ICD-10-CM). ∎

> **SPOTLIGHT** on a Guideline
>
> The ICD guidelines state: "An acute exacerbation is a worsening or a decompensation of a chronic condition. An acute exacerbation is not equivalent to an infection superimposed on a chronic condition, though an exacerbation may be triggered by an infection." ICD-10-CM further defines asthma as mild, moderate, or severe.

COPD and Chronic Bronchitis Chapter-Specific Guidelines

Under the ICD-9-CM guidelines, when acute bronchitis is documented with COPD, code 491.22 would be reported. Code 466, acute bronchitis, would *not* be also reported since the acute bronchitis is included in code 491.22. For acute bronchitis with COPD with an acute exacerbation, only code 491.22 should be reported.

Pneumoconioses and Other Lung Diseases due to External Agents (500–508), ICD-9-CM
Lung Disease due to External Agents (J60–J70), ICD-10-CM

These sections contain codes to be reported for conditions related to occupational or environmental exposure to airborne agents that results in respiratory conditions such as:

- Coal worker's pneumoconiosis (also referred to as *black lung disease, coal worker's lung,* and *miner's asthma*), 500 (J60, ICD-10-CM)
- Asbestosis, 501 (J61, ICD-10-CM)
- Pneumoconiosis due to:
  - Other silica or silicates, 502 (J62.-, ICD-10-CM)
  - Other inorganic dust, 503 (J63.-, ICD-10-CM)
- Pneumonopathy due to inhalation of other dust, 504 (J66, ICD-10)
- Respiratory conditions due to chemical fumes and vapors, 506 (J68.-, ICD-10-CM) (The codes within this category are further defined by the condition resulting from the exposure.)
- Pneumonitis due to solids and liquids, 507 (J69, ICD-10-CM)
- Respiratory condition due to other and unspecified external agents, 508 (J70.-, ICD-10-CM)

> **SPOTLIGHT** on Condition
>
> **Pneumonia** Infectious inflammation of lung tissue.
>
> **Pneumonitis** Noninfectious inflammation of lung tissue.

Other Diseases of the Respiratory System (510–519), ICD-9-CM

Other Respiratory Diseases Principally Affecting the Interstitium (J80–J84), ICD-10-CM

Suppurative and Necrotic Conditions of the Lower Respiratory Tract (J85–J86), ICD-10-CM

Other Diseases of the Pleura (J90–J94), ICD-10-CM

Other Diseases of the Respiratory System (J96–J99), ICD-10-CM

These sections contain codes to be reported for conditions such as:

- Empyema, a condition that results in pus in the pleural space, is coded to category 510 (J86.-, ICD-10-CM).
- Pleurisy is category 511. (R09.1, ICD-10-CM) The conditions included in this category are further defined by the underlying cause.
- Pneumothorax is category 512 (J93, ICD-10-CM), with codes defined by the type of pneumothorax and the underlying cause.
- Abscess of lung and mediastinum is coded to category 513 (J85, ICD-10-CM).
- Pulmonary congestion and hypostasis are category 514 (J81, ICD-10-CM).
- Postinflammatory pulmonary fibrosis is coded to category 515 (J84.10, ICD-10-CM).
- Other alveolar and parietoalveolar pneumonopathy is category 516 (J84.09, ICD-10-CM).
- Lung involvement in conditions classified elsewhere is category 517 Other diseases of the lung are coded to category 518, which includes a variety of conditions affecting the lungs that have not been classified elsewhere, such as:
  - Pulmonary collapse
  - Acute edema of the lung, unspecified (acute pulmonary edema)
  - Pulmonary insufficiency following trauma and surgery
  - Transfusion-related acute lung injury (TRALI)
  - Acute respiratory failure
  - Chronic respiratory failure
- Other diseases of the respiratory system are coded to category 519 (J96–J99, ICD-10-CM), which includes conditions such as:
  - Tracheostomy complications
  - Acute bronchospasm
  - Mediastinitis
  - Disorders of the diaphragm

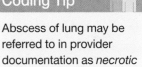

MENTOR
Coding Tip

Abscess of lung may be referred to in provider documentation as *necrotic pneumonia* or *acute necrotizing pneumonia* and is reported as ICD-9-CM code 513.0.

SPOTLIGHT on a Guideline

According to the ICD-9-CM guidelines, the sequencing of respiratory failure codes follows chapter-specific guidelines, with the guidelines for obstetrics, poisoning, HIV, and newborn taking precedence.

1. **a.** Identify what the abbreviation *VAP* stands for, and assign the appropriate ICD-9-CM code.

   b. What instruction is given to the coder by the instructional note included with the ICD-9-CM code?

2. **a.** List the other ways that abscess of the lung may be referred to in provider documentation.

   b. Select the appropriate ICD-9-CM code for this condition.

3. Explain the difference between the definition of pneumonia and that of pneumonitis.

4. Select the appropriate ICD-9-CM code for acute bronchitis with COPD with an acute exacerbation.

5. Define *acute exacerbation*.

6. **a.** Hypoxia is not inherent to COPD and can be reported with an additional code if it is documented in the medical record. Assign the appropriate ICD-9-CM code for documented hypoxia.

   b. Is hypoxia reported in addition to acute respiratory failure?

Also available in

MENTOR Coding Tip

Category 513 states "abscess of lung and mediastinum." The meaning of *and* in ICD is "and/or"; therefore, this category is used for abscess of the lung *and/or* mediastinum.

11.3 Guidelines and Format of the Respiratory Subsection of CPT

The Respiratory System subsection of the CPT manual is formatted by anatomical site from nose to lungs The section has numerous endoscopic codes that are located under specific anatomical subheadings. As with other surgery subsections, there are specific guidelines regarding endoscopic procedures. When a diagnostic procedure is done and then surgical treatment is performed through the scope during the same operative session at the same anatomical site, only the surgical endoscopic procedure is reported.

A coder must be able to translate from the medical documentation the *type of exam,* such as indirect or direct, and the *approach* used, such as internal or external.

SPOTLIGHT on Terminology

Indirect examination Visualization using a mirror.

Direct examination Visualization using a rigid or fiber-optic endoscope.

External approach Through the skin.

Internal approach Through the respiratory system.

external approach Approach through the skin

internal approach Approach through the respiratory system

Table 11.3 Respiratory Subsection General Headings *(Data from CPT 2013. © 2013 American Medical Association. All rights reserved.)*

GENERAL HEADING	CODE RANGE
Nose	30000–30999
Accessory sinuses	31000–31299
Larynx	31300–31599
Trachea and bronchi	31600–31899
Lungs and pleura	32035–32999

There are several questions that a coder needs to ask when reading an operative report and coding a procedure from this section. The following questions will help the coder, when reading through the report, to understand what actually was done and how the procedure should be translated and coded:

- At which anatomical site was the procedure performed?
- Was the treatment for a traumatic injury (acute) or a medical condition (chronic)?
- Was the approach internal or external?
- What was the type of exam (e.g., indirect or direct)?
- Was the procedure performed at a single site or at multiple sites?

Respiratory System Subsection General Heading Code Ranges (30000–32999)

The general headings are listed in Table 11.3.

Respiratory Section Subheadings and Guidelines

The general headings may include the following subheadings:

- Incision
- Excision
- Introduction
- Removal/Removal of Foreign Body
- Repair
- Destruction
- Endoscopy
- Other Procedures

Nose (30000–30999)

Figure 11.5 shows the location of the nasal turbinates.

Incision: 30000–30020

The coder needs to know the approach used in order to use the codes in this section. If an external approach was used, the coder is instructed to use codes from the Integumentary System section (10060, 10140).

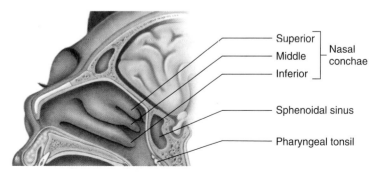

Figure 11.5 Nasal Turbinates

Excision: 30100–30160

Intranasal biopsies are coded 30100. An instructional note below this code refers the coder to the Integumentary System subsection for the appropriate code for biopsy of the skin of the nose.

Excision of nasal polyps is covered by codes 30110 to 30115, with the exact code dependent on whether the procedure is simple or extensive. The instructional notes tell the coder that 30110 (simple) is generally performed in an office setting and 30115 (extensive) is generally performed in a hospital setting.

MENTOR Coding Tip

Determining where the procedure was performed can help the coder toward determining the appropriate code: simple or extensive.

Excision of an inferior turbinate, partial or complete, by any method is coded 30130. This code has an instructional note that informs the coder to use 30999 for excision of a middle or superior turbinate. CPT code 30999 is an unlisted code, and the CPT manual specifically instructs the coder to use this code for procedures performed on the middle and superior turbinates; therefore, this instructional note appears throughout the section.

Introduction: 30200–30220

This subheading includes codes for therapeutic injection into the turbinates, displacement therapy, and insertion of a nasal septal prosthesis.

Removal of Foreign Body: 30300–30320

The distinction for codes is this section is whether the procedure is considered an office-type procedure or requires general anesthesia.

Repair: 30400–30630

Rhinoplasty codes are divided as follows:

- Primary, 30400–30420
- Secondary with:
  - Minor revision (small amount of nasal-tip work), 30430
  - Intermediate revision (bony work with osteotomies), 30435
  - Major revision (nasal-tip work and osteotomies), 30450
- Nasal deformity secondary to congenital cleft lip and/or palate, 30460–30462

Repair of nasal vestibular stenosis, code 30465, excludes obtaining the graft. In order to report the obtaining of the graft(s), see codes 20900 to 20926 and 21210. According to the CPT manual, this code reports a bilateral procedure; therefore, modifier 52 would be appended to 30465 if the procedure was performed unilaterally.

Destruction: 30801–30802

Codes in this subheading are used to report ablation of the soft tissue of inferior turbinates, superficial or intramural (submucosal). For ablation of middle or superior turbinates, the coder is directed to the unlisted code, 30999.

MENTOR
Coding Tip

Insertion of a nasal septal prosthesis could also be documented as *insertion of a septal button*.

Other Procedures: 30901–30999

The codes used to report control of **nasal hemorrhage (nasal bleeding, epistaxis)** are defined by:

Anterior nasal hemorrhage control

- Simple—limited cautery and/or packing
- Complex—extensive cautery and/or packing
  - Control nasal hemorrhage, *anterior, simple,* any method, 30901
  - Control nasal hemorrhage, *anterior, complex,* any method, 30903

Posterior nasal hemorrhage control

- Initial
- Subsequent:
  - Control nasal hemorrhage, *posterior,* with posterior nasal packs and/or cautery, any method; *initial,* 30905
  - Control nasal hemorrhage, *posterior,* with posterior nasal packs and/or cautery, any method; *subsequent,* 30906
- Therapeutic fracture of a nasal inferior turbinate may be performed to enlarge an obstructed nasal airway. The code for this is 30930.

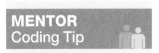

MENTOR Coding Tip

Control of bleeding during a procedure is a normal part of the procedure and is not reported separately. However, if a nasal hemorrhage occurs as a complication of a procedure, report the control procedure with modifier 78.

Accessory Sinuses (31000–31299)

This section includes codes for the paranasal sinuses, which include the:

- Frontal
- Maxillary
- Ethmoid
- Sphenoid

Incision: 31000–31090

Codes under this subheading are defined by these factors:

- Specific sinuses involved.
- With or without removal of polyps.
- With or without biopsy.
- With or without osteoplastic flap, brow or coronal incision.

Excision: 31200–31230

Codes under this subheading include codes for:

- Ethmoidectomy intranasal or extranasal, 31200–31205
- Maxillectomy with or without orbital exenteration, 31225–31230

nasal hemorrhage Nasal bleeding, epistaxis

anterior nasal hemorrhage control Insertion of gauze packing or anterior packing or cauterization.

posterior nasal hemorrhage control Procedure which often requires the use of nasal stents, balloon catheters, or posterior packing.

MENTOR Coding Tip

Orbital exenteration is used for treatment of malignancies of ocular tissues.

Endoscopy: 31231–31297

Codes 31231 to 31235 are used to report diagnostic nasal/sinus endoscopies and are further defined by the specific sinus.

Codes 31237 to 31297 are used to report surgical nasal/sinus endoscopies and are further defined by the specific sinus.

Larynx (31300–31599)

Excision: 31300–31420

The codes under this subheading describe procedures to remove the larynx and are defined by the extent of the procedure:

- Total laryngectomy, without and with radical neck dissection, 31360–31365
- Laryngectomy, subtotal supraglottic, without and with radical neck dissection, 31367–31368
- Partial laryngectomy, horizontal, laterovertical, anterovertical, antero-latero-vertical, 31370–31382:
  - *Laterovertical:* includes resection of vocal cord and adjacent cartilage
  - *Anterovertical:* includes resection of the thyroid cartilage and portions of both vocal cords
  - *Antero-latero-vertical:* includes resection of the vocal cords, thyroid, and a portion of the arytenoids
- Pharyngolaryngectomy with radical neck dissection, without or with reconstruction, 31390–31395

Introduction: 31500–31502

Intubation, endotracheal, as an emergency procedure falls under this subheading and is code 31500. This code is modifier 51 exempt.

Endoscopy: 31505–31579

The codes under this subheading are defined by the method of visualization of the larynx and the procedure performed.

Visualization may be:

Direct: through a scope.

Indirect: with a mirror to view the larynx.

Thus, the code entries include:

- Laryngoscopy, *indirect;* diagnostic, 31505
  with biopsy, 31510
  with removal of foreign body, 31511
  with removal of lesion, 31512
  with vocal cord injection, 31513

> **MENTOR**
> Coding Tip
>
> It is important to carefully read the full description of codes under this subheading.

- Laryngoscopy, *direct,* with or without tracheoscopy; for aspiration, 31515
  diagnostic, newborn, 31520
  diagnostic, except newborn, 31525
  diagnostic, with operating microscope or telescope, 31526
  with insertion of obturator, 31527
  with dilation, initial, 31528
  with dilation, subsequent, 31529

Direct therapeutic laryngoscopy codes are defined by the procedure performed and the use of the operating microscope during the procedure. Included in these codes are:

- Laryngoscopy, *direct,* operative with foreign body removal, 31530–31531
- Laryngoscopy, *direct,* operative with biopsy, 31535–31536
- Laryngoscopy, *direct,* operative with excision of tumor and/or stripping of vocal cords or epiglottis, 31540–31541
- Laryngoscopy, direct, operative, with operating microscope or telescope, with submucosal removal of nonneoplastic lesion(s) of vocal cord; reconstruction with local tissue flap(s), 31545
  reconstruction with graft(s), includes obtaining autograft, 31546
- Laryngoscopy, flexible fiberoptic; diagnostic, 31575
  with biopsy, 31576
  with removal of foreign body, 31577
  with removal of lesion, 31578
- Laryngoscopy, flexible or rigid fiber optic with stroboscopy, 31579

Repair: 31580–31590

Laryngoplasty codes are included under this subheading and are defined by the condition being treated and the method of the procedure.

Trachea and Bronchi (31600–31899)

Incision: 31600–31614

Tracheostomy codes are included under this subheading and are distinguished by planned, emergency, or fenestration procedure with skin flaps. Tracheal puncture and tracheostoma revision (simple or complex) are also reported using codes under this subheading.

Endoscopy: 31615–31651

Endoscopy performed of the trachea and bronchi involves the use of a scope inserted through the nose or mouth as a means of viewing the airway and as an approach to complete therapeutic procedures. According to CPT guidelines, codes 31622 to 31646 of this subheading include fluoroscopic guidance when performed.

- Bronchoscopy rigid or flexible; diagnostic, with cell washing, 31622
    with brushing or protected brushings, 31623
    with bronchial alveolar lavage, 31624
    with bronchial or endobronchial biopsy(s), single or multiple sites, 31625
    with placement of fiducial markers, single or multiple, 31626
    with computer-assisted, image-guided navigation, 31627
    with transbronchial lung biopsy(s), single lobe, 31628
    with transbronchial needle aspiration biopsy(s), trachea, main stem and/or lobar bronchus (i), 31629
    with tracheal/bronchial dilation or closed reduction of fracture, 31630
    with placement of tracheal stent(s), 31631
    with transbronchial lung biopsy(s), each additional lobe, 31632
    with transbronchial need aspiration biopsy(s), each additional lobe, 31633
    with balloon occlusion, 31634
    with removal of foreign body, 31635
    with placement of bronchial stents, 31636
    with revision of tracheal or bronchial stent inserted at previous session, 31638
    with excision of tumor, 31640
    with destruction of tumor or relief of stenosis by any method other than excision, 31641
    with placement of catheter(s) for intracavity radioelement, 31643
    with therapeutic aspiration of tracheobronchial tree, initial, 31645
    with therapeutic aspiration of tracheobronchial tree, subsequent, 31646

Introduction: 31717–31730

Codes under this subheading report introduction of a substance, such as a contrast medium or a catheter into or through the trachea or bronchi. Included under this subheading are codes used to report:

- Catheterization with bronchial brush biopsy, 31717
- Catheter aspiration; nasotracheal, 31720
    tracheobronchial with fiberscope, bedside, 31725
- Transtracheal introduction of needle wire dilator/stent or indwelling tube for oxygen therapy, 31730

Excision, Repair: 31750–31830

Procedures reported with codes under this subheading include:

- Tracheoplasty, 31750–31760
- Bronchoplasty; graft repair, 31770
    excision stenosis and anastomosis, 31775
- Excision tracheal stenosis or anastomosis, 31780–31781
- Excision tracheal tumor or carcinoma, 31785–31786

Lungs and Pleura (32035–32999)

Incision: 32035–32225

Thoracotomy procedures with biopsies are reported with codes from this subheading. Thoracotomy procedures with exploration are also described under this subheading.

Excision/Resection: 32310–32405

Percutaneous needle biopsies of the pleura, lung, or mediastinum are reported with codes from this subheading.

Removal: 32440–32540

Pneumocentesis and thoracentesis codes are located under this subheading, along with several codes for removal of a lung (pneumonectomy). There are multiple instructional notes within this subheading.

Introduction and Removal: 32550–32557

- Insertion of indwelling tunneled pleural catheter with cuff, 32550
- Tube thoracostomy, includes water seal, 32551
- Removal of indwelling tunneled pleural catheter with cuff, 32552
- Thoracentesis, needle or catheter, aspiration of the pleural space; without imaging guidance, 32554
- Thoracentesis, needle or catheter, aspiration of the pleural space, with imaging guidance, 32555
- Pleural drainage, percutaneous, with insertion of indwelling cathether; without imaging guidance, 32556
- Pleural drainage, percutaneous, with insertion of indwelling catheter with imaging guidance, 32557

Destruction: 32560–32562

- Instillation, via chest tube/catheter, agent for pleurodesis, 32560
- Instillation(s), via chest tube/catheter, agent for fibrinolysis; initial day, 32561
    subsequent day, 32562

Thoracoscopy (Video-Assisted Thoracic Surgery): 32601–32674

In the CPT manual, surgical thoracoscopy (VATS) always includes diagnostic thoracoscopy.

Lung Transplantation: 32850–32856

According to CPT, lung allotransplantation involves three distinct components of physician work:

- Cadaver donor pneumonectomy(s), 32850

SPOTLIGHT on a Guideline

If imaging guidance is performed, the CPT manual instructs the coder to use code 75989 from the Radiology section.

SPOTLIGHT on a Guideline

Code 32561 is reported only on the initial day of treatment, and 32562 is reported only once per day of each subsequent day of treatment.

- Back-bench work:
    Single lung, 32855
    Double lung, 32856
- Recipient lung allotransplantation, 32851–32854

The more familiar coders become with the format and guidelines, the better prepared they are for selecting the appropriate CPT code to be linked to the medically necessary diagnosis for the patient encounter.

1. What does a plus (+) sign in front of a CPT code mean about the code?
2. **a.** Code 31620 is an add-on code to be reported with which primary CPT codes?

   b. What is the meaning of the abbreviation EBUS as used in this code?
3. Assign the appropriate CPT code(s) for insertion of an indwelling tunneled pleural catheter with cuff with imaging guidance.
4. List the three distinct components of physician work that CPT includes in lung transplantation, and give the code or code ranges.
5. Assign the appropriate CPT code for catheter aspiration, tracheobronchial with fiberscope, bedside.

Also available in McGraw Hill **connect**™ (plus+)

11.4 Modifiers Most Commonly Used with Codes in the Respiratory Subsection

As with all sections of the CPT manual, modifiers are used in the Respiratory subsection to continue or modify the story of the patient's encounter. In the Respiratory subsection, modifiers are most commonly used to indicate bilateral procedures, reduced services, and multiple procedures (see Table 11.4).

The appropriate use of modifiers with the codes from the Respiratory System subsection will help to tell the patient's full story.

Table 11.4 Respiratory Subsection Modifiers *(Data from CPT 2013. © 2013 American Medical Association. All rights reserved.)*

MODIFIER	DEFINITION	EXAMPLE
50	Bilateral procedure	*Code 30115:* excision nasal polyp(s), extensive. To report a bilateral procedure: 30115–50. *Code 30901:* Control nasal hemorrhage anterior, simple, any method. To report a bilateral procedure: 30901–50.
51	Multiple procedures	Several codes in this section are modifier 51 exempt, for example, 31500.
52	Reduced service	*Code 30465:* repair of nasal vestibular stenosis. Since this code reports a bilateral procedure, modifier 52 would be amended to 30465 if the procedure was performed unilaterally.

SPOTLIGHT on a Guideline

Both examples are instructional notations beneath the CPT codes in the CPT manual.

1. Explain modifier 50, and give an example of its use in the Respiratory System subsection of CPT.

2. Explain modifier 51, and give an example of its use in the Respiratory System subsection of CPT.

3. Explain modifier 52, and give an example of its use in the Respiratory System subsection of CPT.

4. Explain modifier 78, and determine whether it is a modifier that would be used with codes from the Respiratory subsection of CPT.

5. Explain modifier 59, and determine whether it is a modifier that would be used with codes from the Respiratory subsection of CPT.

Also available in [Mc Graw Hill] **connect** (plus+)

11.5 Common Medical and Procedural Terms Used in Operative Reports

As with all sections of CPT, the Respiratory subsection includes medical terms and procedural terms that are specific to the system involved. Tables 11.5 and 11.6 list some of these terms and identify some key terms that could appear in a provider's documentation.

indirect laryngoscopy
Visualization of the larynx by means of a mirror positioned at the back of the throat.

direct laryngoscopy
Visualization of the larynx by means of a rigid or fiber optic endoscope.

Table 11.5 Terms for Respiratory System

TERM	DEFINITION	DOCUMENTATION KEYS
Arterial blood gas	Examination of arterial blood for levels of oxygen, carbon dioxide, or other gases	ABG
Aspirate	Foreign material drawn into the lungs or withdrawn from the lungs for diagnostic or therapeutic reasons	Fluid or tissue
Biopsy	Removal of all or part of a lesion for pathologic examination	Incisional, excisional, needle aspiration, punch, shave
Bronchoscopy	Bronch/o = bronchi; scopy = visual examination of a cavity	Direct airway visualization, diagnostic or therapeutic
Carboxyhemoglobin measurement	Test that measures the amount of carbon monoxide and hemoglobin in blood	Diagnosis and management of carbon monoxide poisoning
Incision	Creation of an opening by surgically cutting into the skin or other tissue	-otomy
Laryngoscopy	Visual examination of the larynx with a scope	**Indirect laryngoscopy:** Visualization of the larynx using a mirror positioned at the back of the throat **Direct laryngoscopy:** Visualization using a rigid or fiber-optic endoscope
Oximetry	Ox/o = oxygen -metry = measure	Measurement of oxygen saturation of the blood

(continued)

Table 11.5 Terms for Respiratory System (*concluded*)

TERM	DEFINITION	DOCUMENTATION KEYS
-plasty	Reshaping or replacing by surgical means	Repair, reconstruction, revision, augmentation
Pneumonectomy	Surgical removal of a lung	pneum/o = lung; ectomy = excision
Repair	Restoration of diseased or damaged tissue	Suture, revision, restore
Spirometry	Spir/o = breathing; -metry = measure	Measurement of breathing or lung volume
Ventilation/perfusion scan	Nuclear medicine study pertaining to air and blood flow to the lungs	V/Q scan

Table 11.6 Additional Terms for Respiratory System

TERM	DEFINITION	DOCUMENTATION KEYS
Adult respiratory distress syndrome (ARDS)	Also defined as acute respiratory distress syndrome. Some symptoms are shortness of breath, tachypnea, hypoxia, and confusion. ARDS can be triggered by trauma burns, or acute illness such as sepsis	Capillary leak syndrome. *Spotlight on Guideline:* ARDS is coded to 518.82 if it is unrelated to trauma or procedure. If it is related to trauma or procedure, codes from subcategory 518.5 would be indicated.
Asthma	Condition in which the airways are hypersensitive and react to inhaled irritants by narrowing or obstructing	*Status asthmaticus,* intractable asthma, refractory asthma. Severe intractable wheezing, airway obstruction not relieved by medication. *Mentor Coding Tip:* Do not assume status asthmaticus is present. Conditions of acute exacerbation and *status asthmaticus* are not assigned together.
Atelectasis	Atel/o = incomplete; ectasis = expansion, dilation Incomplete expansion of the lungs	Trauma, disease, and postop complications are some of the common causes.
Chronic obstructive pulmonary disorder (COPD)	Group of conditions, each of which results in obstruction of the airway. *Spotlight on Guideline: Always* check for a more definite diagnosis.	Chronic obstructive bronchitis or emphysema.
Continuous positive airway pressure (CPAP)	CPAP uses mild pressure to keep the airway from collapsing or blocking.	Treatment is often for sleep apnea.
Dyspnea	Difficulty breathing	Exertional dyspnea: Dyspnea brought on by physical effort or exertion. **Functional dyspnea:** Respiratory distress not related to exertion and not related to organic disease; often related to anxiety. Paroxysmal nocturnal dyspnea: Respiratory distress often associated with congestive heart failure with pulmonary edema; usually occurs during reclining at night.

Table 11.6 Additional Terms for Respiratory System (*concluded*)

TERM	DEFINITION	DOCUMENTATION KEYS
Epistaxis	Discharge of blood from the nose	Nosebleed, rhinorrhagia.
Pneumonia	Inflammation of the lungs caused by an organism	Bacteria, viruses, fungi, and parasites are common causes.
Rales	Abnormal chest sounds	Congested or spasmodic bronchi are often the cause.
Severe acute respiratory syndrome (SARS)	Severe viral infection of the lungs	Some symptoms are high fever, a dry cough, and difficulty breathing. Its mode of transmission is airborne.

EXERCISE 11.5

1. What does the abbreviation *ABG* stand for?
2. List the different types of biopsies that can be coded within the Respiratory System subsection of CPT.
3. What is the meaning of the abbreviation *ARDS,* and what is another term for this condition that could be used in the documentation?
4. Break the word *spirometry* into its parts, and define the word.
5. What is a V/Q scan?

Also available in Mc Graw Hill connect™ (plus+)

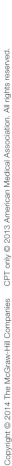

Chapter Eleven Summary

Learning Outcome	Key Concepts/Examples
11.1 Review the anatomy of the respiratory system.	The respiratory system is divided into the upper and lower respiratory tracts. The upper respiratory tract includes the nose, sinuses, pharynx, and larynx, and the lower respiratory system includes the trachea (windpipe), bronchial tubes, and lungs. *Flow of air through the respiratory system:* enters → nose (through the nasal cavities) → paranasal sinuses → pharynx → larynx → trachea → bronchi → lungs
11.2 Understand the chapter-specific ICD guidelines and format for the respiratory system.	Some common diseases coded to the Respiratory chapter of ICD are asthma, bronchitis, COPD, emphysema, influenza, pneumonia, respiratory failure, and TB. When coding these conditions, coders must thoroughly review the provider documentation as well as the guidelines and instructional notes.
11.3 Identify the guidelines and format of the Respiratory subsection of CPT.	The Respiratory System subsection of the CPT manual is formatted by anatomical site from nose to lungs. The section has numerous endoscopic codes that are located under specific anatomical subheadings. A coder must be able to translate from the medical documentation the *type of exam,* such as indirect or direct, and the *approach* used, such as internal or external.
11.4 Apply the modifiers most commonly used with codes in the Respiratory subsection.	Modifiers are used in the Respiratory subsection to continue or modify the story of the patient's encounter. In the Respiratory subsection, modifiers are most commonly used to indicate bilateral procedures, reduced services, multiple procedures, and/or two surgeons performing distinct parts of a single procedure.
11.5 Examine the common medical and procedural terms used in operative reports.	The Respiratory subsection includes medical terms and procedural terms that are specific to the system. There are also some key terms that could appear in a provider's documentation and act as a trigger for the coder to identify the diagnosis and/or procedure for the encounter.

Chapter Eleven Review

Using Terminology

Match each key term to the appropriate definition.

_____ 1. [LO11.1] Alveoli

_____ 2. [LO11.3] Anterior nasal hemorrhage control

_____ 3. [LO11.1] Bronchi

_____ 4. [LO11.5] Direct laryngoscopy

_____ 5. [LO11.1] Ethmoid sinus

A. Visualization of the larynx by means of a mirror positioned at the back of the throat

B. Nasal bleeding, epistaxis

C. Visualization by means of a rigid or fiber-optic endoscope

D. Insertion of gauze packing or anterior packing or cauterization

E. Procedure that often requires the use of nasal stents, balloon catheters, or posterior packing

F. Tiny air sacs that are located at the end of the bronchioles and through which oxygen and carbon dioxide pass

_____ 6. **[LO11.1]** Epiglottis

_____ 7. **[LO11.3]** External approach

_____ 8. **[LO11.5]** Indirect laryngoscopy

_____ 9. **[LO11.3]** Internal approach

_____ 10. **[LO11.1]** Larynx

_____ 11. **[LO11.3]** Nasal hemorrhage

_____ 12. **[LO11.1]** Pharynx

_____ 13. **[LO11.3]** Posterior nasal hemorrhage control

_____ 14. **[LO11.1]** Sphenoid sinus

_____ 15. **[LO11.1]** Trachea

G. Tubular structure that branches into smaller tubes called *bronchioles*

H. Cavity in the skull that opens into the nasal cavity between the nose and the eyes

I. Small flap of cartilage that closes over the trachea

J. Approach through the skin

K. Structure that is also referred to as the *voice box*

L. Approach through the respiratory system

M. Cavity in the skull that opens into the nasal cavity in the center of the skull base

N. Structure that connects the nose and the mouth to the larynx

O. Structure that is also referred to as the *windpipe*

Checking Your Understanding

Choose the most appropriate answer for each of the following questions.

1. [LO11.5] A pneumonectomy involves surgical removal of the:

a. Alveoli

b. Pleura

c. Lungs

d. Trachea

2. [LO11.5] Which test measures the amount of carbon monoxide and hemoglobin in the blood and is used to diagnose and manage carbon monoxide poisoning?

a. CXR

b. Pulmonary function test

c. Oximetry

d. Carboxyhemoglobin

3. [LO11.5] The use of a lighted endoscope to view the pleural spaces and thoracic cavity or to perform a surgical procedure is called:

a. Endoscopy

b. Bronchoscopy

c. Thoracentesis

d. Thoracotomy

4. [LO11.1] The pleura is made up of two layers, and the space between the layers is referred to as the:

a. Glottis

b. Pleural Space

c. Peritoneum

d. None of these

5. [LO11.5] The term that identifies the measurement of oxygen saturation of the blood is:

a. Oximetry

b. Spirometry

c. ABG

d. CPAP

6. [LO11.2] According to ICD guidelines, an acute exacerbation is a worsening or a _____ of a chronic condition. An acute exacerbation is not equivalent to an infection superimposed on a chronic condition, although an exacerbation may be _____ by an infection.

a. deterioration; prompted

b. compensation; enabled

c. decompensation; triggered

d. degeneration; lessened

7. [LO11.2] In coding pharyngitis using the ICD-10-CM manual, the identification of the _____ causing the pharyngitis must be documented and reported.

a. organism

b. cause

c. onset

d. duration

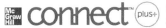 plus+ Enhance your learning by completing these exercises and more at mcgrawhillconnect.com

8. [LO11.3] Assign the correct code for ablation of the soft tissue of the superior turbinate, bilateral by electrocautery, superficial:

a. 30801   c. 30802

b. 30999   d. 30901

9. [LO11.3] Assign the appropriate code for drainage of a nasal abscess by an internal approach:

a. 30000   c. 10140

b. 10060   d. 30020

10. [LO11.3] Assign the appropriate code(s) for a percutaneous needle biopsy of the lung with ultrasound guidance:

a. 32405   c. 32405, 76942

b. 32400   d. 10022

Applying Your Knowledge

Code the following case studies by answering the questions using the process steps as illustrated in Chapter 8.

Case Studies [LO 11.1–11.5] Case 1

Preoperative diagnosis: Tracheal stenosis, subglottic

Postoperative diagnosis: Same

Procedure performed: Fiber-optic bronchoscopy

Surgeon: Stine, Frank, MD

Indications: Tracheal stenosis

Details of the procedure, and potential risks and alternatives, were explained, and patient consent was obtained.

Medications: Xylocaine spray was applied to the throat and Xylocaine gel placed in the nostrils. The patient received 50 mcg of fentanyl and 8 mg of Versed intravenous.

Procedure: The bronchoscope was placed orally once sufficient sedation was obtained. The vocal cords were visualized, and the patient appeared to have some right true vocal cord weakness. Just below the vocal cords, in the subglottic area, scar tissue was noted and moderate narrowing of the upper trachea with almost complete closure of the airway on exhalation. Airways were immediately examined. The trachea; carina; right upper-, middle-, and lower-lobe bronchi; and left main stem bronchus and upper- and lower-lobe bronchi were examined and found to be normal and without significant mucosal abnormalities. The patient tolerated the procedure well. No specimens were collected.

Process 1: CPT

1. What is the procedure?

2. Locate the main term in the index. What additional questions or set of questions can be determined?

3. Upon review of all the code choices identified in the index, what additional questions can be determined?

4. Based on the documentation, what is (are) the correct code(s) for this case?

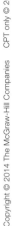

Process 2: ICD

ICD-9-CM

1. Based on the operative report header, what is the preoperative diagnosis?

2. Is the postoperative diagnosis the same as or different from the preoperative diagnosis?

3. Is the postoperative diagnosis supported?

4. What is the main term for this condition?

5. Based on the subterm choices, what question(s) can be developed for this condition?

6. Is any sign, symptom, or additional condition documented?

7. Is the additional condition, sign, or symptom an integral part of the primary (or other) condition coded?

8. Does the additional condition require or affect patient care, treatment, or management?

9. Based on the documentation, what is (are) the correct ICD-9-CM code(s) for this case?

ICD-10-CM

1. Based on the operative report header, what is the preoperative diagnosis?

2. Is the postoperative diagnosis the same as or different from the preoperative diagnosis?

3. Is the postoperative diagnosis supported?

4. What is the main term for this condition?

5. Based on the subterm choices, what question(s) can be developed for this condition?

6. Based on the information in the Tabular List, is additional information needed to determine the appropriate diagnosis code?

7. Is any sign, symptom, or additional condition documented?

8. Is the additional condition, sign, or symptom an integral part of the primary (or other) condition coded?

9. Does the additional condition require or affect patient care, treatment, or management?

10. Based on the documentation, what is (are) the correct ICD-10-CM code(s) for this case?

Process 3: Modifiers

1. Was the procedure performed different from that described by the nomenclature of the code?

2. Was the procedure performed at an anatomical site that has laterality?

3. Was the procedure performed in the global period of another procedure?

4. Were additional procedures performed during the operative session, and does the documentation support them?

5. Did the surgeon have help from another surgeon or another appropriate person?

6. Did a physician different from the surgeon provide the preoperative or postoperative portion of the procedure?

7. What modifier(s) should be appended to the CPT code for this case?

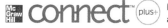
Enhance your learning by completing these exercises and more at mcgrawhillconnect.com

Preoperative diagnosis: Pulmonary infiltrates, bilateral

Postoperative diagnoses: Bilateral pneumonia and tracheobronchitis, diffuse

Procedure performed: Bronchoscopy with biopsy

Surgeon: Harold Potter, MD

Anesthesia: Conscious sedation was provided and monitored by Dr. H. Granger, anesthesiologist

Specimens gathered and sent to pathology include:

Bronchoalveolar lavage and bronchial brushings sent for cytology.

Bronchial washings sent to pathology for culture, Gram stain, C&S, and DFA for Legionella.

Transbronchial biopsies for pathology.

Findings: Trachea of this 61-year-old man was within normal limits. There appeared to be mild diffuse tracheobronchitis from the level of the carina and extending throughout the right and left bronchial trees. No endobronchial lesions or mucosal irregularities were found. During lavage of the left lower lobe, yellow purulent mucous plugs were aspirated. All mucous plugs were cleared upon completion of the lavage procedure.

Procedure: The patient was brought to the endoscopy suite, and local anesthesia of the left naris and posterior pharynx was administered, followed by conscious sedation. After adequate conscious sedation was achieved, the Olympus bronchofiberscope was inserted into the left naris and advanced to the posterior pharynx through the vocal cords and into the trachea. The entire tracheobronchial tree was then systematically inspected. The bronchoscope was advanced to the left upper lobe, and the bronchoscope was wedged into the apical segment. Bronchoalveolar lavage was then performed at this segment, utilizing 80 mL of saline. The bronchoscope was then pulled back at the level of the carina and advanced into the left lower lobe. Bronchial brushings were obtained from the medial and lateral segments of the left lower lobe under fluoroscopic guidance. Under fluoroscopic guidance, transbronchial biopsies ×3 were obtained from various subsegments of both the left lower lobe and the left upper lobe. The areas were then inspected for any acute hemorrhage; none was seen. The bronchoscope was withdrawn. The patient tolerated the procedure well, without complications.

Process 1: CPT

1. What is the procedure?

2. Locate the main term in the index. What additional questions or set of questions can be determined?

3. Upon review of all the code choices identified in the index, what additional questions can be determined?

4. Based on the documentation, what are the correct codes for this case?

   a. 31628 × 3, 31632 × 3, 31624, 31623

   b. 31628, 31632, 31717, 31624

   c. 31629, 31633, 31624, 31623

   d. 31628, 31632, 31624, 31623

Process 2: ICD

ICD-9-CM

1. Based on the operative report header, what is the preoperative diagnosis?

2. Is the postoperative diagnosis the same as or different from the preoperative diagnosis?

3. Is the postoperative diagnosis supported?

4. What is the main term for this condition?

5. Based on the subterm choices, what question(s) can be developed for this condition?

6. Is any sign, symptom, or additional condition documented?

7. Is the additional condition, sign, or symptom an integral part of the primary (or other) condition coded?

8. Does the additional condition require or affect patient care, treatment, or management?

9. Based on the documentation, what are the correct ICD-9-CM codes for this case?
   a. 485, 466.0
   b. 486, 490
   c. 486, 466.0
   d. 483.8, 490

ICD-10-CM

1. Based on the operative report header, what is the preoperative diagnosis?

2. Is the postoperative diagnosis the same as or different from the preoperative diagnosis?

3. Is the postoperative diagnosis supported?

4. What is the main term for this condition?

5. Based on the subterm choices, what question(s) can be developed for this condition?

6. Based on the information in the Tabular List, is additional information needed to determine the appropriate diagnosis code?

7. Is any sign, symptom, or additional condition documented?

8. Is the additional condition, sign, or symptom an integral part of the primary (or other) condition coded?

9. Does the additional condition require or affect patient care, treatment, or management?

10. Based on the documentation, what are the correct ICD-10-CM codes for this case?
    a. J18.1, J40
    b. J18.0, J40
    c. J18.9, J20.9
    d. J18.9, J40

Process 3: Modifiers

1. Was the procedure performed different from that described by the nomenclature of the code?

2. Was the procedure performed at an anatomical site that has laterality?

3. Was the procedure performed in the global period of another procedure?

4. Were additional procedures performed during the operative session, and does the documentation support them?

5. Did the surgeon have help from another surgeon or another appropriate person?

6. Did a physician different from the surgeon provide the preoperative or postoperative portion of the procedure?

7. What modifier(s) should be appended to the CPT for this case?
   a. LT
   b. 51
   c. 50
   d. LT, 51

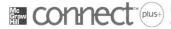

Enhance your learning by completing these exercises and more at mcgrawhillconnect.com

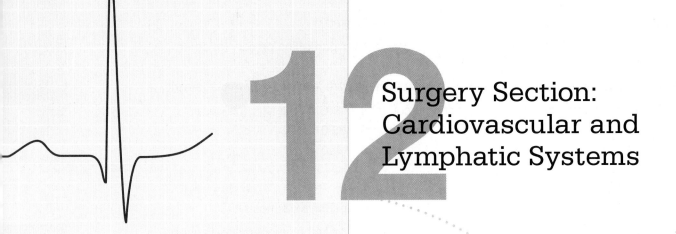

12 Surgery Section: Cardiovascular and Lymphatic Systems

Key Terms

Ablation

Aneurysm

Angina pectoris

Angiography

Aorta

Aortic valve

Arrhythmia

Conduction disorder

Coronary artery bypass graft (CABG)

Deep vein thrombosis (DVT)

Defibrillator

Embolus

Endocardium

Epicardium

Infarction

Irreversible ischemia

Lymph node

Mitral valve

Myocardium

Pericardium

Reversible ischemia

Septum

Stenosis

Thrombus

Tricuspid valve

Learning Outcomes

After completing this chapter, you will be able to:

12.1 Review the anatomy of the cardiovascular system.

12.2 Review the anatomy of the lymphatic system.

12.3 Understand chapter-specific ICD guidelines and format for the circulatory system.

12.4 Identify the guidelines and format of the Cardiovascular subsection of CPT.

12.5 Identify the guidelines and format of the Lymphatic subsection of CPT.

12.6 Apply the modifiers most commonly used with codes in the Cardiovascular subsections.

12.7 Examine the common medical and procedural terms used in operative reports.

Introduction The cardiovascular system's primary function is to nourish the body by transporting nutrients and oxygen to the cells and removing carbon dioxide and other waste products. When coding for services or procedures concerning the cardiovascular system, coders may need to select codes from the Evaluation and Management section, the Surgery section, the Radiology section, and the Medicine section. This chapter focuses on codes from the Surgery section. The lymphatic system's functions are to help maintain fluid balance, defend the body against disease, and absorb and transport liquids from blood vessels.

12.1 Anatomy of the Cardiovascular System

The cardiovascular system consists of the heart, blood, and blood vessels, which include arteries, veins, and capillaries. It includes the pulmonary circulation system, in which blood is pumped away from the heart by the pulmonary artery to the lungs and then returned to the heart by the pulmonary vein. The systemic circulation system transports oxygenated blood away from the heart, to the rest of the body, and returns oxygen-depleted blood back to the heart.

The major structures of the cardiovascular system are the heart, great vessels, coronary vessels, and peripheral blood vessels. (See Figures 12.1 to 12.4 and Table 12.1.)

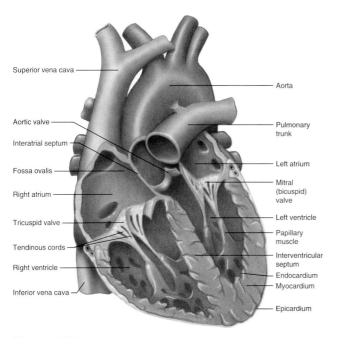

Figure 12.1 Internal Anatomy of the Heart

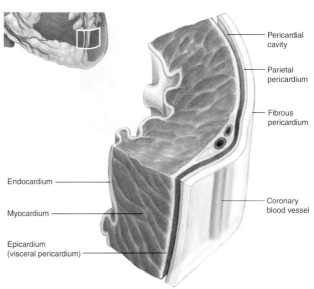

Figure 12.2 Pericardium and Heart Wall

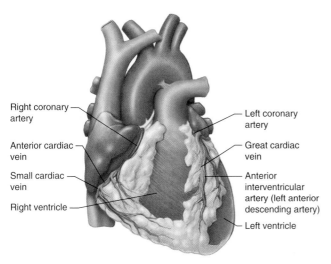

Figure 12.3 Anterior Coronary Circulation

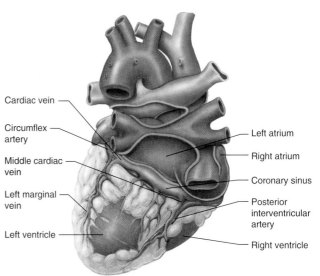

Figure 12.4 Posterior Coronary Circulation

Table 12.1 Structures of the Cardiovascular System

STRUCTURE	DEFINITION/FUNCTION
Heart:	Muscular, cone-shaped organ whose main function is to pump blood
Four chambers:	
Right and left atria Right and left ventricle	Pump deoxygenated blood (from the body) through the right atrium and the right ventricle (to the lungs), and pump oxygenated blood (from the lungs) through the left atrium and the left ventricle (to the body)
Septum	Wall dividing the right and left sides of the heart
Pericardium	Membrane sac that encases the heart
Heart-wall tissue layers:	
Epicardium	Outer layer of heart-wall tissue
Myocardium	Muscle layer of heart-wall tissue
Endocardium	Inner layer of heart-wall tissue
Great vessels:	
Superior vena cava	Largest vein which carries de-oxygenated blood from the head, neck, chest and upper extremities of the body back to the heart
Inferior vena cava	Largest vein which carries de-oxygenated blood from the back, abdomen, and pelvis, and lower extremities of the body back to the heart
Aorta	Largest artery; takes oxygenated blood from the left ventricle to the body
Pulmonary arteries	Carry deoxygenated blood from the right ventricle to the lungs
Pulmonary veins	Take oxygenated blood from the lungs to the left atrium
Peripheral blood vessels:	
Arteries:	Carry blood away from the heart
Layers (tunics) of artery walls:	
Tunica externa	Outer layer
Tunica media	Middle layer
Tunica intima	Inner layer
Arterioles	Smaller branches of arteries
Capillaries	Deliver oxygen and nutrients to cells and carbon dioxide and waste to venules
Veins:	Carry blood to the heart
Superficial veins	Located near the surface of the body
Deep veins	Located closer to arteries

septum The wall dividing the right and left sides of the heart.

epicardium The outer layer of the heart-wall tissue.

endocardium The inner layer of the heart-wall tissue.

aorta The largest artery; carries oxygenated blood from the left ventricle to the body.

MENTOR Coding Tip

Codes are often further defined by whether the vein is superficial or deep, so it is helpful to know which veins are considered superficial and which are considered deep. Often, the coding manual will help with this distinction.

(See Figures 12.5 and 12.6 for the peripheral arteries and veins.)

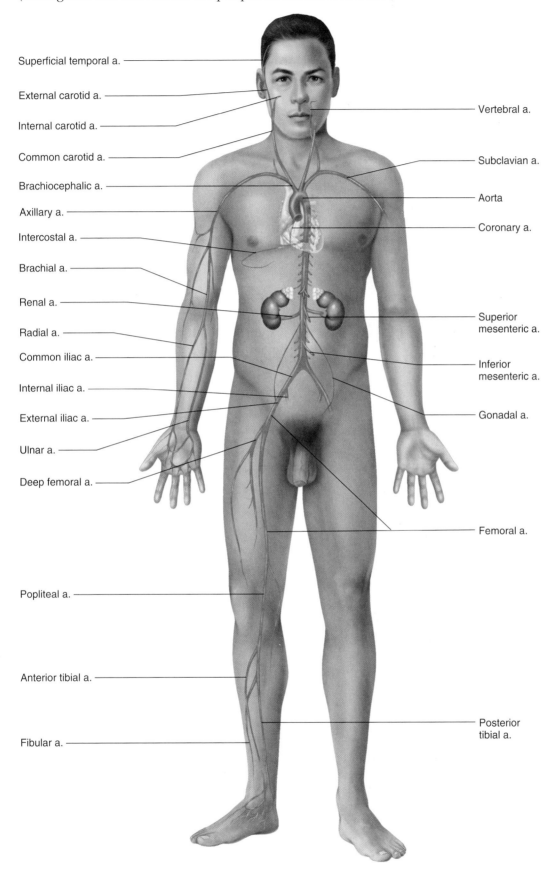

Superficial temporal a.

External carotid a.

Internal carotid a.

Common carotid a.

Brachiocephalic a.

Axillary a.

Intercostal a.

Brachial a.

Renal a.

Radial a.

Common iliac a.

Internal iliac a.

External iliac a.

Ulnar a.

Deep femoral a.

Popliteal a.

Anterior tibial a.

Fibular a.

Vertebral a.

Subclavian a.

Aorta

Coronary a.

Superior mesenteric a.

Inferior mesenteric a.

Gonadal a.

Femoral a.

Posterior tibial a.

Figure 12.5 Peripheral Arteries

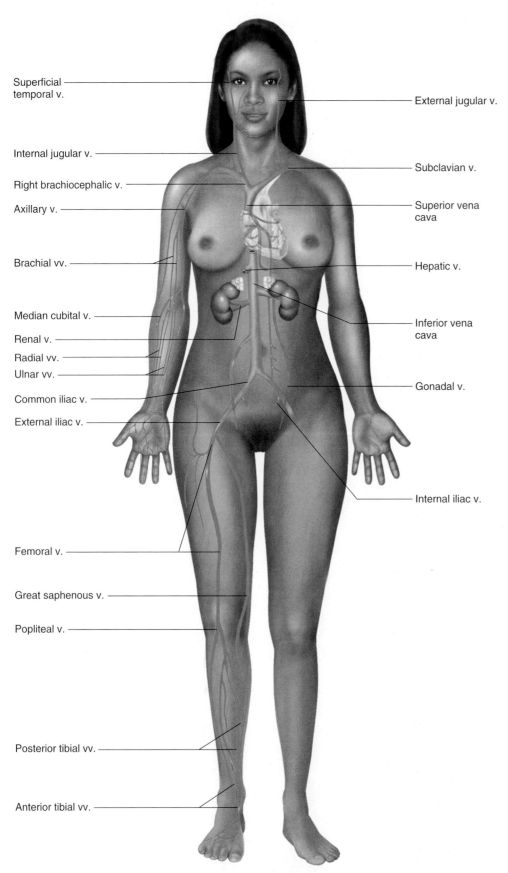

Superficial temporal v.

Internal jugular v.

Right brachiocephalic v.

Axillary v.

Brachial vv.

Median cubital v.

Renal v.

Radial vv.

Ulnar vv.

Common iliac v.

External iliac v.

Femoral v.

Great saphenous v.

Popliteal v.

Posterior tibial vv.

Anterior tibial vv.

External jugular v.

Subclavian v.

Superior vena cava

Hepatic v.

Inferior vena cava

Gonadal v.

Internal iliac v.

Figure 12.6 Peripheral Veins

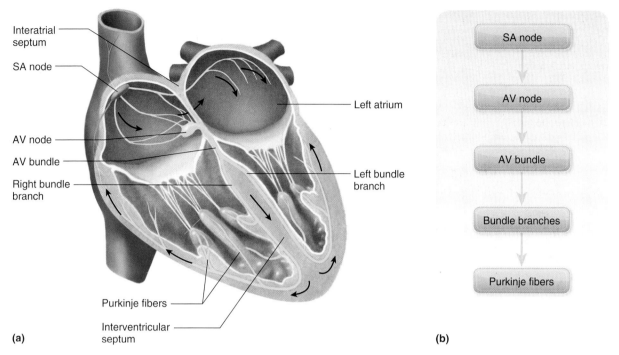

Figure 12.7 Electrical System of the Heart

The electrical system of the heart controls the pumping action of the heart (see Figure 12.7). It creates the signals that instruct the heart to beat and pump blood through the body. The structures of the electrical system are described in Table 12.2.

The chambers of the heart contain the heart valves (see Table 12.3), whose function is the proper flow of blood throughout the heart. When functioning properly, these valves act as one-way valves that permit the blood flow from one chamber to another or the blood flow out of the heart (see Figure 12.8). They control the blood flow by opening and closing during the heart contraction phase.

Table 12.2 Structures of the Heart Electrical System

STRUCTURE	DESCRIPTION
Sinoatrial (SA) node	The heart's natural pacemaker; where the electrical impulses begin
Atrioventricular (AV) node	Bridge between the atria and the ventricles that allows the electrical signals to pass to the bundle of His
His-Purkinje system:	System that carries the electrical signals throughout the ventricles
Bundle of His	Start of the system
Right bundle branch and left bundle branch	Fibers that carry the electrical impulses to the ventricles
Purkinje fibers	End of the system

tricuspid valve Valve located on the right side of the heart between the atrium and the ventricle that stops the backflow of blood between these two chambers.

mitral valve A two-flapped valve that allows blood to flow from the left atrium into the left ventricle. Also called *bicuspid valve.*

aortic valve Valve located between the left ventricle and the aorta; when open, allows the blood to exit the left ventricle and enter the aorta.

Table 12.3 Heart Valves

VALVE	DESCRIPTION
Tricuspid valve	This valve is located on the right side of the heart between the atrium and the ventricle, and its function is to stop the backflow of blood between these two chambers.
Mitral valve	This valve contains two flaps and is also referred to as the *bicuspid valve.* Its function is to allow blood to flow from the left atrium into the left ventricle.
Aortic valve	This valve is located between the left ventricle and the aorta. When the pressure in the left ventricle rises above the pressure in the aorta, the aortic valve opens, allowing blood to exit the left ventricle and flow into the aorta.
Pulmonary valve	This is a semilunar valve located between the right ventricle and the pulmonary artery. It is composed of three cusps that close during heartbeats, preventing the flow of blood back into the right ventricle. When the valve opens, it allows deoxygenated blood to flow through the pulmonary artery into the lungs.

Take a Journey to Heart Town

To understand how the heart works, picture the heart as a city. In this analogy, let's call the city "Heart Town." In this city, the electrical system is the signal lights [the sinoatrial (SA) and atrioventricular (AV) nodes], and the communication system and toll gates between these signals (bundle of His, bundle branches, and Purkinje fibers) control their actions. The vessels of the cardiovascular system are the roadways traveled from (via arterial system) and to (via veins) Heart Town. The major vessels, the aorta, and the superior and inferior venae cavae are the interstate, the lesser veins and arteries are the state highways, and the arterioles and venules are the country roads—connected

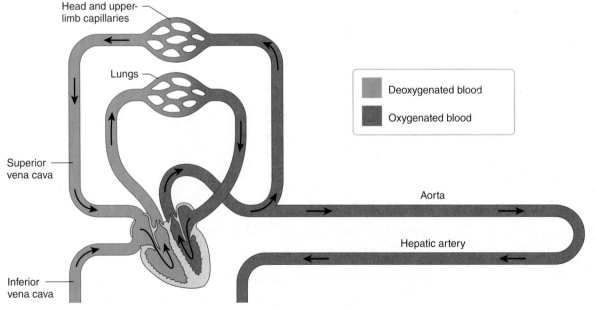

Figure 12.8 Blood Flow Pathway

together, all lead to and from the very small villages of Capillaryville. Let's take a journey to Heart Town to drop off carbon dioxide and pick up oxygen: Begin in Capillaryville, in the south, and head north on Venule Road to Vein Highway and then on to inferior vena cava, the interstate. Head north on vena cava toward Heart Town. Enter Heart Town on the northwest side (upper right), and you will be in the right atrium. Wait for the SA node signal to change, and then pass through the tricuspid gate into the right ventricle. The SA signal is the most important, as it sends the signal on to the atriums to contract and open the gates (tricuspid and mitral valve) on both north sides of Heart Town. The AV signal relays this message to the bundle of His, bundle branches, and Purkinje fibers, which control the remaining gates (pulmonary and aorta) by causing the ventricles on the south side to contract. At the next signal (AV node), pass through the pulmonary valve and onto the pulmonary artery, which will take you to the lungs' Capillaryville, where you can pick up oxygen. Return to Heart Town via the pulmonary vein to the left atrium on the east side of the city. Go through the mitral valve gate to the left ventricle. Once open, travel through the next gate (aortic valve) and onto the Aorta Interstate. Don't take the first exit on the Aorta Interstate or you'll wind up on the outer loop of Heart Town, also known as Coronary Artery Road, where you'll have to go back through Heart Town before you make it back to the Capillaryville in the south. Continue heading south on Aorta Interstate to Artery Highway, and then to Arteriole Road and home to Capillaryville.

---

1. Between which two chambers of the heart is the tricuspid valve located?

2. What is the name of the muscle layer of the heart-wall tissue?

3. What is the name of the heart's natural pacemaker?

4. Which coronary vessel is a branch of the LCA and supplies blood to the left atrium and the back of the left ventricle?

EXERCISE 12.1

Also available in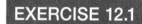

12.2 Anatomy of the Lymphatic System

The lymphatic system is made up of fluid or lymph, lymph vessels, and lymphoid tissue such as lymph nodes, the spleen, and the thymus (see Table 12.4). Fluid is exchanged between the cardiovascular and lymphatic systems (see Figure 12.9.)

Table 12.4 Structures of the Lymphatic System

STRUCTURE	DEFINITION/FUNCTION
Lymph fluid	Contains nutrients, fats, electrolytes, and cellular waste
Lymph vessels	Transport lymph fluids and merge into lymphatic ducts; enable water and other dissolved substances to return to the blood

(continued)

Table 12.4 Structures of the Lymphatic System (*concluded*)

STRUCTURE	DEFINITION/FUNCTION
Lymph nodes	Collections of tissue located along the lymph vessels; act as filters and produce antibodies and lymphocytes
Spleen	Filters blood and is the largest lymph organ
Thymus	Produces T cells, which are important in the functioning of the immune system

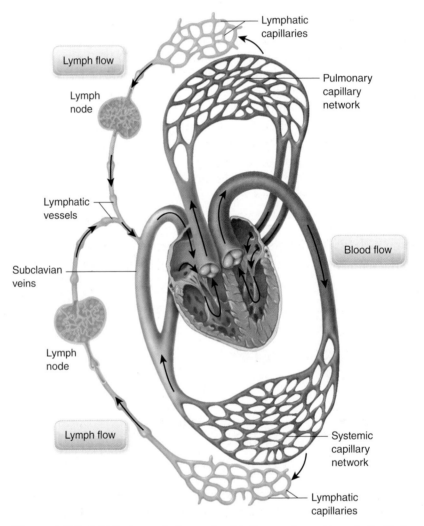

Figure 12.9 Fluid Exchange between the Cardiovascular and Lymphatic Systems

---

EXERCISE 12.2

1. Which structure of the lymphatic system produces T cells?
2. Where are lymph nodes located?
3. What is (are) the function(s) of the lymph nodes?

Also available in Mc Graw Hill connect™ (plus+)

Table 12.5 ICD Circulatory System Subheadings *(Data from ICD-9-CM and ICD-10-CM, Centers for Medicare and Medicaid Services and the National Center for Health Statistics.)*

ICD-9-CM		ICD-10-CM	
SUBHEADING	**CODE RANGE**	**SUBHEADING**	**CODE RANGE**
Acute Rheumatic Fever	390–392	Acute Rheumatic Fever	I00–I02
Chronic Rheumatic Heart Disease	393–398	Chronic Rheumatic Heart Diseases	I05–I09
Hypertensive Disease	401–405	Hypertensive Disease	I10–I15
Ischemic Heart Disease	410–414	Ischemic Heart Diseases	I20–I25
Diseases of Pulmonary Circulation	415–417	Pulmonary Heart Disease and Diseases of Pulmonary Circulation	I26–I28
Other Forms of Heart Disease	420–429	Other Forms of Heart Disease	I30–I52
Cerebrovascular Disease	430–438	Cerebrovascular Disease	I60–I69
Diseases of Arteries, Arterioles, and Capillaries	440–449	Diseases of Arteries, Arterioles, and Capillaries	I70–I79
Diseases of Veins and Lymphatics, and Other Diseases of Circulatory System	451–459	Diseases of Veins, Lymphatic Vessels, and Lymph Nodes, Not Elsewhere Classified	I80–I89
		Other and Unspecified Disorders of the Circulatory System	I95–I99

12.3 ICD Chapter-Specific Guidelines and Format for the Circulatory System

The most common problems patients present with concerning the cardiovascular system are chest pain, hypertension (HTN), edema, murmur, palpitations, congestive heart failure (CHF), arrythmias, syncope, hyperlipidemia, claudication, and rheumatic heart disease. When coding these conditions, coders must thoroughly review the provider documentation as well as the guidelines and instructional notes.

ICD-9-CM: Diseases of the Circulatory System is Chapter 7 in the ICD-9-CM manual, with the code range 390–459.

ICD-10-CM: Diseases of the Circulatory System is Chapter 9 in the ICD-10-CM manual, with the code range I00–I99.

Table 12.5 lists the Circulatory section subheadings and their code ranges.

Acute Rheumatic Fever (390–392), ICD-9-CM
Acute Rheumatic Fever (I00–I02), ICD-10-CM

Rheumatic fever commonly occurs after a throat infection caused by group A streptococci. If not treated promptly or if left untreated, it can lead to complications such as inflammation of the heart.

This section contains codes to be reported for conditions such as:

- Rheumatic fever without mention of heart involvement (390, ICD-9-CM; I00, ICD-10-CM).

- Rheumatic fever with mention of heart involvement (391, ICD-9-CM; I01, ICD-10-CM). Codes in this category are further defined by the type of heart involvement:

  - Acute rheumatic pericarditis (sudden, severe inflammation of the lining of the heart).

- Acute rheumatic endocarditis (sudden, severe inflammation of the inner cavities and chambers of the heart).
- Acute rheumatic myocarditis (sudden, severe inflammation of the heart muscles).
- Rheumatic chorea with and without heart involvement (392, ICD-9-CM; I02, ICD-10-CM).

Chronic Rheumatic Heart Disease (393–398), ICD-9-CM

Chronic Rheumatic Heart Diseases (I05–I09), ICD-10-CM

Codes in this range identify heart valve conditions with rheumatic involvement. Some of the questions a coder must be able to answer from the provider documentation include the two below:

- Which valve or valves were involved?
  - Mitral valve only
  - Aortic valve only
  - Mitral and aortic valves
  - Tricuspid valve

The mitral valve regulates blood flow between the left atrium and the left ventricle.

The aortic valve regulates blood flow from the left ventricle to the aorta.

The tricuspid valve regulates flow of blood from the right atrium to the right ventricle.

- What is the diagnosed disease of the valve or valves?
  - Stenosis only.
  - Insufficiency only (could be documented as incompetence or regurgitation).
  - Stenosis with insufficiency.

SPOTLIGHT on a Guideline

Mitral valve with aortic valve involvement is divided further by the type of disease of each valve:

Stenosis of both valves

Insufficiency of both valves

Stenosis of one valve and insufficiency of the other

There is an *includes* note in ICD-9-CM that tells the coder that codes within this category (396) include involvement of both mitral and aortic valves, whether specified as rheumatic or not.

FOR EXAMPLE Stenosis of mitral valve and insufficiency of aortic valve would be coded with ICD-9-CM 396.1 or ICD-10-CM I08.0. ∎

Hypertensive Disease (401–405), ICD-9-CM
Hypertensive Disease (I10–I15), ICD-10-CM

Hypertension is a cardiovascular disease identified by increased pressure of arterial blood flow. ICD categorizes hypertension as benign or malignant. Benign hypertension (401.1, ICD-9-CM) is classified as arterial pressure that is mildly elevated. In malignant hypertension (401.0, ICD-9-CM), the arterial blood pressure is very high. This severely elevated pressure may lead to necrosis of organs such as the eyes, heart, and kidneys. Malignant hypertension over time may also cause hemorrhage of vessels, which can lead to death.

SPOTLIGHT on a Guideline

ICD-10-CM does not list separate codes for benign, malignant, or unspecified hypertension. Code I10 is for essential primary hypertension and includes high blood pressure and hypertension (arterial, benign, essential, malignant, primary, and systemic). There is also an *includes* note in ICD-10-CM that informs the coder to use an additional code to identify exposure to environmental tobacco smoke, history of tobacco use, occupational exposure to environmental tobacco smoke, tobacco dependence, or tobacco use.

Although malignant hypertension is the more severe form of the two categories of hypertension, either form may lead to complications and associated conditions, including hypertensive heart and hypertensive kidney disease. ICD provides guidance for coding each of these conditions and their associated manifestations.

Hypertensive Heart and/or Kidney Disease: 402–404 (ICD-9-CM), I11–I13 (ICD-10-CM)

As hypertensive heart and hypertensive kidney disease are common complications of hypertension, ICD provides categories for each of these conditions and clarifies the documentation requirements needed to assign codes for each.

Category 402, "Hypertensive heart disease," or 404, "Hypertensive heart and chronic kidney disease," is assigned only when the documentation clearly states or implies the relationship between the heart disease and hypertension.

Category 403, "Hypertensive kidney disease," may be assigned if both hypertension and kidney disease are documented. As the relationship between the kidney disease and hypertension is assumed, the provider's documentation does not need to state the relation. This assumption is also appropriate for category 404 but only as it pertains to the relationship between hypertension and chronic kidney disease (CKD).

When reporting hypertensive heart disease (402 or 404), the coder must use an additional code or codes to identify the type of heart disease, such as myocarditis or cardiomegaly, and the type of heart failure, when present, either congestive, systolic, or diastolic (428.0–428.9).

Likewise, when reporting hypertensive chronic kidney disease (403 or 404), the coder must use an additional code to identify the stage of kidney failure (585.1–585.9).

Table 12.6 lists primary and additional category codes for hypertensive heart disease.

MENTOR
Coding Tip

Look for statements in the documentation such as "heart disease due to hypertension" or "hypertensive heart disease."

Table 12.6 ICD-9-CM Codes for Hypertensive Heart Disease *(Data from ICD-9-CM and ICD-10-CM, Centers for Medicare and Medicaid Services and the National Center for Health Statistics.)*

DIAGNOSIS	PRIMARY CATEGORY CODE	CAUSAL RELATIONSHIP	ADDITIONAL CATEGORY CODES
Hypertension with heart disease	402	Needs to be stated in documentation	428 to identify the type of heart failure when present
Hypertensive chronic kidney disease	403 Requires 5th digit to identify CKD stage	Presumed	585 to identify CKD
Hypertensive heart and chronic kidney disease	404 Requires 5th digit to identify CKD stage	Needs to be stated in documentation	428 to identify the type of heart failure when present 585 to identify CKD

MENTOR Coding Tip

Remember that a primary code from categories 402 to 404 identifies only the relationship between hypertension and heart disease and/or chronic kidney disease. The additional required codes identify the type of hypertensive condition and how far the condition has progressed.

FOR EXAMPLE The patient presents with benign hypertensive chronic kidney disease, stage 1. The appropriate ICD-9-CM codes are 403.10 and 585.1. ■

Secondary hypertension is also reported using codes in this subsection. Secondary hypertension is defined as hypertension due to a primary disease.

Ischemic Heart Disease (410–414), ICD-9-CM
Ischemic Heart Disease (I20–I25), ICD-10-CM

This type of heart disease occurs when the blood supply to the heart is inadequate. This is often caused by a blockage or occlusion of a blood vessel.

Codes within these ranges are used to identify the conditions discussed below.

Acute Myocardial Infarction: 410 (ICD-9-CM), I21–I22 (ICD-10-CM)

Acute myocardial infarction is abbreviated *AMI* and is also called *heart attack*. It occurs when the blood supply to a portion or portions of the heart is insufficient. The codes in this category are further defined by fourth and fifth digits.

Before selecting an appropriate code, the coder needs to review the provider documentation for answers to questions such as the following:

- Which section or sections of heart were involved?
  - Anterolateral wall.
  - Other anterior wall (e.g., anteroseptal).
  - Inferolateral wall.
  - Inferoposterior wall.
  - Other inferior wall (e.g., diaphragmatic wall).

- Other lateral wall (e.g., high lateral).
- True posterior wall (e.g., posterobasal).
- Subendocardial wall.
- Other specified sites (e.g., atrium, septum alone).

The answer to this question will decide the correct fourth digit to be assigned.

- What is the episode of care?
  - **Unspecified:** episode of care not specified.
  - **Initial:** the first episode of care, regardless of facility site, for newly diagnosed MI.
  - **Subsequent:** the episode of care following the initial episode, when patient is admitted for further observation, evaluation, or treatment but MI is less than 8 weeks old.

The answer to this question will decide the correct fifth digit to be assigned.

Other Acute and Subacute Forms of Ischemic Heart Disease: 411 (ICD-9-CM), I20 (ICD-10-CM)

Included in this category is the code for intermediate coronary syndrome, 411.1. Conditions defined by this code are:

- Impending infarction
- Preinfarction angina
- Preinfarction syndrome
- Unstable angina

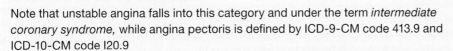

MENTOR Coding Tip

Note that unstable angina falls into this category and under the term *intermediate coronary syndrome*, while angina pectoris is defined by ICD-9-CM code 413.9 and ICD-10-CM code I20.9

Angina pectoris: 413 (ICD-9-CM), I20 and I25 (ICD-10-CM)

Angina pectoris is severe chest pain due to an insufficient blood supply to the heart. The conditions coded in this section are angina decubitus, which is angina occurring when the patient is lying down, and prinzmetal angina, which generally occurs at rest and is often due to spasms of the arteries of the heart.

Other Forms of Chronic Ischemic Heart Disease: 414 (ICD-9-CM), I25 (ICD-10-CM)

Coronary atherosclerosis is included in this category and is further defined by the type of vessel with coronary atherosclerotic involvement:

- Unspecified type of vessel, native or graft.
- Native coronary artery (the patient's natural coronary artery).
- Autologous vein bypass graft (grafted vein taken from the patient's own body).
- Nonautologous biological bypass graft (graft from outside the patient's own body).

angina pectoris Severe chest pain due to insufficient blood supply to the heart.

SPOTLIGHT on a Guideline

ICD-10-CM has combination codes for atherosclerotic heart disease with angina pectoris: I25.11 and I25.7.

- Artery bypass graft (grafted artery taken from the patient's own body).
- Unspecified type of bypass graft.
- Native coronary artery of transplanted heart.
- Bypass graft (artery) (vein) of transplanted heart

Diseases of Pulmonary Circulation (415–417), ICD-9-CM
Pulmonary Heart Disease and Diseases of Pulmonary Circulation (I26–I28), ICD-10-CM

Pulmonary circulation is the circulation between the heart and lungs. Therefore, conditions classified in this category affect both the lungs and the heart.

Pulmonary embolism with infarction is included in this category. This condition involves the closure of the pulmonary artery due to a blood clot and infarction or necrosis (death) of lung tissue.

Chronic pulmonary heart diseases are also included in this category and are reported when the patient has long-term conditions relating to both heart and lungs. There is an instructional note below the code for chronic pulmonary embolism (416.2) which directs the coder to use an additional code, if applicable, for associated long-term (current) use of anticoagulants (V58.61).

Other Forms of Heart Disease (420–429), ICD-9-CM
Other Forms of Heart Disease (I30–I52), ICD-10-CM

Some of the conditions reported with codes from these code ranges are discussed below.

Diseases of the Pericardium, Endocardium, and Myocardium: 420–423 (ICD-9-CM), I30–I41 (ICD-10-CM)

Coders need to determine which area of the heart is involved. Multiple instructional notes in this category direct the coder to code first the underlying disease and to use an additional code to identify an infectious organism, and there are several *includes* and *excludes* notes.

myocardium The muscle layer of the heart-wall tissue.

MENTOR Coding Tip

Remember: The pericardium is the sac around the heart; the endocardium is the inner layer of the heart wall, and the **myocardium** is the muscle layer of the heart wall.

FOR EXAMPLE At the entry "Septic myocarditis" (422.92), a note instructs the coder to identify an infectious organism (e.g., staphylococcus, 041.1). ■

FOR EXAMPLE At the entry "Cardiac tamponade" (423.3), a note instructs the coder to code first the underlying cause. ■

Mitral, Aortic, Tricuspid, and Pulmonary Valve Disorders Not Specified as Rheumatic: 423 (ICD-9-CM), I34–I39 (ICD-10-CM)

Some of the conditions reported using the above range are conduction disorders, AV blocks, dysrhythmias, and heart failure.

Conduction Disorders: 426 (ICD-9-CM), I44–I45 (ICD-10-CM)

Conduction disorders are disturbances in the electrical impulses of the heart. Conditions reported by codes in this category include:

- **Atrioventricular block:** This condition is further defined as complete (third-degree AV block), incomplete (first-degree block), or incomplete (second-degree block).
- **Bundle branch block:** This condition is further defined as left, right, posterior, or anterior.

Cardiac dysrhythmias: 427 (ICD-9-CM), I46–I49 (ICD-10-CM)

Cardiac dysrhythmia is abnormal electrical activity in the heart, such as a heartbeat that is too fast, too slow, or irregular. Atrial and ventricular fibrillation and flutter are conditions reported by codes in this category.

MENTOR
Coding Tip

Be careful when reading the documentation to properly identify the site of the dysrhythmia as atrial or ventricular and the condition as fibrillation or flutter.

Heart Failure: 428 (ICD-9-CM), I50 (ICD-10-CM)

During heart failure the heart cannot pump a sufficient amount of blood throughout the body. The different types of heart failure defined in this category are:

- **Congestive heart failure, unspecified:** The heart is unable to pump blood to the extremities and lungs, resulting in edema of these areas, but the specific area of the heart involved is not specified.
- **Left heart failure:** The left side of the heart fails.
- **Systolic heart failure:** Contraction of the heart muscle does not pump blood adequately.
- **Diastolic heart failure:** The heart does not relax properly after contraction, resulting in decreased blood flow through the heart.

There are codes for combined systolic and diastolic heart failure.

MENTOR
Coding Tip

Right heart failure is included in the code description for congestive heart failure.

FOR EXAMPLE Acute systolic and diastolic heart failure is reported with code 428.41. ■

There is an instructional note at the beginning of the category instructing coders that if the heart failure is due to hypertension, a code from category 402 or 404 should be coded first.

Cerebrovascular Disease (430–438), ICD-9-CM
Cerebrovascular Disease (I60–I69), ICD-10-CM

Subarachnoid hemorrhage (bleeding in the space between the brain and the lining) and intracranial hemorrhage (bleeding within the brain) are reported using codes from these code ranges.

MENTOR Coding Tip

Late effects usually require two codes, one for the late effect and one for the condition or nature of the late effect. Late effects of cerebrovascular disease are reported with a combination code which includes the current condition and the late effect.

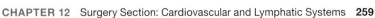

The conditions of occlusion and stenosis of precerebral and cerebral arteries also occur in this code range.

Late effects of cerebrovascular disease are reported using category 438 (ICD-9-CM) or I69 (ICD-10-CM) and include such conditions as aphasia, dysphasia, hemiplagia, and disturbances of vision.

There is a note in the chapter-specific guidelines directing the coder to use V12.54 as an additional code for history of cerebrovascular disease when no neurologic deficits are present.

Diseases of Arteries, Arterioles, and Capillaries (440–449), ICD-9-CM

Diseases of Arteries, Arterioles, and Capillaries (I70–I79), ICD-10-CM

SPOTLIGHT
on a Guideline

Coders should look at the other specified arteries (440.8) for a list of exclusions.

Atherosclerosis of the aorta and of the renal artery are reported by codes from these categories. Atherosclerosis of the extremities is another condition included in these categories, and the codes for this condition are further defined by involvement of native arteries or bypass grafts.

FOR EXAMPLE Atherosclerosis of the pulmonary artery is reported with code 416.0. ■

Aortic aneurysm and dissections are also reported using codes in these ranges, as well as aneurysms of the upper extremity, renal artery, iliac artery, and other lower extremity arteries.

Diseases of Veins and Lymphatics, and Other Diseases of Circulatory System (451–459), ICD-9-CM

Diseases of Veins, Lymphatic Vessels, and Lymph Nodes, Not Elsewhere Classified (I80–I89), ICD-10-CM

Conditions reported by codes in these ranges include those discussed below.

Phlebitis and Thrombophlebitis: 451 (ICD-9-CM) I80, (ICD-10-CM)

This condition is defined as an inflammation of a vein with the development of a thrombus. This category is further defined by superficial (sapheneous) or deep (femoral, popliteal, or tibial) vessels of the lower extremities or superficial (basilic or cephalic) vessels or deep (brachial, radial, or ulnar) vessels of the upper extremities.

There is an instructional note with this category directing the coder to use an additional E code to identify the drug, if the condition is drug-induced.

Acute venous embolism and thrombosis and chronic venous embolism and thrombosis are also conditions assigned to this code category and are further defined as upper or lower extremity and superficial or deep vessel.

deep vein thrombosis (DVT)
Inflammation of a vein with development of a thrombus in a deep vein.

SPOTLIGHT on Condition

Deep Vein Thrombosis (DVT) is a serious condition. After the formation of a blood clot in the vein, usually a vein in the lower extremity, the clot can dislodge, travel through the bloodstream and lodge in the lungs. This resulting pulmonary embolism can then block blood flow.

Varicose Veins of Lower Extremities: 454 (ICD-9-CM), I83 (ICD-10-CM)

Codes in this category are further defined by ulcer, inflammation, and other complications, such as pain, edema, and swelling.

Noninfectious Disorders of Lymphatic Channels: 457 (ICD-9-CM), I89 (ICD-10-CM)

Conditions assigned to this category include postmastectomy lymphedema syndrome (457.0, ICD-9-CM), which is reduced lymphatic circulation following mastectomy. Other lymphedema (457.1, ICD-9-CM), which is fluid retention due to reduced circulation caused by something other than mastectomy, is also included in this category.

---

1. The patient presents with a diagnosis of congestive heart failure (CHF) due to hypertension (HTN). What is (are) the correct ICD-9-CM code(s)?

2. The mitral valve regulates blood flow between the _____ and the _____.

3. The patient is diagnosed with acute rheumatic fever with severe inflammation of the heart muscle. What is the appropriate ICD-9-CM code?

4. A patient presents with a diagnosis of DVT. Assign the appropriate ICD-9-CM code.

5. List the types of heart failure that affect code assignment.

EXERCISE 12.3

Also available in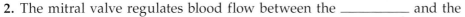

12.4 Guidelines and Format of the Cardiovascular Subsection of CPT

The Cardiovascular System subsection of the CPT manual is formatted from heart and pericardium to the hemic and lymphatic systems and includes code range 33010–39599. (See Table 12.7.)

Table 12.7 Cardiovascular Subsection Headings and Code Ranges *(Data from CPT 2013. © 2013 American Medical Association. All rights reserved.)*

HEADING/SUBHEADING	CODE RANGE
Heart and Pericardium	33010–33999
Pericardium	33010–33050
Cardiac Tumor	33120–33130
Transmyocardial Revascularization	33140–33141
Pacemaker or Pacing Cardioverter-Defibrillator	33202–33249
Electrophysiologic Operative Procedures	33250–33266
Patient Activated Event Recorder	33282–33284
Heart (Including Valves) and Great Vessels	33300–33335
Cardiac Valves	33361–33476
Coronary Artery Anomalies	33500–33507
Endoscopy	33508
Venus Grafting Only for Coronary Artery Bypass	33510–33516
Combined Arterial-Venous Grafting for Coronary Bypass	33517–33530

(continued)

Table 12.7 Cardiovascular Subsection Headings and Code Ranges (*concluded*)

HEADING/SUBHEADING	CODE RANGE
Arterial Grafting for Coronary Artery Bypass	33533–33548
Coronary Endarterectomy	33572
Single Ventricle and Other Complex Cardiac Anomalies	33600–33622
Septal Defect	33641–33697
Sinus of Valsalva	33702–33722
Venus Anomalies	33724–33732
Shunting Procedures	33735–33768
Transposition of the Great Vessels	33770–33783
Truncus Arteriosus	33786–33788
Aortic Anomalies	33800–33853
Thoracic Aortic Aneurysm	33860–33877
Endovascular Repair of Descending Thoracic Aorta	33880–33891
Pulmonary Artery	33910–33926
Heart/Lung Transplantation	33930–33945
Cardiac Arrest	33960–33993
Arteries and Veins	34001–37799
Embolectomy/Thrombolectomy	34001–34490
Venous Reconstruction	34501–34530
Endovascular Repair of Abdominal Aortic Aneurysm	34800–34834
Endovascular Repair of Iliac Aneurysm	34900
Direct Repair of Aneurysm or Excision (partial or total) and Graft Insertion for Aneurysm, Pseuodoaneurysm, Ruptured Aneurysm, and Associated Occlusive Disease	35001–35152
Repair Arteriovenous Fistula	35180–35190
Repair Blood Vessels Other Than for Fistula, with or without Patch Angioplasty	35201–35286
Thromboendarterectomy	35301–35390
Angioscopy	35400
Transluminal Angioplasty	35450–35476
Bypass Graft	35500–35671
Composite grafts	35681–35683
Adjuvant Techniques	35685–35686
Arterial Transposition	35691–35697
Excision, Exploration, Repair	35700–35907
Vascular Injection Procedures	36000–36598
Arterial	36600–36660
Intraosseous	36680
Hemodialysis Access, Intervascular Cannulatin for Extracorporeal Circulation, or Shunt Insertion	36800–36870
Portal Decompression Procedures	37140–37183
Transcatheter Procedures	37184–37216
Endovascular Revascularization (Open or Percutaneous, Transcatheter)	37220–37235
Intravascular Ultrasound Services	37250–37251
Ligation	37565–37785

MENTOR
Coding Tip

Highlight the boldface and italic items in this section of your CPT manual to remind yourself of these tips and guidelines when using the manual.

Heart and Pericardium (33010–33999)

Pericardium: 33010–33050

Conditions coded within this range include pericardiocentesis (surgical puncture into the **pericardium**) and are further defined as initial or subsequent. Pericardiectomy is also coded to this range; to select the appropriate code, the coder must determine whether cardiopulmonary bypass was performed.

pericardium The membrane sac that encases the heart.

Pacemaker or Pacing Cardioverter-Defibrillator: 33202–33249

Pacemakers and cardioverter-defibrillators are electrical devices inserted into the body to shock the heart into regular rhythm. The **defibrillator** generally uses a combination of antitachycardia pacing, low-energy cardioversion, and shocks to treat ventricular tachycardia or ventricular fibrillation. The pacemaker and the cardioverter-defibrillator are both made of two components: the generator (battery) and the electrodes (leads). The generator is placed in a pocket under the skin, usually below the clavicle. It can also be placed underneath the abdominal muscles below the rib cage. This pocket is created by making an incision into the skin and placing the generator in the pocket. The electrodes or leads may be passed into the heart by a vein (transvenous). The electrodes are then placed in only the atrium (single chamber) or in the atrium and ventricle (dual chamber), or they may be placed upon the heart (epicardial), which requires a thoracotomy.

defibrillator An electrical device inserted into the body to shock the heart into regular rhythm.

Before selecting the appropriate code from this code range, the coder must review the provider documentation and answer the following questions:

- Was the device a pacemaker or a cardioverter-defibrillator?
- Was it an initial insertion, a replacement, or a repositioning?
- Was the device permanent or temporary?
- Was it single-chamber or dual-chamber, and where was the lead placed (atrium or ventricle)?
- Was the approach transvenous or epicardial?
- Was the entire system (generator and leads) replaced, or was just the generator or just the leads replaced?
- Was the pacemaker pocket revised?

FOR EXAMPLE

- Insertion of transvenous single lead only without pulse generator:

  Pacemaker = 33216

  Defibrillator = 33216

- Initial pulse generator insertion or replacement plus insertion of transvenous single lead:

  Pacemaker = 33206 (atrial), 33207 (ventricular)

  Defibrillator = 33249 (single or dual chamber)

SPOTLIGHT on a Guideline

In most editions of the CPT manual there is a grid showing the code description of the transvenous procedure and the appropriate pacemaker or defibrillator code. This is a good resource for help with the selection of codes.

There are multiple instructional notes within this code range, and it is important for the coder to fully read the code description and all instructional notes before selecting the code.

MENTOR Coding Tip

It is very helpful to highlight key terms in the description of the codes in this code range, specifically the words *pacemaker* and *cardioverter-defibrillator.* This helps to keep the coding ranges separate when taking the CPC exam. Often, coders will read the scenario and answer quickly, confusing the codes.

Electrophysiologic Operative Procedures: 33250–33266

ablation Ablation works by scarring or destroying cardiac tissue that trigger an abnormal heart rhythm.

These procedures are often referred to as *EP procedures.* Tissue ablation and reconstruction are reported with the codes under this subheading. **Ablation** works by scarring or destroying cardiac tissue that triggers an abnormal heart rhythm. Ablation can, in some cases, prevent abnormal electrical signals from traveling through the heart, thus stopping an arrhythmia.

To select the appropriate code in this range, the coder must know whether the procedure was limited or extensive and whether it was performed with or without cardiopulmonary bypass.

FOR EXAMPLE An operative tissue ablation and reconstruction of atria, extensive (e.g., maze procedure), without cardiopulmonary bypass is coded 33255. ∎

SPOTLIGHT on a Guideline

The guidelines before the range of codes include definitions of limited and extensive operative ablation, and the coder should refer to them before making a code selection.

Heart (Including Valves) and Great Vessels: 33300–33355

Repair of cardiac wounds with or without cardiopulmonary bypass (33300–33305) is included under this subheading. Exploratory cardiotomy, suture repair of aorta or great vessels, and insertion of graft aorta or great vessels are also reported using codes in this range. They also are further defined as with or without cardiopulmonary bypass.

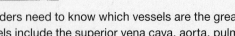

MENTOR Coding Tip

To assign these codes, coders need to know which vessels are the great vessels. *Reminder:* The great vessels include the superior vena cava, aorta, pulmonary arteries, pulmonary veins, and inferior vena cava.

Cardiac Valves: 33361–33478

There is an instructional note at the beginning of this subheading telling the coder that if multiple valve procedures are performed, modifier 51 should be attached to the secondary valve procedure code.

Some of the more common types of conditions treated by codes described in this range are:

- Regurgitation: This is the backflow of blood due to valve prolapse.
- Prolapse: The valvular flaps do not close properly.
- Stenosis: This is the narrowing of a cardiac valve.

Before selecting the appropriate code from this code range, the coder must review the provider documentation and answer the following questions:

- Which valve or valves are involved: aortic, mitral, tricuspid, and/or pulmonary?
- What procedure was performed: valvuloplasty, valvulotomy, or replacement?
- Was the procedure performed with or without cardiopulmonary bypass?

The code ranges for specific cardiac valves are:

Aortic valve	33361–33417
Mitral valve	33420–33430
Tricuspid valve	33460– 33468
Pulmonary valve	33470–33478

FOR EXAMPLE Valvuloplasty, mitral valve, with cardiopulmonary bypass is reported with code 33425. ▪

Transcatheter aortic valve replacement (TAVR/TAVI) with prosthetic valve codes are included in this range. The codes are further defined as to the approach such as percutaneous, open or transaortic and which access artery was used such as femoral, axillary, or iliac

FOR EXAMPLE A transcatheter aortic valve replacement with prosthetic valve; open iliac artery approach is reported with CPT code 33364. ▪

Coronary Artery Bypass Grafting: 33510–33548

When coronary arteries become clogged or occluded with plaque, the flow of blood is reduced. If the heart muscle function is below normal levels, this is termed **reversible ischemia,** and if the heart muscle is denied adequate blood flow for an extended period of time, the muscle may die and this is termed **irreversible ischemia.**

The function of a **coronary artery bypass graft (CABG)** procedure is to bypass the clogged area(s) of the vessels to improve blood flow. This is done by attaching a grafted vessel (artery or vein) to the coronary artery affected, beyond the blockage. There are three types of coronary artery bypass grafting:

- Venous grafting only for coronary artery, 33510–33516
- Combined arterial-venous grafting for coronary bypass, 33517–33530
- Arterial grafting for coronary bypass, 33533–33548

To select the appropriate code from this code range, the coder must review the provider documentation and then answer the following questions:

- What type or types of grafts were used to bypass (e.g., arterial, venous, or combination)?

stenosis Narrowing of an artery or a valve.

There are very specific guidelines in the CPT manual for TAVR/TAVI procedures (TAVR—transcatheter aortic valve replacement; TAVI—transcatheter aortic valve implantation). Coders should become familiar with these guidelines before choosing codes from this code range.

reversible ischemia The heart muscle function is below normal levels.

irreversible ischemia Condition in which heart muscle is denied adequate blood flow for an extended period of time and the muscle dies.

coronary artery bypass graft (CABG) A procedure used to improve blood flow to the heart by bypassing a vessel blockage with a grafted vessel.

All of the codes in range 33517–33530 (combined arterial-venous grafting for coronary bypass) have a plus (+) sign in front of them, indicating that these codes are add-on codes and may not be used alone or as primary codes. When assigning a code from this range, coders should use the appropriate code from range 33533–33548 (arterial grafting for coronary bypass) as the primary code.

- Was the harvested vessel one that can be reported separately (e.g., upper extremity artery, 35600; upper extremity vein, 35500; or femoropopliteal vein segment, 35572)?
- How many of each type of identified graft(s) was used to bypass?
- Was the venous graft harvested endoscopically? If so, 33508 may be used as an additional code.

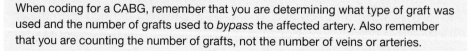

SPOTLIGHT on a Guideline

Open procurement (harvesting) of the saphenous vein or internal mammary artery is included in the code descriptions and is *not* reported separately. This is noted in the guidelines before each section of the grafting code ranges in the CPT manual.

FOR EXAMPLE The right coronary artery (RCA) was blocked and a portion of the harvested saphenous vein was used to bypass the blockage. The type of graft used to bypass was a saphenous vein which was not harvested endoscopically and only a single segment was used. The appropriate CPT code is 33510. ∎

MENTOR Coding Tip

When coding for a CABG, remember that you are determining what type of graft was used and the number of grafts used to *bypass* the affected artery. Also remember that you are counting the number of grafts, not the number of veins or arteries.

FOR EXAMPLE Several portions of the saphenous vein may be used as grafts during a CABG procedure, so the actual number of grafts would be used when determining the appropriate code from range 33510–33516. ∎

Septal Defect: 33641–33697

An atrial septal defect (ASD) occurs when there is a hole in the septum between the upper chambers of the heart. A ventricular septal defect (VSD) occurs when there is a hole in the septum between the two lower chambers of the heart.

A function of the septum is to prevent the mixing of blood from the two sides of the heart.

ASDs and VSDs allow blood to pass from the left side of the heart to the right side, and thus oxygen-rich blood mixes with oxygen-poor blood.

This range of codes is used to report procedures performed to repair these defects.

FOR EXAMPLE Repair of an atrial septal defect and a ventricular septal defect, with direct or patch closure, is reported with CPT code 33647. ∎

There is an instructional note below this code stating that modifier 63 (procedure performed on infants less than 4 kg) should not be reported with code 33647.

Heart/Lung Transplantation: 33930–33945

As with all transplantation code ranges, the code ranges for heart/lung transplantation include three major physician components:

- Cadaver donor cardioectomy with or without pneumonectomy, 33930, 33940 (These codes include harvesting the allograft and cold preservation of the allograft.)
- Backbench work, 33933, 33944
- Recipient heart with or without lung allotransplantation, 33935, 33945 (These codes include the care of the recipient.)

Cardiac Assist: 33960–33993

When a failing heart needs to be partially or completely replaced by a mechanical circulatory device, this can be achieved by the use of a ventricular assist device (VAD). The VAD can be intended for short-term use in patients recovering from heart attacks or heart surgery or for long-term use in patients suffering from CHF. This device is different from an artificial heart.

The insertion of a ventricular assist device can be performed percutaneously (CPT codes 33390–33391) or by a transthoracic approach (CPT codes 33975–33976, 33979). Insertion, removal, and replacement procedures are included in this range of codes.

Aneurysm Repair: 33860–33877, 33880–33891, 34800–34834, 34900, 35001–35152

An **aneurysm** is a bulge or swelling in the wall of a vessel. Aneurysms commonly appear in arteries at the base of the brain or the aorta. As the aneurysm increases in diameter, the wall of the blood vessel weakens and risk of rupture increases. This rupture results in severe hemorrhaging, which can lead to major complications and death.

aneurysm Bulge or swelling in the wall of a vessel. Aneurysms commonly appear in arteries at the base of the brain or the aorta.

Repair of an aneurysm is most commonly accomplished by a direct procedure or by endovascular repair. In a direct procedure, the site of the aneurysm is opened directly, the blood flow is stopped, and a graft is placed. During a endovascular repair, a catheter is guided into the involved artery and the aneurysm, where a balloon is deployed to inflate the graft into place.

- Endovascular repair:
  - Thoracic aorta, 33880–33891
  - Abdominal aorta, 34800–34834
  - Iliac, 34900

There are extensive guidelines before each range of codes that should be reviewed before assigning the appropriate code(s).

FOR EXAMPLE An endovascular repair of an iliac artery aneurysm using an ilio-iliac tube end prosthesis would be assigned code 34900. Based on the guidelines, if fluoroscopic guidance was utilized, code 75954 would be reported in conjunction with 34900. ■

- Direct (open) repair:
  - Thoracic aorta, 33860–33877
  - Other arteries, 35001–35152

Arteries and Veins (34001–34490)

Embolectomy/Thrombectomy: 34001–34203

The codes within this range are determined by:

- The artery/vein involved.
- The incision site: thoracic, arm, abdominal, or leg.

| FOR EXAMPLE | An embolectomy or thrombectomy, femoropopliteal, aortoiliac artery, by leg incision, would be assigned code 34201. ■ |

Vascular Injection Procedures: 36000–36598

CPT coding decisions for vascular injection or introduction procedures are based on whether the physician performed a selective or nonselective catheter placement. If the placement was selective, the codes are then based on the end placement into the first, second, or third order of the vascular family involved.

In nonselective placement, the catheter is left in the access vessel or not advanced beyond the aorta. In selective catheter placement, the catheter is advanced beyond the access vessel or the aorta. CPT codes 36215–36217 pertain to above the diaphragm and 36245–36247 to below the diaphragm.

| FOR EXAMPLE |

Nonselective placement:

- The access vessel for the catheter is the femoral artery, and the catheter does not advance further.
- The access vessel for the catheter is the femoral artery, and the catheter is advanced into the aorta but no further (CPT code 36200).

Selective placement:

- The catheter advances beyond the aorta into the right common carotid artery, which is a second-order vessel of a vascular family (CPT code 36216, above the diaphragm).
- The catheter advances beyond the aorta into the right external iliac artery from a left femoral artery access. This is contralateral (opposite-side) placement of the catheter from the access and advancement to a second order of a vascular family (CPT code 36246). ■

MENTOR Coding Tip

The same rules apply for the venous side, using the vena cava as the point of advancement. Think of the aorta or vena cava as a hallway: If the catheter does not move from the hallway, the placement is considered nonselective. If the catheter moves beyond the hallway through a door and into one of the rooms, or orders, of a vascular family, this is a selective placement.

A code for nonselective catheter placement should not be assigned in addition to a selective catheter placement code unless there are multiple accesses.

There are three orders of arterial or venous vascular family:

- **First order:** This is the first branch of the vascular family.
- **Second order:** The first order bifurcates, or divides, into the second branch.
- **Third order:** The second order bifurcates, or divides, into the third branch.

FOR EXAMPLE

- The right innominate artery is the first branch off the aorta and would be a first-order placement (CPT code 36215, above the diaphragm).
- The right common carotid artery bifurcates, or divides, from the first order and forms the second branch off the aorta and would be a second-order placement (CPT code 36216, above the diaphragm).
- The right internal carotid artery bifurcates, or divides, from the second order and forms the third branch off the aorta and would be a third-order placement (CPT code 36217, above the diaphragm).
- The common iliac artery is the first branch off the aorta and would be a first-order placement (CPT code 36245, below the diaphragm).
- The internal iliac artery bifurcates, or divides, from the first order and forms the second branch off the aorta and would be a second-order placement (CPT code 36246, below the diaphragm).
- The superficial femoral artery bifurcates, or divides, from the second order and forms the third branch off the aorta and would be a third-order placement (CPT code 36247, below the diaphragm). ▪

SPOTLIGHT on a Guideline

Appendix L of the CPT manual outlines the branches and orders of the vascular families.

The selective placement codes are reported by the location at which the catheter ends. If the documentation states that the catheter advanced from the right innominate artery to the right internal carotid artery, only the code for third-order selective placement would be reported, CPT code 36217.

Central Venous Access Procedures: 36555–36598

A central venous access device (CVAD) is a small, flexible tube placed in large veins for patients who require frequent access to their bloodstreams. Some of the common reasons a CVAD would be required are:

- Administration of chemotherapy.
- Administration of medication such as antibiotics.
- Blood transfusions.
- Multiple blood draws.

The guidelines at the beginning of this range of codes instruct the coder that to qualify as a central venous access device, the tip of the catheter must terminate in the subclavian, brachiocephalic (innominate), or iliac veins, the superior or inferior vena cava, or the right atrium.

To select the appropriate code from this code range, the coder must review the provider documentation and then answer the following questions:

- What type of procedure was performed?
  - **Insertion:** placing a catheter through a newly established venous access.
  - **Repair:** fixing a device without replacement of either catheter or port/pump.

- **Partial replacement:** replacing only the catheter component associated with a port/pump device.
- **Complete replacement:** replacing the entire device via the same venous access site.
- **Removal:** removing the entire device.
- Was the catheter inserted centrally or peripherally?
- If the catheter was inserted centrally, was it tunneled or nontunneled?

SPOTLIGHT on a Guideline

A centrally inserted catheter uses the jugular, subclavian, or femoral vein or the inferior vena cava as the entry site. A peripherally inserted catheter is generally placed in the basilic or cephalic vein and then moved forward into the subclavian vein.

MENTOR
Coding Tip

A peripherally inserted catheter is often referred to in documentation as a PICC (peripherally inserted central catheter).

A tunneled catheter is generally inserted for long-term use. The catheter is tunneled through the skin and subcutaneous tissue to a great vein. The documentation should clearly state that a tunnel was created.

- Was a pump or port included?
- What is the age of the patient?

SPOTLIGHT on a Guideline

Many editions of the CPT manual include a central venous access procedures table that should be used as a resource when selecting the appropriate code(s) from this code range.

FOR EXAMPLE If the documentation stated, *"insertion of nontunneled, centrally inserted* central venous catheter" and the patient is *younger than 5 years of age,* the appropriate CPT code would be 36555. If the documentation stated that the nontunneled catheter was *inserted peripherally* in a patient younger than 5 years of age, the appropriate CPT code would be 36568.

Hemodialysis Access: 36800–36870

Creation of an arteriovenous (AV) fistula is the most common method for hemodialysis access. The surgeon connects the artery to the vein, and this abnormal connection between these vessels causes blood to flow from the artery directly to the vein; eventually the vein walls become thicker and stronger and are an ideal placement site for the dialysis needle.

The coder needs to determine whether the fistula was created by vein transposition or direct anastomosis. Codes for vein transposition are defined by the vein used:

- Upper arm (cephalic or brachiocephalic), 36818
- Upper arm basilic vein, 36819
- Forearm vein (radiocephalic), 36820

The direct anastomosis method involves attaching an artery and a vein directly and is reported with code 36821. The surgeon may perform an arteriovenous (AV) graft (36825–36830) to connect the artery to the vein.

1. What are the three types of coronary artery bypass grafting?

2. Identify the code to be assigned for insertion of a PICC without subcutaneous port or pump in a patient younger than 5 years of age.

3. To qualify as a central venous access device, where must the tip of the catheter terminate?

4. Identify the appropriate code for removal of a transvenous electrode only, single lead system, for an implantable cardioverter-defibrillator.

EXERCISE 12.4

Also available in **Mc Graw Hill connect** (plus+)

12.5 Guidelines and Format of the Lymphatic Subsection of CPT

The lymphatic system is a part of the circulatory system, therefore the codes for the lymphatic system are included in the same subsection as the cardiovascular system. Table 12.8 lists code ranges for the hemic and lymphatic systems.

Hemic and Lymphatic Systems (38100–38999)

Spleen: 38100–38200

The spleen is removed for a number of reasons, including:

- Enlargement that becomes destructive to platelets/red blood cells.
- Means of diagnosing certain diseases such as lymphomas.
- Hemorrhaging following physical trauma.
- Spontaneous rupture.

Splenectomy, open or laparoscopic, procedures are included in this code range. Repair of a ruptured spleen with or without a partial appendectomy, code 38115, is also included in this range.

Bone Marrow or Stem Cell Services: 38204–38243

This range of codes is used to identify various procedures to preserve, prepare, and purify bone marrow or stem cells prior to transplantation or reinfusion.

The guidelines at the beginning of this code range inform the coder that each code may be reported only once per day regardless of the quantity of bone marrow or stem cells manipulated.

Table 12.8 Hemic and Lymphatic Subsection Code Ranges *(Data from CPT 2013. © 2013 American Medical Association. All rights reserved.)*

SUBHEADING	CODE RANGE
Spleen	38100–38200
General	38204–38243
Lymph Nodes and Lymphatic Channels	38300–38999

Lymph Nodes and Lymphatic Channels: 38300–38999

Incision, 38300–38382: Included in this code range is drainage of a **lymph node** abscess, either simple or extensive (38300–38305).

Excision, 38500–38555 Included in this code range is biopsy or excision of lymph nodes. The codes in this range are further defined as whether they are cervical or axillary nodes.

The sentinel lymph nodes are the first to receive lymph drainage from the breast and are also the most likely nodes to contain cancer if it has spread. Lymph node biopsies are performed to determine if the cancer has spread to the sentinel node. During these type of biopsies, radioactive tracers are injected as a means of identifiying the sentinel node. The surgeon uses a hand-held Geiger counter to identify radioactive lymph nodes.

FOR EXAMPLE

Partial mastectomy (CPT 19301) with sentinel lymph node biopsy (typically CPT code 38525) and dye injection to identify the sentinel node (CPT code 38792)

The surgeon would use the CPT codes in this example to report the service. ■

EXERCISE 12.5

1. What is the appropriate code for the injection procedure for identification of a sentinel node?
2. Assign the appropriate code for a surgical laparoscopy with multiple retroperitoneal lymph node sampling.

Also available in ![McGraw Hill] **connect** (plus+)

12.6 Modifiers Most Commonly Used with Codes in the Cardiovascular Subsection

As with all sections of the CPT manual, modifiers are used in the Cardiovascular subsection to continue or modify the story of the patient's encounter. Some of the more common modifiers used within this section are 51, multiple procedures; 52, reduced services; 53, discontinued procedure; 57, decision for surgery; 58, staged or related procedure or service by the same physician during the postoperative period; 59, distinct procedural service; 78, unplanned return to the operating/procedure room by the same physician or another qualified healthcare professional following the initial procedure for a related procedure during the postoperative period. (See Table 12.9.)

Table 12.9 Cardiovascular Subsection Modifiers *(Data from CPT 2013. © 2013 American Medical Association. All rights reserved.)*

MODIFIER	DEFINITION	EXAMPLE
50	Bilateral procedure	Injection procedure, lymphangiography, bilateral is reported with CPT code 38790–50.
53	Discontinued procedure	Physician starts a procedure, and the patient experiences an acute or life-threatening condition and the procedure must be terminated. The CPT code for the procedure being performed is assigned along with modifier 53.
57	Decision for surgery	Physician sees the patient in the ER for severe chest pain and determines that a cardioverter-defibrillator needs to be inserted. Modifier 57 is attached to the ER consultation visit since the procedure has a 90-day global period and this modifier indicates the decision for surgery.
59	Distinct procedural service	A right internal carotid angiography and a left vertebral angiography were performed on the same patient during the same session. Modifier 59 is reported to show that a separate and distinct vascular family was imaged.
78	Unplanned return to the operating/procedure room by the same physician or another qualified healthcare professional following the initial procedure for a related procedure during the postoperative period	Physician inserts a pacemaker, which has a 90-day global surgical period attached to the code, and the same physician returns the patient to the operating room during the 90-day period for a related procedure.

EXERCISE 12.6

1. The patient presents in the office today with atrial fibrillation, and the physician decides to insert a dual-chamber pacemaker the next day. Assign the appropriate CPT code along with any needed modifier.

2. Procedures of the atrial and mitral valves were performed. Is a modifier needed? If so, which one would be appropriate?

3. The physician starts a valvuloplasty procedure, and the patient becomes tachycardic and the vavluloplasty is stopped. Which modifier would be used to tell the story of this patient encounter?

Also available in McGraw Hill **connect** (plus+)

12.7 Common Medical and Procedural Terms Used in Operative Reports

As with all sections of CPT, the Cardiovascular and Lymphatic subsections include medical terms and procedural terms that are specific to the system involved. Tables 12.10 and 12.11 list some of these ICD and CPT terms for the cardiovascular and lymphatic systems.

Table 12.10 Terms for Cardiovascular and Lymphatic Systems

TERM	DEFINITION	DOCUMENTATION KEYS
Anastomosis	Surgical connection of two vessels Ana = without; stom/o = mouth or opening; -osis = condition	Seen in reports of an occluded vessel bypass, as in a CABG
Angiography	X-ray exam of the arteries or veins to diagnose conditions of the blood vessels, such as blockage	Arteriography (Remember: *angio* means "vessel," which is an artery or vein.)
Cardioversion	Procedure in which a cardiac arrhythmia is converted to a normal rhythm by using electricity or drugs	*Internal cardioversion:* The shock is delivered from inside the heart, where catheters are placed and the shock is then delivered. *External cardioversion:* The electrodes are placed directly on the chest to deliver the shock.
Coronary artery bypass graft	Procedure used to improve blood flow to the heart by bypassing a blockage of a vessel with a grafted vessel	Many providers refer to this procedure in their documentation as CABG
Endartectomy	Surgical removal of plaque from within a blocked or occluded artery	Carotid endartectomy is the most common way this is reported in provider dictation
Lymphadenectomy	Removal or excision of lymph node(s)	Lymph node dissection or regional lymph node dissection are alternative terms in provider dictation
Percutaneous transluminal coronary angioplasty	Procedure where a catheter with an inflatable balloon attached is inserted into a coronary artery to help dilate the artery and improve the blood flow due to narrowing of the artery caused by blockage	Many providers refer to this procedure in their documentation as PTCA
Stent	Device used to hold open a blood vessel	Dictation will often refer to a stent or a wire mesh tube being placed in an artery to open up a portion of the artery that has been narrowed or block often due to atherosclerosis. The dictation will often refer to the stent being mounted on a balloon which is then advanced through a catheter to the placement site. The balloon is then deflated and removed and the stent is permanently in place. The dictation may refer to the stent being deployed.
Shunt	Tube that diverts or bypasses	For example, during a carotoid endartectomy, a small tube (shunt) maybe be inserted in the carotid artery to deliver blood flow around the area being operated on.

angiography X-ray exam of the arteries or veins to diagnose conditions of the blood vessels, such as blockage.

Table 12.11 Additional Terms for Cardiovascular and Lymphatic Systems

TERM	DEFINITION	DOCUMENTATION KEYS
Temporal arteritis	Inflammation of large blood vessels (e.g., carotid and branches)	Giant cell arteritis, cranial arteritis
Bruit	Abnormal sound heard when listening to the blood flow	Abnormal blowing sounds, vascular murmur
Hypertension (HTN)	Increased pressure in the arterial walls	High blood pressure
Rheumatic chorea	Symptom of rheumatic fever that causes involuntary muscle movements and twitching	Sydenham's, St. Vitus' dance
Arrhythmia	Irregular heartbeat	Dysrhythmia, cardiac arrhythmia
Embolus	Foreign object, such as a detached blood clot, that moves through the bloodstream, lodges in a blood vessel, and occludes the vessel	Difference between embolus and thrombus. Embolus is any foreign object that occludes a vessel such as a thrombus. A thrombus is a clot of blood formed within a blood vessel.
Thrombus	Clot in a blood vessel	clot
Sick sinus syndrome SSS	Group of signs and/or symptoms indicating that the SA node is not functioning adequately	The symptoms may include bradycardia, fatigue, syncope, shortness of breath, confusion, and palpitations.
Lymphedema	Collection of excess fluid in the lymph tissue, which can cause swelling	May also be seen in dictation as lymphatic obstruction.
Portal vein thrombosis	Obstruction of the portal vein that results from a blood clot or narrowing of the vein	Doppler ultrasounds are often used to confirm this diagnosis. Fluid can build up in the stomach, the spleen can enlarge, and severe hemorrhaging can occur in the esophagus. Pressure in the portal vein increases due to the blockage or narrowing of the portal vein. This increased pressure is defined as portal hypertension.

MENTOR
Coding Tip

Documentation of an elevated blood pressure reading without a diagnosis of hypertension is not coded to hypertension.

arrhythmia An irregular heartbeat.

embolus A foreign object, such as a detached blood clot, that moves through the bloodstream, lodges in a blood vessel, and occludes the vessel.

thrombus A clot in a blood vessel.

---

1. An opening or hole between the right and left atriums is a _____.
2. What is the abbreviation for a group of signs and/or symptoms indicating that the SA node is not functioning adequately?
3. An abnormal blowing sound heard on auscultation could be indicated in the documentation as a _____.
4. What are the two types of cardioversion?
5. What is the difference between a shunt and a stent?

EXERCISE 12.7

Also available in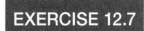

Chapter Twelve Summary

Learning Outcome	Key Concepts/Examples
12.1 Review the anatomy of the cardiovascular system.	The cardiovascular system consists of the heart, blood, and blood vessels which include arteries, veins, and capillaries. It includes the pulmonary circulation system, where blood is pumped away from the heart by the pulmonary artery; to the lungs; and then returned to the heart by the pulmonary vein. The systemic circulation system transports oxygenated blood away from the heart, to the rest of the body, and returns oxygen-depleted blood back to the heart.
12.2 Review the anatomy of the lymphatic system.	The lymphatic system is made up of fluid or lymph, lymph vessels, and lymphoid tissue such as lymph nodes, the spleen, and the thymus.
12.3 Understand chapter-specific ICD guidelines and format for the circulatory system.	The most common problems patients present with concerning this system are chest pain, hypertension, edema, murmur, palpitations, congestive heart failure, arrythmias, syncope, hyperlipidemia, claudication, and congenital heart disease. When coding these conditions, coders must thoroughly review the provider documentation as well as the guidelines and instructional notes.

ICD-9-CM: Diseases of the Circulatory System is Chapter 7 in the ICD-9-CM manual, with the code range 390–459.
ICD-10-CM: Diseases of the Circulatory System is Chapter 9 in the ICD-10-CM manual, with the code range I00–I99.

• Rheumatic fever codes are further defined by the type of heart involvement, such as endocarditis.
• When coding for heart valve conditions, the coder needs to know which valve(s) was (were) involved, such as the mitral valve, and what the diagnosed disease of the involved valve(s) is, such as stenosis.
• The chapter-specific guidelines should be referred to and followed when assigning codes from the hypertensive heart and/or kidney disease range.
• When coding for heart failure, the coder must assign an additional code to identify the specific type of failure.
• Before assigning a code for an AMI, the coder must identify the episode of care and the location of the myocardial infarction. |
| **12.4** Identify the guidelines and format of the Cardiovascular subsection of CPT. | • Before assigning the appropriate codes for a pacemaker or cardioverter-defibrillator procedure, coders must answer several questions, such as whether it was single- or dual-chamber, was an insertion or replacement, and involved a transvenous or epicardial approach.
• There are three types of coronary bypass grafting: venous grafting only, arterial grafting only, and combined arterial-venous grafting.
• Repair of an aneurysm is most commonly accomplished by a direct procedure or by endovascular repair.
• CPT coding decisions for vascular injection or introduction procedures are based on whether the physician performed a selective or nonselective catheter placement. |
| **12.5** Identify the guidelines and format of the Lymphatic subsection of CPT. | • Codes within the hemic and lymphatic ranges include those for procedures involving the spleen, bone marrow or stem cell services, and lymph nodes and lymph channels. |

Learning Outcome	Key Concepts/Examples
12.6 Apply the modifiers most commonly used with codes in the Cardiovascular subsections.	Modifiers are used in the Cardiovascular subsections to continue or modify the story of the patient's encounter. Some of the more common modifiers used in this section are: • Bilateral services, 51 • Discontinued procedure, 53 • Staged or related procedure or service by the same physician during the postoperative period, 58 • Distinct procedural service, 59 • Unplanned return to the operating/procedure room by the same physician or another qualified healthcare professional following the initial procedure for a related procedure during the postoperative period, 78
12.7 Examine the common medical and procedural terms used in operative reports.	The Cardiovascular and Lymphatic subsections include medical terms and procedural terms that are specific to the system involved. There are also some key terms that could appear in a provider's documentation and act as a trigger for the coder to identify the diagnosis and/or procedure for the encounter.

Chapter Twelve Review

Understanding Terminology

Match each key term to the appropriate definition.

_____ 1. [LO12.4] Ablation

_____ 2. [LO12.4] Aneurysm

_____ 3. [LO12.3] Angina pectoris

_____ 4. [LO12.7] Angiography

_____ 5. [LO12.1] Aorta

_____ 6. [LO12.7] Arrhythmia

_____ 7. [LO12.3] Coronary artery bypass graft (CABG)

_____ 8. [LO12.3] Deep vein thrombosis (DVT)

_____ 9. [LO12.4] Defibrillator

_____ 10. [LO12.7] Embolus

_____ 11. [LO12.3] Infarction

_____ 12. [LO12.4] Ischemia

_____ 13. [LO12.4] Lymph node

_____ 14. [LO12.4] Lymph vessel

_____ 15. [LO12.4] Pacemaker

_____ 16. [LO12.7] Thrombus

A. Procedure used to improve blood flow to the heart by bypassing a blockage of a vessel with a grafted vessel

B. Foreign object such as a blood clot in the bloodstream

C. X-ray exam of the arteries or veins used to diagnose the condition of the blood vessels

D. Bulge or swelling in the wall of a vessel

E. Death of a heart muscle

F. Procedure that involves scarring or destroying cardiac tissues that trigger abnormal heart rhythms

G. Severe chest pain due to insufficient blood supply to the heart

H. The largest artery; takes oxygenated blood from the left ventricle to the body

I. Irregular heartbeat

J. A collection of tissue located along the lymph vessels that acts as a filter and produces antibodies and lymphocytes

K. Device that uses a combination of antitachycardia pacing and low-energy cardioversion or shocks to obtain a regular rhythm of the heart

L. Blood clot or thrombus located in a deep vein

M. Irreversible condition in which heart muscle is denied adequate blood flow for an extended period of time and the muscle dies

N. Blood clot

O. Electrical device inserted into the body to shock the heart into a regular rhythm

P. Structure that transports lymph fluids and merges into lymphatic ducts; enables water and other dissolved substances to return to the blood

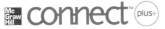 **plus+** Enhance your learning by completing these exercises and more at mcgrawhillconnect.com

Checking Your Understanding

Choose the most appropriate answer for each of the following questions.

1. **[LO12.1]** A mass of undissolved matter that is transported in the blood is called a(an):
   a. Abscess
   b. Clot
   c. Neoplasm
   d. Embolus

2. **[LO12.3]** A 32-year-old patient is admitted for fever, shortness of breath, and night sweats. The patient has just returned from a mission trip for her church during which she traveled to Africa for 3 weeks. Blood tests, cultures, and echocardiograms reveal endocarditis due to blastomycosis. She will remain in the hospital for IV antibiotics. Select the appropriate ICD-9-CM codes:
   a. 116.0, 421.1
   b. 421.0, 116.0
   c. 116.0, 431.0
   d. 431.0, 116.0

3. **[LO12.3, 12.4]** The patient is diagnosed with acute coronary insufficiency and is admitted for CABG using four veins harvested endoscopically from the left saphenous vein. Select the appropriate ICD-9-CM and CPT codes:
   a. 33513, 33508, 411.89
   b. 33513, 411.81
   c. 33536, 411.89
   d. 33536, 411.81

4. **[LO12.7]** Abnormal heart rhythms that are too slow are identified as:
   a. Tachycardia
   b. Dysrhythmia
   c. Bradycardia
   d. Arrythmia

5. **[LO12.3]** A patient is admitted to the cardiac unit with an acute MI of the inferolateral wall and a third-degree AV block. The patient has no history of prior MI. Select the appropriate ICD-9-CM codes:
   a. 410.20, 426.0
   b. 410.21, 426.0
   c. 410.21, 426.4
   d. 410.21, 426.10

6. **[LO12.4]** A physician inserts a single temporary transvenous pacing catheter into the right atrium and connects the electrode to an external pulse generator. How should the physician report these services?
   a. 33214
   b. 33206-52
   c. 33210
   d. 33211-52

7. **[LO12.3]** Choose the appropriate ICD-9-CM code for diagnosis of ataxia due to CVA:
   a. 438.84
   b. 432.0
   c. 438.21
   d. 438.81

8. **[LO12.3, 12.4]** Jack Smith was diagnosed with a thoracic aortic aneurysm. He was admitted to the hospital and underwent transverse arch graft to repair the aneurysm. Cardiopulmonary bypass was provided as well. Select the correct CPT and ICD-9-CM codes:
   a. 33874, 441.2
   b. 33870, 441.2
   c. 33877, 33926, 441.2
   d. 33870, 441.9

9. **[LO12.7]** The heart wall is composed of three layers. They are the epicardium, myocardium, and:
   a. Echocardium
   b. Epithelium
   c. Endocardium
   d. Valves

10. **[LO12.3]** Maria has hypertensive chronic kidney disease, stage III. She also has congestive heart failure and osteoarthritis in her right shoulder. She was seen by her cardiologist for routine maintenance. Reporting only the ICD-9-CM codes, select the correct codes:
    a. 403.10, 585.3, 403.90, 715.91, 428.0
    b. 403.90, 585.3, 428.0, 715,91
    c. 401.9, 585.3, 428.0, 715.91
    d. 401.9, 585.9, 428.0, 715.91

Applying Your Knowledge

Answer the following questions and code the following case study. Be sure to follow the process steps as illustrated in chapter 8

Case Study: Cardio Note

Procedure performed: Placement of permanent pacemaker, dual chamber.

Indications: A definite diagnosis of atrial fibrillation was made, and I determined during the office visit yesterday that a permanent dual-chamber pacemaker device would be inserted today.

Postoperative diagnosis: Atrial fibrillation.

Procedure: The patient was prepped and draped in the usual sterile fashion. A needle was passed into the left subclavian vein, and good blood was noted. The guide wire was passed through the needle, and the needle was removed. The dilator and introducer were then passed over the wire.

Once in position, the dilator and guide wire were removed and leads were placed.

Leads were placed in the right ventricle and atrium, sequentially.

I then turned to placement of the pulse generator. A subcutaneous pacemaker pocket was created in the right anterior chest wall, and the pulse generator was placed in the pocket. A subcutaneous tunnel was made, and the leads were threaded thru and attached to the generator. The pocket was sutured in the usual sterile fashion, and the patient tolerated the procedure well. A chest x-ray was ordered to verify placement of leads and generator upon completion of the procedure.

Process 1: CPT

1. What is the procedure?

2. Locate the main term in the index.

3. What additional questions or set of questions can be determined?

4. Upon review of all the code choices identified in the index, what additional questions can be determined?

5. Based on the documentation, what is (are) the correct code(s) for this case?

    a. 33206

    b. 33249

    c. 33208

    d. 33208, 33217

Process 2: ICD

ICD-9-CM

1. Based on the operative report header, what is the preoperative diagnosis?

2. Is the postoperative diagnosis the same as or different from the preoperative diagnosis?

3. What is the main term for this condition?

4. Based on the subterm choices, what question(s) can be developed for this condition?

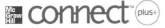

Enhance your learning by completing these exercises and more at mcgrawhillconnect.com

5. Is any sign, symptom, or additional condition documented?

6. Is the additional condition, sign, or symptom an integral part of the primary (or other) condition coded?

7. Based on the documentation, what is the correct ICD-9-CM code for this case?
   a. 427.31
   b. 427.32
   c. 427.41
   d. 427.42

Process 3: Modifiers

1. Was the procedure performed different from that described by the nomenclature of the code?

2. Was the procedure performed on an anatomical site that has laterality?

3. Was the procedure performed in the global period of another procedure?

4. Were additional procedures performed during the operative session, and does the documentation support them?

5. Did the surgeon have help from another surgeon or another appropriate person?

6. Did a physician different from the surgeon provide the preoperative or postoperative portion of the procedure?

7. What modifier should be appended to the CPT for this case?
   a. 57
   b. 50
   c. None
   d. 52

Unit 3 Exam

The questions in this exam cover material in Chapters 9 through 12 of this book.

Choose the most appropriate answer for each question below.

1. **[LO9.4]** Amy presents to the office for destruction of a malignant 2.3-cm lesion of the skin of the neck. Select the appropriate ICD-9-CM and CPT codes for today's encounter:

   a. 17283, 185.0

   b. 17270, 239.2

   c. 17273,173.40

   d. 17280, 216.4

2. **[LO9.4]** Amara presents to the office today as an established patient to have irritated skin tags removed from her neck and shoulders. Dr. Rose prepped her for the procedure and removed 20 skin tags using liquid nitrogen. Select the appropriate CPT code(s) for Amara's visit today:

   a. 11055

   b. 11200 × 15, 11201 × 5 -50

   c. 11200, 11201

   d. 11200, 11202, 99212

3. **[LO9.1]** The form of skin cancer that rarely metastasizes is known as:

   a. Squamous cell carcinoma

   b. Malignant melanoma

   c. Basal cell carcinoma

   d. Cellulitis

4. **[LO9.2]** A female patient had breast cancer 3 years ago, underwent a radical mastectomy, and received radiation and chemotherapy. She has not had treatment in the last 20 months. How is the status of the cancer reported for the patient?

   a. V16.3   **c.** V10.3

   b. V13.2   **d.** V10.4

5. **[LO9.2, 9.3]** **Operation:** Left transaxillary subpectoral mammoplasty with saline-filled implant.

   Preoperative diagnosis: Left hypomastia.

   Postoperative diagnosis: Left hypomastia.

   Anesthesia: General.

   Procedure: After first obtaining a suitable level of general anesthesia with the patient in the supine position, the breasts were prepped with Betadine scrub and solution. Sterile towels, sheets, and drapes were placed in the usual fashion for surgery of the breasts. Following prepping and draping, the anterior axillary folds and the inframammary folds were infiltrated with a total of 20 cc of 0.5 percent Xylocaine with 1:200,000 units of epinephrine.

   After a suitable hemostatic waiting period, transaxillary incisions were made, and dissection was carried down to the edge of the pectoralis fascia. Blunt dissection was then used to form a bilateral subpectoral pocket. Through the subpectoral pocket a sterile suction tip was introduced, and copious irrigation with sterile saline solution was used until the irrigant was clear.

   Following completion of irrigation, 250-cc saline-filled implants were introduced. They were first filled with 60 cc of saline and checked for gross leakage; none was evident. They were overfilled to 300 cc of saline each. The patient was then placed in the seated position, and the left breast needed 10 cc of additional fluid for symmetry.

   Following completion of the filling of the implants and checking the breasts for symmetry, the patient's wounds were closed with interrupted vertical mattress sutures of 4-0 Prolene. Flexan dressings were applied, followed by the patient's bra. She seemed to tolerate the procedure well.

Choose the appropriate CPT and ICD-9-CM codes:

a. 19316-LT, 611.82

b. 19324-LT, 611.82

c. 19325-LT, 611.82

d. 19328-LT, 611.82

6. [LO9.3] A 35-year-old female patient receives biopsies of both breasts. The biopsies are done using fine-needle aspiration without imaging guidance. What is the correct CPT code to use for this procedure?

a. 10021-50

b. 19103-50

c. 10022-50

d. 19102-50

7. [LO10.2] Boris presents to the clinic today for completion of a series of injections into his shoulder for shoulder pain. The physician gives the patient an injection into the left shoulder. Choose the correct CPT and ICD-9-CM codes:

a. 20600-LT, 715.91

b. 20610-LT, 719.41

c. 20610-LT, 719.46

d. 20600-LT, 715.31

8. [LO10.2, 10.3] Gavin presents to the hospital for an outpatient procedure for a diagnostic arthroscopy of the right knee. As the physician is performing the procedure, she identifies a medial meniscal tear and repairs it at that time. Choose the correct CPT and ICD-9-CM codes for this procedure:

a. 29870-RT, 836.1

b. 29871-RT, 836.2

c. 29883-RT, 836.0, 836.1

d. 29882-RT, 836.1

9. [LO10. 3] **Operative Report**

Postoperative diagnosis:

1. Retained hardware, left foot.

2. Decreased range of motion, left ankle.

Procedure: The patient was placed under general anesthesia; her left lower extremity was prepped and draped in a sterile fashion. A time-out procedure was performed.

The patient then had a hardware removal performed on the transcutaneous K-wires, followed by examination of her ankle, which had approximately 5 to 10 degrees lacking of neutral. Gentle manipulation was performed, giving her dorsiflexion to 10 degrees. C- arm fluoroscopy was introduced to the field, taking confirmatory x-ray, and at this point the patient had a sterile dressing applied and was awakened from general anesthesia.

Select the appropriate CPT and ICD-9-CM codes:

a. 20670-LT, 27860-LT, 76000-26

b. 20680-LT, 27899-LT, 76000-26

c. 20690-LT, 27860-LT, 76000-26

d. 20694-LT, 76000-26

10. [LO10.3] Sarah, a 24-year-old female, was walking her dog this morning, and when she wasn't paying attention, she tripped and fell over the curb. The patient states that she fell to the ground using her right hand and arm to brace herself. She states that she heard a "crunch"; the resultant x-ray indicated a compound fracture to the ulna of her right arm. With the patient under general anesthesia, the area was opened and irrigated. The shaft of the ulna was fractured and had to be repaired using screws to hold it into place. The surrounding tissue was repaired, irrigated, and closed in a usual manner. Select the correct CPT code for the repair of the ulna:

a. 25560

b. 25575

c. 25545

d. 25520

11. [LO10.2, 10.3] Jeremy presents to the clinic today for severe wrist pain. After Dr. Wilkins examines it, she diagnoses him with a ganglion cyst of the right wrist. Dr. Wilkins decides to give Jeremy a cortisone injection as a treatment plan. Code the correct CPT and ICD-9-CM:

a. 20605-RT, 727.41   c. 20550-RT × 2, 727.41

b. 20551-RT × 2, 727.42   d. 20612-RT, 727.42

12. [LO10.1] A chronic or acute infection of the bone usually caused by bacteria or fungi is called:

a. Osteoporosis   c. Osteogenesis

b. Osteomalacia   d. Osteomyelitis

13. [LO11.3] A 15-year-old patient has a surgical nasal endoscopy with biopsy of a nasal polyp. What is the correct CPT code for this procedure?

a. 31235   c. 31237

b. 31233   d. 31267

14. [LO11.2, 11.3] Timmy, a 5-year-old, was playing with his toys and decided to stick a bead from his sister's necklace up his nose. The bead was lodged in his nasal passage, and after several unsuccessful attempts by his mother and father to remove it, they took him to the emergency room. After triaging the patient, the physician utilized a surgical instrument to help remove the bead from Timmy's nasal passage. Code the physician services:

a. 30220, 934.9   c. 30310, 932

b. 30400, 932   d. 30300, 932

15. [LO11.2, 11.3] The physician performed thoracentesis with tube insertion to treat pleural effusion caused by small cell cancer of the middle lobe of the right lung. Select the appropriate CPT and ICD codes:

a. 32421, 162.9   c. 32421, 162.4

b. 32422, 162.4   d. 32420, 162.9

16. [LO11.1] Which of the following is the area of the sinus that is located at the top of the nasal cavities between the eyes?

a. Frontal   c. Ethmoid

b. Sphenoid   d. Maxillary

17. [LO11.5] The patient presents to the ED with severe shortness of breath. After testing, the ED physician diagnoses the patient as having ARDS. Select the appropriate ICD-9-CM code:

a. 518.82   c. 518.52

b. 518.81   d. 518.51

18. [LO11.2, 11.3] The patient underwent radical neck dissection with laryngectomy for carcinoma of the larynx and true vocal cords. Choose the correct codes:

a. 31360, 161.0   c. 31360, 163.1

b. 31365, 161.1   d. 31365, 161.0

19. [LO11. 1, 11.3] The patient presents for submucous resection of the middle turbinate, complete. Select the appropriate CPT code:

a. 30140   c. 30999

b. 30520   d. 30130

20. [LO12.3, 12.4] Michael, a 40-year-old male, presented for insertion of a permanent pacemaker by transvenous approach. A pocket was created for the insertion of the generator, and the electrodes were placed in the right atrium and ventricle. Michael is diagnosed with atrial fibrillation. Select the correct codes:

a. 33249, 427.31   c. 33217, 427.32

b. 33208, 427.31   d. 33240, 427.41

21. [LO12.1.] Which of the following great vessels carries deoxygenated blood from the right ventricle to the lungs?

   a. Vena cava

   b. Pulmonary arteries

   c. Pulmonary veins

   d. Aorta

22. [LO12. 4] The patient presents for a direct repair of an aneurysm and graft insertion without a patch graft for an aneurysm of the common iliac artery. Select the appropriate CPT code:

   a. 35122

   b. 35131

   c. 35121

   d. 35103

23. [LO12.4] If the starting point is catheterization of the aorta, to which of the following order branches in the vascular family reporting would the left internal carotid artery belong?

   a. First

   b. Second

   c. Third

   d. Additional third

24. [LO12.6] Gary sees Dr. G on Monday regarding his atrial fibrillation. Gary is a new patient, and Dr. G performs a comprehensive history, an exam, and moderate medical decision making. Dr. G decides to insert a permanent dual-chamber pacemaker. The pacemaker is inserted on Tuesday. Dr. G sees Gary in the hospital on Wednesday and discharges Gary on Thursday. Which of the following is the correct coding of Gary's visits and procedures for Monday through Thursday?

   a. 99204, 33208, 99232, 99238

   b. 99204-57, 33208

   c. 99214, 33207, 99232, 99238

   d. 99204, 33208

25. [LO12.3] A patient is diagnosed with deep vein thrombosis of a lower extremity. Which of the following veins could be involved?

   a. Saphenous

   b. Brachial

   c. Popliteal

   d. Cephalic

Coding for Surgical Procedures on Digestive, Urinary, Male and Female Reproductive Systems, Maternity Care, Nervous System, and Eyes, Ears, and Endocrine System

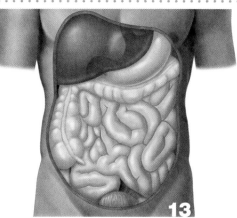

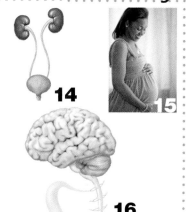

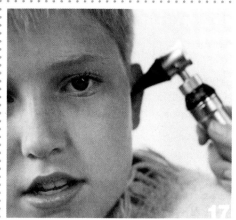

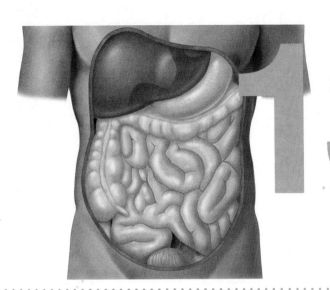

13

Surgery Section: Digestive System

Key Terms

Bolus
Cecum
Choledocholithiasis
Cholelithiasis
Diverticulitis

Diverticulosis
Duodenum
Endoscopic retrograde
  cholangiopancreatography
  (ERCP)

Endoscopy
Gastroesophageal reflux
  disease (GERD)
Ileum
Intussusception

Jejunum
Laparoscopy
Vestibule
Volvulus

Learning Outcomes

After completing this chapter, you will be able to:

13.1 Review the anatomy of the digestive system.

13.2 Understand the chapter-specific ICD guidelines and format for the digestive system.

13.3 Identify the guidelines and format of the Digestive subsection of CPT.

13.4 Apply the modifiers most commonly used with codes in the Digestive subsection.

13.5 Examine the common medical and procedural terms used in operative reports.

Introduction The digestive system is often referred to in documentation as the *gastrointestinal (GI) tract* or *alimentary canal.* The digestive system's primary functions are digestion of food, absorption of nutrients, and elimination of waste products.

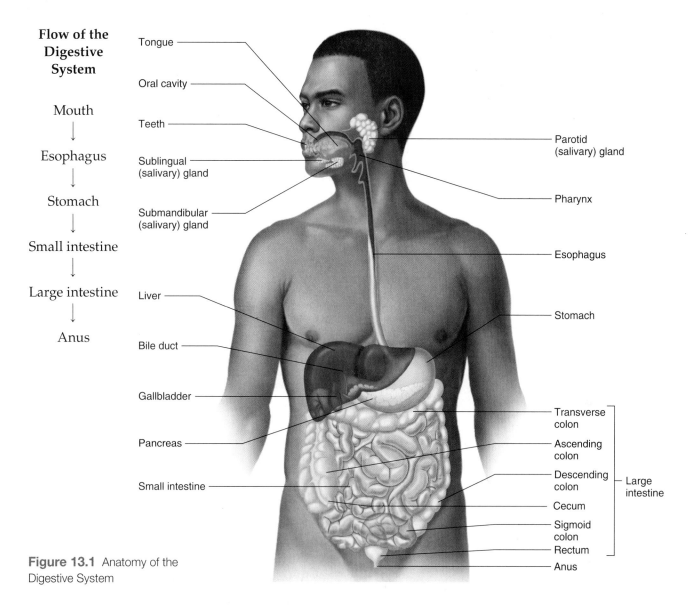

Flow of the Digestive System

Mouth
↓
Esophagus
↓
Stomach
↓
Small intestine
↓
Large intestine
↓
Anus

Tongue

Oral cavity

Teeth

Sublingual (salivary) gland

Submandibular (salivary) gland

Parotid (salivary) gland

Pharynx

Esophagus

Stomach

Liver

Bile duct

Gallbladder

Pancreas

Small intestine

Transverse colon

Ascending colon

Descending colon

Cecum

Sigmoid colon

Rectum

Anus

Large intestine

Figure 13.1 Anatomy of the Digestive System

13.1 Anatomy of the Digestive System

The digestive system consists of the mouth, esophagus, stomach, small intestine, large intestine, and accessory organs consisting of the salivary glands, liver, gallbladder, and pancreas. (See Figure 13.1 and Table 13.1.)

Table 13.1 Structures of the Digestive System

STRUCTURE	DEFINITION/FUNCTION
Mouth	• The oral cavity includes: *Lips:* They form the opening to the oral cavity. *Gums:* They are also called *gingiva*. *Teeth:* Function is to break down food. *Tongue:* Functions are taste and movement of food into the throat. *Hard palate:* This is the roof of the mouth. *Soft palate:* Function is to keep food from entering the nasal cavity. *Uvula:* This triggers the gag reflex and assists in producing sounds and speech.

(continued)

Table 13.1 Structures of the Digestive System (*concluded*)

STRUCTURE	DEFINITION/FUNCTION
Esophagus	• Muscular tube. • Peristaltic action occurs here after food is chewed and swallowed. • Leads to the stomach.
Stomach	• Digestive process continues after the food enters here from the esophagus and mixes with digestive juices and hydrochloric acid. • There are three parts to the stomach: *Fundus:* upper part *Body:* middle part *Antrum/pylorus:* lower part
Small intestine:	• Consists of three main parts: **Duodenum:** first section of small intestine, 10–12 inches in length. Most of digestion occurs here. **Jejunum:** middle section of small intestine, 8 feet in length. **Ileum:** last section of small intestine, 11 feet in length. • This is where another function of the digestive system happens: Nutrients are absorbed into the bloodstream, and the waste is passed into the large intestine.
Large intestine	• Consists of five main parts: **Cecum:** pouch at the beginning of the intestine; links to the ileum Ascending colon Transverse colon Descending colon Sigmoid colon • The colon is a long hollow tube extending from the cecum to the rectum. The main functions of the colon are to remove liquids from digested food and to move the remaining solid waste through the rectum and to the outside of the body through the anus.
Anus	• The opening of the rectum to the outside of the body; solid-waste material exits through the anus.
Accessory organs: Salivary glands	• The three types are: Parotid Sublingual Submandibular • Produce saliva, which when mixed with food starts the digestive process. The mixture of food and digestive enzymes in the saliva is called a **bolus.**
Liver	• Produces bile, which is necessary for the digestion of fats. • Main function is the storage of bile.
Gallbladder	• The gallbladder is small and saclike. • Gallstones, or **cholelithiasis,** form in the gallbladder and can cause cholecystitis, an inflammation of the gallbladder.
Pancreas	• The pancreas functions as both a digestive and an endocrine organ.

duodenum The first section of the small intestine.

jejunum The middle section of the small intestine.

ileum The last section of the small intestine.

cecum Pouch at the beginning of the large intestine that links to the ileum.

MENTOR
Coding Tip

There is a difference between *ilium* and ileum. *Ilium,* with the i, refers to the hip, and *ileum,* with the e, refers to the small intestine. An easy way to remember the distinction between the two is that medical terms relating to the small intestine begin with "e," such as *enteritis*.

bolus A mixture of food and digestive enzymes in the saliva.

cholelithiasis Gallstones.

1. What structure located in the mouth triggers a gag reflex and assists in speech and sound?

2. The mixture of food and digestive enzymes in the saliva is called a _____.

3. Name the accessory organs of the digestive system, and explain their functions.

4. Name the third segment of the small intestine.

5. Which structure connects the small and large intestines?

EXERCISE 13.1

Also available in **connect**™ (plus+)

13.2 ICD Chapter-Specific Guidelines and Format for the Digestive System

Some common diseases coded to the Digestive chapter of ICD are gingivitis, gastroesophageal reflux disease (GERD), jaundice, pancreatitis, cirrhosis, portal hypertension, esophagitis, appendicitis, and hernias. When coding these conditions, coders must thoroughly review the provider documentation as well as the guidelines and instructional notes.

ICD-9-CM: The Digestive subsection is Chapter 9 in the ICD-9-CM manual, with the code range 520–579.

ICD-10-CM: The Digestive subsection is Chapter 11 in the ICD-10-CM manual, with the code range K00–K95.

Table 13.2 lists the Chapter 9 and 11 subheadings and their code ranges.

Table 13.2 ICD Digestive System Subsection Format *(Data from ICD-9-CM and ICD-10-CM, Centers for Medicare and Medicaid Services and the National Center for Health Statistics.)*

ICD-9-CM		ICD-10-CM	
SUBHEADING	**CODE RANGE**	**SUBHEADING**	**CODE RANGE**
Diseases of Oral Cavity, Salivary Glands, and Jaws	520–529	Diseases of Oral Cavity and Salivary Glands	K00–K14
Diseases of Esophagus, Stomach, and Duodenum	530–539	Diseases of Esophagus, Stomach, and Duodenum	K20–K31
Appendicitis	540–543	Diseases of Appendix	K35–K38
Hernia of Abdominal Cavity	550–553	Hernia	K40–K46
Noninfectious Enteritis and Colitis	555–558	Noninfectious Enteritis and Colitis	K50–K52
Other Diseases of Intestines and Peritoneum	560–569	Other Diseases of Intestines	K55–K64
		Diseases of Peritoneum and Retroperitoneum	K65–K68
Other Diseases of Digestive System	570–579	Diseases of Liver	K70–K77
		Diseases of Gallbladder, Biliary Tract, and Pancreas	K80–K87
		Other Diseases of Digestive System	K90–K95

Diseases of Oral Cavity, Salivary Glands, and Jaws (520–529), ICD-9-CM

Diseases of Oral Cavity and Salivary Glands (K00–K14), ICD-10-CM

This section contains codes to be reported for conditions such as:

- Disorders of tooth development and eruption:
  - Anodontia (absence of teeth).
  - Abnormalities of size and form.
  - Disturbances of tooth formation and tooth eruption.
  - Hereditary disturbances in tooth structure.
- Diseases of hard tissues of teeth:
  - Dental caries (521, ICD-9-CM; K02, ICD-10-CM). Codes in this section require a fifth digit that defines the type of dental caries.
  - Cracked tooth.

FOR EXAMPLE

521.03 Dental caries extending into the pulp (ICD-9-CM)

K02.63 Dental caries on smooth surface penetrating into the pulp (ICD-10-CM) ∎

- Diseases of pulp and periapical tissues:
  - Pulpitis.
  - Degeneration and necrosis of the pulp.
- Gingival and periodontal diseases:
  - Gingivitis.
  - Periodontitis.
- Dentofacial anomalies, including malocclusion.

SPOTLIGHT on a Guideline

There are four classifications of malocclusion: normal occlusion, Class 1 malocclusion, Class II malocclusion, and Class III malocclusion. A diagram showing these different classifications is included in some editions of the ICD-9-CM manual. In ICD-10-CM, codes for dentofacial anomalies, including malocclusion, have been moved to the Diseases of the Musculoskeletal chapter.

- Other diseases and conditions of the teeth and supporting structures:
  - Loss of teeth:
    Complete: due to trauma, periodontal diseases, caries, other specified causes, or unspecified causes.
    Partial: due to trauma, periodontal diseases, caries, other specified causes, or unspecified causes.
- Diseases of the jaw.
- Diseases of the salivary glands.
- Diseases and other conditions of the tongue.

SPOTLIGHT on a Guideline

Both ICD-9-CM and ICD-10-CM have a note informing the coder that if the tooth is broken due to trauma, a code from the Injury chapter is reported.

SPOTLIGHT on a Guideline

The sections on diseases of pulp and periapical tissues and on gingival and periodontal diseases contain separate codes for acute and for chronic conditions.

SPOTLIGHT on a Guideline

In ICD-10-CM, several subsections within the subheading "Diseases of the Oral Cavity" require the use of an additional code to identify alcohol abuse, environmental and occupational exposure to tobacco smoke, history of tobacco use, and exposure to tobacco in the perinatal period.

Diseases of Esophagus, Stomach, and Duodenum (530–539), ICD-9-CM

Diseases of Esophagus, Stomach, and Duodenum (K20–K31), ICD-10-CM

Figure 13.2 references the anatomy of the stomach, which is important for the coder to understand when reviewing an operative report.

To report the appropriate codes from these sections, coders must be able to determine whether there were obstructions, perforations, or hemorrhage related to ulcers and inflammatory diseases. These sections contain codes to be reported for conditions such as:

- Diseases of the esophagus. (They are further specified as to reflux, acute, and eosinophilic.)
- Ulcer of the esophagus. (The codes in this section are further defined as to with or without bleeding. There is an instructional note telling the coder to use an additional code if the ulcer was induced by a chemical or drug.)
- Stricture and stenosis of the esophagus. (This includes compression and obstruction of the esophagus.)
- Perforation of the esophagus.
- Other specified disorders of the esophagus:
  - Esophageal reflux.
  - Esophageal hemorrhage.
- Infection of esophagostomy.
- Gastric ulcer (an ulcer occurring in the stomach).
- Duodenal ulcer (an ulcer occurring in the first, or upper, section of the small intestine).
- Peptic ulcer. A peptic ulcer often occurs in the lining of the stomach or the duodenum. A peptic ulcer in the stomach is called a gastric ulcer. An ulcer in the duodenum is called a duodenal ulcer.

> **SPOTLIGHT** on a Guideline
>
> Some *excludes* notations in ICD-9-CM for this range of codes include congenital conditions and traumatic perforations.

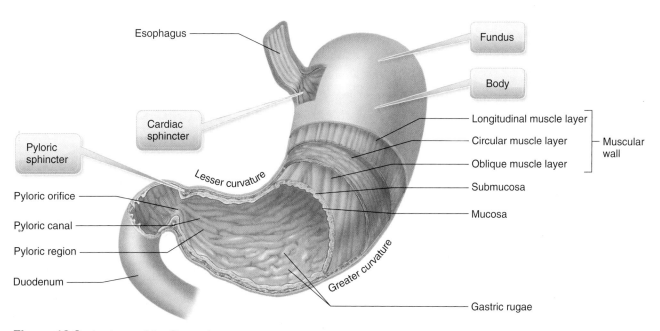

Figure 13.2 Anatomy of the Stomach

- Gastrojejunal ulcer (an ulcer occurring in the stomach and the jejunum—the second section of the small intestine).
- Gastritis and duodenitis.
- Disorders of function of the stomach.
- Gastrostomy complications.
- Other disorders of the stomach and duodenum.
- Complications of gastric band procedures and other bariatric procedures.

Appendicitis (540–543), ICD-9-CM
Diseases of Appendix (K35–K38), ICD-10-CM

These sections contain codes to be reported for conditions such as:

- Acute appendicitis:
  - With generalized peritonitis
  - With peritoneal abscess
  - Without mention of peritonitis
- Appendicitis unqualified
- Other appendicitis
  - Recurrent, chronic
- Other diseases of the appendix

Hernia of Abdominal Cavity (550–553), ICD-9-CM
Hernia (K40–K46), ICD-10-CM

To code the appropriate hernia ICD codes, a coder needs to find answers in the medical documentation to questions such as:

- Where is the hernia located?
- Is gangrene present?
- Is there an obstruction?
- Was it bilateral or unilateral?
- Was it recurrent?

These sections contain codes to be reported for the various types of hernias, which are explained in Table 13.3.

Noninfectious Enteritis and Colitis (555–558), ICD-9-CM
Noninfectious Enteritis and Colitis (K50–K52), ICD-10-CM

Figures 13.3 and 13.4 reference the anatomy of the small and large intestines. A good knowledge of the anatomy of these structures benefits the coder in accurate translation and coding of an operative report.

These sections contain codes to be reported for conditions such as:

- Regional enteritis (Crohn's disease):
  - Excludes ulcerative colitis.
  - Further specified as involving small intestine, large intestine, small intestine with large intestine, or unspecified site.
- Ulcerative colitis.

Table 13.3 Hernias

TYPE OF HERNIA	DEFINITION
Hernia	• Protrusion through the wall of the cavity in which it is normally located.
Inguinal hernia	• Protrusion through a weak point or tear in the lower abdominal wall. • *Direct:* protrusion in the groin area. • *Indirect:* protrusion has moved to the scrotum area.
Femoral hernia	• Similar to inguinal hernia. • Appears as a slightly lower bulge.
Umbilical hernia	• Appears as a bulge at the navel or umbilicus. • Often caused by a weakening of the area or an imperfect closure of the area.
Ventral hernia	• Also called *incisional hernia*. • Often occurs as a bulge in the abdomen at the site of an old surgical scar.
Diaphragmatic hernia	• Also referred to as *hiatal hernia*. • It is not visible on the outside of the body. Part of the abdomen protrudes up through the diaphragm into the chest.

- Vascular insufficiency of intestine (specific to acute or chronic).
- Other and unspecified noninfectious gastroenteritis and colitis:
  - Due to radiation
  - Toxic (Assign an additional code to identify the toxin.)
  - Allergic (Assign an additional code to identify the type of food allergy.)

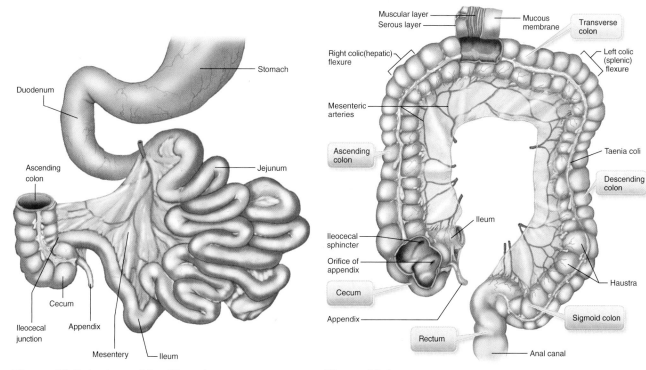

Figure 13.3 Anatomy of Small Intestine

Figure 13.4 Anatomy of Large Intestine

Other Diseases of Intestines and Peritoneum (560–569), ICD-9-CM

Other Diseases of Intestines (K55–K63), ICD-10-CM

Diseases of Peritoneum and Retroperitoneum (K65–K68), ICD-10-CM

These sections contain codes to be reported for conditions such as:

- Intestinal obstruction without mention of hernia
- Intussusception
- Paralytic ileus
- **Volvulus** knotting, strangulation, torsion, or twisting of the intestine, bowel, or colon
- Impaction of intestine
- Diverticula
  - Small intestine
  - Colon

volvulus Knotting, strangulation, torsion, or twisting of the intestine, bowel, or colon.

diverticulitis Inflammation of the diverticula.

diverticulosis A condition of the diverticula.

- Functional digestive disorders, not classified elsewhere:
  - Constipation (excludes fecal impaction).
  - Irritable bowel syndrome (IBS) spastic colon.
  - Postgastric surgery syndromes: dumping syndrome, jejunal syndrome.
- Anal fissure and fistula.
- Abscess of anal and rectal regions.
- Peritonitis and retroperitoneal infections.

Other Diseases of Digestive System (570–579), ICD-9-CM

Diseases of Liver (K70–K77), ICD-10-CM

Diseases of Gallbladder, Biliary Tract, and Pancreas (K80–K87), ICD-10-CM

Other Diseases of Digestive System (K90–K95), ICD-10-CM

Figures 13.5 and 13.6 review the anatomy of the gallbladder and the liver, which is helpful when interpreting an operative report concerning the digestive system.

These sections contain codes to be reported for conditions such as:

- Acute and subacute necrosis of the liver:
  - Acute hepatic failure.

- Chronic liver disease and cirrhosis:
  - Alcoholic cirrhosis of the liver.
  - Chronic hepatitis.
  - Cirrhosis of the liver without mention of alcohol.
- Other disorders of the liver.
- Cholelithiasis.

SPOTLIGHT on Diagnosis

Cholelithiasis calculus (gallstone) located in the gall bladder

Choledocholithiasis A condition in which stones form in the biliary duct and gallbladder.

choledocholithiasis A condition in which stones form in the biliary duct and gallbladder.

MENTOR Coding Tip

The coder must be very careful when coding from these sections to determine whether the calculus is located in the gallbladder alone, biliary tract alone, or both the gallbladder and the biliary tract. The coder must also determine whether there is mention of acute cholecystitis.

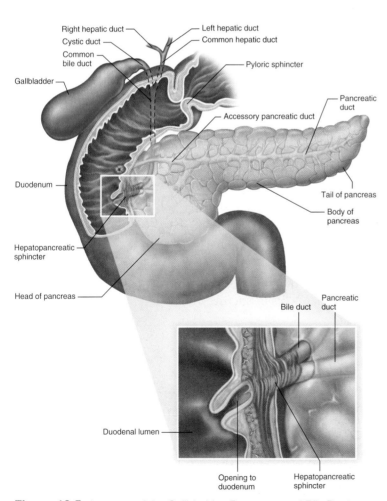

Figure 13.5 Anatomy of the Gallbladder, Pancreas, and Bile Ducts

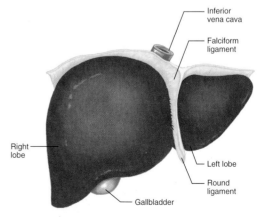

Figure 13.6 Anatomy of the Liver

- Other disorders of the gallbladder:
  - Acute cholecystitis.
  - Other cholecystitis.
  - Obstruction of the gallbladder.
  - Perforation of the gallbladder.
- Other disorders of the biliary tract:
  - Cholangitis.
  - Obstruction of a bile duct.
  - Perforation of a bile duct.
- Diseases of the pancreas:
  - Pancreatitis, specified as acute or chronic.
  - Cyst and pseudocyst.
- Gastrointestinal hemorrhage.
- Intestinal malabsorption.

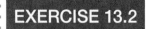

EXERCISE 13.2

1. What questions should be asked before selecting the appropriate ICD code for a hernia diagnosis?
2. What are the four classifications used for dentofacial malocclusions?
3. Which type of hernia is defined as a protrusion through a tear in the lower abdominal wall and can be direct or indirect?
4. If a tooth is broken due to trauma, a code would be selected from which chapter in ICD-9-CM and in ICD-10-CM?
5. Codes for digestive system ulcers in both ICD-9-CM and ICD-10-CM have a high degree of specificity assigned to them such as whether they are _____.

Select the appropriate ICD-9-CM code for the following:

6. A patient with a history of gastric ulcers presents to the ER with nausea, vomiting, and rectal bleeding. The discharge diagnosis is acute gastric ulcer perforation with bleeding.

    ICD-9-CM code: _____

7. The patient presents with severe abdominal pain, fever, and vomiting. This has been occurring for the past 2 days. The final diagnosis is acute cholecystitis.

    ICD-9-CM code: _____

8. The patient presents to the dental office complaining of pain within a dental implant. The final diagnosis is fracture of a dental implant.

    ICD-9-CM code: _____

Also available in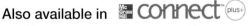

13.3 Guidelines and Format of the Digestive Subsection of CPT

The Digestive System subsection of the CPT manual is formatted by anatomical site from mouth to anus. It has numerous endoscopic codes that are located within specific anatomical subheadings. **Endoscopy** is the visual examination of a cavity.

endoscopy The visual examination of a cavity.

The subsection includes specific guidelines regarding endoscopic or laparoscopic procedures. When a diagnostic procedure is done and then surgical treatment is performed through the scope during the same operative session at the same anatomical site, only the surgical endoscopic or laparoscopic procedure is reported.

There are several questions a coder needs to ask when reading an operative report and coding a procedure from this section. The following questions will help the coder, when reading through the report, to understand what actually was done and how the procedure should be translated and coded:

- Where is the anatomical site at which the procedure was performed ?
- Was the treatment for a traumatic injury (acute) or for a medical condition (chronic)?
- Was the approach internal or external?
- Was the type of the exam open, endoscopic, or laparoscopic?
- Was the procedure performed at a single site or multiple sites?

Digestive System Subsection General Heading Code Ranges (40490–49999)

The general headings and their code ranges are shown in Table 13.4.

Table 13.4 Digestive General Headings and Code Ranges *(Data from CPT 2013. © 2013 American Medical Association. All rights reserved.)*

HEADING	CODE RANGE
Lips	40490–40799
Vestibule of Mouth	40800–40899
Tongue and Floor of Mouth	41000–41599
Dentoalveolar Structures	41800–41899
Palate and Uvula	42000–42299
Salivary Gland and Ducts	42300–42699
Pharynx, Adenoids, and Tonsils	42700–42999
Esophagus	43020–43499
Stomach	43500–43999
Intestines	44005–44799
Meckel's Diverticulum and the Mesentry	44800–44899
Appendix	44900–44979
Rectum	45000–45999
Anus	46020–46999
Liver	47000–47399
Biliary Tract	47400–47999
Pancreas	48000–48999
Abdomen, Peritoneum, and Omentum	49000–49999

Digestive Section Subheadings and Guidelines

The general headings may include the following subheadings:

- Incision
- Excision
- Introduction, Revision, Removal
- Transplantation
- Repair
- Destruction
- Endoscopy
- Laparoscopy
- Other Procedures

SPOTLIGHT on Terminology

Endoscopy is the visualization of a cavity through a scope

Laparascopy is the the process of inserting a scope through the skin of the abdominal wall for examination.

Lips (40490–40799)

Excision: 40490–40530

The coder is instructed to use codes from the Integumentary System section for procedures performed on the skin of the lips.

Biopsy and excision of the lip procedures are reported with codes from this range. The excision codes are further defined by the following:

- Transverse wedge excision, 40510
- V excision, 40520
- Full thickness, with local flap, 40525
- Full thickness, with cross flap, 40527

Resection of the lip without reconstruction, CPT code 40530, is also in this code range.

An instructional note attached to this code leads the coder to 13131 for reconstruction.

Repair: 40650–40761

Plastic repair of cleft lip and/or nasal deformity is reported with codes 40700–40761. This code range is further defined as to whether the procedure is:

- Primary, unilateral
- Primary, bilateral, 1 stage
- Primary, bilateral 1 of 2 stages
- Secondary, recreation and closure

MENTOR Coding Tip

Repair of the lip can also be documented in the medical record as cheiloplasty.

An instructional note with this range of codes refers the coder to a different range of codes for repair of a cleft palate.

Vestibule of Mouth (40800–40899)

The CPT manual (2013) informs the coder that the **vestibule** is the part of the oral cavity outside the dentoalveolar structures; it includes the mucosal and submucosal tissue of lips and cheeks.

Incision: 40800–40806

This subheading includes codes for drainage of an abscess, cyst, or hematoma; removal of an embedded foreign body; and incision of the labial frenum. The codes are distinguished by whether the procedure is simple or complicated.

Excision, Destruction: 40808–40820

The codes in this subheading range are used to report a biopsy of the vestibule of the mouth (CPT code 40808) and excision of lesions of the mucosa and submucosa. The latter are further defined as without repair or with simple or complex repair and, if complex, whether the excision involved underlying muscle (CPT codes 40810–40816).

Repair: 40830–40845

Codes in this subheading are defined by the following:

- Closure of laceration of the vestibule of the mouth, defined by size as less than or greater than 2.5 cm, 40830–40831.
- Vestibuloplasty, which involves rearrangement of the mucosal tissue and/or grafting of soft tissue into the vestibule to increase the height of the bony ridge of the jaw, which contains the teeth. The codes are defined by the site and extent of the repair:
  - Anterior, 40840
  - Posterior, unilateral, 40842
  - Posterior, bilateral, 40843
  - Entire arch, 40844
  - Complex, 40845 (ridge extension, muscle repositioning)

Tongue and Floor of the Mouth (41000–41599)

Incision: 41000–41019

Codes under this subheading include incision and drainage of an abscess, cyst, or hematoma of the tongue or floor of the mouth. They are defined by the site and extent of the procedure:

- Intraoral:
  - Lingual, 41000
  - Sublingual, superficial, 41005
  - Sublingual, deep, 41006
  - Submental space, 41007
  - Submandibular space, 41008
  - Masticator space, 41009

MENTOR Coding Tip

Both ICD and CPT have codes specific to cleft lip and cleft palate.

vestibule The part of the oral cavity outside the dentoalveolar structures; it includes the mucosal and submucosal tissue of lips and cheeks.

MENTOR Coding Tip

Be sure to watch for definitions throughout the CPT manual. This can help during the CPC exam if you get stuck on medical terminology or anatomy.

MENTOR Coding Tip

The codes for repair of the mouth are dependent on size, site, anterior/ posterior, laterality, entire arch, and complexity. Look for these elements in the documentation.

MENTOR Coding Tip

When coding for an I&D in this area, first determine whether the approach is intraoral or extraoral. For intraoral, look for documentation describing manipulation of the tongue.

- Extraoral:
  - Sublingual, 41015
  - Submental, 41016
  - Submandibular, 41017
  - Masticator space, 41018
- Placement of needles, catheters, or other device(s) into the head and/or neck region (percutaneous, transoral, or transnasal) for subsequent interstitial radioelement application, 41019

> **MENTOR** Coding Tip
>
> Review the documentation for the specific anatomical site, such as tongue, below tongue, below the jaw, cheek, or tongue base.

Excision: 41100–41155

This range of codes includes biopsy and excision of the tongue and floor of the mouth or base of the tongue. The codes for biopsy are defined by the anatomical site of the biopsy:

- Anterior two-thirds, 41100
- Posterior one-third, 41105
- Floor of mouth, 41108

Codes for the excision of lesions of the tongue and floor of the mouth are defined by the site of the lesion and extent of the surrounding structures removed and by whether closure was performed at the time of excision:

- Excision of a lesion of the tongue, 41100–41114
  - Without closure, 41110
  - With closure, anterior two-thirds, 41112
  - With closure, posterior one-third, 41113
  - With local tongue flap, 41114
- Excision of the lingual frenum, 41115
- Excision of a lesion of the mouth, 41116
- Glossectomy, 41120–41155; distinguished by the following:
  - Less than one-half of the tongue, 41120
  - Hemiglossectomy, 41130
  - Partial, with unilateral radical neck dissection, 41135
  - Complete or total with or without tracheostomy, without radical neck dissection, 41140
  - Complete or total with or without tracheotomy, with unilateral radical neck dissection, 41145
  - Composite procedure with resection of the floor of the mouth and mandibular resection, without radical neck dissection, 41150
  - Composite procedure with resection of the floor of the mouth, with suprahyoid neck dissection, 41153
  - Composite procedure with resection floor of mouth, mandibular resection, and radical neck dissection, 41155

Repair: 41250–41252

Codes under this subheading are for repairs of lacerations of the mouth and are defined by the size, site, and extent of the repair:

- 2.5 cm or less, anterior two-thirds of tongue, 41250
- 2.5 cm or less, posterior one-third of tongue, 41251
- Over 2.6 cm or complex repair, 41252

Complex closures involve tissue rearrangement, repair of lacerations through the tongue, and extensive layered closure.

Other Procedures: 41500–41599

Codes in this subheading include:

- Fixation of the tongue, 41500
- Suture of the tongue to the lip, 41510
- Tongue base suspension, 41512
- Frenoplasty, 41520
- Submucosal ablation of the tongue base, radiofrequency, 41530

Dentoalveolar Structures (41800–41899)

Incision: 41800–41806

This subheading includes codes for drainage of an abscess, cyst, or hematoma from dentoalveolar structures and removal of an embedded foreign-body soft tissue or bone.

Excision, Destruction: 41820–41850

Codes under this subheading include incision and excision of the dentoalveolar structures, which are the structures related to the gum and tooth socket. Procedures include:

- Excision of the gingival tissue, pericoronal tissue, and fibrous or osseous tuberosities.
- Excision of lesions or tumors, dentoalveoloar structures other than gingival, pericoronal, or fibrous tissues, without repair or with simple or complex repair.
- Destruction of a lesion (except excision) dentoalveolar structure.

Palate and Uvula (42000–42299)

Incision: 42000

The only code listed under this subheading reports drainage of an abscess of the palate or uvula

Excision, Destruction: 42100–42160

Codes within this subheading are used for the following procedures:

- Biopsy of the palate or uvula, 42100
- Excision, lesion of the palate or uvula, without closure, with simple closure, or with local flap closure, 42104–42107
- Resection of the palate or extensive resection of a lesion, 42120 (An instructional note below this code instructs the coder to use a range of codes in the Integumentary subsection for resection of the palate with extraoral tissue.)
- Uvulectomy, 42140
- Destruction of a lesion on the palate or uvula, 42160

Repair: 42180–42281

Codes under this subheading include several codes for palatoplasty for cleft palate, lengthening of the palate, repair of the anterior palate and nasolabial fistula, maxillary impression for a palatal prosthesis, and insertion of a pin-retained palatal prosthesis.

Salivary Gland and Ducts (42300–42699)

Incision: 42300–42340

As with the other incision subheadings within the Digestive System subsection, drainage of an abscess is included in this subheading. The codes are further defined by location, such as parotid, submaxillary, or sublingual, and by simple or complicated.

Excision: 42400–42450

Codes under this subheading include biopsy of the salivary gland, differentiated by needle or incisional. An instructional note guides the coder to a code from the Integumentary subsection if the procedure is a fine-needle aspiration. There is an additional instructional note about the appropriate codes to be assigned if imaging guidance is performed (76942 for ultrasound guidance; 77002, fluoroscopic guidance; 77012, CT guidance; 77021, MR guidance)

Excisions included in this range of codes include:

- Excision of a sublingual salivary cyst, 42408
- Excision of a parotid tumor or parotid gland:
  - Lateral lobe, without nerve dissection, 42410
  - Lateral lobe, with dissection and preservation of the facial nerve, 42415
  - Total, with dissection and preservation of the facial nerve, 42420
  - Total, en bloc removal with sacrifice of the facial nerve, 42425
  - Total, with unilateral radical neck dissection, 42426
- Excision of submandibular gland, 42440
- Excision of sublingual gland, 42450

Repair: 42500–42510

Codes under this subheading cover plastic repair of a salivary duct, which is differentiated by primary or simple and secondary or complicated. Also included are codes for parotid duct diversion, bilateral; these codes are further defined by the excision of one submandibular gland, excision of both submandibular glands, or ligation of both submandibular ducts.

Pharynx, Adenoids, and Tonsils (42700–42999)

Incision: 42700–42725

Codes under this subheading are used for incision and drainage of a peritonsillar abscess and are further defined by the approach: intraoral or external.

Excision, Destruction: 42800–42894

Biopsy of the oropharynx, hypopharynx, and nasopharyx are included under this subheading. An instructional note refers coders to the Respiratory subsection for laryngoscopic biopsy.

Excision or destruction of a lesion of the pharynx and removal of a foreign body from the pharynx are also included under this subheading. The excision codes cover removal of the adenoids and tonsils. The codes are defined by the tissue excised and the age of the patient:

- Tonsillectomy and adenoidectomy:
  - Younger than age 12, 42820
  - Age 12 or over, 42821
- Tonsillectomy, primary or secondary:
  - Younger than age 12, 42825
  - Age 12 or over, 42826
- Adenoidectomy, primary:
  - Younger than age 12, 42830
  - Age 12 or over, 42831
- Adenoidectomy, secondary:
  - Younger than age 12, 42835
  - Age 12 or over, 42836
- Radical resection of a tonsil, tonsillar pillars, and/or a retromolar trigone:
  - Without closure, 42842
  - Closure with local flap (e.g., tongue, buccal), 42844
  - Closure with another flap, 42845
- Excision of tonsil tags, 42860

Repair: 42900–42953

Codes under this subheading are assigned for suture of the pharynx for wound or injury, pharyngoplasty, and pharyngoesophageal repair.

Other Procedures: 42955–42999

Codes for control of oropharyngeal and nasopharyngeal hemorrhage are included in this subheading. They are differentiated by primary or secondary, complicated, requiring hospitalization, and secondary surgical intervention.

Esophagus (43020–43499)

Incision: 43020–43045

Esophagotomy with removal of a foreign body by either cervical or thoracic approach is assigned to this subheading.

Excision: 43100–43135

Procedures under this subheading include removal of the esophagus or esophagectomies. Esophagectomies performed without thoracotomy, codes 43107 and 43108 are completed through two smaller incisions: one cervical and the other in the upper midline abdominal area. The esophagus is removed, and the stomach and pharynx are anastomosed through the cervical incision. When reviewing the documentation, watch for these incision sites to guide you in code selection.

Codes in this subheading are often defined by the following:

- **Approach:** cervical, thoracic, or abdominal
- **Amount of tissue excised:** total, near total, or partial
- **Method:** with or without thoracotomy

An instructional note attached to code 43116 tells the coder to *not* use the operating microscope code, 69990, in conjunction with code 43116. There is another instructional note with this code about the use of modifier 52. Refer to Section 13.4 (Modifiers Most Commonly Used with Codes from the Digestive Subsection) for additional information.

Endoscopy: 43200–43273

When coding from this subheading concerning endoscopic procedures of the esophagus, coders must find answers in the documentation to the following questions:

- Was the procedure diagnostic, surgical, or both during the same session?
- Was the procedure an esophagoscopy (CPT code range 43200–43232), an upper gastrointestinal endoscopy (CPT range 43235–43259), or an **endoscopic retrograde cholangiopancreatography (ERCP)** (CPT range 43260–43272)?
- Was one of the following also performed:
  - Biopsy
  - Injection
  - Removal of a foreign body
  - Ligation
  - Removal of a tumor by forceps or by snare
  - Insertion of a plastic tube or stent
  - Balloon dilation (need to know the size of the balloon)
  - Image guidance (requires code from the Radiology section)
  - Endoscopic ultrasound examination

Laparoscopy: 43279–43289

The descriptions of most of the codes under this subheading include eponym procedures such as the Heller type, Nissen procedure, Toupet's procedure, and Collis gastroplasty. If this information is included in the operative report, use the eponym to help locate the appropriate CPT code.

Instructional notes below codes 43279 and 43280 guide the coder for procedures performed with an open approach.

Repair: 43300–43425

When coding from this subheading for repair procedures of the esophagus, coders must find answers in the documentation to the following questions:

- What approach was used: cervical, thoracic, or abdominal?
- Was there a repair of the tracheoesophageal fistula, and was the fistula congenital or acquired?

endoscopic retrograde cholangiopancreatography (ERCP) X-ray exam of the pancreatic and biliary ducts.

MENTOR
Coding Tip

The terms listed to the right further define code selection and should be identified when reviewing the documentation of the procedure.

- Was there a repair of a paraesophageal hiatal hernia (CPT code range 43332–43337)?
- Was there implantation of mesh or another prosthesis?

An instructional note below code range 43332–43337 specifies the use of CPT code 39503 for neonatal diaphragmatic hernia.

Some other procedures assigned to this subheading are:

- Gastrointestinal reconstruction, 43360–43361
- Ligation, direct, esophageal varices, 43400
- Ligation or stapling at the gastroesophageal junction for preexisting esophageal perforation, 43405

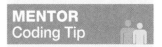

> **MENTOR Coding Tip**
>
> To determine the correct code for gastrointestinal reconstruction procedures, review the documentation for additional sites and procedures that are components of each procedure code.

Manipulation: 43450–43460

Codes under this subheading are used for dilation of the esophagus and are divided by anatomical site and by method and/or device. Instructional notes direct the coder to CPT code 74360 in the Radiology section for radiological supervision and interpretation.

Stomach (43500–43999)

Incision: 43500–43520

Gastrotomy and pyloromyotomy procedures are assigned to this subheading. Codes are differentiated by patient condition and definitive procedure, that is, foreign-body removal or repair. An instructional note below CPT code 43520 states that modifier 63 (procedure performed on an infant less than 4 kg) is not to be attached to this code.

Excision: 43605–43641

Included under this subheading are:

- Biopsy of stomach, by laparotomy, 43605
- Excisions, defined by the reason for the excision:
  - Ulcer or benign tumor of the stomach, 43610
  - Malignant tumor of the stomach, 43611

Gastrectomy codes are defined first by the extent of the stomach removed and then by the method of and points of reconnection of the anastomosis. For example, esophagoenterostomy is the connection of the esophagus to the small intestine. To connect these two anatomical sites, a total gastrectomy is performed.

- Total gastrectomies are included in code range 43620–43622, and partial gastrectomies are reported with codes 43631 to 43634.
- Vagotomy involves the transection of the vagus nerve and may be performed in addition to gastrectomy procedures or alone. It is reported with codes in the range 43635–43641.

laparoscopy Process of inserting a scope through the skin of
the abdomen for examination.

Laparoscopy: 43644–43659

Laparoscopy codes are located below the Stomach subheading and include gastrectomy, vagotomy, and gastric banding. An instructional note at the beginning of this range of codes states, For upper gastrointestinal endoscopy including esophagus, stomach, and either the duodenum and/or jejunum, see 43235–43259.

Introduction: 43752–43761

This subheading includes procedures such as the following:

- Nasogastric or orogastric tube placement, requiring a physician's skill and fluoroscopic guidance (includes fluoroscopy, image documentation, and report), 43752 (Instructional notes below this code specific the use of CPT 49440 for percutaneous placement of a gastrostomy tube and CPT codes 44500 and 74340 for enteric tube placement.).
- Change of gastrostomy tube, percutaneous, without imaging or endoscopic guidance, 43760 (An instructional note below this code states that CPT 49450 is to be used for fluoroscopic-guided replacement.)
- Repositioning of a nasogastric or orogastric feeding tube, through the duodenum for enteric nutrition, 43761 (Instructional notes below this state that CPT code 76000 is used if imaging guidance is performed, CPT 44373 is used for endoscopic conversion of a gastrostomy tube to a jejunostomy tube, and CPT 44500 is used for placement of a long gastrointestinal tube into the duodenum.)

The procedures in this code range may involve the stomach, duodenum, jejunum, and/or ileum and are divided based on placement, revision, removal, and removal and replacement. The codes for removal and replacement are further divided based on the components removed.

Intestines, Except Rectum (44005–44799)

Incision: 44005–44055

The procedures below for entry into the intestines are assigned to this range of codes. These codes are first divided by anatomical site of the intestines and then by the definitive procedure, such as lysis or foreign-body removal. When coding for entry by incision into the intestines, coders need an understanding of the anatomy of these sites.

- Enterolysis, 44005
- Duodenotomy, 44010
- Enterotomy, 44020
- Colotomy, 44025

Excision: 44100–44160

Intestinal transplantation codes are assigned to this code range. As with all transplantation codes, there are three distinct components of physician work for this type of transplantation:

- Cadaver donor, 44132 (This code includes the harvesting of the intestine graft and cold preservation of the graft.)

  or

Living donor, 44133 (This code includes the harvesting of the intestine graft and cold preservation of the graft as well as the care of the donor.)

- Backbench work, 44715, 44720–44721 (These codes include preparation and reconstruction of the graft prior to transplantation.)
- Recipient intestinal allotransplantation with or without recipient enterectomy, 44135–44136 (These codes include the actual transplantation of the graft and care of the patient following the procedure.)

Laparoscopy: 44180–44227

Codes within this range are for laparoscopic procedures performed on the intestines, excluding the rectum. These codes are grouped by base procedure and divided by definitive procedures within these groups:

- Incision, enterolysis, 44180
- Enterostomy, 44186–44188
- Excision, 44202–44213 (by site and amount resected, small intestine or colon, partial or total)
- Repair, 44227

Codes 44186 and 44187 describe a jejunostomy. The primary difference is that in code 44187 the loop of the intestine is exteriorized through the skin (opened and sutured to the skin) and in 44186 a tube is inserted through the skin into the jejunum.

SPOTLIGHT on a Guideline

Multiple instructional notes in the intestinal laparoscopy range of codes (44180–44227) guide the coder to the appropriate CPT code for an open procedure.

Endoscopy, Small Intestine and Stomal: 44360–44397

The codes in this range describe procedures performed through an endoscope on the small intestine. Because these codes state "with," it is appropriate to code as many separate codes as needed to fully describe the procedures performed. Also, all of the codes in this range include the use of moderate sedation when done by the surgeon.

These codes are divided by extent or location of the scope and by inclusion or noninclusion of the ileum or colon. These procedures are further divined by:

- Diagnostic or evaluation only, 44360, 44376, 44380, 44388
- Biopsy, 44361, 44377, 44382, 44386, 44389
- Removal of a foreign body, 44363, 44390
- Removal of tumor(s), polyp(s), or lesion(s):
  - By snare 44364, 44394
  - By hot forceps or bipolar cautery, 44365, 44392
  - By ablation, 44369, 44393
- Control of bleeding, 44366, 44378, 44391

- Placement of devices:
  - Stent, 44370, 44379, 44383, 44397
  - Jejunostomy tube (J tube), 44372
  - Conversion of a Gastrostomy tube (G tube) to a jejunostomy tube (J tube), 44373

Appendix (44900–44979)

Incision: 44900–44901

Incision and drainage of an abscess of the appendix are assigned to this code range and are further defined by whether the approach is open or percutaneous.

Excision: 44950–44960

Appendectomy codes are defined by the reason for the procedure and the condition of the appendix:

- Appendectomy, 44950
- Appendectomy done for a condition of the appendix at the time of another major procedure, 44955
- Appendectomy for a ruptured appendix with an abscess or generalized peritonitis, 44960
- Appendectomy done laparoscopically, 44970

Rectum (45000–45999)

Incision: 45000–45020

Incision and drainage of an abscess are included in this range.

Excision: 45100–45172

Biopsy, proctectomy, and excision of rectal tumors are assigned to this code range.

Destruction: 45190

Destruction of rectal tumors is assigned to code 45190.

    Note the difference between the codes for excision of rectal tumors (45160-45172) and destruction of rectal tumors (45190). An instructional note directs the coder to assign CPT 0184T for a TEMS (transanal endoscopic microsurgical) excision of a rectal tumor.

Endoscopy: 45300–45392

Procedures assigned to this code range are proctosigmoidoscopy, sigmoidoscopy, and colonoscopy.

MENTOR Coding Tip

The guideline at the beginning of this subheading section contains information regarding the *extent* and *anatomical location* of the scope. Be sure to highlight this information as these terms directly relate to the first division of these codes.

When coding from this subheading concerning endoscopic procedures, coders must find answers in the documentation to the following questions:

- Was the procedure diagnostic, surgical, or both during the same session?
- Where did the scope start and end?
- Was one of the following also performed:
  - Biopsy.
  - Removal of a foreign body.
  - Ablation.
  - Ligation.
  - Removal of a tumor by forceps or by snare.
  - Insertion.

Anus (46020–46999)

Incision: 46020–46083

Abscess incision and drainage codes are assigned to this code range.

Excision: 46200–46320

Fissurectomy and hemorrhoidectomy procedures are assigned to this code range. Some specific procedures include:

- Incision of thrombosed external hemorrhoid, 46083
- Ligation of internal hemorrhoid, 46221, 46945, 46946
- Excision of internal and/or external hemorrhoids, 46250–46262, 46320
- Injection of hemorrhoids, 46500
- Destruction of internal hemorrhoids by thermal energy, 46930
- Hemorrhoidopexy, 46947

Liver (47000–47399)

Incision: 47000–47015

Procedures listed under this subheading include open and percutaneous approaches for biopsies or drainage of an abscess or cyst of the liver. Percutaneous procedures include conscious sedation, which is not reported in addition to the procedure. Specific procedures include:

- Biopsy of the liver, by needle:
  - Percutaneous, 47000
  - When done for indicated purpose at time of another major procedure, +47001
- Hepatotomy:
  - Open drainage of an abscess or cyst, 1 or 2 stages, 47010
  - Percutaneous drainage of an abscess or cyst, 1 or 2 stages, 47011

Excision: 47100–47130

- Biopsy of the liver, wedge, 47100

Codes for resection of the liver are also assigned to this range and are further defined as partial lobectomy, trisegmentectomy, and total left or total right lobotomy.

Transplantation: 47133–47147

Liver allotransplantation codes are assigned to this code range. As with all transplantation codes, there are three distinct components of physician work for this type of transplantation:

- Cadaver donor, 47133 (This code includes the harvesting of the graft and cold preservation of the graft.)

  or

  Living donor, 47140–47142 (This code includes the harvesting of the graft and cold preservation of the graft as well as the care of the donor.)

- Backbench work, 47143–47147
- Recipient liver allotransplantation, 44135–44136

Repair: 47300–47362

Management of liver hemorrhage is assigned to this code range and further defined by simple or complex suture, with or without hepatic artery ligation, and exploration or reexploration of the wound.

Biliary Tract (47400–47999)
Introduction: 47490–47530

Injection procedures for cholangiography are assigned to this range. Introduction of precautious transhepatic catheters and stents for biliary drainage is also included in this code range. Multiple instructional notes refer the coder to the Radiology section for the appropriate codes for radiological supervision and interpretation.

Excision: 47600–47715
- Cholecystectomy, 47600
  - With cholangiography, 47605 (An instructional note refers the coder to CPT codes 47562–47564 for laparoscopic approach.)
- Cholecystectomy with exploration of common duct, 47610 (An instructional note refers the coder to use CPT code 47550 with 47610 for cholecystectomy with exploration of the common duct with biliary endoscopy.)
- Biliary duct stone extraction, 47630

Pancreas (48000–48999)
Incision: 48000–48020

This code range includes codes for placement of drains for acute pancreatitis and removal of pancreatic calculus.

Excision: 48100–48160

Procedures assigned to this code range include:

- Biopsy of pancreas:
  - Open, 48100
  - Percutaneous, 48102
- Excision of a lesion of the pancreas, 48120

- Pancreatectomy, 48140–48155
  - Distal or proximal
  - Subtotal, near total, or total
  - With or without pancreatojejunostomy
- Transplantation of islet cells, 48160

Abdomen, Peritoneum, and Omentum (49000–49999)
Incision: 49000–49084

Included in the procedures assigned to this code range are drainage of peritoneal and retroperitoneal abscesses and of subdiaphragmatic or subphrenic abscesses. Abdominal paracentesis (CPT code 49082) is also included in this range.

Introduction, Revision, Removal: 49400–49436

Initial placement, 49440–49442: Insertion of gastrostomy, duodenostomy, jejunostomy, or colostomy tube percutaneously is assigned to codes 49440–49442.

Conversion, 49446: For conversion of a gastrostomy tube (G tube) to a gastrojejunostomy tube (G-J tube), CPT code 49446 is the appropriate code to use. An instructional note informs the coder that when a G tube is converted to a G-J tube at the time of the initial gastrostomy tube placement, codes 49446 and 49440 should be reported.

Replacement, 49450–49452: Included in this range of codes are procedures for gastrostomy, duodenostomy, jejunostomy, gastrojejunostomy, and cecostomy tube replacements.

SPOTLIGHT on a Guideline

The guidelines before the replacement range of codes state if an existing gastrostomy, duodenostomy, jejunostomy, gastrojejunostomy, or colostomy tube is removed and then a new tube is placed via a *separate access site*, the placement of the new tube is not considered a replacement and would be reported using a code from the initial-placement range, 49440–49442.

Repair: 49491–49659

Hernioplasty, herniorrhaphy, and herniotomy are included in this code range.
  When coding from this range, coders must find answers in the documentation to the following questions:

- What type of hernia was being treated? Example: Was it inguinal, femoral, or incisional?
- Was the hernia initial or recurrent? Example: Was the hernia previously repaired?
- What is the patient's age? (This includes postconception age, which equals the gestational age at birth plus the age in weeks at the time of the hernia repair.)
- Was the hernia reducible versus incarcerated or strangulated?
- If the hernia repair was incisional, was mesh or another prosthesis used?

EXERCISE 13.3

1. For conversion of a gastrostomy tube (G tube) to a gastrojejunostomy tube (G-J tube), CPT code _____ is the appropriate code to use.

2. What are the three common components for physician work involving transplantation?

3. During an open abdominal procedure, exploration of the surgical field is routinely performed. In this case, should an exploratory laparoscopy, CPT code 49000, be reported along with the open procedure?

4. What is the code range for an ERCP?

Also available in connect plus+

13.4 Modifiers Most Commonly Used with Codes in the Digestive Subsection

As with all sections of the CPT manual, modifiers are used in the Digestive subsection to continue or modify the story of the patient's encounter. Some of the more common modifiers used in this section are 52, reduced services; 53, discontinued procedure; 58, staged or related procedure or service by the same physician and/or other qualified healthcare professional during the postoperative period; 59, distinct procedural service; and 78, unplanned return to the operating/procedure room by the same physician or another qualified healthcare professional following the initial procedure for a related procedure during the postoperative period. (See Table 13.5.)

Table 13.5 Digestive Subsection Modifiers (*Data from CPT 2013. © 2013 American Medical Association. All rights reserved.*)

MODIFIER	DEFINITION	EXAMPLE
52	Reduced service	If an intestinal or free jejunal graft with microvascular anastomosis is performed by another physician, modifier 52 is reported with code 43116 (CPT 2013).
53	Discontinued procedure	When performing an endoscopy on a patient who is scheduled and prepped for a total colonoscopy, if the physician is unable to advance the scope beyond the splenic flexure due to unforeseen circumstances, modifier 53 is appended to the colonoscopy code (CPT 2013).
58	Staged or related procedure or service by the same physician during the postoperative period	When an endoscopy is performed to determine the need for a more extensive open procedure, modifier 58 is appended to identify that the scope and more extensive procedure were staged.
59	Distinct procedural service	If an abscess is drained during treatment of hemorrhoids and the I&D is at a separate site unrelated to the hemorrhoids, modifier 59 is appended to the incision and drainage code.
78	Unplanned return to the operating/procedure room by the same physician or another qualified healthcare professional following the initial procedure for a related procedure during the postoperative period	If the patient is returned to the operating room by the same physician following the initial procedure for an unplanned procedure and this happens during the postoperative period for a procedure which has a 90-day global period, modifier 78 is appended.

1. The patient is returned to the operating room by the same physician following the initial procedure for an unplanned procedure and this happens during the postoperative period for a procedure that has a 90-day global period. The coder should append modifier_____ to the appropriate CPT code from the Digestive System section.

2. An incidental appendectomy during intra-abdominal surgery is usually not reported separately. If it is necessary to report, modifier_____ should be appended to CPT code 44900, appendectomy.

3. An esophagogastroduodenoscopy (EGD) performed for a separate condition should be reported with modifier_____ to let the payer know that it was a distinct procedure.

Also available in ■ connect (plus+)

13.5 Common Medical and Procedural Terms Used in Operative Reports

As with all sections of CPT, the Digestive subsection includes medical terms and procedural terms that are specific to the system involved. Tables 13.6 and 13.7 list some of these terms and identify some key terms that could appear in a provider's documentation.

Table 13.6 Terms for Digestive System

TERM	DEFINITION	DOCUMENTATION KEYS
Abdominocentesis	Surgical puncture of the abdomen	Diagnostic, therapeutic
Cholelithotomy	Cholelith/o = gall stone -otomy = incision	Surgical removal of a gall stone through an incision into the gall bladder.
Cholelithotripsy	Cholelith/o = gall stones -tripsy = crushing	May be referenced in provider documentation as Extracorporeal Shock Wave Therapy
Colonoscopy	Examination of the entire colon, rectum to cecum; may include examination of the terminal ileum	A colonoscopy can be used as a screening or diagnostic test generally used to identify ulcers, polyps, tumors, or to recognize areas of bleeding.
Endoscopic retro-grade cholangio-pancreatography (ERCP)	X-ray exam of pancreatic and bile ducts	The provider documentation will refer to the scope being inserted into the mouth and then gradually moved through the esophagus, stomach, and duodenum into the pancreatic and bile ducts.
Esophagoplasty	Surgical repair of the esophagus	Plastic repair reconstruction
Fundoplication	Mobilization of the lower end of the esophagus and plication or folding of the fundus of the stomach around it.; This is a procedure often used in the treatment of GERD, and hiatial hernias.	Fundic wrapping

(continued)

Table 13.6 Terms for Digestive System (*concluded*)

TERM	DEFINITION	DOCUMENTATION KEYS
Gastroplasty	Surgical treatment of the stomach or lower esophagus; used to decrease the size of the stomach, mainly in the treatment of morbid obesity, and to correct defects in the lower esophagus or the stomach	Banded gastroplasty, silicone elastomer ring, vertical gastroplasty, horizontal banded gastroplasty
Sigmoidoscopy	Examination of the entire rectum and sigmoid colon; may include examination of a portion of the descending colon	Provider documentation may discuss the insertion of a length of flexible tube connected to a fiberoptic camera with a light attached to the scope. This type of exam may be performed as a screening or diagnostic examination.

Table 13.7 Additional Terms for Digestive System

TERM	DEFINITION	DOCUMENTATION KEYS
Ascites	Abnormal accumulation of fluid in the peritoneal cavity	May be referenced in documentation as peritoneal cavity fluid
Crohn's disease	Chronic inflammatory disease primarily of the bowel	May also be referred to in provider documentation as regional enteritis
Dysphagia	Difficulty swallowing	Often related to GERD
Esophageal varices	Bulging, enlarged veins in the walls of the esophagus that are at risk of tearing, resulting in severe, possibly fatal, bleeding	Portal hypertension (increased pressure in the veins of the liver) contributes to the formation of esophageal varices. Some conditions which can cause portal hypertension and then esophageal varices are cirrhosis, portal and hepatic vein blood clots, certain drugs and infections, and severe heart failure.
Gastroesophageal reflux disease (GERD)	Weakness of the valve between the esophagus and the stomach that can cause stomach acid to reflux (regurgitate, backup) into the esophagus and irritate and inflame the lining	Severe heartburn
Intussusception	The sliding of one part of the intestine into another	Provider documentation may refer to telescoping instead of sliding.
Peritonitis	Inflammation of the lining of the abdominal cavity	Peritoneal signs (indications of peritonitis), tender abdomen, rebound pain (i.e., pain when manual pressure is applied)
Portal hypertension	Increase in blood pressure in the veins between the GI tract and the liver, causing enlargement of the veins; can be a complication of chronic alcoholism, resulting in liver damage and obstruction of venous blood flow through the liver	Caput medusae

gastroesophageal reflux disease (GERD) Weakness of the valve between the esophagus and stomach that can cause stomach acid to reflux.

intussusception The sliding of one part of the intestine into another.

1. The patient presents with abdominal pain and a swollen belly. The physician is concerned about bleeding into the abdomen and orders a procedure in which the abdomen will be punctured and fluid will be drained. This procedure is called a(an)_____.

2. The physician orders an examination of the entire rectum and sigmoid colon and a possible examination of a portion of the descending colon. A _____ has been ordered.

3. The patient presents with difficult and painful swallowing. The diagnosis on the chart could be_____.

4. Symptoms of tender abdomen and rebound pain could be indications of _____.

Also available in connect (plus+)

Chapter Thirteen Summary

Learning Outcome	Key Concepts/Examples
13.1 Review the anatomy of the digestive system.	The digestive system consists of the mouth, esophagus, stomach, small intestine, large intestine, and accessory organs consisting of the salivary glands, liver, gallbladder, and pancreas. *Flow of the digestive system:* mouth → esophagus → stomach → small intestine → large intestine → anus.
13.2 Understand the chapter-specific ICD guidelines and format for the digestive system.	Some common diseases coded to the Digestive chapter of ICD are gingivitis, GERD, jaundice, pancreatitis, cirrhosis, portal hypertension, esophagitis, appendicitis, and hernias. When coding these conditions, coders must thoroughly review the provider documentation as well as the guidelines and instructional notes. *ICD-9-CM:* The Digestive subsection is Chapter 9 in the ICD-9-CM manual, with the code range 520–579. *ICD-10-CM:* The Digestive subsection is Chapter 11 in the ICD-10-CM manual, with the code range K00–K94.
13.3 Identify the guidelines and format of the Digestive subsection of CPT.	The Digestive System subsection of the CPT manual is formatted by anatomical site from mouth to anus. It has numerous endoscopic codes that are located within specific anatomical subheadings. The subsection includes specific guidelines regarding endoscopic procedures. When a diagnostic procedure is done and then surgical treatment is performed through the scope during the same operative session at the same anatomical site, only the surgical endoscopic procedure is reported. There are several questions a coder needs to ask when reading an operative report and coding a procedure from this section. The following questions will help the coder, when reading through the report, to understand what actually was done and how the procedure should be translated and coded: • Where is the anatomical site at which the procedure was performed? • Was the treatment for a traumatic injury (acute) or a medical condition (chronic)? • Was the approach internal or external? • Was the type of the exam open, endoscopic, or laparoscopic? • Was the procedure performed at a single site or multiple sites?
13.4 Apply the modifiers most commonly used with codes in the Digestive subsection.	Modifiers are used in the Digestive subsection to continue or modify the story of the patient's encounter. Some of the more common modifiers used in this subsection are: • Reduced services, 52 • Discontinued procedure, 53 • Staged or related procedure or service by the same physician and/or other qualified healthcare professional during the postoperative period, 58 • Distinct procedural service, 59 • Unplanned return to the operating/procedure room by the same physician or another qualified healthcare professional following the initial procedure for a related procedure during the postoperative period, 78
13.5 Examine the common medical and procedural terms used in operative reports.	The Digestive subsection includes medical terms and procedural terms that are specific to the system involved. There are also some key terms that could appear in a provider's documentation and act as a trigger for the coder to identify the diagnosis and/or procedure for the encounter.

Chapter Thirteen Review

Using Terminology

Match each key term to the appropriate definition.

_____ 1. [LO13.1] Bolus

_____ 2. [LO13.1] Cecum

_____ 3. [LO13.1] Choledocholithiasis

_____ 4. [LO13.5] Cholelithiasis

_____ 5. [LO13.1] Diverticulitis

_____ 6. [LO13.1] Diverticulosis

_____ 7. [LO13.1] Duodenum

_____ 8. [LO13.5] Endoscopic
retrograde
cholangiopan-
creatography
(ERCP)

_____ 9. [LO13.5] Gastroesophageal reflux dis-
ease (GERD)

_____ 10. [LO13.1] Ileum

_____ 11. [LO13.5] Intussusception

_____ 12. [LO13.1] Jejunum

_____ 13. [LO13.3] Laparoscopy

_____ 14. [LO13.2] Volvulus

A. X-ray exam of the pancreatic and biliary ducts
B. The sliding of one part of the intestine into another
C. Gallstones
D. Pouch at the beginning of the intestine that links to the ileum
E. Visualization of the abdominal wall through a scope
F. Mixture of food and digestive enzymes in the saliva
G. Stones that form in the biliary duct and gallbladder
H. Inflammation of diverticula
I. A condition of diverticula
J. First section of the small intestine
K. Last section of the small intestine
L. Weakness of the valve between the esophagus and the stomach that can cause stomach acid to reflux
M. Knotting, strangulation, torsion, or twisting of the intestine, bowel, or colon
N. Middle section of the small intestine

Checking Your Understanding

Choose the most appropriate answer for each of the following questions.

1. [LO13.2, 13.3] The patient was brought to the operating room for a diaphragmatic hernia. A transthoracic repair was performed. Select the appropriate CPT and ICD-9-CM code:

   a. 43334, 553.3
   b. 39503, 756.6
   c. 43336, 553.3
   d. 39540, 756.6

2. [LO13.5] An operative report states in the header that an EGD was performed. What type of procedure was performed?

   a. Esophagogastric
   b. Esophagogastroduodenoscopy
   c. Endoscopic retrograde cholangiopancreatography
   d. Enterocolostomy

3. [LO13.2] Which one of the following statements best describes a hiatal hernia?

   a. A protrusion of part of the stomach through the diaphragm
   b. A protrusion of part of the esophagus through the larynx
   c. A protrusion of part of the stomach through the rectum
   d. A protrusion of part of the esophagus through the oropharynx

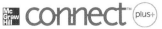

Enhance your learning by completing these exercises and more at mcgrawhillconnect.com

4. **[LO13.2, 13.3]** A 60-year-old man is brought to the operating room for a biopsy of the liver. A wedge biopsy is taken and sent to pathology. The report comes back the same day as surgery indicating that primary malignant cells are present. The decision is made to perform a total left lobotomy. Code the operative procedure and diagnosis:

   a. 47100, 47125–51, 197.7

   b. 47130, 155.0

   c. 47125, 47100–51, 155.0

   d. 47132, 197.7

5. **[LO13.2, 13.3]** A patient was brought back to the operating room 60 days after an initial surgical repair on a strangulated inguinal hernia; this procedure was performed by the physician who previously performed the initial surgery. The surgical decision was made due to the patient's presenting to the ER for lower abdominal pain and radiological testing that confirmed a restrangulation of the hernia. Select the appropriate ICD-9-CM and CPT codes:

   a. 49521–78, 550.11

   b. 49501, 550.10

   c. 49507–78, 550.11

   d. 49525–58, 550.11

6. **[LO13.2, 13.3]** A 45-year-old patient presents for a flexible sigmoidoscopy for three rectal polyps; the procedure involved the use of hot biopsy forceps. Select the appropriate ICD-9-CM and CPT codes:

   a. 45315, 569.2

   b. 45320, 569.0

   c. 45317, 569.49

   d. 45333, 569.0

7. **[LO13.2, 13.3]** Emily had been complaining of abdominal pain for the past 4 months. It seemed to be worse after she ate fatty foods or ice cream. She was diagnosed with gallbladder disease and underwent a laparoscopic cholecystectomy that revealed chronic cholecystitis and cholelithiasis. Select the appropriate ICD-9-CM and CPT codes to report Emily's encounter:

   a. 47562, 575.11, 574.10

   b. 47563, 575.11, 592.9

   c. 47562, 574.10

   d. 47563, 575.10, 574.10

8. **[LO13.2, 13.3]** A patient presented in the office with symptoms of severe upper gastric pain. After the examination and blood tests, the physician diagnosed hepatitis resulting from infectious mononucleosis. Select the ICD-9-CM codes:

   a. 573.1, 070.12

   b. 573.3, 070.30

   c. 075, 573.1

   d. 573.2, 070.51

9. **[LO13.1]** Which of the following is *not* a part of the stomach?

   a. Fundus

   b. Antrum/pylorus

   c. Body

   d. Ileum

10. **[LO13.1]** Which type of ulcer occurs in the first, or upper, section of the intestine?

   a. Gastric ulcer   **c.** Peptic ulcer

   b. Duodenal ulcer   **d.** Gastrojejunal ulcer

Applying Your Knowledge

Answer the following questions and code the following case study. Be sure to follow the process steps as illustrated in Chapter 8

Case Studies [LO 13.1–13.5] Case 1

Preoperative diagnosis: Chronic tonsillitis and enlarged adenoids

Postoperative diagnosis: Chronic tonsillitis and enlarged adenoids

Procedure: Tonsillectomy with adenoidectomy

The patient, a 6-year-old male, was placed under general anesthesia for bilateral removal of tonsils with adenoids. The tonsils were grasped with an Allis forceps, and the incision made around the anterior tonsillar pillar. The tonsillar capsule was identified, and the tonsils bluntly dissected free. Next we turned our attention to the nasopharynx, which was viewed indirectly. There was a considerable amount of hypertrophic adenoids present; they were removed by curette, and all nubbins of adenoid tissue were removed. All bleeding was controlled with pressure sponges, and several small bleeding areas were touched with electrocoagulation. At the close of both procedures, there was no bleeding present. Blood loss was minimal, and the postoperative condition of the patient was good.

Process 1: CPT

1. What is the procedure?

2. Locate the main term in the index.

3. What additional questions or set of questions can be determined?

4. Upon review of all the code choices identified in the index, what additional questions can be determined?

5. Based on the documentation, what is the correct code for this case?
   a. 42830
   b. 42831
   c. 42820
   d. 42825

Process 2: ICD

ICD-9-CM

1. Based on the operative report header, what is the preoperative diagnosis

2. Is the postoperative diagnosis the same as or different from the preoperative diagnosis?

3. Is the postoperative diagnosis supported?

4. What is the main term for this condition?

5. Based on the subterm choices, what question(s) can be developed for this condition?

6. Is any sign, symptom, or additional condition documented?

7. Is the additional condition, sign, or symptom an integral part of the primary (or other) condition coded?

8. Does the additional condition require or affect patient care, treatment, or management?

9. Based on the documentation, what is (are) the correct ICD-9-CM code(s) for this case?
   a. 474.02   c. 474.00, 474.01
   b. 474.00   d. 474.00, 474.12

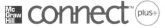 **plus+** Enhance your learning by completing these exercises and more at mcgrawhillconnect.com

ICD-10-CM

1. Based on the operative report header, what is the preoperative diagnosis?

2. Is the postoperative diagnosis the same as or different from the preoperative diagnosis?

3. Is the postoperative diagnosis supported?

4. What is the main term for this condition?

5. Based on the subterm choices, what question(s) can be developed for this condition?

6. Based on the information in the Tabular List, is additional information needed to determine the appropriate diagnosis code?

7. Is any sign, symptom, or additional condition documented?

8. Is the additional condition, sign, or symptom an integral part of the primary (or other) condition coded?

9. Does the additional condition require or affect patient care, treatment, or management?

10. Based on the documentation, what is (are) the correct ICD-10-CM code(s) for this case?
    - **a.** J35.01, J35.2
    - **b.** J35.01, J35.02
    - **c.** J35.2
    - **d.** J35.3

Process 3: Modifiers

1. Was the procedure performed different from that described by the nomenclature of the code?

2. Was the procedure performed at an anatomical site that has laterality?

3. Was the procedure performed in the global period of another procedure?

4. Were additional procedures performed during the operative session, and does the documentation support them?

5. Did the surgeon have help from another surgeon or another appropriate person?

6. Did a physician different from the surgeon provide the preoperative or postoperative portion of the procedure?

7. What modifier should be appended to the CPT code for this case?
    - **a.** 50
    - **b.** 58
    - **c.** 51
    - **d.** None

[LO 13.1–13.5] Case 2

Procedure: Small bowel enteroscopy

Anesthesia: Premedication: Versed slow IV push, Blucagon 0.2 mg in increments during the procedure

Indications: The patient is a 77-year-old woman admitted for recurrent anemia and angina pectoris related to her anemia.

The patient has profound microcytic, hypochromic anemia, initially presenting with a hemoglobin of 6.5. A few weeks ago, she was transfused, discharged, and then returned with a hemoglobin of 6.4 with recurrent anginal symptoms and marked fatigue. Most recent stool Hemoccults have been negative. She did, however, report having black tarry stool immediately prior to admission.

Operative procedure: The instrument was passed through the oropharynx into the stomach. The esophagus was well seen and was normal. On retroversion, the cardia and fundus were well seen and were unremarkable. There was a small hiatal hernia but no evidence of erosions in the gastric mucosa and nothing to suggest a lesion. The body of the stomach distended well and had normal rugal pattern. The antrum was well seen and was normal, as was the duodenal bulb. The instrument was withdrawn into the stomach at this point, and the overtube, which had been premounted on the scope, was then passed into the antrum. The enteroscope was then passed into the duodenal bulb, the descending duodenum, distal duodenum to the ligament of Traits, and the jejunum to what was felt to be the midjejunum, which at least was well seen. The patient was given Glucagons to facilitate visualization of the small bowel. No abnormalities were noted specifically, with nothing to suggest inflammatory change, AVMs, or neoplasia.

Impression: Unremarkable enteroscopy and upper gastrointestinal tract

Plans: Will discuss the situation with Dr. Smith. An option will be to follow the patient and consider reassessing her distal bowel in the event of recurrent bleeding. The patient did, however, have a significant drop in hemoglobin and hematocrit just this past week from reasons that are still entirely unclear.

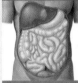

Process 1: CPT

1. What is the procedure?

2. Locate the main term in the index.

3. What additional questions or set of question can be determined?

4. Upon review of all the code choices identified in the index, what additional questions can be determined?

5. Based on the documentation, what is the correct code for this case?
   a. 44376
   b. 44376-52
   c. 44360
   d. 44366

Process 2: ICD

ICD-9-CM

1. Based on the operative report header, what is the preoperative diagnosis?

2. Is the postoperative diagnosis the same as or different from the preoperative diagnosis?

3. Is the postoperative diagnosis supported?

4. What is the main term for this condition?

5. Based on the subterm choices, what question(s) can be developed for this condition?

6. Is any sign, symptom, or additional condition documented?

7. Is the additional condition, sign, or symptom an integral part of the primary (or other) condition coded?

8. Does the additional condition require or affect patient care, treatment, or management?

9. Based on the documentation, what are the correct ICD-9-CM codes for this case?
   a. 280.0, 578.9, 413.9
   b. 280.9, 578.1, 413.9
   c. 280.0, 578.1, 413.9
   d. 578.9, 413.9

ICD-10-CM

1. Based on the operative report header, what is the preoperative diagnosis?

2. Is the postoperative diagnosis the same as or different from the preoperative diagnosis?

3. Is the postoperative diagnosis supported?

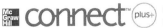

Enhance your learning by completing these exercises and more at mcgrawhillconnect.com

4. What is the main term for this condition?

5. Based on the subterm choices, what question(s) can be developed for this condition?

6. Based on the information in the Tabular List, is additional information needed to determine the appropriate diagnosis code?

7. Is any sign, symptom, or additional condition documented?

8. Is the additional condition, sign, or symptom an integral part of the primary (or other) condition coded?

9. Does the additional condition require or affect patient care, treatment, or management?

10. Based on the documentation, what are the correct ICD-10-CM codes for this case?
    a. D50.9, K92.1, I20.9   c. D50.9, K92.1, I20.0
    b. D50.0, K92.1, I20.9   d. D50.0, K92.1, I20.9

Process 3: Modifiers

1. Was the procedure performed different from that described by the nomenclature of the code?

2. Was the procedure performed at an anatomical site that has laterality?

3. Was the procedure performed in the global period of another procedure?

4. Were additional procedures performed during the operative session, and does the documentation support them?

5. Did the surgeon have help from another surgeon or another appropriate person?

6. Did a physician different from the surgeon provide the preoperative or postoperative portion of the procedure?

7. What modifier should be appended to the CPT code for this case?
   a. 51   c. 58
   b. 78   d. None

Surgery Section: Urinary System and Male Reproductive System

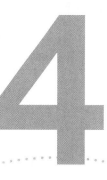 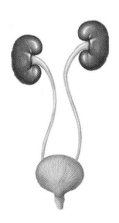

Key Terms

Benign prostatic hyperplasia (BPH)
Cowper's glands
Epididymis
Erythropoiesis

Erythropoietin
Glomerulus
Male reproductive system
Micturition
Nephrons

Prepuce
Seminal vesicle
Seminiferous tubules
Spermatic cord
Testes

Ureters
Urethra
Urinary system
Vas deferens

Learning Outcomes

After completing this chapter, you will be able to:

14.1 Review the anatomy of the urinary system.

14.2 Review the anatomy of the male reproductive system.

14.3 Understand chapter-specific ICD guidelines and format for the genitourinary system.

14.4 Identify the CPT guidelines and format for the urinary system.

14.5 Identify the CPT guidelines and format for the male reproductive system.

14.6 Apply the modifiers most commonly used with codes for the genitourinary system.

14.7 Examine the common medical and procedural terms used in operative reports.

Introduction

The genitourinary system consists of the urinary system and the genitalia and reproductive system. This chapter concentrates on the urinary system and the male reproductive system

The **urinary system** consists of the kidneys, ureters, urinary bladder, and urethra (see Table 14.1). Their combined functions filter the blood, create and maintain the balance of water and chemicals such as sodium and potassium, and remove waste (urea) and excess fluids from the body.

The **male reproductive system** consists of the testes, epididymis, vas deferens, seminal vesicle, ejaculatory duct, prostate gland, Cowper's glands, urethra, and penis. The functions of this system include production of male hormones and production and transportation of sperm.

To assign the appropriate codes for these body systems, a coder must not only be aware of the medical terminology, anatomy, and functions of these systems but also understand and apply the urinary and male reproductive system coding guidelines.

14.1 Anatomy of the Urinary System

The two kidneys, two ureters, the urinary bladder, and the urethra are the structures of the urinary system. The main functions of the kidneys are to filter blood and create urine. The main function of the ureters, bladder, and urethra are to eliminate urine from the body. (See Figures 14.1 to 14.3.)

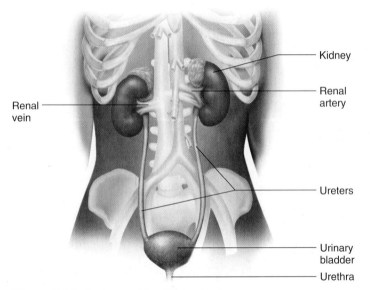

Figure 14.1 Anatomy of the Urinary System

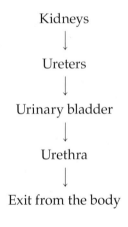

Flow of Urine through the Urinary System

Kidneys
↓
Ureters
↓
Urinary bladder
↓
Urethra
↓
Exit from the body

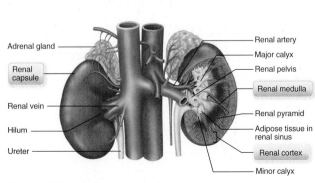

Figure 14.2 Anatomy of the Kidney

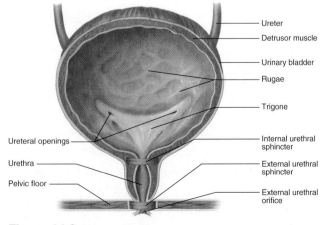

Figure 14.3 Urinary Bladder

Table 14.1 Structures of the Urinary System

STRUCTURE	DEFINITION/FUNCTION
Kidneys:	• There are two kidneys, located on the posterior wall of the abdominal cavity below the ribs. • They perform the following functions: *Filter the blood and produce urine*: This is the primary function of the urinary system. *Regulate blood pressure and blood volume:* The volume of blood is regulated by the kidneys' conservation or elimination of fluid. Blood pressure is regulated when the volume of blood in the body is adjusted. *Regulate the PH in the blood* *Produce red blood cells:* This is done by the release of the hormone **erythropoietin,** which stimulates **erythropoiesis** (production of red blood cells). *Excrete waste products and foreign substances:* This is done by the formation of urine to be released from the body, carrying foreign substances such as drugs or environmental toxins.
Regions of the kidneys	• *Cortex:* outer layer. • ***Nephrons:*** kidney cells whose function is to filter blood and form urine. • ***Glomerulus:*** region through which blood passes as it enters the kidney; filters the blood, removing water and waste products (urea, creatinine, ammonia, and mineral salts). • *Renal tubules:* capture water and waste products to form urine and deposit the urine into the renal pelvis. • *Medulla:* inner layer. • *Renal pelvis:* upper extended part of the ureters. Urine collects here and passes to the urinary bladder via the ureters.
Ureters	• There are two ureters, and each one transports urine from the kidney to the urinary bladder. • The ureters pass beneath the urinary bladder where the urinary bladder compresses the ureters, preventing the backflow of urine. This prevention of backflow is important because it reduces the chance of cystitis, inflammation of the ureter/urinary bladder, which can develop into a kidney infection.
Urinary bladder:	• This structure stores urine as a result of the bladder walls relaxing and expanding. When the walls contract and flatten, the urine empties into the urethra. • *Incontinence* is the lack of voluntary control over this process.
Sphincter muscles	• These are two circular muscles which assist in keeping urine from leaking. They close tightly like a rubber band around the bladder opening.
Nerves	• Their function is to indicate the necessity to urinate and empty the bladder.
Urethra	• This is a passageway, or tube, through which urine passes from the urinary bladder to the outside of the body. • The female urethra's only function for the urinary system is as an outlet for urine to exit the body. • The male urethra functions as a reproductive outlet as well as a urinary system outlet.

erythropoietin Hormone that stimulates erythropoiesis.

erythropoiesis Production of red blood cells.

nephrons Kidney cells whose functions are to filter blood and form urine.

glomerulus A region of the kidney through which blood passes as it enters the kidney and which filters the blood, removing water and waste products.

ureters Two structures that transport urine from the kidney to the urinary bladder.

urethra Tube that carries urine from the urinary bladder to the outside of the body; in the male, also functions as a reproductive outlet.

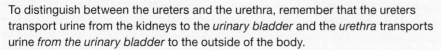

MENTOR Coding Tip

To distinguish between the ureters and the urethra, remember that the ureters transport urine from the kidneys to the *urinary bladder* and the *urethra* transports urine *from the urinary bladder* to the outside of the body.

EXERCISE 14.1

1. What hormone released by the kidneys stimulates the production of red blood cells?
2. Illustrate the flow of urine through the urinary system.
3. List the functions of the kidneys.
4. Explain the functions of the female urethra and male urethra.
5. If the ureters and urinary bladder are not able to prevent the backflow of urine, what condition can develop?

Also available in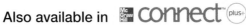

14.2 Anatomy of the Male Reproductive System

The male reproductive system consists of external and internal structures (see Figure 14.4 and Table 14.2). The external structures are the penis, scrotum, and testes. The internal structures are the vas deferens, ejaculatory ducts, urethra, seminal vesicles, prostate gland, and Cowper's glands. The combined functions of these structures are the production and transportation of sperm. It is important for the coder to be able to identify these structures and their specific functions in order to assign the appropriate ICD and CPT codes.

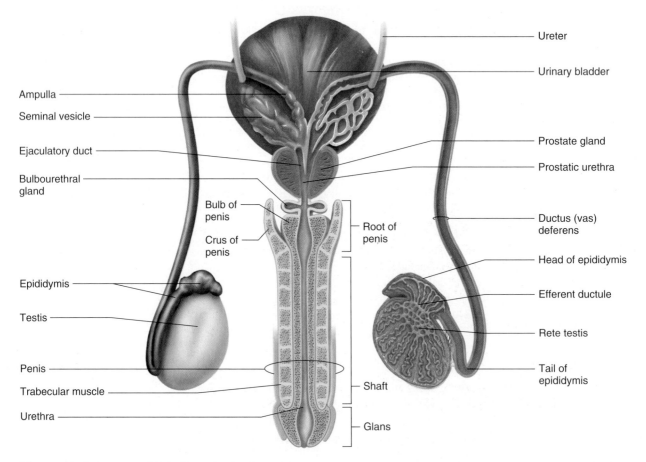

Figure 14.4 Anatomy of Male Reproductive System

Table 14.2 Structures of Male Reproductive System

STRUCTURE	DEFINITION/FUNCTION
External structures:	
Penis	• This is the male sex organ. • It has three parts: *Root:* attaches to the wall of the abdomen. *Body:* shaft of the penis. *Glans:* cone-shaped end, or head, of the penis, where the opening of the urethra is located. • The **prepuce,** or foreskin, surrounds and protects the head of the penis.
Scrotum	• This pouchlike sac contains the testicles (testes). • Many nerves and blood vessels are located here. • The functions of the scrotum are protection and climate control for the testes.
Testes	• These are also called *testicles.* • They are oval organs located in the scrotum, secured by the **spermatic cord.** • The function of the testes is production of testosterone and sperm. Within the testes are coiled masses of tubes called **seminiferous tubules.** These tubules are responsible for producing sperm cells through a process called *spermatogenesis.*
Epididymis	• Long, coiled tube located on the back of the testicle. • Functions of the epididymis are transportation, storage, and maturation of sperm cells produced by the testes.
Internal structures:	
Vas deferens	• This is a tube traveling from the epididymis to the pelvic cavity. • The function of the vas deferens is to transport mature sperm to the urethra.
Ejaculatory ducts	• The vas deferens and the seminal vesicles fuse to form the ejaculatory ducts, which empty into the urethra.
Urethra	• This tube carries urine from the urinary bladder to the outside of the body. • In males, the urethra also has the function of ejaculating semen.
Seminal vesicles	• These are saclike pouches attached to the vas deferens. • The function of the seminal vesicles is production of seminal fluid, which is a source of energy that aids sperm motility.
Prostate gland	• This walnut-size structure is located below the urinary bladder. • One of the functions of the prostate gland is to produce additional fluid that aids in the nourishment of the sperm.
Cowper's glands	• These glands are also called *bulbourethral glands.* • They are pea-size structures on the sides of the urethra, below the prostate. • The function of these glands is production of fluid that empties into the urethra and acts as a lubricant for the urethra and as a neutralizer for urine.

prepuce Foreskin that surrounds and protects the head of the penis.

testes Oval organs that are located in the scrotum and produce testosterone and sperm. Also called *testicles.*

spermatic cord Cord that secures the testes in the scrotum.

seminiferous tubules Coiled masses of tubes that are responsible for producing sperm cells through a process called *spermatogenesis.*

epididymis A long, coiled tube located on the back of the testicle.

vas deferens Tube from the epididymis to the pelvic cavity that transports mature sperm to the urethra.

seminal vesicle A saclike pouch that is attached to the vas deferens and produces seminal fluid.

Cowper's glands Pea-size structures on the sides of the urethra, below the prostate. Also called *bulbourethral glands.*

1. Which structure of the male reproductive system has the functions of transportation, storage, and maturation of sperm cells?
2. List the three parts of the penis.
3. Which structure of the male reproductive system protects and controls the climate for the testes?
4. List the external and internal structures of the male reproductive system.

Also available in 🅜 connect (plus+)

14.3 Chapter-Specific ICD Guidelines and Format for the Genitourinary System (Urinary and Male Reproductive ICD Codes)

Conditions of the urinary system can be caused by illness, injury, and aging (due to changes in the structure of the kidneys and the urinary bladder muscles). Any of these causes can interfere with a kidney's ability to filter blood and/or block the flow of urine. Some common diseases coded to the Genitourinary chapters of ICD are hematuria, cystitis, renal failure, and nephropathy.

Conditions of the male reproductive system can also be caused by illness, injury, and aging. Some common diseases coded to the Genitourinary chapters of ICD for the male reproductive system include prostate disease, orchitis, male infertility, and disorders of the penis and testes.

When coding these conditions, coders must thoroughly review the provider documentation as well as the guidelines and instructional notes.

ICD-9-CM: Diseases of the Genitourinary System (urinary system and male reproductive system) is Chapter 10 of the ICD-9-CM manual, with the code range 580–608.

ICD-10-CM: Diseases of the Genitourinary System (urinary system and male reproductive system) is Chapter 14 of the ICD-10-CM manual, with the code range N00–N51.

Table 14.3 lists the relevant Chapter 10 and 14 subheadings and their code ranges.

> **MENTOR**
> Coding Tip
>
> Highlight the instructional notes in this section of your ICD manual to remind yourself of these tips and guidelines when using the manual.

Table 14.3 Urinary System and Male Reproductive System Subsection Format *(Data from ICD-9-CM and ICD-10-CM, Centers for Medicare and Medicaid Services and the National Center for Health Statistics.)*

ICD-9-CM		ICD-10-CM	
SUBHEADING	**CODE RANGE**	**SUBHEADING**	**CODE RANGE**
Nephritis, Nephrotic Syndrome, and Nephrosis	580–589	Glomerular Diseases	N00–N08
		Renal Tubulo-interstitial Diseases	N10–N16
Other Diseases of the Urinary System	590–599	Acute Kidney Failure and Chronic Kidney Disease	N17–N19
Diseases of Male Genital Organs	600–608	Urolithiasis	N20–N23
		Other Diseases of Kidney and Ureter	N25–N29
		Other Diseases of the Urinary System	N30–N39
		Diseases of Male Genital Organs	N40–N51

Nephritis, Nephrotic Syndrome, and Nephrosis (580–589), ICD-9-CM

Glomerular Diseases (N00–N08), ICD-10-CM

Renal Tubulo-interstitial Diseases (N10–N16), ICD-10-CM

Acute Kidney Failure, Chronic Kidney Disease (N17–N19), ICD-10-CM

Nephritis is inflammation of the kidney. Glomerulonephritis, inflammation of the round filters (glomeruli) found in the kidneys, is the most common form of acute nephritis.

Nephrotic syndrome is a group of symptoms or disorders that can damage the kidney, resulting in too much protein in the urine. Some of the contributing causes are diabetes, infection, glomerulonephritis, and certain types of drugs. Primary nephritic syndrome is limited to the kidney, while secondary nephritic syndrome affects the kidney and other parts of the body.

Nephrosis is often defined as a noninflammatory condition of the kidneys, degenerative disease of the renal tubules, and kidney disease affecting function of the nephrons.

The codes within this range are further defined by the following conditions:

- Acute glomerulonephritis, 580, ICD-9-CM (N00, ICD-10-CM)

In this condition, the filtering system becomes inflamed and often scarred, and the ability to remove waste from the blood is compromised. The codes within this category require a fourth digit that specifies the condition as a proliferative or progressive lesion or other specified pathologic lesion.

SPOTLIGHT on Condition

A lesion of proliferative glomerulonephritis is a condition in which there is unchecked growth of tissue, which affects the ability of the kidney to filter the blood. A lesion of rapidly progressive glomerulonephritis is a condition in which the kidney function has been progressively and rapidly destroyed, and it can result in end-stage renal disease (ESRD).

FOR EXAMPLE Acute glomerulonephritis with a lesion of proliferative glomerulonephritis is assigned ICD-9-CM code 580.0. An instructional note under the code for other specified pathologic lesion (580.81) directs the coder to code first the underlying disease. ▪

- Nephrotic syndrome, 581, ICD-9-CM (N00, ICD-10-CM)

The codes within this category are further defined by specific type of glomerulonephrotic lesion, such as membranous, or by other specified pathologic lesion in the kidney.

FOR EXAMPLE Nephrotic syndrome with a lesion of membranous glomerulonephritis is assigned ICD-9-CM code 581.1. ▪

- Chronic glomerulonephritis, 582, ICD-9-CM (N00.1, ICD-10-CM)

This is an advanced stage of kidney disease in which the glomeruli are destroyed over time, affecting the ability of the kidneys to filter blood. The codes in this category are also defined by the type of glomerulonephrotic lesion or other specified pathologic lesion.

FOR EXAMPLE Chronic glomerulonephritis with a lesion of rapidly progressive glomerulonephritis is assigned ICD-9-CM code 582.4. (N03.8, ICD-10-CM) ■

- Nephritis and nephropathy not specified as acute or chronic, 583, ICD-9-CM; N05, ICD-10-CM

According to the *includes* instructional note located under category 583, Renal disease, so stated, not specified as acute or chronic but with stated pathology or cause describes codes assigned to this category.

- Acute kidney failure, 584, ICD-9-CM; N17, ICD-10-CM

When renal function is interrupted suddenly, acute kidney failure can occur. Often, renal function returns with treatment. If renal function does not return after treatment of acute kidney failure, the condition progresses to chronic kidney disease. Some causes of acute kidney failure include calculi obstructing the flow of urine, tumors, congestive heart failure, or surgical complications.

The codes within this category are further defined as to acute kidney failure with a specific type and location of lesion, such as tubular necrosis, renal cortical necrosis, and renal medullary necrosis.

FOR EXAMPLE Acute kidney failure with a lesion of tubular necrosis is assigned 584.5 (ICD-9-CM) or N17.0 (ICD-10-CM). ■

- Chronic kidney disease, 585, ICD-9-CM; N18, ICD-10-CM

SPOTLIGHT on a Guideline

Acute kidney failure, unspecified (nontraumatic), is included in category 584 with an *excludes* instructional note directing the coder to code range 866.00–866.13 if the documentation describes a traumatic kidney injury.

Chronic kidney disease (CKD) is a progressive loss of kidney function. There are multiple instructional notes at the beginning of this category that need to be reviewed before assigning a code from this section. They direct the coder to code first hypertensive chronic disease, to use an additional code to identify kidney transplant status (V42.0, ICD-9-CM; Z94.0, ICD-10-CM), and to use an additional code to identify a manifestation such as neuropathy (357.4, ICD-9-CM; G63, ICD-10-CM).

Chronic kidney disease consists of five different stages and end-stage renal disease:

Stage 1—some kidney damage.

Stage 2—mild form of kidney disease.

Stage 3—moderate form of kidney disease; patient may be experiencing some anemia and bone loss.

Stage 4—severe form of kidney disease; symptoms are progressively more pronounced.

Stage 5—very severe form of kidney disease; often, patients require dialysis.

An *excludes* instructional note with the code for chronic kidney disease, stage 5 (585.5, ICD-9-CM; N18.5 ICD-10-CM) informs the coder that this code is not to be used if the documentation describes the condition as chronic kidney disease, stage 5, requiring chronic dialysis.

End-stage renal disease (ESRD)—defined in ICD as chronic kidney disease requiring chronic dialysis.

- Renal failure, unspecified, 586, ICD-9-CM; N19, ICD-10-CM

Uremia, NOS (not otherwise specified), is assigned a code from this category. There are several *excludes* instructional notes with this code category.

FOR EXAMPLE Uremia following labor and delivery is assigned code 669.3–. ∎

Other Diseases of the Urinary System (590–599), ICD-9-CM
Other Diseases of the Urinary System (N30–N39), ICD-10-CM

The codes within these ranges are further defined by the following conditions:

- Infections of kidney, 590, ICD-9-CM; N11, ICD-10-CM

Acute pyelonephritis and chronic pyelonephritis are assigned codes from this category. They are further defined by whether the condition is with or without a lesion of renal medullary necrosis.

SPOTLIGHT on a Guideline

Patients can experience some signs and symptoms that involve the urinary system but are not coded to the Diseases of the Genitourinary System chapter of ICD. They include renal colic or kidney pain, dysuria, retention of urine, urinary incontinency, urinary frequency, and polyuria. They are coded in Chapter 16 of ICD-9-CM, under "Symptoms Involving the Urinary System" (category 788), and Chapter 18 of ICD-10-CM, under "Symptoms and Signs Involving the Genitourinary System (category R30–R39).

FOR EXAMPLE Chronic pyelonephritis with a lesion of renal medullary necrosis is assigned 590.01 (ICD-9-CM). ∎

- Calculus of kidney and ureter, 592, ICD-9-CM; N20, ICD-10-CM
- Other disorders of the kidney and ureter, 593, ICD-9-CM

Conditions in this category include floating kidney or nephroptosis (593.0, ICD-9-CM), hypertrophy of a kidney (593.1, ICD-9-CM), acquired cyst of a kidney (593.2, ICD-9-CM; congenital cyst of a kidney is assigned ICD-9-CM code 753.1), stricture (kinking) of a ureter (593.3, ICD-9-CM), and hydroureter (593.5, ICD-9-CM).

Vascular disorders of the kidney, such as renal artery embolism or hemorrhage or renal infarction, are also assigned codes from this category (593.81, ICD-9-CM).

SPOTLIGHT on a Guideline

Other conditions listed under this code description include nephrolithiasis, renal calculus, kidney stone, and staghorn calculus for the kidney and ureteric stone and ureterolithiasis for the ureter.

- Calculus of the lower urinary tract, 594, ICD-9-CM; N21.0, ICD-10-CM

  Calculi occurring in the urinary bladder and urethra are assigned codes from this category.

- Cystitis, 595, ICD-9-CM; N30, ICD-10-CM

  Cystitis is inflammation of the urinary bladder. An instructional note at the beginning of this category directs the coder to use an additional code to identify the organism (such as *E. coli*).

  Irradiation cystitis, which is inflammation of the bladder due to the effects of radiation, is included in this category (595.82, ICD-9-CM; N30.4, ICD-10-CM), and an instructional note directs the coder to use an additional E code to identify the cause.

- Other disorders of the bladder, 596, ICD-9-CM; N32, ICD-10-CM

  Bladder neck obstruction (596.0, ICD-9-CM; N32.0, ICD-10-CM) is one of the conditions in this category of codes. Some other terms used to describe this condition are *contracture* or *stenosis*.

  Diverticulum of the bladder (596.3, ICD-9-CM) is also included in this category; an instructional note with this code excludes calculus in diverticulum of the bladder.

  Overactive bladder (596.51, ICD-9-CM; N32.81, ICD-10-CM) and neutrogenic bladder NOS (596.54, ICD-9-CM; N31.9, ICD-10-CM) are also included in this code category.

- Other disorders of the urethra and urinary tract, 599, ICD-9-CM; N39, ICD-10-CM

  Urinary tract infection, site not specified (599.0, ICD-9-CM; N39.0, ICD-10-CM), is included in this code category. An instructional note directs the coder to use an additional code to identify the organism.

  Hematuria, which is further defined as unspecified, gross, or microscopic, is included in this category.

SPOTLIGHT on a Guideline

In ICD-9-CM hematuria is included in category 599 (other disorders of the urethra and urinary tract), while in ICD-10-CM hematuria, unspecified, is included in R31.9 (symptoms and signs of the genitourinary system).

Diseases of Male Genital Organs (600–608), ICD-9-CM
Diseases of Male Genital Organs (N40–N51), ICD-10-CM

Conditions involving the prostate, penis, and testes are assigned codes from these categories:

- Hyperplasia of the prostate, 600, ICD-9-CM; N40, ICD-10-CM

  Benign prostatic hypertrophy is assigned a code from this category (600.0, ICD-9-CM; N40.0, ICD-10-CM).

- Inflammatory diseases of the prostate, 601, ICD-9-CM; N40.41, ICD-10-CM

  Acute and chronic prostatitis and abscess of the prostate are some of the conditions assigned codes in this category. An additional code is needed to

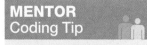

MENTOR
Coding Tip

Benign prostatic hypertrophy is most commonly documented as BPH.

identify an organism, such as streptococcus. The codes in this category have an age and gender edit as designated by the use of the letter A (adult age 15–124) and the male symbol (♂) located to the right of the codes in the ICD manual.

- Disorders of the penis, 607, ICD-9-CM

Leukoplakia, a condition characterized by white thick patches on the glans penis, is listed in this category of codes. Balantis (607.1, ICD-9-CM; N48.1, ICD-10-CM), an inflammation of the glans penis and prepuce, is also included in this category. Abscess, boil, carbuncle, and cellulitis are included in subcategory 607.2 (ICD-9-CM; N48.29, ICD-10-CM), "Other Inflammatory Disorders of Penis."

- Other disorders of male genital organs, 608, ICD-9-CM; N50, ICD-10-CM

Conditions of the testes and spermatic cord are included in this category.

FOR EXAMPLE Torsion of a testis, unspecified, is assigned code 608.20, ICD-9-CM; N44.00, ICD-10-CM. ▪

EXERCISE 14.3

1. Both CKD and ESRD are documented in the report. Assign the appropriate code.
2. Chronic glomerulonephritis is an advanced stage of kidney disease in which the glomeruli are destroyed over time, affecting the ability of the kidneys to filter blood. How are the codes in the relevant range further defined?
3. Assign the appropriate code for a diagnosis of staghorn calculus.
4. Encysted hydrocele of the spermatic cord is diagnosed. Assign the appropriate code(s).
5. The diagnosis is an abscess of the epididymis with streptococcus identified as the organism. Assign the appropriate code(s).

Also available in 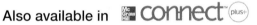 connect (plus+)

14.4 Guidelines and Format of the Urinary System Subsection of CPT

General Guidelines for Urinary System Subsection of CPT

- Insertion of a urinary bladder catheter is part of the global surgical package.
- Placement of a catheter for postoperative drainage is not reported separately.
- Cystourethroscopy with one or more biopsies includes all biopsies performed during the procedure.
- Irrigation or drainage procedures integral to the primary procedure are not reported separately.
- When an endoscopic procedure is performed as part of an open procedure, only the open procedure is coded.

The endoscopic procedure is confirmatory or is used to evaluate the surgical field. ■

- A surgical endoscopic or laparoscopic procedure includes the diagnostic procedure.
- When multiple endoscopic approaches are attempted during the same procedure, only the completed approach is coded.

There are several questions a coder needs to ask when reading an operative report and coding a procedure from this section. The following questions will help the coder, when reading through the report, to understand what actually was done and how the procedure should be translated and coded:

- At which anatomical site was the procedure performed?
- What approach was used?
- What type of exam, such as endoscopic, laparoscopic, or open, was performed?
- Does the documentation describe a procedure done at a single site or multiple sites?

Urinary System Subsection General Heading Code Ranges (50010–53899)

The general headings and code ranges are listed in Table 14.4.

Section Subheadings and Guidelines

The general headings may include the following subheadings:

- Incision
- Excision
- Introduction
- Removal/Removal of Foreign Body
- Repair
- Laparoscopy
- Endoscopy
- Other Procedures

Kidney (50010–50593)

Incision: 50010–50135

Drainage of a perirenal or renal abscess is reported with codes in this range (50020–50021). The codes for this drainage are further defined as open or percutaneous.

Table 14.4 Urinary System General Headings and Code Ranges *(Data from CPT 2013. © 2013 American Medical Association. All rights reserved.)*

HEADING	CODE RANGE
Kidney	50010–50593
Ureter	50600–50980
Bladder	51020–52700
Urethra	53000–53899

Nephrostomy with drainage or with exploration is within this code range (50040–50045). An instructional note associated with the nephrostomy codes directs the coder to see CPT codes 50570 to 50580 if renal endoscopy was also performed.

Nephrolithotomy has several codes in this range. To assign the appropriate code, the coder must review the documentation and be able to identify the following:

- Removal of calculus.
- Secondary surgical operation for calculus.
- Complicated by congenital kidney abnormality.
- Removal of large staghorn calculus filling renal pelvis and calyces.

FOR EXAMPLE If the nephrolithotomy was complicated by a congenital kidney abnormality, code 50070 is reported. ◼

Excision: 50200–50290

Renal biopsies are reported with codes from this code range. Coders need to know whether the biopsy was performed percutaneously by trocar or needle (50200) or by surgical exposure of the kidney (50205). If the procedure was a fine-needle aspiration, code 10022 from the integumentary system would be assigned.

Nephrectomy procedures are within code range 50220–50240. A nephrectomy is most often performed to remove a seriously damaged or diseased kidney. This procedure is performed as an open procedure through a large incision (open nephrectomy) or as a laparoscopic procedure either through a single large incision in the abdomen or side or through a series of small incisions in the abdomen (laparoscopic nephrectomy).

The medical documentation needs to be reviewed to determine the following:

- Did the procedure include a partial or total ureterectomy?
- Was the procedure complicated because of previous surgery on the same kidney?
- Was it a radical procedure with regional lymphadenectomy and/or vena cava thrombectomy?
- Was there vena caval resection with reconstruction?
- Was it an open or a laparoscopic procedure?

FOR EXAMPLE A nephrectomy including partial ureterectomy, with any open approach including rib resection, and complicated because of previous surgery on the same kidney is assigned CPT code 50225. ◼

Renal Transplantation: 50300–50380

As with all transplantation code ranges, the code ranges for renal transplantation include three major physician components:

- Cadaver donor nephrectomy, unilateral or bilateral, 50300

  or

  Living donor nephrectomy, 50320, 50547 (These codes include harvesting and cold preservation of grafts.)

- Backbench work, 50323–50329
- Recipient renal allotransplantation, 50360, 50365 (These codes include the care of the recipient.)

Instructional notes direct the coder to use CPT code 50547 for laparoscopic donor nephrectomy.

Introduction: 50382–50389

Renal pelvis catheter procedures are included in this code range and are further defined as internally dwelling (50382–50386) or externally accessible (50387–50389) for removal and replacement procedures.

As outlined in the anatomy discussion earlier in this chapter, the function of the ureter is the flow of urine from the kidney to the urinary bladder. Often, an obstruction caused by a calculus or tumor occurs and a stent is placed to allow the urine to flow. An internal placement has no part of the stent protruding from the body, whereas an externally accessible stent protrudes outside the body and is attached to a drainage tube.

Repair: 50400–50540

Pyeloplasty (surgical repair of the renal pelvis) is included in this code range and is further defined as simple or complicated.

Nephrorrhaphy of a kidney wound or injury and fistula closures are also included in this code range.

Laparoscopy: 50541–50549

Surgical laparoscopic ablation of renal cysts and renal mass lesions are included in this range. An open procedure is coded to 50250, and percutaneous ablation of renal tumors is reported with code 50592 or 50593.

Surgical laparoscopic partial and radical nephrectomies are also included in this code range. The radical nephrectomy code (50545) includes the removal of Gerota's fascia and surrounding fatty tissue, removal of regional lymph nodes, and adrenalectomy.

Ureter (50600–50980)

Incision: 50600–50630

Ureterotomy for insertion of an indwelling stent is assigned to this range. Ureterolithotomy is defined further by location, such as upper, middle, or lower one-third of the ureter.

There is an instructional note directing the coder to use CPT code 51065 for cystotomy with stone basket extraction of ureteral calculus.

Repair: 50700–50940

To assign the appropriate code from this range, the coder must determine from the medical documentation what type of procedure was performed, such as ureteroplasty, ureterolysis, or ureterostomy. The -ostomy codes are further defined by the location of the anastomosis.

FOR EXAMPLE

Ureteropyelostomy, anastomosis of ureter and renal pelvis, 50740

Ureterocalycostomy, anastomosis of ureter to renal calyx, 50750

Ureteroenterostomy, direct anastomosis of ureter to intestine, 50800 ■

Bladder (51020–52700)

Incision, removal, and excision are subsections within this subheading and include codes for cystotomy, aspiration of the bladder, and cystectomy.

A cystectomy is a surgical procedure to remove all or part of the urinary bladder and is often performed to treat malignant neoplasms of the bladder. The cystectomy codes (51550–51596) are further defined by whether the procedure is partial or complete. In a partial or segmental cystectomy, part of the bladder is removed; in a complete or radical cystectomy, the bladder is removed along with other pelvic organs and/or structures. The complete cystectomy is often performed for treatment of a malignant neoplasm that has invaded the bladder muscle.

Urodynamics: 51725–51798

Urodynamic studies are performed to evaluate the bladder's function and efficiency. Urodynamic testing provides volume and pressure information.

Some abbreviations to be familiar with when assigning codes from this code range are:

CMG Cystometrogram (measures how much fluid the bladder can hold and how much pressure builds up inside the bladder)

UPP Ureteral pressure profile (records the resistance of the urethra to fluid flow with measurements taken of the pressure at various points)

EMG Electromyography (records pelvic muscle activity)

UFR Uroflowmetry (measures the amount of urine and the flow)

Endoscopy: 52000–52010

Procedures in this code range include cystoscopy, urethroscopy, and cystourethroscopy. The removal of a temporary ureteral catheter during a diagnostic or therapeutic endoscopic procedure is included in CPT codes 52320 to 52355 and is not reported.

Cystoscopy is the visualization of the urinary bladder by the use of a scope, and the primary code reported for this is 52000. Other procedures and codes related to cystourethroscopy include the following:

- Basic cystourethroscopy procedures, 52001–52010
- Cystoscopy with urethra or bladder procedures, 52205–52318
- Cystoscopy with ureter and pelvic procedures, 52320–52355
- Cystoscopy and associated prostate surgery, 52400–52640

Therapeutic cystourethroscopy always includes the diagnostic cystourethroscopy.

Urethra (53000–53899)

Incision: 53000–53085

Urethrotomy, keratotomy, and drainage codes are assigned to this code range.

Repair: (53400–53520)

Urethroplasty procedures are included in this code range and are further defined as first or second stage and as male or female urethra.

Urethroplasty, first-stage reconstruction of a male anterior urethra, is reported with CPT code 53410.

Urethroplasty, reconstruction of female urethra, is reported with CPT code 53430. ■

Removal codes, urethrorrhaphy, and closure codes are also included in this code range.

The more familiar coders become with the format and guidelines, the better prepared they are for selecting the appropriate CPT code for the medically necessary diagnosis for the patient encounter.

EXERCISE 14. 4

1. What is the difference between an indwelling ureteral stent and an externally accessible ureteral stent?

2. Describe a nephrectomy procedure and the different approaches.

3. Define *urodynamic procedure*.

4. The cystectomy codes (51550–51596) are further defined by whether the procedure is partial or complete. Explain the difference between a partial cystectomy and a complete cystectomy.

Also available in ![McGraw Hill] connect (plus+)

14.5 Guidelines and Format of the Male Reproductive System Subsection of CPT

General Guidelines for Male Reproductive System Subsection of CPT

- Placement of a catheter for postoperative drainage is not reported separately.
- Irrigation or drainage procedures integral to the primary procedure are not reported separately.
- A surgical laparoscopic procedure includes the diagnostic procedure.
- Exploration of the surgical field is not reported separately.

There are several questions a coder needs to ask when reading an operative report and coding a procedure from this section. The following questions will help the coder, when reading through the report, to understand what actually was done and how the procedure should be translated and coded:

- At which anatomical site was the procedure performed?
- What approach was used?
- What type of exam was performed?
- Does the documentation describe a procedure done at a single site or multiple sites?

Table 14.5 Male Reproductive System General Headings and Code Ranges *(Data from CPT 2013. © 2013 American Medical Association. All rights reserved.)*

HEADING	CODE RANGE
Male reproductive system	**54000–55899**
Penis	54000–54450
Testis	54500–54699
Epididymis	54700–54901
Tunica Vaginalis	55000–55060
Scrotum	55100–55180
Vas Deferens	55200–55450
Spermatic Cord	55500–55559
Seminal Vesicles	55600–55680
Prostate	55700–55899

Male Reproductive System Subsection General Heading Code Ranges (54000–55899)

The general headings and their code ranges are listed in Table 14.5.

Section Subheadings and Guidelines

The general headings may include the following subheadings:

- Incision
- Excision
- Introduction
- Exploration
- Laparoscopy
- Repair

Penis (54000–54450)

Incision: 54000–54015

Incision and drainage of the penis, deep, is included in this code range. An instructional note directs the use of codes from the Integumentary System section to report I&D of skin and subcutaneous abscesses.

Excision: 54100–54164

Circumsion is reported with codes in this range. These codes are further defined by the specific method used, such as a clamp or another device, a regional dorsal penile or ring block, or surgical excision other than a clamp, device, or dorsal slit.

FOR EXAMPLE Circumcision, using a clamp or another device, with a regional dorsal penile or ring block is assigned CPT code 54150. ■

An instructional note below code 54150 directs the use of modifier 52 when circumcision is performed without a dorsal penile or ring block.

Repair: 54300–54440

Urethroplasty procedures are identified by codes in this range. They are further defined by the following:

- First, second, or third stage
- Size of lesion
- With or without skin flaps

FOR EXAMPLE A urethroplasty for second-stage hypospadias repair (including urinary diversion), less than 3 cm, is assigned CPT code 54308. ■

Insertion, removal, and replacement of a penile prosthesis are included in this code range.

Testis (54500–54699)

Excision: 54500–54535

Biopsy of a testis, either by needle or incision, is assigned to this code range. Orchiectomy procedures are further defined as simple, partial, or radical.

A surgical laparoscopic orchiectomy is reported with CPT codes 54690 to 54699.

Prostate (55700–55899)

Incision: 55700–55725

Biopsy of the prostate by needle, punch, or incision is reported with CPT code 55700 or 55705. A transperineal stereotactic template–guided saturation prostate biopsy is assigned CPT code 55706. (This code's description includes imaging guidance.)

Excision: 55801–55865

Prostatectomy codes are included in this range. It is important to note that the codes' description includes control of postoperative bleeding, vasectomy, keratotomy, urethral calibration, and dilation.

EXERCISE 14.5

1. How are orchiectomy codes further defined?
2. What code range covers urethroplasty procedures, and how are the codes further defined?

Also available in 📊 connect (plus+)

14.6 Modifiers Most Commonly Used with Codes in the Urinary and Male Reproductive Subsections

As with all sections of the CPT manual, modifiers are used in the Urinary and Male Reproductive subsections to continue or modify the story of the patient's encounter. Some of the more common modifiers used in these subsections are 50, bilateral procedure; 58, staged or related procedure or service by the same physician or other qualified healthcare professional during the postoperative period; 59, distinct procedural service; and 78, unplanned

Table 14.6 Urinary and Male Reproductive Subsection Modifiers *(Data from CPT 2013. © 2013 American Medical Association. All rights reserved.)*

MODIFIER	DEFINITION	EXAMPLE OF USE
50	Bilateral procedure	Code 50382 is used for removal and replacement of an internally dwelling ureteral stent via percutaneous approach. For a bilateral procedure, append modifier 50 to code 50382.
51	Multiple procedures	For renal autotransplantation extracorporeal (bench) surgery, CPT directs the coder to use autotransplantation as the primary procedure and report secondary procedures such as partial nephrectomy or nephrolithotomy with modifier 51.
58	Staged or related procedure or service by the same physician or other qualified healthcare professional during the postoperative period	For cystourethroscopic removal of a self-retaining indwelling ureteral stent, code 52310 or 52315 could have modifier 58 appended if appropriately documented.
59	Distinct procedural services	When a diagnostic antegrade pyelogram is performed prior to the stent placement, it can be reported separately with modifier 59.
78	Unplanned return to the operating/procedure room by the same physician or another qualified healthcare professional following the initial procedure for a related procedure during the postoperative period	If transurethral fulguration of the prostate for postoperative bleeding is performed by the same physician, modifier 78 would be appended.

return to the operating/procedure room by the same physician or another qualified healthcare professional following the initial procedure for a related procedure during the postoperative period. (See Table 14.6.)

The appropriate use of modifiers with the codes from the system subsection helps to tell the patient's full story.

EXERCISE 14.6

1. A bilateral procedure was performed, but the CPT code description does not define the code as unilateral or bilateral. Which modifier would be assigned?

2. The patient is being taken back to the operating room during the postoperative period for an unplanned procedure of the urinary system or male reproductive system. Which modifier would be used?

3. When multiple procedures are performed in the same investigative session of urodynamic procedures, which modifier would be reported?

Also available in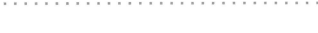

14.7 Common Medical and Procedural Terms Used in Operative Reports

As with all sections of CPT, the Urinary and Male Reproductive subsections include medical terms and procedural terms that are specific to the system involved. Tables 14.7 and 14.8 list some of these terms and identify some key terms that could appear in a provider's documentation concerning the genitourinary system.

Table 14.7 Terms for Urinary and Male Reproductive Systems

TERM	DEFINITION	DOCUMENTATION KEYS
Cystography	X-ray of the urinary bladder	Retrograde cystography (x-ray of the bladder after contrast dye is placed into the bladder through the urethra)
Lithotripsy	Noninvasive treatment of calculi (stones) by crushing	Extracorporeal shock wave lithotripsy (ESWL)
Nephrolithotomy	Removal of kidney stones by a small puncture wound through the skin	Removal of kidney stone through a tube
Orchiopexy	Procedure in which an undescended testicle is lowered into the scrotum and fixed in place	Laparoscopic orchidopexy
Prostate-specific antigen (PSA) test	Screening test for prostate cancer	If the screening test shows an elevated PSA level and the patient is asymptomatic, the provider may order another PSA as confirmation of the original findings.
Pyelography	Imaging of the renal pelvis and ureter	IVP, or intravenous pyelography; RP, or retrograde pyelography
Transurethral resection of the prostate (TURP)	Surgical removal of all or part of the prostate gland.	This procedure is usually done to relieve symptoms caused by an enlarged prostate by trimming away excess prostate tissue.
Urethroplasty	Surgical repair of the urethra	Provider documentation may also refer to this as urethral reconstruction
Vasectomy	Surgical procedure in which the vas deferens (the tube that carries sperm to the urethra) is cut	Male sterilization
Voiding cystourethrogram (VCUG)	X-ray examination of the bladder and urethra that is performed while the bladder is emptying	Micturating cystourethrogram (MCUG))

Table 14.8 Additional Terms for Urinary and Male Reproductive Systems

TERM	DEFINITION	DOCUMENTATION KEYS
Anorchism	Absence of one or both testes	Abnormality of testes
Benign prostatic hyperplasia (BPH)	Enlargement of the prostate gland, which can interfere with urinary function	Provider documentation may also refer to this condition as prostate gland enlargement, benign prostatic hypertrophy, or benign enlargement of the prostate.
Calculi	Stones that can occur in any of the structures of the urinary system	Stones, lithiasis
Cryptorchidism	Failure of one or both testes to descend into the scrotum	Undescended testes
Cystocele	Hernial protrusion of the urinary bladder	Herniation of the bladder
Hypospadias	Condition in which the urethra opens on the underside of the penis	Congenital defect or anomaly

benign prostatic hyperplasia (BPH) Enlargement of the prostate gland, which can interfere with urinary function.

Table 14.8 Additional Terms for Urinary and Male Reproductive Systems (*concluded*)

TERM	DEFINITION	DOCUMENTATION KEYS
Micturition	Process in which the bladder contracts and expels urine	Urination, voiding
Nephrolithiasis	Condition in which stones, or calculi, occur in the kidney	Kidney stone, kidney calculus
Nephroptosis	Downward displacement of the kidney	Floating kidney, prolapse of the kidney
Proteinuria	Abnormal amount of protein in the urine	Albuminuria
Pyelonephritis	Inflammation of the kidney and renal pelvis	Acute, chronic
Renal failure	Inability of the kidneys to regulate water and chemicals in the body or remove waste products from the blood	*Acute renal failure (ARF):* the sudden onset of kidney failure from causes such as accidents that injure the kidneys, the loss of a lot of blood, or some drugs or poisons *Chronic kidney disease (CKD):* the gradual reduction of kidney function, which may lead to permanent kidney failure or end-stage renal disease (ESRD)
Urinary tract infection (UTI)	Bacteria in the urinary tract	Cystitis (infection in the urinary bladder)

micturition Urination.

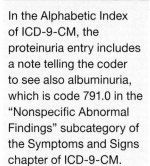

MENTOR
Coding Tip

In the Alphabetic Index of ICD-9-CM, the proteinuria entry includes a note telling the coder to see also albuminuria, which is code 791.0 in the "Nonspecific Abnormal Findings" subcategory of the Symptoms and Signs chapter of ICD-9-CM.

1. List three types of renal failure and define each.
2. The process in which the bladder contracts and expels urine can be defined three different ways. List these three different ways.
3. What is the term used to describe a congenital defect in which the urethra opens on the underside of the penis?
4. Define *TURP procedure*.
5. What is the procedure in which an undescended testicle is lowered into the scrotum and fixed in place?
6. Describe ESWL.

EXERCISE 14.7

Also available in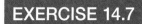

Chapter Fourteen Summary

Learning Outcome	Key Concepts/Examples
14.1 Review the anatomy of the urinary system.	*Kidneys:* regulate blood volume and composition, help to regulate blood pressure and pH, participate in red blood cell production, and excrete waste products and foreign substances. *Ureters:* transport urine from the kidneys to the urinary bladder. *Urinary bladder:* stores urine and expels urine into the urethra. *Urethra:* discharges urine from the body.
14.2 Review the anatomy of the male reproductive system.	External structures: • *Penis:* three parts—root, body, and glans • *Scrotum:* protective pouch for the testes • *Testes:* function is the production of testosterone and sperm Internal structures: • *Vas deferens:* transports mature sperm to the urethra • *Ejaculatory ducts:* formed by fusion of the vas deferens and the seminal vesicles; empty into the urethra • *Urethra:* carries urine from the urinary bladder to the outside of the body • *Seminal vesicles:* produce seminal fluid • *Prostate gland:* produces additional fluid that aids in the nourishment of the sperm • *Cowper's glands:* produce fluid that empties into the urethra and acts as a lubricant for the urethra and neutralizer for urine.
14.3 Understand chapter-specific ICD guidelines and format for the genitourinary system.	*ICD-9-CM:* Diseases of the Genitourinary System (urinary system and male reproductive systems) is Chapter 10 of the ICD-9-CM manual, with the code range 580–608. *ICD-10-CM:* Diseases of the Genitourinary System (urinary system and male reproductive systems) is Chapter 14 of the ICD-10-CM manual, with the code range N00–N51.
14.4 Identify the CPT guidelines and format for the urinary system.	General guidelines for the Urinary System subsection of CPT: • Insertion of a urinary bladder catheter is part of the global surgical package. • Placement of a catheter for postoperative drainage is not reported separately. • Cystourethroscopy with one or more biopsies includes all biopsies performed during the procedure. • Irrigation or drainage procedures integral to the primary procedure are not reported separately. • When an endoscopic procedure is performed as part of an open procedure, only the open procedure is coded. (E.g., the endoscopic procedure is confirmatory or is used to evaluate the surgical field.) • A surgical endoscopic or laparoscopic procedure includes the diagnostic procedure. • When multiple endoscopic approaches are attempted during the same procedure, only the completed approach is coded.
14.5 Identify the CPT guidelines and format for the male reproductive system.	General guidelines for the Male Reproductive System subsection of CPT: • Placement of a catheter for postoperative drainage is not reported separately. • Irrigation or drainage procedures integral to the primary procedure are not reported separately. • A surgical laparoscopic procedure includes the diagnostic procedure. • Exploration of the surgical field is not reported separately.

Learning Outcome	Key Concepts/Examples
14.6 Apply the modifiers most commonly used with codes for the genitourinary system.	Modifiers are used in the Genitourinary subsection to continue or modify the story of the patient's encounter. Some of the more common modifiers used in this subsection are: • Bilateral services, 50 • Multiple procedures, 51 • Staged or related procedure or service by the same physician or other qualified healthcare provider during the postoperative period, 58 • Distinct procedural service, 59 • Unplanned return to the operating/procedure room by the same physician or other qualified healthcare professional following the initial procedure for a related procedure during the postoperative period, 78
14.7 Examine the common medical and procedural terms used in operative reports.	*Acute renal failure (ARF):* the sudden onset of kidney failure from causes such as accidents that injure the kidneys, the loss of a lot of blood, or some drugs or poisons *Chronic kidney disease (CKD):* the gradual reduction of kidney function, which may lead to permanent kidney failure or end-stage renal disease (ESRD) *Nephrolithiasis:* a condition of stones, or calculi, in the kidney *TURP:* transurethral resection of the prostate *Vasectomy:* male sterilization

Chapter Fourteen Review

Understanding Terminology

Match each key term to the appropriate definition.

_____ 1. **[LO14.7]** BPH

_____ 2. **[LO14.2]** Cowper's glands

_____ 3. **[LO14.2]** Epididymis

_____ 4. **[LO14.1]** Erythropoiesis

_____ 5. **[LO14.1]** Glomerulus

_____ 6. **[LO14.2]** Reproductive system

_____ 7. **[LO14.7]** Micturition

_____ 8. **[LO14.1]** Nephrons

_____ 9. **[LO14.2]** Prepuce

_____10. **[LO14.2]** Testes

_____11. **[LO14.1]** Ureters

_____12. **[LO14.1]** Urethra

_____13. **[LO14.1]** Urinary system

_____14. **[LO14.2]** Vas deferens

A. Kidneys, ureters, urinary bladder, and urethra

B. Kidney cells whose function is to filter blood and form urine

C. System whose functions include production of male hormones and production and transportation of sperm

D. Urination

E. Structure into which urine flows from the urinary bladder and then to the outside of the body

F. Structure through which blood passes as it enters the kidney and which filters the blood, removing water and waste products

G. Enlargement of the prostate gland, which can interfere with urinary function

H. Long, coiled tube located on the back of the testicle

I. Production of red blood cells

J. Transports urine from the kidney to the urinary bladder

K. Also called *bulbourethral glands*

L. The foreskin that surrounds and protects the head of the penis

M. Oval organs located in the scrotum, secured by the spermatic cord

N. Tube from the epididymis to the pelvic cavity

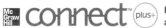

Enhance your learning by completing these exercises and more at mcgrawhillconnect.com

Checking Your Understanding

Choose the most appropriate answer for each of the following questions.

1. **[LO14.3, 14.5]** A 1-year-old boy has a midshaft hypospadias with a very mild degree of chordee. He also has a persistent right hydrocele. The surgeon brought the boy to the operating room to perform a right hydrocele repair and one-stage repair of the hypospadias with a preputial onlay flap. Select the appropriate CPT and ICD-9-CM codes:

   a. 54322, 55040, 752.62, 752.63

   b. 54322, 55041-51, 752.61, 752.63, 603.9

   c. 54324, 55060-51, 752.61, 752.63, 603.9

   d. 54324, 55060, 752.63, 603.9

2. **[LO14.3, 14.4]** An acute or chronic inflammation that is located in the glomeruli of the kidney is called:

   a. Nephritis   c. Nephrosis

   b. Bright's disease   d. Pyelitis

3. **[LO14.3]** A 31-year-old male presents with chronic glomerulonephritis due to type 2 diabetes. Select the appropriate ICD-9-CM codes:

   a. 583.81, 250.41   c. 250.40, 582.81

   b. 250.40, 250.00, 582.81   d. 250.40, 582.9

4. **[LO14.3]** A 63-year-old female with chronic kidney disease, stage V, presents for kidney dialysis. Select the appropriate ICD-9-CM codes:

   a. V56.8, 585.9   c. V56.0, 585.5

   b. V56.0, 585.9   d. 585.5, V56.0

5. **[LO14.6]** An elderly gentleman has worsening bilateral hydronephrosis. He did not have much of a postvoid residual on a bladder scan. The physician performed a bilateral cystoscopy and retrograde pyeloram. The results came back as gross prostatic hyperplasia. Select the appropriate CPT and ICD-9-CM codes:

   a. 52005, 600.3   c. 52005-50, 600.91, 591

   b. 52000, 591, 600.9   d. 52000-50, 591, 600.9

6. **[LO14.7]** Kidney stones are also called:

   a. Cholelithiasis   c. Nephrolithiasis

   b. Renal calculi   d. Both renal calculi and nephrolithiasis

7. **[LO14.1]** A capillary tuft that performs the first step in filtering blood to form urine is called the:

   a. Medulla   c. Ureter

   b. Cortex   d. Glomerulus

8. **[LO14.3, 14.5]**

   Procedure: Meatotomy infant

   Diagnosis: Congenital meatal stenosis

   Operative note: The patient was taken to the operating room and was placed in the supine position on the operating table. A general inhalation anesthesia was administered. The patient was prepped and draped in the usual sterile fashion. The urethral meatus was calibrated with a small mosquito hemostat and was gently dilated. Next, a midline ventral-type incision was made, opening the meatus. This was done after clamping the tissue to control bleeding. The meatus was opened to about 3 mm. Next, the meatus was easily calibrated from 8 to 12 French with bougis sounds. Next, the mucosal edges were everted and reapproximated to the glans skin edges with approximately five interrupted 6-0 Vicryl sutures. The meatus still calibrated between 10 and 12 French. Antibiotic ointment was applied. The procedure was terminated. The patient was awakened and returned to the recovery room in stable condition.

Select the appropriate CPT and ICD-9-CM codes:

a. 53025, 598.9   **c.** 53025, 753.29

b. 53020-63, 753.29   **d.** 53025-63, 598.9

9. **[LO14.3]** The patient was diagnosed with cystitis due to *Escherichia coli.* Choose the appropriate ICD-9-CM codes:

a. 595.9   **c.** 595.9, 041.49

b. 595.89, 041.49   **d.** 595.4, 041.49

10. **[LO14.5]** A nephrolithotomy after ESWL for staghorn calculus would be coded with which of the following ICD-9-CM and CPT codes?

a. 50075, 50590, 592.0   **c.** 50060, 50590, 592.0

b. 50590, 50075, 592.0   **d.** 50075, 592.0

Applying Your Knowledge

Answer the following questions and code the following case study. Be sure to follow the process steps as illustrated in Chapter 8

Case Studies [LO 14.1–14.7] Case 1

Preoperative diagnosis: Spontaneous rupture of the bladder

Postoperative diagnosis: Same

Procedure: Repair of bladder tear

Indications for procedure: 2.7-cm tear of the bladder dome. During surgical inspection no other injuries were found.

    The patient was prepped and draped in the usual fashion. A Pfannenstiel incision was made at a previous cesarean section scar. Inspection of the bladder showed no other injury. The tear was a 2.7-cm transverse tear in the dome of the bladder.

    A two-layer closure was done of the mucosa using 4-0 continuous Vicryl. The muscularis was closed using interrupted 2-0 Vicryl. Postrepair inspection revealed good hemostasis. No other tears were noted. Minimal blood loss was noted.

Process 1: CPT

1. What is the procedure?

2. Locate the main term in the index.

3. What additional questions or set of questions can be determined?

4. Upon review of all the code choices identified in the index, what additional questions can be determined?

5. Based on the documentation, what is the correct code for this case?

a. 51860   **c.** 51865

b. 51880   **d.** 51940

Process 2: ICD
ICD-9-CM

1. Based on the operative report header, what is the preoperative diagnosis?

2. Is the postoperative diagnosis the same as or different from the preoperative diagnosis?

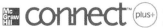

3. Is the postoperative diagnosis supported?

4. What is the main term for this condition?

5. Based on the subterm choices, what question(s) can be developed for this condition?

6. Is any sign, symptom, or additional condition documented?

7. Is the additional condition, sign, or symptom an integral part of the primary (or other) condition coded?

8. Does the additional condition require or affect patient care, treatment, or management?

9. Based on the documentation, what is the correct ICD-9-CM code for this case?
   a. 639.2
   b. 596.6
   c. 596.7
   d. 596.89

ICD-10-CM

1. Based on the operative report header, what is the preoperative diagnosis?

2. Is the postoperative diagnosis the same as or different from the preoperative diagnosis?

3. Is the postoperative diagnosis supported?

4. What is the main term for this condition?

5. Based on the subterm choices, what question(s) can be developed for this condition?

6. Based on the information in the Tabular List, is additional information needed to determine the appropriate diagnosis code?

7. Is any sign, symptom, or additional condition documented?

8. Is the additional condition, sign, or symptom an integral part of the primary (or other) condition coded?

9. Does the additional condition require or affect patient care, treatment, or management?

10. Based on the documentation, what is the correct ICD-10-CM code for this case?
    a. N33   c. N32.89
    b. N32.9   d. N32.81

Process 3: Modifiers

1. Was the procedure performed different from that described by the nomenclature of the code?

2. Was the procedure performed at an anatomical site that has laterality?

3. Was the procedure performed in the global period of another procedure?

4. Were additional procedures performed during the operative session, and does the documentation support them?

5. Did the surgeon have help from another surgeon or another appropriate person?

6. Did a physician different from the surgeon provide the preoperative or postoperative portion of the procedure?

7. What modifier(s) should be appended to the CPT code for this case?
   a. 50   c. 62
   b. 58   d. None of these

[LO 14.1–14.7] Case 2

Procedure: Bilateral segmental vasectomy, transscrotal

Preoperative diagnosis: Elective vasectomy

Postoperative diagnosis: Same

Indications: This 32-year-old father of three requested sterilization via vasectomy.

Anesthesia: Local with 1 percent Xylocaine infiltration

Procedure: The patient was placed in the supine position, prepped, and draped in routine fashion for a scrotal procedure. The right vas deferens was identified and isolated adjacent to the scrotal skin. Local anesthesia was obtained using infiltration of 1 percent Xylocaine without epinephrine.

An incision was made overlying the vas deferens. The vas deferens was identified and delivered to the operative field. A 2.1-cm segment of the vas deferens was then excised between hemostats. The ends of the vasa were then cauterized with Bovie electrocautery. The distal end was suture-ligated and folded back upon itself with 3-0 chromic. The proximal end was suture-ligated. Hemostasis was obtained using a suture of 3-0 chromic. The distal end was then buried in the surrounding adventitia with a figure-of-eight suture of 3-0 chromic. Next, attention was directed to the left side, and the procedure was repeated.

After confirming adequate hemostasis, the vasa deferentia were returned to the normal locations within the scrotum. The skin was closed using interrupted sutures of 3-0 chromic. After confirming adequate hemostasis, the patient was returned to the recovery room in good condition.

No complications were noted, with minimal blood loss.

CHAPTER FOURTEEN REVIEW

Answer the following questions, and code the case above. Be sure to follow the process steps as illustrated in Chapter 8.

Process 1: CPT

1. What is the procedure?

2. Locate the main term in the index.

3. What additional questions or set of questions can be determined?

4. Upon review of all the code choices identified in the index, what additional questions can be determined?

5. Based on the documentation, what is the correct code for this case?

   a. 55200

   b. 55300

   c. 55450

   d. 55250

Process 2: ICD

ICD-9-CM

1. Based on the operative report header, what is the preoperative diagnosis?

2. Is the postoperative diagnosis the same as or different from the preoperative diagnosis?

3. Is the postoperative diagnosis supported?

4. What is the main term for this condition?

5. Based on the subterm choices, what question(s) can be developed for this condition?

6. Is any sign, symptom, or additional condition documented?

7. Is the additional condition, sign, or symptom an integral part of the primary (or other) condition coded?

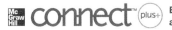 **Enhance your learning** by completing these exercises and more at mcgrawhillconnect.com

8. Does the additional condition require or affect patient care, treatment, or management?

9. Based on the documentation, what is the correct ICD-9-CM code for this case?

    a. V26.51   **c.** V26.52

    b. V26.21   **d.** V26.82

ICD-10-CM

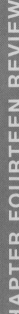

1. Based on the operative report header, what is the preoperative diagnosis?

2. Is the postoperative diagnosis the same as or different from the preoperative diagnosis?

3. Is the postoperative diagnosis supported?

4. What is the main term for this condition?

5. Based on the subterm choices, what question(s) can be developed for this condition?

6. Based on the information in the Tabular List, is additional information needed to determine the appropriate diagnosis code?

7. Is any sign, symptom, or additional condition documented?

8. Is the additional condition, sign, or symptom an integral part of the primary (or other) condition coded?

9. Does the additional condition require or affect patient care, treatment, or management?

10. Based on the documentation, what is the correct ICD-10-CM code for this case?

    a. Z98.52   **c.** Z30.2

    b. Z98.51   **d.** Z30.8

Process 3: Modifiers

1. Was the procedure performed different from that described by the nomenclature of the code?

2. Was the procedure performed on an anatomical site that has laterality?

3. Was the procedure performed in the global period of another procedure?

4. Were additional procedures performed during the operative session, and does the documentation support them?

5. Did the surgeon have help from another surgeon or another appropriate person?

6. Did a physician different from the surgeon provide the preoperative or postoperative portion of the procedure?

7. What modifier(s) should be appended to the CPT code for this case?

    a. 50   **c.** 51

    b. 58   **d.** None of these

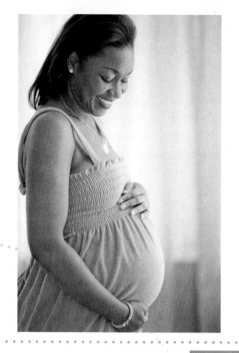

Surgery Section: Female Reproductive System and Maternity Care and Delivery

Key Terms

Amenorrhea	Colposcopy	Labia majora	Peripartum
Antepartum	Corpus uteri	Labia minora	Postpartum
Bartholin's glands	Dystocia	Myometrium	Puerperium
Cerclage	Endometrium	Ovary	Vagina
Cervix uteri	Fimbriae	Oviduct	Vulva

Learning Outcomes

After completing this chapter, you will be able to:

15.1 Review the anatomy of the female reproductive system.

15.2 Understand chapter-specific ICD guidelines and format for complications of pregnancy, childbirth, and the puerperium.

15.3 Identify the guidelines and format of the Female Genital System and Maternity Care and Delivery subsections of CPT.

15.4 Apply the modifiers most commonly used with codes in the Female Genital System and Maternity Care and Delivery subsections.

15.5 Examine the common medical and procedural terms used in operative reports.

Introduction
The primary function of the female genital system is reproduction. Its functions include production of female egg cells (oocytes), transportation of the oocytes to the uterus for implantation, and production of estrogen and progesterone. An associated and secondary function is to enable sperm to enter the body for reproduction.

15.1 Anatomy of the Female Genital System

The female reproductive system includes both internal and external organs and structures (see Figures 15.1 and 15.2 and Table 15.1). The internal organs and tissue include the vagina, uterus, ovaries, and fallopian tubes, including the fimbriae of each. The external structures include the vulva, labia majora, labia minora, Bartholin's glands, and clitoris.

Flow of the Female Reproductive System (Path of the Oocyte)

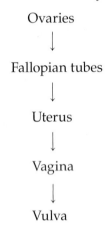

Ovaries

↓

Fallopian tubes

↓

Uterus

↓

Vagina

↓

Vulva

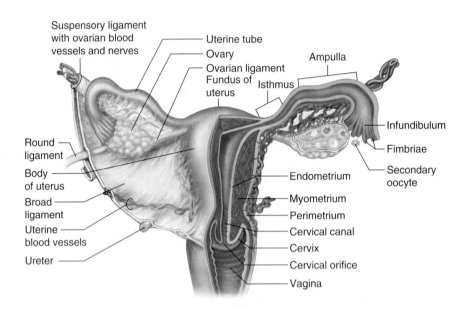

Figure 15.1 Anatomy of Female Reproductive System

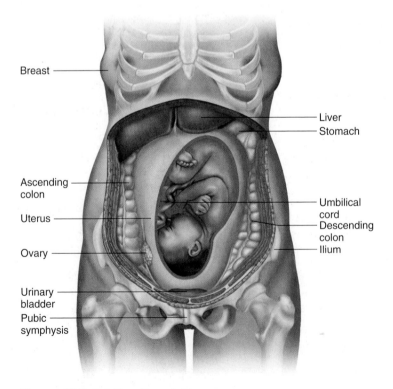

Figure 15.2 Full-Term Fetus in Uterus

Table 15.1 Structures of Female Reproductive System

STRUCTURE	DEFINITION/FUNCTION
Ovaries	Small oval-shaped glands. Functions are production of the oocyte and ovum, and production of the female hormones, estrogen and progesterone.
Fallopian tubes	Also known as **oviducts.** Primary function is transportation of the oocyte. Conception normally occurs within one or both of these tubes: • *Fimbriae:* Fingerlike structures at the end of each tube that capture and sweep the egg into the tube. • *Cilia:* Hairlike projections within each tube that aid in the movement of the egg through the tube.
Uterus: **Corpus uteri**	Main body of the uterus. Functions are to nourish and protect a developing fetus. Consists of three layers: • *Endometrium:* innermost layer; functions as a lining and prevents adhesions between the opposite walls of the uterus. During pregnancy, it forms the placenta. • *Myometrium:* smooth muscle that forms the wall of the uterus. Functions are to expel the fetus and placenta and reduce blood loss during labor and delivery. • *Perimetrium:* outermost layer; covers the fundus (top) ventral and dorsal aspects.
Cervix uteri	Also called *neck of the uterus.* Lower, narrow part of the uterus where it joins with the vagina. Consists of three main portions: • *Endocervical canal:* passageway between the uterine cavity and external os that terminates at the internal os. • *Portio vaginalis:* portion projecting into the vagina (also called *exocervix*). • *External os:* opening in the portio vaginalis that dilates during labor.
Vagina	Hollow muscular tube extending from the cervix to the labia. Its functions are to receive sperm during intercourse and provide a passageway for birth and for expulsion of the intrauterine tissue during menstruation.
Vulva	Also known as *pudendum.* External genitalia. Its functions are to protect the internal reproductive organs from infectious organisms and to enable sperm to enter the body. Consists of three main parts: • *Labia majora:* outermost structure; contains sweat- and oil-secreting glands. • *Labia minora:* inside the labia majora; contains the vaginal and urethral openings and the clitoris. • *Clitoris:* small, sensitive protrusion located at the upper ends of the labia minor.
Bartholin's glands	Located next to the vaginal opening. Their function is to produce mucous secretions.

ovary Small oval-shaped gland that produces the oocyte, ovum, and female hormones.

oviduct Also known as fallopian tubes. Primary function is transportation of the oocyte.

fimbriae Fingerlike structures at the end of each fallopian tube that capture and sweep the egg into the tube.

corpus uteri The main body of the uterus; function is to protect a developing fetus.

endometrium Innermost layer of the uterus; functions as a lining.

myometrium Smooth muscle that forms the wall of the uterus; functions to expel the fetus and placenta and reduce blood loss during labor and delivery.

cervix uteri The lower, narrow part of the uterus where it joins with the vagina. Also called *neck of the uterus.*

vagina Hollow muscular tube extending from the cervix to the labia; functions are to receive sperm and provide a passageway for births.

vulva Female external genitalia that protects internal reproductive organs and enables sperm to enter the body.

labia majora Outermost structure of the vulva; contains sweat- and oil-secreting glands.

labia minora Structure that lies inside the labia majora; contains the vaginal and urethral openings and the clitoris.

Bartholin's glands Glands that are located next to the vaginal opening; function is to produce mucous secretions.

1. What are the primary functions of the ovaries?
2. The portion of the cervix that projects into the vagina is known as the _____.
3. What is the myometrium?
4. Name the parts of the pudendum.
5. The lowest, narrow part of the uterus where it joins with the vagina is known as the _____.

Also available in Mc Graw Hill **connect** (plus+)

15.2 ICD Chapter-Specific Guidelines and Format for the Female Reproductive System and Complications of Pregnancy, Childbirth, and the Puerperium

Some common diseases coded to these chapters of ICD are endometriosis, uterine prolapse, menstrual disorders, infertility, and pregnancy and pregnancy-related disorders and complications. When coding these conditions, coders must thoroughly review the provider documentation as well as the guidelines and instructional notes.

ICD-9-CM: The Female Reproductive subsection is found in Chapter 10 of the ICD-9-CM manual, with the code range 614–629.9.

ICD-9-CM: Complications of Pregnancy, Childbirth, and the Puerperium is Chapter 11 of the ICD-9-CM manual, with the code range 630–679

ICD-10-CM: The Female Reproductive subsection is found in Chapter 14 of the ICD-10-CM manual, with the code range N70–N99.89.

ICD-10-CM: Pregnancy, Childbirth, and the Puerperium subsection is found in Chapter 15 of the ICD-10-CM manual, with the code range O00–O9A.23-

Tables 15.2 and 15.3 list the relevant chapter subheadings and their code ranges.

Table 15.2 Female Reproductive System Subsection Format *(Data from ICD-9-CM and ICD-10-CM, Centers for Medicare and Medicaid Services and the National Center for Health Statistics.)*

ICD-9-CM		ICD-10-CM	
SUBHEADING	CODE RANGE	SUBHEADING	CODE RANGE
Inflammatory Disease of Female Pelvic Organs	614–616	Inflammatory Disease of Female Pelvic Organs	N70–N77
Other Disorders of Female Genital Tract	617–629	Noninflammatory Disease of Female Genital Tract	N80–N98
		Intraoperative Postprocedural Complications and Disorders of Genitourinary System, Not Elsewhere Classified	N99

Table 15.3 Complications of Pregnancy, Childbirth, and the Puerperium Subsection Format *(Data from ICD-9-CM and ICD-10-CM, Centers for Medicare and Medicaid Services and the National Center for Health Statistics.)*

ICD-9-CM		ICD-10-CM	
SUBHEADING	CODE RANGE	SUBHEADING	CODE RANGE
Ectopic and Molar Pregnancy	630–633	Pregnancy with Abortive Outcome	O00–O08
Other Pregnancy with Abortive Outcome	634–639		
Complications Mainly Related to Pregnancy	640–649	Supervision of High-Risk Pregnancy	O09
		Edema, Proteinuria, and Hypertensive Disorders in Pregnancy, Childbirth, and the Puerperium	O10–O16
		Other Maternal Disorders Predominantly Related to Pregnancy	O20–O29
Normal Delivery and Other Indications for Care in Pregnancy, Labor, and Delivery	650–659	Maternal Care Related to the Fetus and Amniotic Cavity and Possible Delivery Problems	O30–O48
		Encounter for Delivery	O80–O82
Complications Occurring Mainly in the Course of Labor and Delivery	660–669	Complications of Labor and Delivery	O60–O77
Complications of the Puerperium	670–677	Complications Predominantly Related to the Puerperium	O85–O92
Other Maternal and Fetal Complications	678–679	Other Obstetric Conditions, Not Elsewhere Classified	O94–O9A

Inflammatory Disease of Female Pelvic Organs (614–616), ICD-9-CM

Inflammatory Disease of Female Pelvic Organs (N70–N77), ICD-10-CM

These sections contain codes to be reported for conditions such as salpingitis and oophoritis, peritoneal adhesions, endometritis, intrauterine infections, vaginitis, and cyst or abscess of a Bartholin's gland. The codes for these conditions are divided based on the anatomical site of the condition and on the status of the condition as chronic or acute.

Also included in these sections is acute myometritis of the uterus, 615.0 (ICD-9-CM, inflammatory disease of uterus, acute) or N71.0 (ICD-10-CM, acute inflammatory disease of uterus).

SPOTLIGHT on a Guideline

When coding for several of these conditions, coders must use additional codes to identify infectious organisms, associated infertility, associated or underlying conditions, or external causes.

Other Disorders of Female Genital Tract (617–629), ICD-9-CM

Noninflammatory Disease of Female Pelvic Organs (N80–N98), ICD-10-CM

These sections contain codes to be reported for conditions such as endometriosis, genital prolapse, and disorders of the ovaries, fallopian tubes, uterus, cervix, vagina, or vulva. Also located in these sections are codes for menstruation disorders, including menopause, pain associated with the female genital organs, and female infertility.

The codes in these sections are first grouped by condition and then divided by anatomical site.

Stricture and stenosis of cervix, 622.4 (ICD-9-CM)

Stricture and stenosis of cervix uteri, N88.2 (ICD-10-CM)

Stricture and atresia of vagina, 623.2 (ICD-9-CM)

Stricture and atresia of vagina, N89.5 (ICD-10-CM) ▪

SPOTLIGHT on Condition

Menopause has four stages:

Premenopause Early beginning of menopause, marked by shorter or longer periods but no other classic menopausal symptoms.

Perimenopause Marked by irregular periods, hot flashes, vaginal dryness, and reduction of estrogen.

Menopause Begins with the woman's final period and lack of a menstrual period, for 1 year.

Postmenopause Begins after the woman has been without a period for at least 1 year.

Complications of Pregnancy, Childbirth, and the Puerperium (630–679), ICD-9-CM

Pregnancy, Childbirth, and the Puerperium (O00–O9A), ICD-10-CM

Chapter 11 is used to report conditions, disorders, diseases, and complications that take place during pregnancy, childbirth, and the postpartum period, or 6 weeks after delivery.

The ICD-9-CM guidelines for Chapter 11, Complications of Pregnancy, Childbirth, and the Puerperium, provide direction and guidance regarding sequencing of pregnancy as well as non-pregnancy-related conditions, appropriate use of the normal-delivery code, and a description of the postpartum and peripartum periods.

Several of the guidelines for this chapter focus on specific conditions or complications of pregnancy. Two of the guidelines encompass all codes from this chapter. First, codes from Chapter 11 take sequencing priority over codes from all other chapters. This means that when a patient is receiving care for a condition, disease, or disorder related to pregnancy, birth, or the postpartum period (6 weeks following delivery), the condition and first-listed code are selected from this chapter. Additional codes may be needed from other chapters to further define the condition.

MENTOR
Coding Tip

The descriptions of *postpartum* and *peripartum* periods are located in Section 1,C 11,I,1 of the ICD-9-CM Official Coding Guidelines. Highlighting the description of these terms allows the coder to quickly locate this information when using codes from this chapter.

FOR EXAMPLE 30-week pregnancy complicated by morbid obesity due to excessive caloric intake.

The first code describes the complication: obesity complicating pregnancy, childbirth, or the puerperium, 649.13 (ICD-9-CM) or O99.21 (ICD-10-CM).

The second code further describes the obesity: morbid obesity, 278.01 (ICD-9-CM) or E66.01 (ICD-10-CM). ▪

The second general chapter guideline explains that codes from Chapter 11 are only reported on the maternal, or mother's, record and never on the newborn's record.

There are many different terms used to describe the stages of pregnancy. Providers may use any of the terms listed below, and conditions may be classified according to these terms:

Trimesters

First: Less than 14 weeks

Second: 14 weeks to 28 weeks

Third: 28 weeks to delivery

Early pregnancy Less than 22 weeks' gestation.

Antepartum Prenatal period beginning with conception and ending at the time of delivery.

Peripartum Period beginning 30 days prior to delivery and extending to 5 months after delivery.

Puerperium Period beginning with delivery of the placenta and extending to 6 weeks after delivery.

Postpartum 6 weeks following delivery.

antepartum The period beginning with conception and ending at the time of delivery.

peripartum The period that begins 30 days prior to delivery and extends to 5 months after delivery.

puerperium The period that begins with the delivery of the placenta and extends through 6 weeks after delivery.

postpartum The period of 6 weeks following delivery.

Many of the codes in this chapter require an additional digit to indicate the current episode of care in which the condition is diagnosed, treated, or managed. In ICD-9-CM, the episode of care is identified by the fifth digit:

0 Unspecified episode of care or the episode is not applicable to the care.

1 Delivery episode of care, with or without documentation of an antepartum condition.

2 Delivery episode of care with documentation of a postpartum condition that develops while the patient is still in the hospital from the delivery.

3 Antepartum condition or complication, no delivery during this episode of care.

4 Postpartum condition or complication that develops after the mother has been discharged from the hospital after delivery.

A fifth digit of 2 equates to "while patient is still in the hospital from the delivery and there is documentation of a *postpartum* complication during the stay."

Review Figure 15.3 which provides a visual representation of these fifth digit guidelines.

Understanding the episodes of care is particularly important when coding from this chapter as many of the guidelines use this concept to identify appropriate sequencing and use of multiple codes.

When multiple codes from ICD-9-CM ranges 630–648 and 651–676 are required to completely code a single episode of care, the fifth digit of each code should match.

FOR EXAMPLE

The normal-delivery code is appropriate when a complication of the pregnancy was addressed and resolved during an episode of care prior to the episode of care for delivery.

When the episode of care for pregnancy during an admission does not end in delivery, the first-listed diagnosis should be the condition that led to the admission.

If delivery occurs prior to admission and the mother is admitted for postpartum care without complication, code V24.0, postpartum care and examination immediately after delivery (Z39.0, ICD-10-CM), is assigned. ▪

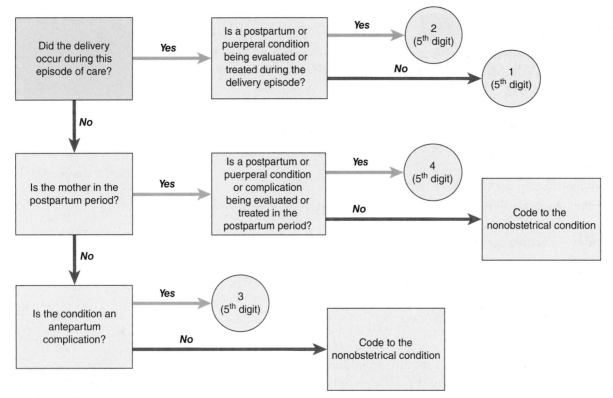

Figure 15-3 Episode of care, fifth-digit decision tree

Ectopic and Molar Pregnancy (630–633), ICD-9-CM
Pregnancy with Abortive Outcome (O00–O08), ICD-10-CM

Codes in these sections include conditions that are the result of abnormal products of conception (630–631.8), missed abortion (632), or conception in abnormal anatomical sites, ectopic pregnancy (633.00–633.91). The codes for ectopic pregnancy are divided by the anatomical site of the pregnancy and by whether the condition was with or without intrauterine pregnancy.

Ectopic pregnancy sites may be:

- Abdominal, 633.0-, ICD-9-CM; O00.0, ICD-10-CM (The ovum implants in the peritoneal cavity.)
- Tubal, 633.1-, ICD-9-CM; O00.1, ICD-10-CM (The ovum implants in a fallopian tube and may cause rupture of the tube.)
- Ovarian, 633.2-, ICD-9-CM; O00.2, ICD-10-CM (The ovum implants on an ovary.)
- Other ectopic, 633.8-, ICD-9-CM; O00.8, ICD-10-CM [The ovum implants on the cervix, uterine horn (cornual), or muscle of the uterus (mesometric).]

Other Pregnancy with Abortive Outcome (634–639), ICD-9-CM

Pregnancy with Abortive Outcome (O00–O08), ICD-10-CM

Codes in these sections report complications associated with abortion. The codes are divided by the nature of the abortion:

- Spontaneous, also known as a *miscarriage*, 634.0- to 634.9, ICD-9-CM; O03.0–O03.9, ICD-10-CM
- Legally induced, 635.0x–635.9, ICD-9-CM; no ICD-10-CM equivalent

- Illegally induced, 636.0x–636.9, ICD-9-CM; no ICD-10-CM equivalent
  - Induced (O04.5–O04.89, ICD-10-CM *(ICD-10-CM does not classify induced abortions as legal or illegal.)*
- Unspecified, 637.0- to 637.9, ICD-9-CM; no ICD-10-CM equivalent
- Failed attempted, 638.0–638.9, ICD-9-CM; O07.0–O07.4, ICD-10-CM
- Ectopic and molar, O08.0–O08.9, ICD-10-CM

The fourth digit of these codes further defines the condition by its associated complication(s): infection, hemorrhage, damage to organs and/or tissue, renal failure, metabolic disorder, shock, embolism, and other or unspecified complications.

When required, the fifth digit of the ICD-9-CM code further defines the abortion as incomplete (1), complete (2), or unspecified in the documentation as a complete abortion (0). An incomplete abortion is one in which all of the products of conception have not been removed or expelled from the uterus.

Codes from category 639, ICD-9-CM (O08, ICD-10-CM), "Complications following abortion and ectopic and molar pregnancy," are used to report conditions that are the result of or due to the abortion, either immediately following the abortion or leading to a subsequent encounter for treatment.

Should an attempted abortion result in the birth of a live-born fetus, do not use a code from this section. Code the birth as early onset of delivery (644.21). An additional code to identify the outcome of the delivery is also needed to provide the complete diagnostic story.

MENTOR Coding Tip

As with other chapters of the ICD further clarification or breakdown of the fourth or fifth digit can be found at the beginning of the section. Coders should make it a habit to return to the beginning of each section or chapter to locate this information to aid in correct coding of the condition.

Complications Mainly Related to Pregnancy (640–649), ICD-9-CM
Supervision of High-Risk Pregnancy (O09), ICD-10-CM
Edema, Proteinuria, and Hypertensive Disorders in Pregnancy, Childbirth, and the Puerperium (O10–O16), ICD-10-CM
Other Maternal Disorders Predominantly Related to Pregnancy (O20–O29), ICD-10-CM

The codes in this code range identify complications related to or due to the pregnancy and include complications that develop during labor, delivery, or the puerperium.

The conditions identified by these codes are categorized first by the condition complicating the pregnancy. Additional specificity for each of these conditions is provided at the subclassification level. Conditions include hemorrhage, hypertension, excessive vomiting, early or threatened labor, late pregnancy, infections and parasitic disease, and other conditions in the mother that complicate the pregnancy.

Included in these sections are the codes for gestational diabetes (abnormal glucose tolerance, 648.8-, ICD-9-CM; O24.429, ICD-10-CM) and diabetes mellitus complicating pregnancy (648.0-, ICD-9-CM; O24.32, ICD-10-CM). Diabetes mellitus complicating pregnancy (648.0-) is used to indicate that the mother had diabetes prior to the pregnancy. An additional code from category 250 is needed to identify the type of diabetes. Gestational diabetes (648.8-) arises during and due to the pregnancy and may or may not continue after the pregnancy.

In either of these conditions, if the mother manages her diabetes with the use of insulin, an additional code is needed: associated long-term (current) insulin use, V58.67 (Z79.4, ICD-10-CM). However, do not list V58.67 if the preexisting diabetes was type 1 diabetes mellitus.

Normal Delivery and Other Indications for Care in Pregnancy, Labor, and Delivery (650–659), ICD-9-CM
Maternal Care Related to the Fetus and Amniotic Cavity and Possible Delivery Problems (O30–O48), ICD-10-CM
Encounter for Delivery (O80–O82), ICD-10-CM

The codes in these sections identify conditions that may complicate labor and delivery. Also included in this code range is the code for a normal uneventful delivery. Most of the codes from these sections are only used for the episode of care resulting in delivery.

Normal Delivery: 650, ICD-9-CM; O80, ICD-10-CM

ICD defines a normal delivery as one that requires no additional intervention or treatment during the delivery and meets the following criteria:

- Full term.
- Single, live-born infant.
- Spontaneous labor and delivery.
- Head-first presentation (cephalic).
- Vaginal delivery.
- No rotation or manipulation of the baby due to fetal position or presentation.

Normal delivery may be preceded by induction of labor; however, the delivery must meet the criteria above. Normal delivery (650 or O80) should not be listed if any other code for a complication of the prenatal, delivery, or perinatal period from this chapter is needed to fully describe and code the delivery episode of care.

As with all delivery codes, an additional code is needed to identify the outcome of delivery on the mother's medical record (V27.0–V27.9, ICD-9-CM; Z37.0–Z37.9, ICD-10-CM).

MENTOR
Coding Tip

The bracketed numbers below each code identify the appropriate fifth digit for each code. The numbers 0, 1, and 3 are used only during the delivery episode.

FOR EXAMPLE For vaginal delivery with cephalic presentation of a single male infant without antepartum or postpartum complications, the codes are:

Normal delivery, 650, ICD-9-CM; O80, ICD-10-CM

Single live-born infant, V27.0, ICD-9-CM; Z37.0, ICD-10-CM

The code V27.0 (single live-born infant) is the only appropriate outcome-of-delivery code when code 650, normal delivery, is used to identify the episode of delivery.

ICD-9-CM categories 655 and 656 (O35 and O36, ICD-10-CM) describe conditions of the fetus that affect how the provider manages the pregnancy in the mother. This change in management may include diagnostic tests or studies, more frequent visits, additional observation, special care, and, if necessary, termination of the pregnancy. Do *not* use these codes if the fetal condition does not affect how the provider manages the pregnancy.

Included in these conditions is spina bifida (655.0-, ICD 9-CM; O35.0xx-, ICD-10-CM), which may lead to in utero surgery to correct the condition prior to delivery. When in utero surgery is performed and the coder is coding for treatment of the mother, do *not* list codes from the perinatal chapter to describe the fetal condition. Codes from the perinatal chapter are assigned only to the baby's record and should never be listed to describe a maternal condition.

Complications Occurring Mainly in the Course of Labor and Delivery (660–669), ICD-9-CM

Complications of Labor and Delivery (O60–O77), ICD-10-CM

These sections include:

- Physical conditions in the mother or fetal positions that may lead to obstructed labor, 660.-, ICD-9-CM; O64.- to O66.- , ICD-10-CM
- Inability of the uterine muscle to contract adequately during labor and delivery, 661.-, ICD-9-CM; O62.-, ICD-10-CM
- Abnormally long labor, 662.-, ICD-9-CM; O63.-, ICD-10-CM
- Malposition of umbilical cord leading to complications, 663.-, ICD-9-CM; O69.-, ICD-10-CM
- Injuries and trauma resulting from complications of labor and delivery, 664.- and 665.-, ICD-9-CM; O70.- and O71.-, ICD-10-CM
- Hemorrhage, with and without retained placenta, after delivery, 666.-, ICD-9-CM; O72.-, ICD-10-CM
- Retained placenta without hemorrhage, 667.-, ICD-9-CM; O73.-, ICD-10-CM
- Complications related to the use of an anesthetic or sedation during labor and delivery, 668.-, ICD-9-CM; O74.-, ICD-10-CM
- Other complications such as shock, low blood pressure (hypotension), acute kidney failure, and manual extractions, 669.-, ICD-9-CM; O75–O77.9, ICD-10-CM

The codes for labor and delivery injury and trauma are further divided based on anatomical site:

- Category 664, "Trauma to perineum and vulva during delivery," is further defined by the degree of the perineal laceration (O70, ICD-10-CM).
- Category 665, "Other obstetrical trauma," includes damage from instruments during labor and delivery. This category is divided by anatomical site, the episode of care, and the nature of the injury (O71, ICD-10-CM).

FOR EXAMPLE

Rupture of uterus before onset of labor, 665.0- , ICD-9-CM; O71.0-, ICD-10-CM

Rupture of uterus during labor, 665.1-, ICD-9-CM; O71.1, ICD-10-CM ■

SPOTLIGHT on a Guideline

Labor is divided into three stages:

Stage 1   From onset of labor to complete dilation and effacement of cervix.

Stage 2   From complete dilation to birth.

Stage 3   Directly following birth until the placenta is expelled.

In prolonged labor **(dystocia)** or labor that fails to progress, the total of these stages may last many hours to days.

Complications of the Puerperium (670–677), ICD-9-CM
Complications Predominantly Related to the Puerperium (O85–O92), ICD-10-CM

Conditions that arise during the postpartum period, beginning with delivery of the placenta, and are directly related to the delivery are included in these sections. However, many of the conditions listed in categories 671, ICD-9-CM (O87, ICD-10-CM) and 673, ICD-9-CM (O88, ICD-10-CM) to 676 may also occur during pregnancy, and these codes should be used to identify the condition when it occurs.

MENTOR Coding Tip

At the beginning of the complications of the puerperium section is an instructional note. Highlighting this note and each of the categories relating to the note provides coders with a visual cue for which codes of this section are appropriate for use during the antepartum period.

SPOTLIGHT
on Condition

Puerperal infection is a bacterial infection that follows delivery. The onset of symptoms begins with a fever at approximately 10 days after delivery, and if left untreated, the condition may lead to puerperal sepsis.

Conditions included in this section are:

- Major puerperal infections, 670.-, ICD-9-CM; O85–O86.-, ICD-10-CM
- Varicose veins, thrombophlebitis, phlebothrombosis, and other venous complications, 671.-, ICD-9-CM; O87.-, ICD-10-CM
- Postpartum fevers, 672, ICD-9-CM
- Pulmonary embolisms related to pregnancy, childbirth, or the puerperium, 673.-, ICD-9-CM; O88.-, ICD-10-CM
- Disruption or dehiscence of perineal or cesarean wounds, 674.-, ICD-9-CM; O90.-, ICD-10-CM
- Infections and disorders of the breast related to childbirth and lactation, 675.- and 676.-, ICD-9-CM; O91.- and O92.-, ICD-10-CM

As with coding sepsis in other chapters of ICD, multiple codes are needed to complete the diagnostic description of the condition. The first-listed code identifies the pregnancy-related condition, puerperal sepsis (670.2-, ICD-9-CM; O85, ICD-10-CM), followed by a code for the specific type of infection (041.-, ICD-9-CM; B95.- or B96.-, ICD-10-CM). As the primary code already describes the condition as sepsis, do *not* use an additional sepsis code from Chapter 1 of ICD. If organ failure is also present, use additional codes to identify severe sepsis and the associated organ dysfunction.

Also included in this section of ICD-9-CM is the code for late effect of complications of pregnancy, childbirth, and puerperium (677). To use this code, the documentation should clearly state that the current condition is the direct result of a complication that occurred during pregnancy, delivery, or the postpartum period. This code should be sequenced after the code that identifies the condition for which the patient is being seen.

Other Maternal and Fetal Complications (678–679), ICD-9-CM

Other Obstetric Conditions, Not Elsewhere Classified (O94–O9A), ICD-10-CM

The last section of this chapter includes complications for the mother (679.0-) or fetus (679.1-) due to an in utero procedure performed on the fetus during pregnancy. These codes are used to report only a complication of the in utero procedure and not a history of the procedure. To indicate a maternal history of an in utero procedure, the coder would report code V23.86, ICD-9-CM (O09.8-, ICD-10-CM) maternal history of in utero procedure during previous pregnancy.

Supervision of Normal Pregnancy (V22.0–V22.2), ICD-9-CM

Encounters for Supervision of Normal Pregnancy (Z34.00–Z34.93), ICD-10-CM

Supervision of High-Risk Pregnancy (V23.0–V23.9), ICD-9-CM

Supervision of High-Risk Pregnancy (O09.00–O09.93), ICD-10-CM

Routine prenatal visits are encounters with the provider when no complication of or due to the pregnancy is the primary reason for the encounter. The ICD codes for this service are categorized by the type of pregnancy: normal (V22.-, ICD-9-CM; Z34.-, ICD-10-CM) or high risk (V23.-, ICD-9-CM; O09.-, ICD-10-CM). Each of these categories is further defined by the number of pregnancies or type of risk.

EXERCISE 15.2

1. List and define the three stages of labor.
2. Which categories in ICD-9-CM and ICD-10-CM describe conditions of the fetus that affect how the provider manages the pregnancy in the mother?
3. Conditions coded in categories 614 to 616 (ICD-9-CM) and N70 to N77 (ICD-10-CM), which encompass inflammatory diseases of female pelvic organs, are further divided based on _____ and _____.
4. Define the time frame of each trimester.
5. Delivery occurred prior to admission, and the mother is admitted for postpartum care without any complications. Assign the appropriate ICD-9-CM codes.

Also available in ![McGraw-Hill] **connect** (plus+)

15.3 Guidelines and Format of the Female Genital System and Maternity Care and Delivery Subsections of CPT

The Female Genital System subsection of the CPT manual is formatted by anatomical site from the vulva to the ovaries and includes in vitro fertilization. The Maternity Care and Delivery subsection is formatted based on the episode and type of care or delivery.

There are several questions a coder needs to ask when reading an operative report and coding a procedure from this section. The following questions will help the coder, when reading through the report, to understand what actually was done and how the procedure should be translated and coded:

- At which anatomical site was the procedure performed?
- Was the treatment obstetrical or nonobstetrical?
- What approach was used, such as internal or external?
- What was the extent of the surgical procedure?
- Read the code description carefully to determine if the code describes a procedure done at a single site or multiple sites.

General Subsection Guidelines

Included in all gynecologic procedures are the following:

- Diagnostic pelvic examinations and routine evaluation of the surgical field.
- Vaginal or cervical dilation for procedures done by vaginal approach unless the CPT code states "without cervical dilation."
- Diagnostic scopes (laparoscopy, peritoneoscopy, colposcopy, and hysteroscopy) are included in the surgical scope procedure.
- Surgical laparoscopic procedures include lysis of adhesions.
- Anesthesia when performed by the surgeon.

Nonscope surgical procedures do not include diagnostic scopes. When a diagnostic scope leads to an open surgical procedure, list the codes for both the surgical and the diagnostic procedures and append modifier 58 to the diagnostic scope code.

Female Genital System Subsection Subheadings and Guidelines (56405–58999)

The subheadings and code ranges are listed in Table 15.4.

Table 15.4 Female Genital Subheadings and Code Ranges *(Data from CPT 2013. © 2013 American Medical Association. All rights reserved.)*

SUBHEADING	CODE RANGE
Vulva, Perineum, and Introitus	56405–56821
Vagina	57000–57426
Cervix Uteri	57452–57800
Corpus Uteri	58100–58579
Oviduct/Ovary	58600–58770
Ovary	58800–58960
In Vitro Fertilization	58970–58999

Vulva, Perineum, and Introitus (56405–56821)

Anatomical sites included under this subheading are the labia majora, labia minora, mons pubis, greater and lesser vestibular glands, bulb of the vestibule, vestibule of the vagina, vaginal orifice (vulva), the area located between the anus and the vulva (perineum), hymen, and Bartholin's glands.

Procedures included in this subheading are incision, destruction, excision, repair, and endoscopy.

Each of these categories is further divided by extent or method of the procedure.

FOR EXAMPLE The codes for excision (56620–56640) are defined by the extent of the vulva excised. Extent for these codes is defined as simple, radical, partial, or complete. ■

MENTOR Coding Tip

The definitions of each of these terms are listed at the beginning of this subheading. Highlight this guideline and the corresponding terms in each of the codes in range 56620–56640 to aid in selection of the correct code when coding for this procedure.

Vagina (57000–57426)

Procedures listed under this subheading include incision, destruction, excision, introduction, repair, manipulation, and endoscopy/laparoscopy.

Incision: 57000–57023

The incision category lists codes describing both colpotomy and colpocentesis procedures. Both of these procedures provide access to the space between the rectum and the uterus. In colpotomy, an incision is made in the posterior wall of the vagina behind the cervix to enter the posterior pelvic cavity. In colpocentesis, access to the posterior pelvic cavity is accomplished with a needle to aspirate fluid from this area.

Destruction: 57061–57065

CPT divides the codes for destruction of vaginal lesions by the terms *simple* (57061) and *extensive* (57065). Simple destruction is defined as a few smaller lesions that are simple to destroy. Extensive involves numerous large lesions that are difficult to destroy.

Excision: 57100–57135

Codes listed in the excision category are divided based on the extent of the vaginal wall removed. Vaginectomies may be partial (57106), or partial excision may be more extensive by including surrounding diseased or damaged tissue and some of the area lymph nodes (57107) or very extensive by removing the pelvic lymph nodes in addition to the surrounding diseased or damaged tissue (57109). Biopsies may also be performed of the aortic lymph nodes. Likewise, a total vaginectomy may involve complete excision of the vagina only (57110) or of the vagina and surrounding tissue and excision of lymph nodes (57111 or 57112).

Introduction: 57150–57180

Codes under this subheading include services and procedures for irrigation, insertion, and fitting of devices such as a pessary, diaphragm, cervical cap or radiation ovoids, tandems, and apparatus.

Repair: 57200–57335

Included in this range of codes is suturing of nonobstetrical vaginal injuries (57200–57210), plastic and other repairs of the urethral sphincter, cystoceles, or rectoceles (57220–57270).

Many of the remaining codes in this category are further defined by the different surgical approaches of each.

FOR EXAMPLE

Paravaginal defect repair; open abdominal approach, 57284

Paravaginal defect repair; vaginal approach, 57285 ■

All of the codes listed in the manipulation category (57400–57415) are reportable only when the procedure or service was performed under anesthesia. These codes include removal of a foreign body, vaginal dilation, and a pelvic exam and are reportable only when the procedure is performed in the absence of another procedure at the same anatomical site and surgical session.

The endoscopy/laparoscopy category (57420–57426) includes CPT codes for diagnostic and surgical scope procedures of the vagina. Inspection of the vagina, exposure and washing of the cervix, and, when needed to improve visualization, application of acetic acid to the columnar villi and any lesion are included in the scope procedures and not separately reportable.

Cervix Uteri (57425–57800)

This subheading lists diagnostic and therapeutic procedures performed on the cervix and upper adjacent vagina. There are only four categories included in this subheading: endoscopy, excision, repair and manipulation.

Endoscopy: 57452–57461

The endoscopy category lists colposcopic examinations and procedures including biopsies and curettage. The codes for biopsy of the cervix are divided based on the method of biopsy and whether the biopsy was done at the same time as endocervical curettage.

When the procedure is completed using a loop electrode to excise tissue from the cervix, either CPT code 57460 or 57461 is reported: Code 57460 identifies a procedure done to obtain one or more biopsies of the cervix, while code 57461 is used to identify loop electrode conization of the cervix and is performed to remove a lesion from the cervix.

Excision: 57500–57558

The excision category also lists codes for biopsy, curettage, and conization of the cervix; however, the method of approach is direct (without a scope). Other procedures listed in this category include removal of the cervix.

CPT divides the codes for cervical removal first by the presence of the uterus and then by approach. Trachelectomy is amputation of the cervix, leaving the uterus in place. The codes for trachelectomy are divided based on the extent of the procedure. CPT code 57530 describes a simple amputation of the cervix, while code 57531 describes a radical trachelectomy.

The codes for excision of the cervical stump (57540–57556) are divided based on approach and whether additional procedures were performed at the time of excision.

Corpus Uteri (58100–58579)

The Corpus Uteri subheading is the largest in this subsection and includes categories for excision, introduction, repair, and surgical laparoscopy/hysteroscopy.

58100–58294

The excision category lists CPT codes for biopsies of the uterus (58100–58110), nonobstetrical D&C (58120), and excision of tumors of the uterus (myomectomy). CPT further defines the codes for myomectomy by weight of the tumor, more or less than 250 grams, and approach, either vaginal or abdominal (58140–58146).

The hysterectomy codes are divided in a similar method. The codes for hysterectomy are first divided by approach: abdominal (58150–58240), vaginal (58260–58294), or laparoscopic (58541–58544, 58548–58554, and 58570–58573). CPT further defines vaginal and laparoscopic hysterectomy codes by the weight of the excised uterus and by whether the tubes and ovaries are excised during the same operative session.

Introduction: 58300–58356

Procedures listed in the introduction category include insertion and removal of an intrauterine device (58300–58301) and artificial insemination (58321–58322). Also listed in this category is the procedural component of a sonohysterography or hysterosalpingography (58340). A parenthetical note included directly below this code indicates the additional Radiology section codes needed to report the complete procedure.

Other procedures included in this category are insertion of devices for brachytherapy (58346) and procedures to diagnose and aid in the repair of fallopian tubes (58345 and 58350). The remaining two codes in this category describe endometrial ablation by heat (58353) or cold (58356).

Repair: 58400–58540

The repair category lists procedures for nonobstetrical repairs of the uterus, which are divided based on the type of repair: suspension (58400–58410), suturing of a rupture (58520), and plastic repairs of anomalies (58540).

Laparoscopy/Hysteroscopy: 58541–58579

In addition to the CPT codes for laparoscopic hysterectomy, the laparoscopy/hysteroscopy category lists procedures for laparoscopic myomectomies. The codes for myomectomies (58545–58546) are divided based on the number and total weight of the lesions excised.

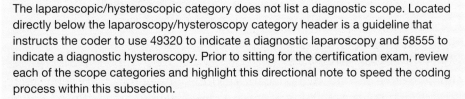

MENTOR Coding Tip

The laparoscopic/hysteroscopic category does not list a diagnostic scope. Located directly below the laparoscopy/hysteroscopy category header is a guideline that instructs the coder to use 49320 to indicate a diagnostic laparoscopy and 58555 to indicate a diagnostic hysteroscopy. Prior to sitting for the certification exam, review each of the scope categories and highlight this directional note to speed the coding process within this subsection.

The hysteroscopy codes (58558–58565) are divided based on the procedure performed through the scope. As with scope procedures in other subsections of the CPT described as "with," use as many hysteroscopy codes as needed to fully describe the procedure(s).

SPOTLIGHT on Procedure

Many coders believe that a "total hysterectomy" is the removal of the uterus, tubes, and ovaries. However, a total hysterectomy is the complete removal of the uterus and cervix, with or without the tubes and ovaries.

MENTOR Coding Tip

Many student coders find that highlighting only the approach and uterine weight in each of the hysterectomy codes speeds location of the correct code. When coding for radical hysterectomy procedures, as with other *radical* procedures, this term means that the organ, surrounding tissue, and lymph nodes at that site are removed.

Oviduct/Ovary (58600–58770)

Incision: 58600–58615

The incision category under the Oviduct/Ovary subheading includes codes for transection of the fallopian tube. The codes for such procedures are divided based on the episode of care during which the procedure was performed. If the transection is not completed during the admission for delivery, the service is identified by CPT code 58600. When the transection of fallopian tubes is performed postpartum, the coder must determine whether the transection was completed as part of a cesarean delivery or other intra-abdominal surgery (58611) or as a separate procedure after a vaginal birth (58605).

Laparoscopy: 58660–58679

Surgical laparoscopic oviduct procedures include excision and fulguration of lesions of the ovary (58662) or oviducts (58670), band, clip or ring occlusion of the oviducts (58671), plastic repair of the fimbriae (58672), and creation of a new opening in the oviduct at the fimbrial end (58673).

Excision: 58700–58720

Removal of one or both fallopian tubes only (58700) and removal of one or both fallopian tubes and ovaries (58720) are listed under the excision category. Both of these codes are considered separate procedures and are reported only when the procedure is the only one performed at this anatomical site. When excision of the oviducts or ovaries takes place during a hysterectomy or another procedure on the female genital system, it is included in the primary procedure.

Repair: 58740–58770

The last category under this subheading lists procedures for repairs of the oviduct, fimbriae, (58760), and open salpingostomy (58770). The codes for oviduct repair include tube-to-tube reanastomosis (58750) and tube-to-uterus implantation (58752).

Ovary (58800–58960)

Incision: 58800–58825

Codes for drainage of an ovarian cyst, ovarian abscess, and pelvic abscess due to ovarian conditions are included in the ovary incision category. These drainage codes are divided based on the condition being treated and the approach.

FOR EXAMPLE

Drainage of ovarian abscess; vaginal approach, open, 58820

abdominal approach, 58822 ■

Excision: 58900–58960

Although there are only two categories included under the Ovary subheading, the excision category contains multiple codes related to the treatment of ovarian malignancy (58950–58960). The codes are divided first based on the stage of treatment and then by the extent of the procedure. The initial resection of ovarian, tubal, or primary peritoneal malignancy is indicated by code range 58950–58952. Codes used to identify procedures for debulking of the malignancy are defined by initial (58953–58956) or recurrent malignancy (58957).

The last code in this range is used to indicate that the procedure was performed for a surgical evaluation for recurrence of the malignancy (58960).

Maternity Care and Delivery Subsection Subheadings and Guidelines (59000–59899)

The subheadings and code ranges are listed in Table 15.5.

As many of the services and procedures in the Maternity Care and Delivery subsection may be packaged into the global delivery codes of this subsection, the subsection can be divided into three main segments:

- Antepartum services that are not included in the delivery package
- Delivery
- Other services and procedures

Antepartum and Fetal Invasive Services (59000–59076)

Services and procedures listed under the Antepartum and Fetal Invasive Services subheading include diagnostic and therapeutic amnio procedures such as:

- Diagnostic amniocentesis, 59000
- Amniotic fluid reduction, 59001
- Infusing an underhydrated amniotic sac, 59070
- Obtaining blood and tissue samples from the umbilical cord, 59012, or placenta, 59015, for diagnostic examination
- Occlusion of the umbilical cord for fetal termination, 59072
- Drainage of fetal pleural effusions or pulmonary cysts, 59074

Excision: 59100–59160

Introduction: 59200

Repair: 59300–59350

The excision category lists procedures related to treatment of ectopic pregnancy (59120–59151). These codes are divided based on the approach, the location of the ectopic pregnancy, and excision/resection of tubes or the uterus.

Also included in this category is postpartum curettage. In contrast to the code for dilation and curettage located in the Female Genital System subsection (58120), CPT code 59160 is used for an obstetrical D&C procedure.

Table 15.5 Maternity Care and Delivery Subheadings and Code Ranges *(Data from CPT 2013. © 2013 American Medical Association. All rights reserved.)*

HEADING	CODE RANGE
Antepartum and Fetal Invasive Services	59000–59076
Excision	59100–59160
Introduction	59200
Repair	59300–59350
Vaginal Delivery, Antepartum and Postpartum Care	59400–59430
Cesarean Delivery	59510–59525
Delivery after Previous Cesarean Delivery	59610–59622
Abortions	59812–59857
Other Procedures	59866–59899

When an episiotomy or vaginal repair is performed during the delivery admission by a physician other than the attending (delivering) physician, report code 59300, episiotomy or vaginal repair by other than attending physician, from the repair category. Other procedures listed in this category include suture repair of a ruptured uterus (59350) and threaded suture or banding of an incompetent cervix, a procedure called *cerclage*. CPT divides the codes for cerclage based on approach: vaginal (59320) or abdominal (59325).

Delivery Services and Procedures

Each of the global delivery subheadings—Vaginal Delivery, Antepartum and Postpartum Care (59400–59430), Cesarean Delivery (59510–59525), and Delivery after Previous Cesarean Delivery (59610–59622)—covers codes for the global delivery by type of delivery and codes for individual components of the global delivery package.

The normal global delivery package includes:

Antepartum care
- Monthly visits to 28 weeks.
- Biweekly visits to 36 weeks.
- Weekly visits until delivery.

  Each antepartum visit should include:

- Initial and subsequent history and physical exam.
- Recording of weight and blood pressure.
- Fetal heart tones.
- Routine chemical urinalysis.

  Additional visits (high-risk pregnancy) are reported separately and in addition to the global delivery package.

Delivery
Services included in the delivery and not separately reportable are:

- Admission services.
- Fetal monitoring during labor.
- Episiotomy.
- Delivery of placenta.

MENTOR Coding Tip

The services and procedures listed above are included in the delivery whether or not the delivery is part of a global delivery package or reported separately.

Postpartum care
- Hospital and outpatient postpartum visits up to 6 weeks postpartum.

  CPT provides codes to indicate when antepartum services consisting of fewer than the typical number of visits are provided. CPT divides the antepartum visit codes based on the number of visits: four to six visits (59425) and seven or more visits (59426). In cases where three or fewer antepartum visits are provided, do not report the visits as antepartum care visits. Instead, report them with the appropriate E/M code for the location and type of service provided.

As with the antepartum visit codes, CPT provides individual component codes to indicate when a provider may have participated in only a portion of the delivery package: delivery only, delivery and postpartum, delivery of placenta only, and postpartum care only. These component codes are divided and listed under the corresponding delivery type.

FOR EXAMPLE An expecting 16-year-old presented to the ED in active labor. The patient was unaware that she was pregnant and had received no prenatal care. The OB physician on call examined the patient and admitted her to labor and delivery. At 12:37 p.m. the patient vaginally delivered a viable male infant. The patient agreed to see the delivering OB for all postpartum care. The appropriate code is 59410. ▪

In addition, the division of components of the delivery package provides a means of coding for delivery of multiple babies and by multiple methods.

FOR EXAMPLE Global care and delivery of triplets, one vaginal and two by cesarean, is coded as:

Routine obstetric care including antepartum care cesarean delivery and postpartum care, 59510

Cesarean delivery only, 59514

Vaginal delivery only, 59409 ▪

Abortion (59812–59857)

The services and procedures included in this category are for the treatment of incomplete, missed, or induced abortions. A parenthetical note instructs the coder to use an E/M code to identify services provided after a complete spontaneous abortion.

Treatment of an incomplete abortion (59812) involves removal of any remaining products of conception that were not expelled during spontaneous abortion. The codes for missed abortion are divided based on the trimester the fetus completed (59820–59821). Missed abortions occur when the fetus remains in the uterus for up to 8 weeks after intrauterine death.

Should infection of the endometrium and uterus also be present, the abortion is considered septic (59830).

The procedures for induced abortions (59850–59857) are divided based on the method used to induce and complete the abortive procedures.

1. Describe a total hysterectomy.
2. CPT defines the codes for myomectomy by _____ and _____.
3. CPT codes in the ectopic pregnancy code range (59120–59151) are determined based on what criteria?
4. What is included in the normal global delivery package?
5. CPT defines codes of a destruction of vaginal lesions as simple (57061) and extensive (57065). Explain the difference between simple destruction and extensive destruction.

EXERCISE 15.3

Also available in 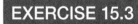 connect plus+

15.4 Modifiers Most Commonly Used with Codes in the Female Genital and Maternity Care and Delivery Subsections

As with all sections of the CPT manual, modifiers are used in the Female Genital and Maternity Care and Delivery subsections to continue or modify the story of the patient's encounter. Some of the more common modifiers used in these subsections are 50, bilateral procedure; 52, reduced services; 58, staged or related procedure or service by the same physician during the postoperative period; 59, distinct procedural service; and 78, unplanned return to the operating/procedure room by the same physician or another qualified healthcare professional following the initial procedure for a related procedure during the postoperative period. (See Table 15.6.)

The appropriate use of modifiers with the codes from the system subsection helps to tell the patient's full story.

Table 15.6 Female Genital and Maternity Care and Delivery Subsection Modifiers *(Data from CPT 2013. © 2013 American Medical Association. All rights reserved.)*

MODIFIER	DEFINITION	EXAMPLE OF USE
50	Bilateral procedure	A vulvectomy, radical, complete, with inguino-femoral, iliac, and pelvic lymphadenectomy performed bilaterally is reported as 56640–50.
52	Reduced services	Code 58565 describes the procedure as hysteroscopy, surgical, with bilateral fallopian tube cannulation to induce occlusion by placement of permanent implants. An instructional note directs the use of modifier 52 for a unilateral procedure.
58	Staged or related procedure or service by the same physician or other qualified healthcare provider during the postoperative period	When a diagnostic scope leads to an open surgical procedure, list the codes for both the surgical and the diagnostic procedures and append modifier 58 to the diagnostic scope code.
59	Distinct procedural service	Hernia repair is often included in the code description for several genitourinary services and is not reported separately. However, if the hernia repair is performed at a different site, it can be separately reported with modifier 59, indicating that the service occurred at a different site (i.e., via a different incision).
78	Unplanned return to the operating/procedure room by the same physician or another qualified healthcare professional following the initial procedure for a related procedure during the postoperative period	An example for use of this modifier would be a return to the operating room for debridement of an incision site infection during the postoperative period of a related procedure by the same physician.

1. When a procedure such as a vulvectomy is performed bilaterally and the code is not inherently bilateral or there is no specific code for the bilateral procedure, which modifier should be appended to the report?

2. What does appending modifier 52 to a code such as 58565, which is inherently bilateral, tell the payer?

3. How would you indicate to the payer that the diagnostic procedure led to an open procedure and should be reported separately?

Also available in 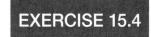 connect (plus+)

15.5 Common Medical and Procedural Terms Used in Operative Reports

As with all sections of CPT, the Female Genital and Maternity Care and Delivery subsections include medical terms and procedural terms that are specific to the system involved. Tables 15.7 and 15.8 list some of these terms and identify some key terms that could appear in a provider's documentation.

Table 15.7 Terms for Female Genital System and Maternity Care and Delivery

TERM	DEFINITION	DOCUMENTATION KEYS
Amniocentesis	Surgical puncture into the amniotic sac	Diagnostic, therapeutic
Cerclage	Suturing of the opening of the cervix	Treatment for incompetent cervix when the cervix is unable to contain the pregnant uterus
Cephalic version	Procedure used to turn a fetus from a breech position	Version
Colposcopy	Visualization of the vagina and cervical tissue by means of a scope	Scope examination of vagina
Conization	Removal of cone-shaped tissue or a segment of the cervix; can be diagnostic or therapeutic	Cone biopsy
Dilation and curettage (D&C)	Dilation, or widening, and curettage, or surgical removal, of part of the lining of the uterus	D&C
Episiotomy	Incision on the perineum and posterior vaginal wall during labor ***Mentor Coding Tip:*** Episiotomy is part of the normal delivery code, 650.	Perineotomy
Hysterosalpingography	X-ray of the uterus and fallopian tubes	Radiologic exam of female genital tract

cerclage The suturing of the opening of the cervix—treatment for incompetent cervix (i.e., the cervix is unable to contain the pregnant uterus).

colposcopy Visualization of the vagina and cervical tissue through a scope.

Table 15.8 Additional Terms for Female Genital System and Maternity Care and Delivery

TERM	DEFINITION	DOCUMENTATION KEYS
Amenorrhea	Lack menstruation	Without menses
Abruptio placentae	Premature separation of the placenta from the uterus	Placental abruption
Conception	Union of the sperm and the ovum	Fertilization
Dystocia	Difficult or painful labor	Prolonged labor *Shoulder dystocia:* specific type of dystocia in which the shoulder of the infant becomes lodged after delivery of the fetal head and requires manipulation
Endometriosis	Growth or presence of tissue outside the uterus that normally grows inside the uterus	Implants, lesions, nodules
Hydatidiform mole	Abnormality during the early stages of pregnancy in which tissue around a fertilized egg develops into an abnormal cluster of grapelike cells instead of a normal embryo.	Molar pregnancy
Salpingitis	Inflammation of one or both fallopian tubes	Inflammation of oviducts
Uterine fibroids	Fibrous-like tumors in the smooth muscles of the uterus	Leiomyomas, uterine fibromyomas
Uterine prolapse	Falling or sliding of the uterus from its normal position	Pelvic organ prolapse

amenorrhea Lack of menustration.

dystocia Difficult or painful labor.

EXERCISE 15.5

1. Premature separation of the placenta could be documented in a medical record as _____.
2. An x-ray of a patient's uterus and fallopian tubes was ordered. How would this be documented on the medical record?
3. A procedure that is performed during labor to prevent perineal laceration or tearing and is considered part of the normal-delivery ICD code is called a(n) _____.
4. What procedure is performed as treatment for an incompetent cervix?
5. When indexing the condition uterine fibroid the Alphabetic Index of ICD directs the coder to see also _____.

Also available in **connect** (plus+)

Chapter Fifteen Summary

Learning Outcome	Key Concepts/Examples
15.1 Review the anatomy of the female reproductive system.	The female reproductive system includes both internal and external organs and structures. The internal organs and tissue include the vagina, uterus, ovaries, and fallopian tubes, including the fimbriae of each. The external structures include the vulva, labia majora, labia minora, Bartholin's glands, and clitoris. *Flow of the female reproductive system (path of the oocyte):* ovaries → fallopian tubes → uterus → vagina → vulva
15.2 Understand chapter-specific ICD guidelines and format for complications of pregnancy, childbirth, and the puerperium.	Some common diseases coded to these chapters of ICD are endometriosis, uterine prolapse, menstrual disorders, infertility, and pregnancy and pregnancy-related disorders and complications. ICD-9-CM: The Female Reproductive subsection is found in Chapter 10 of the ICD-9-CM manual, with the code range 614–629.9. ICD-9-CM: Complications of Pregnancy, Childbirth, and the Puerperium is Chapter 11 of the ICD-9-CM manual, with the code range 630–676.14. ICD-10-CM: The Female Reproductive subsection is found in Chapter 14 of the ICD-10-CM manual, with the code range N70–N99.89. ICD-10-CM: Pregnancy, Childbirth, and the Puerperium is Chapter 15 of the ICD-10-CM manual, with the code range O00–O9A.212.
15.3 Identify the guidelines and format of the Female Genital System and Maternity Care and Delivery subsections of CPT.	The following questions will help a coder, when reading through an operative report, to understand what actually was done and how the procedure should be translated and coded: • At which anatomical site was the procedure performed? • Was the treatment obstetrical or nonobstetrical? • Was the approach internal or external? • What was the extent of the surgical procedure? • Was the procedure done at a single site or multiple sites? **General Subsection Guidelines** Included in all gynecologic procedures: • Diagnostic pelvic examinations and routine evaluation of the surgical field. • Vaginal or cervical dilation for procedures done by vaginal approach unless the CPT code states "without cervical dilation." • Diagnostic scopes (laparoscopy, peritoneoscopy, colposcopy, and hysteroscopy) are included in the surgical scope procedure. • Surgical laparoscopic procedures include lysis of adhesions. • Anesthesia when performed by the surgeon.
15.4 Apply the modifiers most commonly used with codes in the Female Genital System and Maternity Care and Delivery subsections.	Modifiers are used in the Female Genital System and Maternity Care and Delivery subsections to continue or modify the story of the patient's encounter. Some of the more common modifiers used in these subsections are 50, bilateral procedure; 52, reduced services; 58, staged or related procedure or service by the same physician during the postoperative period; 59, distinct procedural service; and 78, unplanned return to the operating/procedure room by the same physician or another qualified healthcare professional following the initial procedure for a related procedure during the postoperative period.

(continued)

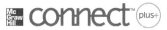

Enhance your learning by completing these exercises and more at mcgrawhillconnect.com

Learning Outcome	Key Concepts/Examples
15.5 Examine the common medical and procedural terms used in operative reports.	*Episiotomy:* an incision on the perineum and posterior vaginal wall during labor *Conization:* removal of cone-shaped tissue or a segment of the cervix for diagnostic or therapeutic purposes; also referred to as *cone biopsy* *Colposcopy:* visualization of the vagina and cervical tissue by means of a scope *Endometriosis:* growth or presence of tissue outside the uterus that normally grows inside the uterus *Dystocia:* difficult, painful, or prolonged labor

Chapter Fifteeen Review

Using Terminology

Match each key term to the appropriate definition.

_____ 1. [LO15.2] Antepartum

_____ 2. [LO15.1] Bartholin's glands

_____ 3. [LO15.5] Colposcopy

_____ 4. [LO15.1] Cervix uteri

_____ 5. [LO15.1] Corpus uteri

_____ 6. [LO15.1] Endometrium

_____ 7. [LO15.1] Fimbriae

_____ 8. [LO15.1] Labia majora

_____ 9. [LO15.1] Labia minora

_____10. [LO15.1] Myometrium

_____11. [LO15.1] Ovary

_____12. [LO15.2] Peripartum

_____13. [LO15.2] Puerperium

_____14. [LO15.2] Vagina

_____15. [LO15.1] Vulva

A. Lower part, or neck, of the uterus where it joins the vagina

B. Period that begins with the delivery of the placenta and extends through 6 weeks after delivery

C. Main body of the uterus

D. Fingerlike structures at the end of each tube that capture and sweep the egg into the tube

E. Structure that is located next to the vaginal opening and functions to produce mucous secretions

F. Innermost layer of the uterus

G. Functions are to produce the oocyte and female hormones

H. Hollow muscular tube extending from the cervix to the labia

I. Smooth muscle that forms the wall of the uterus

J. Visualization of the vagina and cervical tissue by means of a scope

K. Outermost structure of the vulva, containing sweat- and oil-secreting glands

L. External genitalia, with the function of protecting the internal productive organs

M. Structure that is located inside the labia majora and contains the vaginal and urethral openings

N. Period that begins 30 days prior to delivery and extends to 5 months after delivery

O. Perinatal period beginning with conception and ending at the time of delivery

Checking Your Understanding

Choose the most appropriate answer for each of the following questions.

1. [LO15.3] **Preoperative diagnosis:** Ovarian cyst, right

   Postoperative diagnosis: Ovarian cyst, right

   Anesthesia: General

   Procedure: Open, drainage of cyst

   The patient was taken to the operating room, prepped, and draped in the usual manner, and adequate anesthesia was induced. An infraumbilical incision was made, and an abdominal entrance was made.

The abdomen was visualized. The cyst was noted on the right, a 4-cm ovarian cyst. This was needled, and a hole was cut in it with scissors and the cyst was drained. Instruments were removed. The patient was awakened and taken to the recovery room in good condition.

Select the appropriate CPT codes for this scenario:

a. 58800, 620.2

c. 58820, 620.2

b. 58805, 620.2

d. 58822, 620.2

2. **[LO15.2]** A patient who is 32 weeks' pregnant is admitted because of an HIV-related illness. The patient spent 3 days in the hospital and was sent home in stable condition. The baby was not delivered during the hospital stay. Select the appropriate ICD-9-CM codes for this encounter:

a. 042, 647.60

c. 647.83, 042

b. 042, 647.83

d. 647.63, 042

3. **[LO15.2]** The patient is 25 weeks' pregnant with her first child. She undergoes a routine prenatal examination without complications. Select the appropriate ICD-9-CM code:

a. V22.0

c. V22.2

b. V23.0

d. 624.41

4. **[LO15.3]** A 32-year-old female presents with an ectopic pregnancy. The physician performs a laparoscopic salpingectomy. Select the appropriate CPT and ICD-9-CM codes for this encounter:

a. 59120, 633.90

c. 59120, 633.80

b. 58943, 633.10

d. 59151, 633.90

5. **[LO15.2, 15.3]** Total obstetrical care does *not* include:

a. Antepartum care

c. Diagnostic procedures such as ultrasounds

b. Delivery of the baby

d. Postpartum care

6. **[LO15.5]** The term salpingo-oophorectomy describes:

a. The removal of a fallopian tube

b. The removal of a fertilized egg

c. An incision into a fallopian tube and ovary for a surgical procedure

d. The removal of a fallopian tube and ovary

7. **[LO15.3]** The patient had a cesarean section delivery 2 years ago and presented today for an attempted vaginal delivery, which resulted in a repeat cesarean section delivery. Select the appropriate CPT code for the delivery only:

a. 59618

c. 59620

b. 59612

d. 59514

8. **[LO15.4]** Hernia repair is often included in the code description for several genitourinary services and is not reported separately. However, if a hernia repair is performed at a different site, it can be separately reported. Which of the following modifiers is used to indicate that the service occurred at a different site (via a different incision)?

a. 51

c. 22

b. 59

d. A modifier is not required.

9. **[LO15.2]** Menopause consists of four stages. Which one of the following stages is actually the stage of menopause?

a. This stage is the early beginning of menopause, marked by shorter or longer periods but no other classic menopausal symptoms.

b. This stage is marked by irregular periods, hot flashes, vaginal dryness, and reduction of estrogen.

c. This stage begins after the woman has been without a period for at least 1 year.

d. This stage begins with a woman's final period and continued lack of a menstrual period, for 1 year.

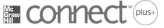

Enhance your learning by completing these exercises and more at mcgrawhillconnect.com

10. [LO15.5] A perineotomy, when performed, is considered part of the normal delivery ICD-9-CM code, 650. Which one of the following terms is the more common term for this procedure?

a. Episiotomy

b. Conization

c. Cerclage

d. Dilation and curettage

Applying Your Knowledge

Answer the following questions and code the following case study. Be sure to follow the process steps as illustrated in Chapter 8

Case Studies [LO 15.1–15.5] Case 1

Maternal labor and delivery note: Patient is a 38-year-old female with estimated date of conception 10/09 and estimated gestational age of +41 weeks. Her prolonged labor began with uterine contractions for the past 2 days, mild this a.m. and increasingly more severe this evening, with contractions now every 2 to 4 minutes. Cervix is 1 cm/20 percent/=1 station, EFW3, 500 g, 7/21.

Patient did progress to 7 cm; however, she was exhausted due to labor and loss of sleep for the past 2 nights due to her labor pain.

Delivery of a single viable female infant was performed vaginally with vacuum assistance. Episiotomy with fourth-degree laceration was repaired with 2-0 and 3-0 Vicryl.

Process 1: CPT

1. What is the procedure?

2. Locate the main term in the index.

3. What additional questions or set of questions can be determined?

4. Upon review of all the code choices identified in the index, what additional questions can be determined?

5. Based on the documentation, what is the correct code for this case?

a. 59409

b. 59412

c. 59400

d. 59410-22

Process 2: ICD

ICD-9-CM

1. Based on the operative report header, what is the preoperative diagnosis?

2. Is the postoperative diagnosis the same as or different from the preoperative diagnosis?

3. Is the postoperative diagnosis supported?

4. What is the main term for this condition?

5. Based on the subterm choices, what question(s) can be developed for this condition?

6. Is any sign, symptom, or additional condition documented?

7. Is the additional condition, sign, or symptom an integral part of the primary (or other) condition coded?

8. Does the additional condition require or affect patient care, treatment, or management?

9. Based on the documentation, what are the correct ICD-9-CM codes for this case?

   a. 669.51, 660.9, V27.0   **c.** 669.51, 661.01, V27.0

   b. 669.51, V27.0   **d.** 669.51, 661.01, 664.34, V27.0

ICD-10-CM

1. Based on the operative report header, what is the preoperative diagnosis?

2. Is the postoperative diagnosis the same as or different from the preoperative diagnosis?

3. Is the postoperative diagnosis supported?

4. What is the main term for this condition?

5. Based on the subterm choices, what question(s) can be developed for this condition?

6. Based on the information in the Tabular List, is additional information needed to determine the appropriate diagnosis code?

7. Is any sign, symptom, or additional condition documented?

8. Is the additional condition, sign, or symptom an integral part of the primary (or other) condition coded?

9. Does the additional condition require or affect patient care, treatment, or management?

10. Based on the documentation, what are the correct ICD-10-CM codes for this case?

   a. O66.5, O66.9, Z37.0   **c.** O66.5, O62.0, Z37.0

   b. O66.5, Z37.0   **d.** O66.5, O62.0, O70.3, Z37.0

Process 3: Modifiers

1. Was the procedure performed different from that described by the nomenclature of the code?

2. Was the procedure performed at an anatomical site that has laterality?

3. Was the procedure performed in the global period of another procedure?

4. Were additional procedures performed during the operative session, and does the documentation support them?

5. Did the surgeon have help from another surgeon or another appropriate person?

6. Did a physician different from the surgeon provide the preoperative or postoperative portion of the procedure?

7. What modifier should be appended to the CPT code for this case?

   a. 59   **c.** 51

   b. No modifier   **d.** 22

Case 2 [LO 15.1–15.5]

Preoperative diagnosis: Uterine fibroids and menometrorrhagia

Postoperative diagnosis: Same

Operation: Total abdominal hysterectomy

Pathology specimen: Uterus, approximately 240 grams; tubes and ovaries

Approach and surgical procedure: The patient was placed in the dorsal supine position, prepped, and draped in the routine fashion. A lower abdominal midline incision was made through the skin, subcutaneous tissue, and anterior rectus fascia.

The retractor was placed, and the bowel retracted laterally. Kelly clamps were placed on the round

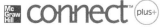

ligaments. The round ligaments were divided, and the anterior peritoneum was entered. The contents of the abdomen were explored; the liver, gallbladder, kidneys, and aorta were noted as grossly normal in appearance. The appendix was in place. The bladder was retracted anteriorly. Clamps were placed across the adnexa, and the pedicles were sutured with figure-of-eight #1 chromic and a free tie of #1 chromic. The infundibulopelvic ligament, broad ligament, and cardinal ligament were clamped, transected, and ligated bilaterally.

The posterior peritoneum was entered, and the uterine vessels were grasped with an Allis clamp and sutured with #1 chromic. Clamps were placed on either side of the ligature; the vessels were divided and again suture-ligated with #1 chromic.

The vagina was entered anteriorly, and the cervix was removed. Figure-of-eight #1 chromic sutures were placed to the lateral vaginal cuff. The cuff was then reefed using continuous interlocking #1 chromic. Hemostasis was noted as good, and the posterior peritoneum was closed with continuous catgut. The retractor and packs were removed. Sponge and instrument counts were correct. The abdominal peritoneum was closed with continuous 0 chromic gut.

The fascia was closed with continuous interlocking 0 Vicryl. The fat was closed with continuous #2-0 plain and the skin closed with staples. The patient tolerated the procedure well and left the operating suite in satisfactory condition.

Answer the following questions, and code the case above. Be sure to follow the process steps as illustrated in Chapter 8.

Process 1: CPT

1. What is the procedure?

2. Locate the main term in the index.

3. What additional questions or set of questions can be determined?

4. Upon review of all the code choices identified in the index, what additional questions can be determined?

5. Based on the documentation, what is the correct code for this case?
   a. 58150   **c.** 58275
   b. 58260   **d.** 58570

Process 2: ICD

ICD-9-CM

1. Based on the operative report header, what is the preoperative diagnosis?

2. Is the postoperative diagnosis the same as or different from the preoperative diagnosis?

3. Is the postoperative diagnosis supported?

4. What is the main term for this condition?

5. Based on the subterm choices, what question(s) can be developed for this condition?

6. Is any sign, symptom, or additional condition documented?

7. Is the additional condition, sign, or symptom an integral part of the primary (or other) condition coded?

8. Does the additional condition require or affect patient care, treatment, or management?

9. Based on the documentation, what are the correct ICD-9-CM codes for this case?
   a. 218.1, 626.4   **c.** 218.9, 626.2
   b. 219.9, 626.6   **d.** 220, 626.5

ICD-10-CM

1. Based on the operative report header, what is the preoperative diagnosis?

2. Is the postoperative diagnosis the same as or different from the preoperative diagnosis?

3. Is the postoperative diagnosis supported?

4. What is the main term for this condition?

5. Based on the subterm choices, what question(s) can be developed for this condition?

6. Based on the information in the Tabular List, is additional information needed to determine the appropriate diagnosis code?

7. Is any sign, symptom, or additional condition documented?

8. Is the additional condition, sign, or symptom an integral part of the primary (or other) condition coded?

9. Does the additional condition require or affect patient care, treatment, or management?

10. Based on the documentation, what are the correct ICD-10-CM codes for this case?

   a. D25.1, N92.6   **c.** D25.9, N92.6

   b. D26.9, N92.1   **d.** D27.9, N92.3

Process 3: Modifiers

1. Was the procedure performed different from that described by the nomenclature of the code?

2. Was the procedure performed at an anatomical site that has laterality?

3. Was the procedure performed in the global period of another procedure?

4. Were additional procedures performed during the operative session, and does the documentation support them?

5. Did the surgeon have help from another surgeon or another appropriate person?

6. Did a physician different from the surgeon provide the preoperative or postoperative portion of the procedure?

7. What modifier should be appended to the CPT code for this case?

   a. 22   **c.** 51

   b. None   **d.** 57

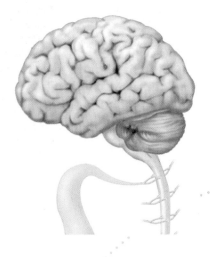

16

Surgery Section: Nervous System

Key Terms

Alzheimer's disease
Autonomic nervous system
Central nervous system (CNS)
Cerebellum
Cerebrum
Corpectomy
Craniectomy

Craniotomy
Encephalitis
Facetectomy
Foraminotomy
Hemiparesis
Hemiplegia
Hydrocephalus
Hypothalamus
Intracerebral

Intracranial
Laminectomy
Laminotomy (hemilaminectomy)
Meningitis
Mononeuritis
Nerve plexus
Neurorrhapy
Parkinson's disease

Peripheral nervous system (PNS)
Somatic nervous system
Status migrainous
Stereotactic
Syringobulbia
Syringomyelia
Vertebral interspace
Vertebral segment

Learning Outcomes

After completing this chapter, you will be able to:

16.1 Review the anatomy of the nervous system.

16.2 Understand chapter-specific ICD guidelines and format for the nervous system.

16.3 Identify the guidelines and format of the Nervous System subsection of CPT.

16.4 Apply the modifiers most commonly used with codes in the Nervous System subsection.

16.5 Examine the common medical and procedural terms used in operative reports.

Introduction

The nervous system is one of the most complex organ systems of the human body. It is responsible for control and communication between all parts of the body and the brain, controlling all thought and movement. Just as this system is complex, so too is coding for the various conditions, procedures, and services associated with the nervous system.

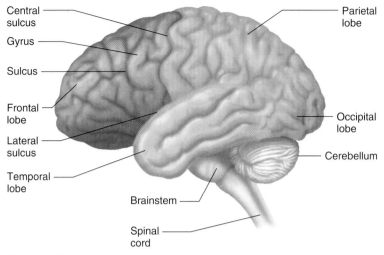

Figure 16.1 Lobes of the Brain

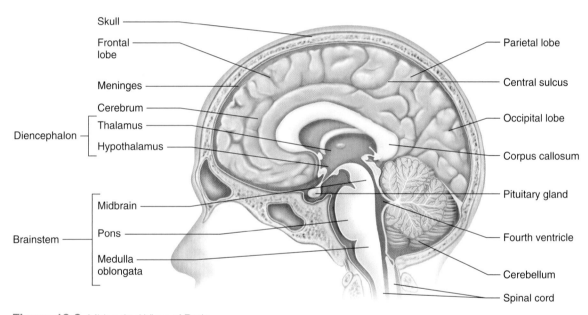

Figure 16.2 Midsagittal View of Brain

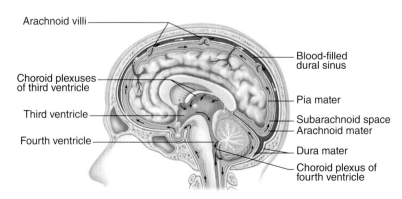

Figure 16.3 Ventricles and Circulation of CSF

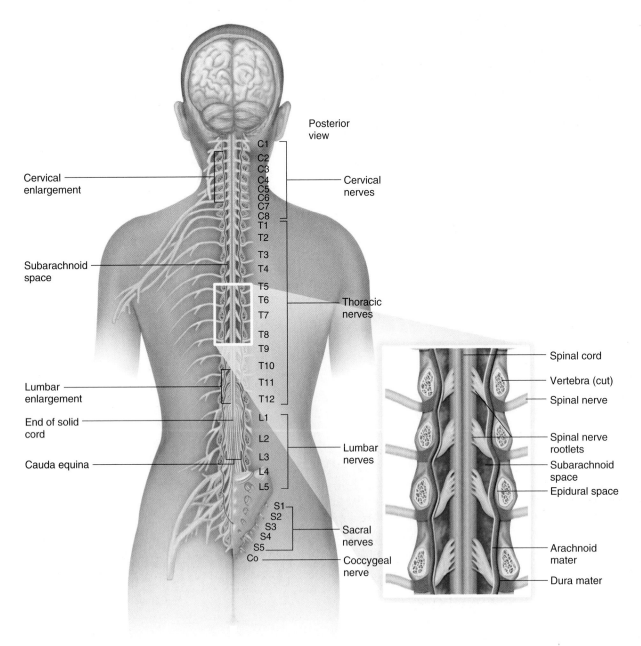

Figure 16.4 Spinal Cord

Posterior view

Cervical enlargement

C1
C2
C3
C4
C5
C6
C7
C8

Cervical nerves

T1
T2
T3
T4
T5
T6
T7
T8
T9
T10
T11
T12

Subarachnoid space

Thoracic nerves

Lumbar enlargement

L1
L2
L3
L4
L5

End of solid cord

Lumbar nerves

Cauda equina

S1
S2
S3
S4
S5

Sacral nerves

Co

Coccygeal nerve

Spinal cord
Vertebra (cut)
Spinal nerve
Spinal nerve rootlets
Subarachnoid space
Epidural space
Arachnoid mater
Dura mater

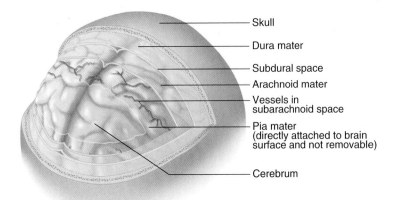

Figure 16.5 Meninges of Brain

Skull
Dura mater
Subdural space
Arachnoid mater
Vessels in subarachnoid space
Pia mater (directly attached to brain surface and not removable)
Cerebrum

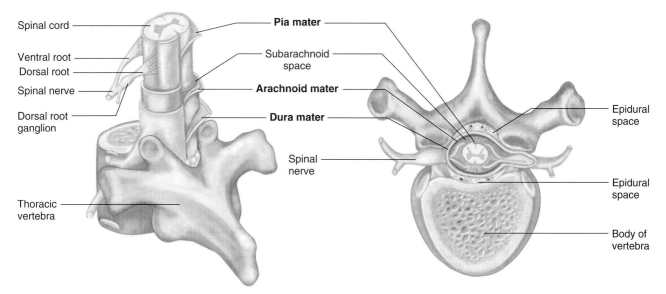

Figure 16.6 Meninges of Spinal Cord

16.1 Anatomy of the Nervous System

The primary function of the nervous system is to send and receive messages via nerve pathways made up of neurons. The human body has approximately 1,000 billion neurons sending messages to the brain and spinal cord to process information received from the sensory organs, peripheral nerves, and endocrine system. The brain or spinal cord processes and uses this information to control and coordinate the body's actions and reactions.

The nervous system is divided into two major systems: the **central nervous system (CNS),** which includes the brain and spinal cord, and the **peripheral nervous system (PNS),** which connects all body parts to the central nervous system. The peripheral nervous system is subdivided into two systems: the **autonomic** and **somatic nervous systems.**

The flow of information within the nervous system is very complex. However, the basic information in Table 16.1 regarding this system's message transmission and reception is sufficient for medical coding purposes.

Flow of the Nervous System
Stimuli may begin externally, from peripheral nerves or sense organs, or it may begin internally, at the cellular level (endocrine system)

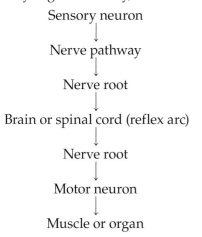

Sensory neuron
↓
Nerve pathway
↓
Nerve root
↓
Brain or spinal cord (reflex arc)
↓
Nerve root
↓
Motor neuron
↓
Muscle or organ

central nervous system (CNS) System that includes the brain and spinal cord and is responsible for coordination and communication within the entire body.

peripheral nervous system (PNS) System that consists of nerves only and connects the brain and spinal cord to the body.

somatic nervous system System that regulates body movement through control of skeletal or voluntary muscles.

cerebellum Brain structure that is located posterior to the brainstem and inferior to the cerebrum; responsible for fine motor coordination and movement, posture, and balance. Also called *hindbrain*.

hypothalamus Structure that links the nervous system to the endocrine system, regulates hormone secretion, and is the control center for many autonomic functions of the peripheral nervous system.

Table 16.1 Structures of the Nervous System

STRUCTURE	DEFINITION/FUNCTION
Central nervous system	Includes the brain and spinal cord and is responsible for coordination and communication within the entire body. See Figure 16.4.
Peripheral nervous system:	Made up of nerves only and connects the brain and spinal cord to the body.
Autonomic nervous system	Controls muscles of internal organs and is divided into two parts: • *Sympathetic nervous system:* responsible for fight-or-flight response (increased heart and respiratory rate; dilated pupils; constriction of blood vessels to skin, kidneys, and digestive tract; and release of endorphins). • *Parasympathetic nervous system:* responsible for relaxation, bringing all systems back to normal after a fight-or-flight reaction.
Somatic nervous system	Part of the peripheral nervous system and controls voluntary movement and carries sensory information.
Brain:	Controls the body's functions, thoughts, and actions.
Cerebrum	Directs conscious motor functions, processes sensory input, and governs intelligence and reasoning, allowing for speech, memory, and learning. • *Corpus callosum:* structure that divides the left and right hemispheres of the cerebrum. • *Frontal lobes:* largest lobes of the brain and prone to injury because they sit just inside the front of the skull and near rough bony ridges; involved in planning, organizing, problem solving, memory, impulse control, decision making, selective attention, and control of behavior and emotions. The left frontal lobe plays a large role in speech and language. The motor cortex lies at the posterior portion of the frontal lobe and controls voluntary movement. It receives information from other lobes of the brain and uses this information to carry out body movements. • *Parietal lobes:* located posterior to the frontal lobes and superior to the occipital lobes; integrate sensory information from various parts of the body, and map objects perceived visually into body coordinate positions, telling us which way is up and helping to keep us from bumping into things when we walk. They also allow for knowledge of numbers and their relations. They contain the primary sensory cortex, which controls sensation (touch, hot or cold, pain). • *Temporal lobes:* located on the sides of the brain under the parietal lobes and behind the frontal lobes at about the level of the ears: involved in auditory perception and contain the primary auditory cortex. They allow for processing of semantics in both speech and vision, recognizing and processing sound, and understanding and producing speech, as well as various aspects of memory, comprehension, naming, verbal memory, and other language functions. Parts of the temporal lobes are involved in high-level visual processing of complex stimuli (e.g., faces and scenes), object perception, and recognition.
Amygdala	Located in the frontal portion of the temporal lobe and just above the hypothalamus gland; responsible for processing and memory of emotions. • *Occipital lobes:* located at the lower back of the head; contain the primary visual cortex, which receives and processes visual information such as color and motion, and contain areas that help in perceiving and interpreting shapes and colors. See Figure 16.1.
Cerebellum	Located posterior to the brainstem and inferior to the cerebrum; responsible for fine motor coordination and movement, posture, and balance. Also called *hindbrain.* See Figure 16.2. • *Tentorium*: An extension of the dura mater that forms a tentlike structure enclosing the cerebellum.
Brainstem	Located at the base of the brain and continues on with the spinal cord. It regulates basic involuntary functions necessary for survival, such as breathing, heart rate, blood pressure, and swallowing. See Figure 16.2. • *Medulla oblongata:* closest structure to the spinal cord; regulates breathing, heartbeat, and centers for reflexes such as hiccupping, coughing, and vomiting. *Pons:* Responsible for communication and coordination between the two hemispheres of the brain.

Table 16.1 Structures of the Nervous System (*concluded*)

STRUCTURE	DEFINITION/FUNCTION
Hypothalamus	Links the nervous system to the endocrine system and regulates hormone secretion, and is the control center for many autonomic functions of the peripheral nervous system and sleep-wake cycles
Thalamus	Acts as a central relay for incoming messages to the nervous system.
Hippocampus	Plays a key role in the formation of long-term memory.
Spinal cord:	Carries sensory information from the peripheral nerves to the brain and from the brain to the peripheral nerves; divided into four regions: cervical, thoracic, lumbar, and sacral.
Nerve roots	Beginning segments of the peripheral nerves leaving the central nervous system as they exit the spine through the foramina. See Figure 16.6.
Peripheral nerves	Carry sensory information from the body to the spinal cord and from the brain and spinal cord to the body; consist of: • 12 pair of cranial nerves • 31 pair of spinal nerves
Meninges	System of membranes surrounding the central nervous system; primary functions are to contain cerebrospinal fluid and protect the central nervous system. The meninges consist of three membranes (see Figure 16.5): • *Dura mater:* Outermost and most fibrous of the three membranes covering the brain and spinal cord; consists of two layers: the periosteal and the meningeal. • *Arachnoid mater:* Middle serous membrane lying between and connected to both the dura and pia maters, but much more closely to the pia mater. • *Pia mater:* Innermost layer of the membranes, and the vascular membrane of the brain; carries the tiny branches of the internal carotid and vertebral arteries around and into the brain.
Ventricles	Four cavities filled with cerebrospinal fluid: See Figure 16.3 • Two large lateral ventricles are in the cerebrum. • One lies between the two thalami. • One is between the cerebellum and the brainstem. Primary functions are: • Production of cerebrospinal fluid • Transport of CSF • Regulation of CSF pressure within the central nervous system
Cerebrospinal fluid (CSF)	The CSF has several functions including: • *Protection:* cushions the brain and lessens the impact of a blow to the head. • *Buoyancy:* reduces the weight of the brain and reduces pressure at the base of the brain. • *Excretion of waste products:* takes potentially harmful metabolites, drugs, and other substances away from the brain and into the bloodstream for elimination. • *Endocrine medium:* transports hormones to other areas of the brain.

1. The CNS consists of what anatomical parts?
2. What are the location and function of the brainstem?
3. Name the four lobes of the brain, and explain the function of one.
4. Name the structure that divides the left and right hemispheres of the cerebrum.
5. What is the function of the spinal cord?

EXERCISE 16.1

Also available in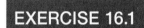

16.2 ICD Chapter-Specific Guidelines and Format for the Nervous System

Some common diseases coded to the Nervous System chapter of ICD related to the central nervous system are meningitis, organic sleep disorders, hydrocephalus, multiple sclerosis, paralysis, and Parkinson's disease. Common diseases and conditions of the peripheral nervous system include trigeminal and facial nerve disorders, carpal tunnel syndrome, mononeuropathy and polyneuropathy, and Guillain-Barré syndrome.

When coding these conditions, coders must thoroughly review the provider documentation as well as the guidelines and instructional notes.

ICD-9-CM: Diseases of the Central Nervous System and Sense Organs is Chapter 6 of the ICD-9-CM manual, with the code range 320–359.9. (ICD-9-CM coding for sense organs is discussed in Chapter 17 of this text.)

ICD-10-CM: Diseases of the Nervous System is Chapter 6 of the ICD-10-CM manual, with the code range G00–G99.0.

Table 16.2 lists the Chapter 6 subheadings and their code ranges.

Inflammatory Diseases of the Central Nervous System (320–326), ICD-9-CM

Inflammatory Diseases of the Central Nervous System (G00–G09), ICD-10-CM

meningitis Inflammation of the meninges of the brain and/or spinal cord.

encephalitis Inflammation of the brain tissue and spinal cord. Also called *myelitis*.

These sections contain codes to be reported for conditions such as **meningitis, encephalitis,** myelitis, and abscess within the spine or cranium as the cause of

Table 16.2 Nervous System Subsection Format *(Data from ICD-9-CM and ICD-10-CM, Centers for Medicare and Medicaid Services and the National Center for Health Statistics.)*

ICD-9-CM		ICD-10-CM	
SUBHEADING	**CODE RANGE**	**SUBHEADING**	**CODE RANGE**
Inflammatory Diseases of the Central Nervous System	320–326	Inflammatory Diseases of the Central Nervous System	G00–G09
Organic Sleep Disorders	327	Episodic and Paroxysmal Disorders	G40–G47
Hereditary and Degenerative Diseases of the Central Nervous System	330–337	Systemic Atrophies Primarily Affecting the Central Nervous System	G10–G14
		Extrapyramidal and Movement Disorders	G20–G26
		Other Degenerative Diseases of the Nervous System	G30–G32
Pain	338	Other Disorders of the Nervous System	G89–G99
Other Headache Syndromes	339	Episodic and Paroxysmal Disorders	G40–G47
Other Disorders of the Central Nervous System	340–349	Demyelinating Disease of the Central Nervous System	G35–G37
		Episodic and Paroxysmal Disorders	G40–G47
		Cerebral Palsy and Other Paralytic Syndromes	G80–G83
Disorders of the Peripheral Nervous System	350–359	Nerve, Nerve Root, and Plexus Disorders	G50–G59
		Polyneuropathies and Other Disorders of the Peripheral Nervous System	G60–G65
		Diseases of Myoneural Junction and Muscle	G70–G73

inflammation within the brain or spine. The first division of this section is based on the condition or the manifestation of the underlying condition. Each subcategory is then further categorized and grouped by the underlying condition.

The codes for meningitis, 320–322 (G00.0–G03.9, ICD-10-CM), are further defined as bacterial or due to other infectious organisms. Many of these codes are combination codes that do not require an additional code to identify the bacterium or other organism.

FOR EXAMPLE

Pneumococcal meningitis, 320.1, ICD-9-CM; G00.1, ICD-10-CM ▪

However, there are also many combination codes within this category that require that the underlying disease be coded first when coders are reporting these conditions.

FOR EXAMPLE

Cryptococcosis, 117.5, ICD-9-CM; B45.1, ICD-10-CM

Cryptococcal meningitis, 321.0 ICD-9-CM; G02, ICD-10-CM ▪

The encephalitis, myelitis, and encephalomyelitis category, 323 (G04–G05, ICD-10-CM), differs from the meningitis category as most of the underlying conditions listed in this category are the result of viral or parasitic diseases or are due to a complication of immunizations or previous systemic infections.

SPOTLIGHT on Condition

Meningitis and encephalitis/myelitis are often confused by coders as both result in the inflammation of tissues of the central nervous system. The distinction between the two is the specific tissue inflamed:

Meningitis The inflammation of the meninges of the brain and/or spinal cord.

Encephalitis/myelitis The inflammation of the brain tissue and spinal cord.

Organic Sleep Disorders (327), ICD-9-CM

Episodic and Paroxysmal Disorders (G40–G47), ICD-10-CM

These sections list sleep disorders that are the result of a disease process, anatomical anomaly, or physiologic abnormality. Sleep disorders related or due to substance abuse or behavioral disorders are coded to Chapter 5 or 16 of the ICD-9-CM. Conditions listed under ICD-9-CM category 327 (G47, ICD-10-CM) are subdivided by the nature of the sleep disorder and its underlying or root cause. Organic insomnia, 327.0- (G47.0-, ICD-10-CM), identifies conditions in which the patient has difficulty falling asleep or staying asleep. Hypersomnolence or excessive somnolence, 327.1- (G47.1-, ICD-10-CM) indicates that the patient suffers from excessive sleepiness or longer-than-normal sleep times. Organic sleep apnea, 327.2- (G47.3-, ICD-10-CM) identifies patients with sleep

Bruxism A movement disorder that results in clenching of the jaw or grinding of the teeth.

apnea due to a physiologic disorder or disease origin, such as obesity or alveolar dysfunction, resulting in fragmented sleep. Disorders in the sleep-wake cycle, or circadian rhythm, are coded to subcategory 327.3- (G47.2-, ICD-10-CM) and are divided based on the specific rhythm disorder. Subcategory 327.4- (G47.5-, ICD-10-CM) categorizes parasomnia, or disruptive sleep patterns due to abnormal behavior or physiologic events. The last subcategory in the Organic Sleep Disorders section identifies abnormal movements during sleep, such as bruxism, muscle cramps, and limb movement.

Hereditary and Degenerative Diseases of the Central Nervous System (330–337), ICD-9-CM

Systemic Atrophies Primarily Affecting the Central Nervous System (G10–G14), ICD-10-CM

Extrapyramidal and Movement Disorders (G20–G26), ICD-10-CM

Other Degenerative Diseases of the Nervous System (G30–G32), ICD-10-CM

Some of the common conditions located in these sections include Alzheimer's disease, hydrocephalus, Reye's syndrome, and Parkinson's disease. ICD-9-CM categorizes the codes for these conditions first by the age of the patient (childhood and other) and then by either the underlying cause or the manifestation as it relates to the anatomical site that is degenerating. For example, **Alzheimer's disease** is due to the destruction of subcortical white matter of the brain, and **Parkinson's disease** is due to the degeneration of nigral neurons that are responsible for creating dopamine (a neurotransmitter).

Alzheimer's disease Disease due to the destruction of subcortical white matter of the brain.

Parkinson's disease Disease due to the degeneration of nigral neurons, which are responsible for creating dopamine (a neurotransmitter).

cerebrum Brain structure that directs conscious motor functions, processes sensory input, and governs intelligence and reasoning, allowing for speech, memory, and learning.

hydrocephalus A disorder of the ventricle and/or cerebrospinal fluid that leads to increased intracranial pressure.

The first division of this ICD-9-CM section reports degenerative conditions that typically occur during childhood (330.-). A *use additional code* instructional note asks the coder to also code for associated intellectual disabilities when listing codes from this category.

Subcategory 331.1 identifies forms of dementia related to degeneration of the **cerebrum** or lobes of the brain, such as Alzheimer's, 331.0 (G30.-, ICD-10-CM), and Pick's disease, 331.11 (G31.01, ICD-10-CM).

Code range 331.3–331.5 (G91-, ICD-10-CM) identifies various types of hydrocephalus. **Hydrocephalus** is a disorder of the ventricle causing disruption of and/or decrease in the flow of cerebrospinal fluid (CSF) that leads to increased intracranial pressure. Conditions in this subcategory are divided by the underlying cause of the hydrocephalus.

Chapter 6 of the ICD-9-CM manual includes three types of hydrocephalus:

Communicating Occurs when another condition prevents the absorption of CSF through the normal ventricular channels.

Obstructive Caused by a blockage within the CSF channels.

Idiopathic normal pressure Caused by an increase in the volume of CSF within the ventricles.

Mild cognitive impairment or age-associated memory impairment, 331.83, ICD-9-CM (G31.84, ICD-10-CM), indicates a patient with impairment in memory or cognition that is greater than normal for the person's age but does not meet the definition of dementia.

Category 332, "Parkinson's disease," is divided by primary, 332.0 (G20, ICD-10-CM), and secondary, 332.1 (G21.-, ICD-10-CM), Parkinson's, which is Parkinson's due to an underlying cause such as drugs. Parkinson's is the degeneration of the basal ganglia of the brain, leading to symptoms that include tremors, rigidity, dragging, and a shuffling gate.

Category 333 (G20–G26, ICD-10-CM) lists codes for diseases of the extrapyramidal nerve system that lead to tremors, tics, muscle contractions, and other abnormal movement disorders. This category includes codes for:

- Huntington's chorea, 333.4 (G10, ICD-10-CM)
- Torsion dystonia, genetic, 333.6 (G24.1, ICD-10-CM)
- Torsion dystonia, acquired, 333.7- (G24.8, ICD-10-CM):
  - Caused by athetoid cerebral palsy, 333.71 (G80.3, ICD-10-CM)
  - Due to drugs, 333.72 (G24.02, ICD-10-CM)
- Restless legs syndrome 333.94 (G25.81, ICD-10-CM)

Spinocerebellar diseases are categorized to code 334.- (G10–G14, ICD-10-CM) and are divided based on the type, such as Friedreich's ataxia, 334.0 (G11.1, ICD-10-CM), or the underlying cause of the condition.

Anterior horn cell diseases are a group of conditions that affect the anterior nerve root—the nerve root responsible for communication between the central nervous system and the motor neurons. Conditions coded to category 335 include Werdnig-Hoffmann disease, 335.0 (G12.0, ICD-10-CM), and amyotrophic lateral sclerosis (ALS), 335.20 (G12.21, ICD-10-CM).

Category 336 (G95.-, ICD-10-CM) includes conditions affecting the nerve sheath of the spinal cord (myelopathy), and they are divided based on the underlying cause of the condition.

Pain (338), ICD-9-CM

Other Disorders of the Nervous System (G89–G99), ICD-10-CM

The ICD-9-CM chapter-specific guidelines provide instruction in the use and sequencing of codes listed in category 338. These codes, 338.0–338.4 (G89.0–G90.9, ICD-10-CM), are used when:

- The encounter is for pain management or a procedure to control pain (e.g., insertion of a neurostimulator or pain pump), and treatment is *not* directed at the underlying cause of the pain. (List a code from this category first, followed by a code for the underlying cause if known.)
- The addition of the pain code further clarifies the condition as chronic or acute.

This category is divided by the type of pain (central, acute, or chronic) and the underlying cause of the pain, such as trauma, surgery, or neoplasm. Pain related to neoplasms, 338.3 (G89.3, ICD-10-CM), may be caused by the neoplasm or by treatment of the neoplasm regardless of whether the neoplasm is benign or malignant.

Other Headache Syndromes (339), ICD-9-CM

Episodic and Paroxysmal Disorders (G40–G47), ICD-10-CM

Various types of headaches other than migraines are classified to category 339 and are subcategorized based on the type or underlying cause of the condition. The types include cluster, tension, post-traumatic, drug-induced, and complicated syndrome headaches. The subcategories for cluster- and tension-type headaches, 339.00–339.12 (G44.00–G44.89, ICD-10-CM), are further classified based on whether the condition is episodic or chronic. Cluster headaches are defined further by pain that occurs on one or both sides of the head.

> **MENTOR** Coding Tip
>
> When coding for drug-induced headaches, 339.3, be sure to code also for the drug when it is stated in the provider's documentation. A *code also* note does not appear at the 339.3 code level, so coders should write this note by the code as a reminder.

> **MENTOR**
> Coding Tip
>
> If the type of headache is not stated in the provider's documentation, it is coded as a symptom from Chapter 16 of the ICD-9-CM manual: 784.0, headache.

Complicated headache syndromes, subcategory 339.4, includes the condition hemicrania continua, 339.41 (G44.51, ICD-10-CM), which may also be documented as a persistent or continual primary unilateral headache. Other conditions in this subcategory include new daily persistent headache, 339.42 (G44.52, ICD-10-CM), and primary thunderclap headache, 339.43 (G44.53, ICD-10-CM).

Other Disorders of the Central Nervous System (340–349), ICD-9-CM

Demyelinating Disease of the Central Nervous System (G35–G37), ICD-10-CM

Episodic and Paroxysmal Disorders (G40–G47), ICD-10-CM

Cerebral Palsy and Other Paralytic Syndromes (G80–G83), ICD-10-CM

These sections of ICD list conditions that stem from disorders or diseases of the central nervous system and its associated structures and includes conditions such as multiple sclerosis, paralysis, cerebral palsy, epilepsy, and various types of migraines.

hemiplegia Loss of the ability to move one side of the body; total paralysis.

hemiparesis Weakness on one side of the body.

Demyelinating disease refers to a disease that damages the myelin sheath, leading to disruption of the nerve pathways and communication. Demyelinating diseases of the CNS are divided into two distinct categories: multiple sclerosis, 340 (G35, ICD-10-CM), and other demyelinating diseases of the CNS, 341 (G36–G37, ICD-10-CM). Category 341 is further subcategorized by the type of acute transverse myelitis.

> **MENTOR** Coding Tip
>
> Transverse myelitis not stated as acute is coded as 323.82. The directional note for this is listed with subcategory code 341.2; however, since many coders miss this guidance, coders should highlight the note to find it quickly and aid in accurate coding of this condition during the exam.

Various types of **hemiplegia** and **hemiparesis** are coded to category 342 (G81, ICD-10-CM) and are primarily divided based on the type of hemiplegia: flaccid, 342.0- (G81.0-, ICD-10-CM), or spastic, 342.1- (G81.1, ICD-10-CM). In addition, a fifth digit is needed to identify the affected side of the paralysis as dominant or nondominant. Selection of the correct fifth digit requires that the documentation state the affected side, right or left, and the patient's laterally dominant side, either left, right, or ambidextrous.

MENTOR
Coding Tip

The fifth digit for ambidextrous patients is always considered the dominant side, or a 1.

FOR EXAMPLE A right-hand-dominant patient suffers a right hemisphere CVA affecting the left-side flaccid hemiplegia, 342.02 (G81.04, ICD-10-CM). The correct fifth digit for this scenario is 2 as the hemiplegia is affecting the patient's nondominant side. ■

Category 343 (G80, ICD-10-CM) identifies various types of infantile cerebral palsy and is divided based on the level or extent of the body affected by the condition. Infantile cerebral palsy is due to damage to the motor function of the brain during birth and may also be referred to as *congenital.* Code range 343.0–343.3 is used to identify conditions present at birth, and code range 343.4–343.9 (infantile) identifies conditions that develop during the first 2 years after birth.

"Other paralytic syndromes," category 344 (G83, ICD-10-CM), classifies paralysis of unspecified cause and/or paralysis that has been present for some duration. The codes are divided based on the level or extent of the body paralyzed or the nature of the condition, such as cauda equine syndrome, 344.6- (G83.4, ICD-10-CM).

The various forms of epilepsy are listed under category 345 (G40, ICD-10-CM) and are categorized first by the type of epilepsy:

- Generalized nonconvulsive, 345.0-, ICD-9-CM (G40.301, G40.311, ICD-10-CM)
- Generalized convulsive, 345.1-, ICD-9-CM (G40.301, G40.311, ICD-10-CM)
- Petit mal status, 345.2-, ICD-9-CM (G40.301, ICD-10-CM)
- Grand mal status 345.3, ICD-9-CM (G40.301, G40.4, ICD-10-CM)
- Localization related, 345.4–345.5, ICD-9-CM (G40.0–G40.2-, ICD-10-CM)
- Infantile spasms, 345.6-, ICD-9-CM (G40.4-, ICD-10-CM)
- Epilepsia partialis continua, 345.7-, ICD-9-CM (G40.5-, ICD-10-CM)

All of these subcategories require the addition of a fifth digit to indicate whether or not the epilepsy is intractable. The term *intractable* refers to a condition that fails to respond to treatment or is poorly controlled by treatment.

Category 346 (G43, ICD-10-CM) identifies migraines and is divided based on the type and nature of the condition. Each of the listed subcategories requires an additional fifth digit to identify the intractability of the migraine and the presence of **status migrainous,** a severe migraine that lasts for 72 hours or more and may lead to hospitalization.

status migrainous A severe migraine that lasts for 72 hours or more and may lead to hospitalization.

Category 348 (G93, ICD-10-CM), "Other conditions of the brain," includes a variety of conditions not listed in the previous, specific CNS categories. Common conditions included in this category are anoxic brain damage, 348.1 (G93.1, ICD-10-CM), benign intracranial hypertension, 348.2 (G93.2, ICD-10-CM), and encephalopathy, 348.3- (G93.4-, ICD-10-CM).

MENTOR Coding Tip

To aid in accurate selection of the required fifth digit when coding for migraines, coders should highlight the term *with* in the description of each fifth digit. As the term *without* equates to "not stated," coders would not find this information documented. Targeting in on only what is documented when selecting a code speeds up the coding process during the exam.

Category 349, "Other and unspecified disorders of the nervous system," includes conditions related to previous medical procedures but not considered a complication of the previous procedure. For example, 349.0 identifies the patient's reaction following a spinal or lumbar puncture, such as a headache, but not a complication of the procedure, such as a cerebrospinal fluid leak following a lumbar spine puncture, 997.09 (G97.0, ICD-10-CM).

Disorders of the Peripheral Nervous System (350–359), ICD-9-CM

Nerve, Nerve Root, and Plexus Disorders (G50–G59), ICD-10-CM

Polyneuropathies and Other Disorders of the Peripheral Nervous System (G60–G65), ICD-10-CM

Diseases of Myoneural Junction and Muscle (G70–G73), ICD-10-CM

Codes within these sections list conditions or disorders affecting the peripheral nerves. The categories in these sections are subdivided either by the nerve or by the nature of the condition (i.e., neuritis, neuropathy, or muscle/nerve disorders).

The first division within this section involves conditions affecting the trigeminal nerve, 350 (G50, ICD-10-CM), facial nerve, 351 (G51, ICD-10-CM), and 5 of the 12 cranial nerves, 352 (G52, ICD-10-CM). Conditions specific to the nerves related to functions of the eyes and ears are included in the ICD sections for each of those anatomical sites.

nerve plexus A network of intersecting nerves and blood and lymph vessels; named for the area of the body in which it is located.

A **nerve plexus** is a network of intersecting nerves and blood and lymph vessels named for the area of the body in which it is located. Category 353 (G54, ICD-10-CM) identifies disorders of the nerve root and plexus and specifically lists only two anatomical sites of neural plexus lesions: brachial, 353.0 (G54.0, ICD-10-CM), and lumbosacral, 353.1 (G54.1, ICD-10-CM). Neural plexus lesions of other sites are coded to 353.8 (G54.2–G54.4, ICD-10-CM).

mononeuritis Inflammation of a single nerve; may affect the body along the entire nerve path.

Mononeuritis is the inflammation of a single nerve and may affect the body along the entire nerve path. Mononeuritis multiplex is the inflammation of at least two unrelated nerves and is coded to 354.5 (G56–G57-, ICD-10-CM). Coding of mononeuritis is categorized anatomically by upper limb, 354 (G56, ICD-10-CM), and lower limb, 355 (G57, ICD-10-CM). Each of these categories is subdivided based on the nerve affected. A very common condition included in these categories is carpal tunnel syndrome, 354.0 (G56.0-, ICD-10-CM).

Category 356 identifies hereditary peripheral neuropathy, which is a genetic disorder of the peripheral nerves themselves (G60, ICD-10-CM). Also included in this category is idiopathic peripheral neuropathy, which identifies genetic disorders of other body systems that in turn impact the peripheral nerves (356.3–356.8, ICD-9-CM; G60.3, ICD-10-CM).

Inflammatory and toxic neuropathy is due to the body's response to another disease or toxin, leading to pain, swelling, and loss of peripheral nerve function. Category 357 identifies inflammatory and toxic neuropathy and is divided based on the underlying condition or disease or the toxin, such as alcohol or a drug. A common condition coded to this category is Guillain-Barré syndrome, 357.0 (G61.0, ICD-10-CM).

Myoneural disorders, in category 358 (G70, ICD-10-CM), are a group of diseases affecting the junction or connection between the nerve and the muscle at the muscle. This category is divided based on the underlying disease, condition, or cause. The ICD manual provides instruction on identifying the underlying disease or toxic agent with an additional code.

Category 359, ICD-9-CM (G71, ICD-10-CM) includes muscular dystrophy and is divided based on the type. Congenital hereditary muscular dystrophy, which may or may not be progressive, involves degeneration of both the nerve and the muscle (359.0, ICD-9-CM; G71.0, ICD-10-CM). Hereditary progressive muscular dystrophy involves degeneration of the muscle without nerve degeneration (359.1, ICD-9-CM; G71.0, ICD-10-CM).

Also included in category 359 (G71.1, ICD-10-CM) are myotonic disorders. Myotonic disorders are due to abnormalities of the muscle membrane that cause delayed muscle relaxation, leading to spasmatic or rigid muscles. Myotonic disorders are classified by the type and underlying cause of the condition.

---

1. Define *bruxism*.
2. How does the encephalitis, myelitis, and encephalomyelitis category differ from the meningitis category?
3. Define *mononeuritis* and *mononeuritis multiplex*, and explain how these conditions are further defined in ICD.
4. Six months after insertion of a neurostimulator, the patient is experiencing uncomfortable stimulation of the original pain site. What is the correct code?

Also available in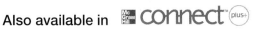

16.3 Guidelines and Format of the Nervous System Subsection of CPT

The Nervous System subsection of the CPT manual is formatted anatomically from the brain through the spinal cord to the peripheral nerves.

The nervous system is considered one of the most difficult areas of procedural coding due to its complexity. However, while the system itself is complex, a thorough understanding of the anatomy of both the nervous system and the skeletal support structures will enable coders to understand the approaches and definitive procedures included in this subsection of CPT. Therefore, coders are strongly encouraged to use anatomical charts while coding procedures for the nervous system.

There are several questions a coder needs to ask when reading an operative report and coding a procedure from this section. The following questions will help the coder, when reading through the report, to understand what actually was done and how the procedure should be translated and coded:

- At which anatomical site was the procedure performed?
- Was the treatment for a traumatic injury (acute) or a medical condition (chronic)?
- What was the approach (e.g., open, closed, epidural, subdural, supratentorial, infratentorial, with or without laminectomy)?
- Was the procedure primary or a reexploration of a surgical site?
- Was the procedure done at a single site or multiple sites?

Table 16.3 Nervous System General Headings and Code Ranges *(Data from CPT 2013. © 2013 American Medical Association. All rights reserved.)*

HEADING	CODE RANGE
Skull, Meninges, and Brain	61000–62258
Spine and Spinal Cord	62263–63746
Extracranial Nerves, Peripheral Nerves, and Autonomic Nervous System	64400–64999

Nervous System Subsection General Heading Code Ranges (61000–64999)

The general headings and code ranges are listed in Table 16.3.

Skull, Meninges, and Brain (61000–62258)

Procedures included in this subsection are specific to the portion of the central nervous system contained within the skull and are primarily divided by the approach to this anatomical site.

CPT divides codes for injection, drainage, or aspiration (61000–61070) first by the anatomical site in which the needle is placed, such as subdural, for infants only, ventricular, or cistern. These codes are further identified as initial or subsequent and with or without injection of a substance at the time of puncture.

Code range 61105–61253 includes approach by means of a twist drill, burr hole, or trephine and is divided by the method of entry into the skull. The codes are further divided based on the reason for the procedure, such as puncture or implantation of a catheter or pressure recording device or drainage of a hematoma, abscess, or cyst. Many of these codes are also defined by the anatomical site of the procedure, such as **intracerebral** (within the cerebrum), **intracranial** (within the skull), ventricular, supratentorial, or infratentorial.

Burr holes are commonly used to begin a craniotomy or craniectomy and are not coded in addition to the more extensive approach when performed for this purpose.

Craniectomy/Craniotomy: 61304–61576

There is one distinct difference between the terms *craniectomy* and *craniotomy*:

Craniectomy: Bone flap is removed without return to the original site.

Craniotomy: Bone flap is removed with return to the original site.

The bone flap may be returned immediately or at a later time (delayed). If the return is delayed, the surgeon will place the bone flap somewhere else in the body, such as the abdomen, under fatty tissue to maintain is viability until it is returned to its original location (+61316).

The numerous procedures listed within the craniectomy/craniotomy code range are primarily divided and grouped based on the nature of or reason for the procedure and on the approach through the skull. Primary groupings are:

- Exploration, 61304–61305
- Evacuation, 61312–61315
- Drainage, 61320–61321
- Decompression/exploration, 61322–61480
- Lobotomy, 61490
- Excision, 61500–61530

intracerebral Within the cerebrum.

intracranial Within the skull.

craniectomy An excision of the cranium in which a bone flap is removed and not returned to the original site.

craniotomy An incision into the cranium in which a bone flap is removed and then returned either immediately or at a later time (delayed) to the original site.

- Implantation, 61531
- Hypophysectomy, 61546–61548
- Osteotomy/osteoectomy, 61550–61564
- Craniotomy with bone flap:
  - Electrode implantation/removal and/or electrocorticography, 61531–61536
  - Resection/transection (lobectomy, hemispherectomy), 61537–61545, 61566–61567
- Transoral approach (skull base), 61575–61576

Each grouping is then subdivided by the anatomical site of the condition.

FOR EXAMPLE

Craniectomy, trephination, bone flap craniotomy;

    For excision of brain tumor, supratentorial, except meningioma, 61510

    For excision of meningioma, supratentorial, 61512

    For excision of brain abscess, supratentorial, 61514

    For excision or fenestration of cyst, supratentorial, 61516

Surgery of Skull Base: 61580–61619

Skull base surgery involves treatment of lesions located at the base of the inferior portion of the brain adjacent to the base of the cranial vault. Due to the nature and complexity of skull base procedures, multiple surgeons may be needed to complete the operation. CPT divides the total skull base procedure into three component procedures:

- **Approach procedures:** These are divided by entry point through the skull—anterior, middle, and posterior (61580–61598).
- **Definitive procedures:** These are also divided by the approach—anterior, middle, and posterior. These procedures are further divided by the nature of the procedure (excision, transection, obliteration) and by definitive anatomical site, either extramural or intramural (61600–61616).
- **Repair and/or reconstruction:** When these procedures are performed, the codes report extensive dual, cranial, muscle, or skin repairs, including grafting when required (61618–61619).

MENTOR Coding Tip

As the anatomical sites for the approach and the definitive procedure should match up, many coders find that identifying the correct definitive procedure first also identifies the correct approach grouping and allows for an easier process of elimination and selection of the approach code.

When multiple surgeons perform the complete skull base procedure (approach procedure, definitive procedure, reconstruction/repair), each surgeon reports only the code for the specific procedure he or she performed. If one surgeon performs all of the procedures, then all the applicable codes are reported, with modifier 51 added to the secondary procedure(s).

Endovascular Therapy: 61623–61642

The procedures within this range of codes are performed in the same manner as those located in the Medicine and Cardiovascular subsections of CPT except for the anatomical vascular site at which the procedure is performed: the central nervous system, namely, intracranial or spinal cord vessels. The codes within this section are further defined by the reason for the procedure:

- Occlusion/remobilization, 61623–61626
- Angioplasty/stent placement, 61630–61635
- Dilation, 61640–61642

CPT code 61623 is reported for a temporary occlusion, which is performed to control blood flow during a surgical procedure carried out on the intracranial or extracranial vessels.

Surgery for Aneurysm, Arteriovenous Malformation, or Vascular Disease: 61680–61711

Procedures within this code range identify procedures performed via an open approach, intracranial or extracranial. The procedures are grouped by the condition or reason for the procedure and further defined by the anatomical site or vascular circulation (e.g., carotid circulation).

FOR EXAMPLE

Surgery of intracranial arteriovenous malformation;
    supratentorial, simple, 61680
    supratentorial, complex, 61682
    infratentorial, simple, 61684
    infratentorial, complex, 61686 ■

SPOTLIGHT on Procedure

Arteriovenous malformation resections are divided based on complexity of the resection. Simple resections are easily accessible. Complex resections are arteriovenous malformations (AVMs), which are difficult to access and excise.

Stereotaxis: 61720–61791

stereotactic Medical imaging technique that creates a 3-D image of a specific anatomical site for therapeutic surgical or diagnostic interventions or localization of a tumor prior to radiation therapy.

Stereotactic refers to a technique or method using medical imaging to create a three-dimensional image of a specific anatomical site within the body for therapeutic surgical or diagnostic interventions or localization of a tumor prior to radiation therapy. The procedures in the stereotaxis code range are divided based on the surgical or diagnostic intervention and include:

- Creation of a lesion (globus pallidus or thalamus), 61720–61735
  - (gasserian ganglion or trigeminal medullary tract), 61790–61791
- Biopsy, aspiration or excision of intracranial lesions, 61750–61760
- Implantation of depth electrodes, 61760
- Insertion of catheters, 61770
- Navigation (used in conjunction with other surgical procedures), 61781–61783

Stereotactic Radiosurgery (Cranial): 61796–61800

Procedures in this code range involve the use of stereotactic imaging to locate and map intracranial lesions and isolate the tumor from surrounding healthy tissue, allowing for precise targeting of radiation delivery. The listed services and procedures include application of the stereotactic head frame (61800) and mapping of a lesion to be dosed with radiation. Actual radiation delivery is coded using codes from the Radiation Oncology section of CPT. Stereotactic radiosurgery services are divided based on complexity and number of cranial lesions treated.

Neurostimulators: 61850–61888

The procedures listed in this code range include placement, revision, or removal of neurostimulation devices. The codes within this section are divided first by the approach: twist drill, burr hole, or craniectomy. The codes are further defined by the depth of the placement, cortical versus subcortical, and by whether the placement is initial or a revision/replacement of a previous array. Add-on codes are provided to list additional arrays after the initial array. CPT provides codes for the placement/replacement of the neurostimulator's pulse generator and defines these codes by the number of electrode arrays to which the stimulator is connected (61885–61886).

Neuroendoscopy: 62160–62165

As in other scope approach procedures, the surgeon uses a neuroendoscope to complete a minimally invasive intracranial therapeutic procedure through the skull or skull base for the dissection of adhesions, fenestration of the septum pellucidum or intraventricular cysts, retrieval of a foreign body, or excision of tumors.

CPT code 62160 is an add-on code that identifies the use of a neuroendoscopy technique for the placement/replacement of a ventricular catheter for a CSF shunt.

Cerebrospinal Fluid (CSF) Shunt: 62180–62258

Procedures within this code range identify interventions in the treatment of hydrocephalus and other disorders causing obstruction to the flow of CSF through and out of the ventricles. These codes identify the surgeon's work to create or insert a shunt or form a duct from the lateral ventricles to the atria, jugular veins, auricular processes, pleural space, peritoneal space, or another area to allow excess CSF to drain.

The codes for initial insertion are divided based on the location of the distal end of the shunt:

- 62220 if the distal end is located at the atria, jugular veins, or auricular processes.
- 62223 if it is located at the pleural space, peritoneal space, or another area.
- 62190–62192 for creation of a shunt, subarachnoid/subdural.

Procedures for replacement/revision or removal of a CSF shunt are defined by the portion of the shunt system being replaced/revised or removed. The codes for CSF removals are divided as to with or without replacement.

Spine and Spinal Cord (62263–63746)

As with coding for procedures performed on the brain, an understanding of the anatomy of the spinal cord and its supporting structures will aid the coder in accurate code selection for the procedures performed.

Injection, Drainage, or Aspiration: 62263–62319

Procedures listed in this range of codes include a variety of diagnostic and therapeutic procedures completed percutaneously via a needle or catheter. The codes are divided based on the method or type of procedure and subdivided based on the condition, nature of the procedure (diagnostic versus therapeutic), anatomical site of the procedure, or number of days on which the procedure is performed. Procedures include:

- Lysis, 62263–62264
- Aspiration, 62267–62268
- Biopsy, 62269
- Puncture, 62270–62272
- Injection/infusion, therapeutic, 62280–62282, 62292–62294, 62310–62311
- Injection/infusion, diagnostic, 62284, 62290–62291
- Injection via catheter, 62318–62319

> **MENTOR** Coding Tip
>
> CPT includes detailed guidelines and parenthetical notes regarding the correct use of the codes within this subheading. Many of these codes are component codes and require the radiological supervision and interpretation code to completely report the procedure. Coders need to be aware of this pairing and watch for cases on the exam in which both codes are needed to complete the coding sequence.

Catheter Implantation: 62350–62355

The codes for implantation of catheters within this range of codes identify catheters that are tunneled under the skin and left for an extended period of time. Implantation-of-catheter codes are divided as to with or without laminectomy.

Reservoir/Pump Implantation: 62360–62370

The codes for implantation of a reservoir or pump are primarily defined by the type of device and by whether the encounter is for implantation or removal of the device or analysis/programming of the device.

Decompressive Spine Procedures: 63001–63615

Procedures within this range of codes include various methods and approaches designed to decompress the spinal cord. Accurate coding of these procedures requires a working knowledge of not only the spinal cord but also its supporting structures, the spinal column and intervertebral discs, and the terms in the CPT manual that describe these structures.

Corpectomy: removal or resection of the anterior portion of the vertebra (spinal column).

Foraminotomy: enlargement of the foramen or hole through which the nerve root exits the spinal canal. The foramen is formed by the inferior and superior facets of two articulating vertebral segments.

corpectomy The removal or resection of the anterior portion of the vertebra (spinal column).

foraminotomy Enlargement of the foramen, or hole, through which the nerve root exits the spinal canal.

Facetectomy: removal of the facet or bony overgrowth from the facet that leads to compression of the nerve root.

Laminectomy: removal of the lamina of a vertebral segment (multiple levels are counted by segment).

Laminotomy: removal of the superior or inferior half of the lamina (multiple levels are counted by interspace). Also called **hemilaminectomy.**

Vertebral segment: one complete vertebral bone, including laminae and articulating processes.

Vertebral interspace: the nonbony area between two vertebral segments, including the intervertebral disc (nucleus pulposus, annulus fibrosus, and cartilaginous end plates).

MENTOR Coding Tip

The surgeon's documentation will identify whether the procedure was performed on a vertebra or a vertebral interspace. Typically, this information is provided by identifying the anatomical site as L2 or as L2–3. These notations mean two very different things:

- L2 identifies the second lumbar *vertebra*, the vertebral segment.

- L2–3 is used to identify the *interspace* between the second and third lumbar vertebrae.

Think of the dash between the two vertebrae as the intervertebral disc. This association will also help when trying to determine the number of interspaces treated.

All decompressive spine procedures are divided primarily by the approach and the method in which decompression is achieved, such as with or without facetectomy, foraminotomy, or discectomy. The approaches and code ranges are listed in Table 16.4.

Table 16.4 Decompressive Spine Procedures *(Data from CPT 2013. © 2013 American Medical Association. All rights reserved.)*

APPROACH	GROUPING FURTHER DEFINED BY:	CODE RANGE
Posterior extradural for exploration/decompression of neural elements or excision of herniated intervertebral disc	*Procedure:* Laminectomy or laminotomy with or without facetectomy and foraminotomy Initial or reexploration *Level:* cervical, thoracic, or lumbar	63001–63051
Posterolateral extradural for exploration or decompression	*Approach:* transpedicular or costovertebral *Level:* thoracic or lumbar Add on codes for additional levels	63055–63066
Anterior or anterolateral for extradural exploration/ decompression	*Procedure:* discectomy or corpectomy *Approach:* anterior, transthoracic, thoracolumbar, transperitoneal, or retroperitoneal *Level:* cervical, thoracic, or lumbar	63075–63091
Lateral extracavitary for extradural exploration/ decompression	*Level:* thoracic or lumbar Add on codes for additional levels	63101–63103

Incision: 63170–63200

This range of codes identifies procedures performed on the spinal cord and includes drainage of a syrinx, rhizotomy, and cordotomy. The approach for all of the procedures listed under this subheading is posterior, by laminectomy.

Excision by Laminectomy of Lesion Other Than Herniated Disc: 63250-63295

Excision, Anterior or Anterolateral Approach, Intraspinal Lesion: 63300-63308

Excision of intraspinal lesions is divided into two groupings by approach: posteriorly by laminectomy (63250–63295) and anteriorly by vertebral corpectomy (63300–63308). The procedures within the posterior approach are further defined by the condition or reason for the procedure and the anatomical site of the lesion, such as extradural, intradural, and level of the spine.

Implantation of Neurostimulator Electrodes: 63655–63688

Procedures within this code range identify the percutaneous or open placement and removal of spinal neurostimulators. The codes are divided based on the placement, removal, or revision of the stimulator or pulse generator. Each code is further defined by the approach as percutaneous or open via laminectomy.

Repair: 63700–63710

The spine and spinal cord Repair subheading includes procedures for repair of meningoceles, myelomeningoceles, and dura. Most of these codes are specific regarding the size of the repair and/or the approach, via laminectomy.

Shunt, Spinal CSF: 63740–63746

Similar in nature to the ventricular shunt, spinal shunts allow for management of cerebrospinal fluid pressure by creating a shunt system within the spinal canal at the lumbar level. The codes under this subheading are divided based on the nature of the procedure, either creation, replacement, or removal, and the approach, open or percutaneous.

Extracranial Nerves, Peripheral Nerves, and Autonomic Nervous System (64400–64999)

Introduction/Injection of Anesthetic Agent (Nerve Block), Diagnostic or Therapeutic (64400–64530)

Regional nerve blockades or nerve blocks involve the injection of an anesthetic agent along a nerve pathway for temporary control of pain or to alleviate pain. These ranges of codes are first categorized by the type of nerves affected: somatic, paravertebral spinal nerves and branches, and autonomic. The procedures within each of these categories are then further defined by the nerve treated and the method of treatment, via single injection or infusion by catheter.

Neurostimulators (Peripheral Nerves): 64550–64595

Peripheral neurostimulators may be used to decrease pain in an area of the body or to augment the function of a dysfunctioning body part such as the bladder or digestive tract. The codes within this range are categorized based on the method of electrode placement: external or surface, percutaneous, or implanted electrodes. Codes are further defined based on the nerve or nerve pathway in which the electrode is implanted.

---

autonomic nervous system System that controls the muscles of internal organs; divided into the sympathetic nervous system and the parasympathetic nervous system.

MENTOR
Coding Tip

Several parenthetical notes inform the coder that daily hospital management of an epidural or subarachnoid pain catheter (01996) is not reportable on the same day as placement of the catheter. Writing the description of code 01996 on this page of your manual will speed coding of these services.

This code range includes the code for removal and revision or replacement of the pulse generator or electrode array, and the codes are again divided based on the specific nerve affected by the neurostimulator.

Destruction by Neurolytic Agent: 64600–64681

Nerve destruction, like a regional nerve blockade, is performed for control of or to alleviate pain. Nerve destruction differs from regional blocks in two ways: effect and method. The effect (i.e., pain relief) lasts for a considerably longer period of time. The method in which the procedure is performed may involve injection of a neurolytic agent or chemical (e.g., botox), thermal (heat), electrical, or radiofrequency. Regardless of the method of destruction the codes are divided based on the nerve targeted for destruction. The CPT manual includes numerous parenthetical notes that instruct the coder regarding the use of additional codes for imaging guidance.

Neuroplasty: 64702–64727

The procedures under this subheading describe the decompression of peripheral nerves by release or transposition of the nerve. A commonly used code within this category is 64721, which is the CPT code for carpal tunnel surgery. The codes are divided based on the specific nerve or body area in which the nerve is released.

Neurorrhaphy: 64831–64911

Neurorrhaphy is the repair of transected nerves by suturing. The procedures within this code range are categorized by whether repairs are completed without a nerve graft (64831–64876) or with a graft (65885–64911). Repairs completed without a graft are further divided by suturing of the transected nerve and anastomosis of two nerves. The codes for suturing are further defined by the nerve repaired. Codes for repair by anastomosis are further defined by the two nerves used to complete the repair.

neurorrhapy Repair of transected nerves by suturing.

> **FOR EXAMPLE** *Anastomosis; facial-spinal accessory* means the joining by anastomosis of the facial nerve to the spinal accessory nerve. ∎

Nerve repair procedures completed with the use of grafts are divided by the type of graft used: nerve or synthetic conduit or vein. The codes are further defined by the nerve grafted and the size of the graft needed to complete the procedure.

EXERCISE 16.3

1. Burr holes are commonly used to begin a craniotomy or craniectomy. Is this procedure coded in addition to the more extensive approach when it is performed for this purpose?

2. Regional nerve blockades or nerve blocks involve the injection of an anesthetic agent along a nerve pathway for temporary control or alleviation of pain. Discuss the further differentiation of code choices in this range.

3. What is the commonly used code for carpal tunnel surgery?

4. Excision of intraspinal lesions is divided into two groupings by approach. List these approaches and their code ranges.

5. Laminotomy is also known as _____ .

Also available in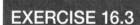

Table 16.5 Nervous System Subsection Modifiers *(Data from CPT 2013. © 2013 American Medical Association. All rights reserved.)*

MODIFIER	DEFINITION	EXAMPLE OF USE
50	Bilateral procedure	Hemilaminectomies performed at both the right and left laminae of the L4–5 interspace
51	Multiple procedures	Costovertebral decompression of spinal cord, T12 and L1
59	Distinct procedural service	Laminectomy for decompression of L3, laminotomy of L1–2: codes 63017, 63030-59
62	Two surgeons (cosurgeons)	Anterior T2–3 discectomy for decompression of spinal cord, in which the approach to the spinal column was performed by a thoracic surgeon and decompression was completed by a neurosurgeon: code 63077-62 for each surgeon
RT, LT	Right side or left side	Carpal tunnel release of right median nerve: code 64721-RT

16.4 Modifiers Most Commonly Used with Codes in the Nervous System Subsection

As with all sections of the CPT manual, modifiers are used in the Nervous System subsection to continue or modify the story of the patient's encounter. In this subsection, modifiers 50, 51, 59, 62, RT, and LT are the most commonly used to indicate the rest of the story of the patient encounter. (See Table 16.5.)

The appropriate use of modifiers with the codes from the system subsection helps to tell the patient's full story.

EXERCISE 16.4

1. Which modifier is used to identify that a procedure normally bundled into another procedure is actually a separate procedure and is medically necessary?
2. The approach to the spinal column was performed by a thoracic surgeon, and decompression was completed by a neurosurgeon. What modifier is appended to both surgeons' codes?
3. Which modifier identifies that a procedure was performed bilaterally?

Also available in **Mc Graw Hill connect** (plus+)

16.5 Common Medical and Procedural Terms Used in Operative Reports

As with all sections of CPT, the Nervous System subsection includes medical terms and procedural terms that are specific to the system involved. Tables 16.6 and 16.7 list some of these terms and identify some key terms that could appear in a provider's documentation.

Table 16.6 Terms for Nervous System

TERM	DEFINITION	DOCUMENTATION KEYS
Cerebrospinal fluid analysis	Removal of a small amount of the fluid that protects the brain and spinal cord. The fluid is tested to detect any bleeding or brain hemorrhage, diagnose infection to the brain and/or spinal cord, and measure intracranial pressure.	Spinal tap, lumbar puncture.
Echoencephalography	Radiographic study of the intracranial structures of the brain.	Ultrasound. Diagnose conditions that cause a shift in the midline structures of the brain.
Electroencephalography	Recording and analysis of the electrical activity in the brain.	Cells emit distinct patterns of rhythmic electrical impulses.
Neurorrhaphy	Repair of transected nerves by suturing.	Suturing of the transected nerve and anastomosis of two nerves.
Polysomnogram	Recording that measures brain and body activity during sleep.	Sleep study recording
Stereotactic	Medical imaging technique or method that creates a 3-D image of a specific anatomical site within the body.	Therapeutic surgical or diagnostic interventions or localization of a tumor prior to radiation therapy.

Table 16.7 Additional Terms for Nervous System

TERM	DEFINITION	DOCUMENTATION KEYS
Ataxia	Lack of muscle coordination in the execution of voluntary movement	Friedreich's ataxia
Anterior horn cell diseases	A group of conditions that affect the anterior nerve root, which is responsible for communication between the central nervous system and the motor neurons	Werdnig-Hoffmann disease Amyotrophic lateral sclerosis (ALS)
Complicated headache syndrome	A primary persistent unilateral headache.	Hemicrania continua May also be documented as a persistent or continual unilateral headache
Dementia	Cognitive deficit	Memory impairment
Syncope	Temporary loss of consciousness due to the sudden decline of blood flow to the brain	Fainting

1. The patient record documents diagnosis of vertigo. Would the ICD code for syncope be the appropriate code to report? If not, why?

EXERCISE 16.5

2. Werndig-Hoffman disease, a _____ disease which affects communication between the CNS and the _____.

3. What test is performed to record electrical activity of the brain?

Also available in McGraw Hill connect™ plus+

Chapter Sixteen Summary

Learning Outcome	Key Concepts/Examples
16.1 Review the anatomy of the nervous system.	The primary function of the nervous system is to send and receive messages via nerve pathways made up of neurons. The nervous system is divided into two major systems: the central nervous system (CNS), which includes the brain and spinal cord, and the peripheral nervous system (PNS) which connects all body parts to the central nervous system. *Flow of the nervous system:* Stimuli: external, from peripheral nerves or sense organs, or internal, at the cellular level (endocrine system) → sensory neuron → nerve pathway → nerve root → brain or spinal cord (reflex arc) → nerve root → motor neuron → muscle or organ
16.2 Understand chapter-specific ICD guidelines and format for the nervous system.	*ICD-9-CM:* Diseases of the Nervous System and Sense Organs is Chapter 6 of the ICD-9-CM manual, with the code range 320–359.9. *ICD-10-CM:* Diseases of the Nervous System is Chapter 6 of the ICD-10-CM manual, with the code range G01–G99.0.
16.3 Identify the guidelines and format of the Nervous System subsection of CPT.	The following questions will help a coder, when reading through an operative report, to understand what actually was done and how the procedure should be translated and coded: • At which anatomical site was the procedure performed? • Was the treatment for a traumatic injury (acute) or a medical condition (chronic)? • What was the approach (e.g., open, closed, epidural, subdural, supratentorial, infratentorial, with or without laminectomy)? • Was the procedure primary or a reexploration of a surgical site? • Was the procedure done at a single site or multiple sites?
16.4 Apply the modifiers most commonly used with codes in the Nervous System subsection.	Modifiers are used in the Nervous System subsection to continue or modify the story of the patient's encounter. In this subsection, modifiers 50, 51, 59, 62, RT, and LT are most commonly used.
16.5 Examine the common medical and procedural terms used in operative reports.	Corpectomy: removal or resection of the anterior portion of the vertebra (spinal column) Discectomy: removal of all or a part of the intervertebral disc Foraminotomy: enlargement of the foramen or hole through which the nerve root exits Facetectomy: removal of the facet or bony overgrowth from the facet to decompress the nerve root Laminectomy: Removal of the lamina of a vertebral Hemilaminectomy/Laminotomy: removal of the superior or inferior half of the lamina Craniectomy: Bone flap is removed without return to the original site Craniotomy: Bone flap is removed with return to the original site

Chapter Sixteen Review

Using Terminology

Match each key term to the appropriate definition.

_____ 1. [LO16.2] Alzheimer's disease

_____ 2. [LO16.1] Central nervous system (CNS)

_____ 3. [LO16.2] Encephalitis

_____ 4. [LO16.3] Facetectomy

_____ 5. [LO16.2] Hemiparesis

_____ 6. [LO16.2] Hemiplegia

_____ 7. [LO16.2] Hydrocephalus

_____ 8. [LO16.1] Meninges

_____ 9. [LO16.2] Meningitis

_____ 10. [LO16.2] Parkinson's disease

_____ 11. [LO16.1] Peripheral nervous system (PNS)

_____ 12. [LO16.3] Stereotactic

_____ 13. [LO16.3] Vertebral interspace

_____ 14. [LO16.3] Vertebral segment

A. Includes the brain and spinal cord and is responsible for coordination and communication with the entire body

B. System that connects all body parts to the central nervous system

C. System of membranes that surround the central nervous system and whose primary functions are to contain cerebrospinal fluid and protect the central nervous system

D. The degeneration of the basal ganglia of the brain, leading to symptoms that include tremors, rigidity, dragging, and a shuffling gate

E. Disease due to the destruction of subcortical white matter of the brain

F. Disorder of the ventricle and/or cerebrospinal fluid (CSF) that leads to increased intracranial pressure

G. Inflammation of the brain tissue and spinal cord

H. Inflammation of the meninges of the brain and/or spinal cord

I. Loss of the ability to move one side of the body; total paralysis

J. Medical imaging technique or method that creates a three-dimensional image of a specific anatomical site within the body for therapeutic surgical or diagnostic interventions or localization of a tumor prior to radiation therapy

K. Removal of the facet or bony overgrowth from the facet that leads to compression of the nerve root

L. Weakness affecting one side of the body

M. One complete vertebral bone, including laminae and articulating processes

N. The nonbony area between two vertebral segments that includes the intervertebral disc (nucleus pulposus, annulus fibrosus, and cartilaginous end plates)

Checking Your Understanding

Choose the most appropriate answer for each of the following questions.

1. [LO16.1] The name of the entire motor nervous system is:

a. Autonomic nervous system

b. Peripheral nervous system

c. Parasympathetic nervous system

d. Sympathetic nervous system

2. [LO16.1] Which type of hydrocephalus occurs when another condition prevents the absorption of CSF through the normal ventricular channels?

a. Obstructive

b. Communicating

c. Idiopathic normal pressure

d. Ventricular

3. [LO16.2, 16.3] Callie has been a medical transcriptionist for 25 years and has been complaining of a tingling sensation in her right arm. She was diagnosed with carpal tunnel syndrome and underwent an open procedure that included neuroplasty and transposition of the median nerve at the carpal tunnel. Select the appropriate ICD and CPT codes from the following:

a. 64721-RT, 354.0

b. 25210, 354.10

c. 64721-RT, 354.1

d. 64721-RT, 354.0, 354.1

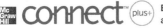 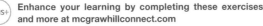 Enhance your learning by completing these exercises and more at mcgrawhillconnect.com

4. **[LO16.3]** A patient has a cranial bone flap removed and placed under fatty tissue in the abdomen for return to the original site later. This procedure is a(n):

    a. Craniectomy

    b. Craniotomy

    c. Lobotomy

    d. Implantation

5. **[LO16.3]** A patient presents to the operating room for enlargement of the foramen, or hole, through which the nerve root exits the spinal canal. This type of procedure would be identified on an operative report as a:

    a. Laminectomy

    b. Foraminotomy

    c. Facetectomy

    d. Corpectomy

6. **[LO16.2]** A patient's CT scan shows inflammation of the meninges of the brain and spinal cord. The diagnosis on the report would be:

    a. Meningitis

    b. Myelitis

    c. Encephalitis

    d. Pneumococcal meningitis

7. **[LO16.3]** A patient presents for reprogramming of a programmable CSF shunt. Select the appropriate CPT code:

    a. 62256

    b. 62230

    c. 62252

    d. 61070

8. **[LO16.2]** The patient is diagnosed with peripheral neuropathy in diabetes. Select the appropriate ICD-9-CM code(s):

    a. 249.60, 337.1   **c.** 337.1, 250.60

    b. 356.9   **d.** 250.60, 337.1

9. **[LO16.4]** In an anterior C2–3 discectomy for decompression of the spinal cord, the approach to the spinal column was performed by a thoracic surgeon and decompression was completed by a neurosurgeon. Select the appropriate CPT code with the appropriate modifier, if needed, for both surgeons:

    a. 63077-62   **c.** 63076-62

    b. 63077   **d.** 63081-62

10. **[LO16.5]** A patient's diagnosis in the medical record is hemicrania continua. Which of the following also identifies this diagnosis?

    a. Complicated headache syndrome

    b. Continual primary unilateral headache

    c. Migraine

    d. Complicated headache syndrome and continual primary unilateral headache

Applying Your Knowledge

Answer the following questions and code the following case study. Be sure to follow the process steps as illustrated in Chapter 8.

Case Studies [LO 16.1–16.5] Case 1

Preoperative diagnosis: Herniated disk left L4–5 interspace, with sequestered fragment, left L5 radiculopathy

Postoperative diagnosis: Herniated disk left L4–5 interspace, with sequestered fragment, left L5 radiculopathy

Procedure: Left L4–5 partial hemilaminectomy, medial facetectomy, removal of herniated disk and sequestered far lateral disk

Anesthesia: General anesthesia

Estimated blood loss: 30 ml

Endotracheal anesthesia was administered, and the back was prepped and draped in the usual fashion. We used intraoperative x-ray to approximate the location of the L4–5 interspace such that we could center the incision over this area. An incision was made over the L4–5 interspace, and the incision carried down through the subcutaneous tissues, which in this lady were quite considerable. The lumbosacral fascia was opened on the left side only, and the paraspinal muscles were stripped subperiosteally to expose the spinous processes and laminae of L4 and L5. We obtained an x-ray with our marker at the L5 lamina. Once this was done, the L4–5 interspace was identified and a left L4–5 partial hemilaminectomy and medial facetectomy were performed. Verifying that was inferior enough sufficiently to be able to reach the L5 nerve root and sequestered fragment. Partially, the bony removal was accomplished also, in addition to the Midas Rex drill. It was performed using curettes and Kerrisons. The yellow ligament was removed, exposing the common dural sac, and I was able to identify the L4–5 interspace, which appeared to be indurated and consistent with a previous disc herniation. The L5 nerve root was identified and was gently mobilized medially, and I was able to identify the sequestered disc, which was actually in three large fragments. These were mobilized with a blunt hook and then delivered with a small pituitary punch. Perhaps the largest of the fragments actually appeared to extend out the foramina along with the L5 nerve root. After the fragments were released, the dura and nerve root appeared to be much more relaxed and I probed out the foramina using both a blunt hook and then a Woodson. No additional fragments were uncovered. I inspected the L4–5 disk with an Epstein curette. There were no additional rents that appeared to be scarred, and rather than risk a second disc herniation through an area that appeared to be already healed, this was left alone. The common dural sac was well decompressed en route. The area was irrigated with an antibiotic saline solution. A small autologous fat graft was harvested and placed over the root and dura and then covered with a Gelfoam thrombin slurry. The wound was infiltrated with 25 percent Marcaine with epinephrine, and the wound was closed by reapproximating the muscles and fascia with O Vicryl: a 2-0 Vicryl subcutaneous closure and a running 4-0 subcuticular stitch in the skin. The wound was reinforced with Steri-Strips. A sterile dressing was applied. Throughout the case the patient remained hemodynamically stable.

Process 1: CPT

1. What is the procedure?

2. Locate the main term in the index.

3. What additional questions or set of questions can be determined?

4. Upon review of all the code choices identified in the index, what additional questions can be determined?

5. Based on the documentation, what is (are) the correct code(s) for this case?
   a. 63030
   b. 63030, 63035
   c. 63042, 63043
   d. 63042

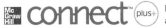

Process 2: ICD

ICD-9-CM

1. Based on the operative report header, what is the preoperative diagnosis?

2. Is the postoperative diagnosis the same as or different from the preoperative diagnosis?

3. Is the postoperative diagnosis supported?

4. What is the main term for this condition?

5. Based on the subterm choices, what question(s) can be developed for this condition?

6. Is any sign, symptom, or additional condition documented?

7. Is the additional condition, sign, or symptom an integral part of the primary (or other) condition coded?

8. Does the additional condition require or affect patient care, treatment, or management?

9. Based on the documentation, what is (are) the correct ICD-9-CM code(s) for this case?
   - **a.** 722.52
   - **b.** 722.10
   - **c.** 722.10, 724.4
   - **d.** 722.11

ICD-10-CM

1. Based on the operative report header, what is the preoperative diagnosis?

2. Is the postoperative diagnosis the same as or different from the preoperative diagnosis?

3. Is the postoperative diagnosis supported?

4. What is the main term for this condition?

5. Based on the subterm choices, what question(s) can be developed for this condition?

6. Based on the information in the Tabular List, is additional information needed to determine the appropriate diagnosis code?

7. Is any sign, symptom, or additional condition documented?

8. Is the additional condition, sign, or symptom an integral part of the primary (or other) condition coded?

9. Does the additional condition require or affect patient care, treatment, or management?

10. Based on the documentation, what is (are) the correct ICD-10-CM code(s) for this case?
   - **a.** M51.17
   - **b.** M51.16
   - **c.** M51.06
   - **d.** M51.26, M54.16

Process 3: Modifiers

1. Was the procedure performed different from that described by the nomenclature of the code?

2. Was the procedure performed at an anatomical site that has laterality?

3. Was the procedure performed in the global period of another procedure?

4. Were additional procedures performed during the operative session, and does the documentation support them?

5. Did the surgeon have help from another surgeon or another appropriate person?

6. Did a physician different from the surgeon provide the preoperative or postoperative portion of the procedure?

7. What modifier should be appended to the CPT code for this case?
   - **a.** None
   - **b.** 78
   - **c.** LT
   - **d.** 58

[LO 16.1–16.5] Case 2

Preoperative diagnosis: Acute/chronic subdural hematoma, headaches, and right-sided weakness

Postoperative diagnosis: Acute/chronic subdural hematoma, headaches, and right-sided weakness

Procedure: Left-sided burr hole evacuation of subdural hematoma

Anesthesia: General anesthesia

Estimated blood loss: Less than 10 ml

Description of procedure: Following a thorough discussion of the risk, benefits, and alternative treatments with the patient and verifying that she has sufficient information to make an informed decision, we proceeded. The patient received preoperative antibiotics and had sequential compression devices that were operating prior to the induction of the general anesthetic. Under general endotracheal anesthesia, the patient was placed supine on the operating table and prepped and draped in the usual fashion. The CT scan of the head was verified. Following our last time-out, two incisions were made over the left convexity, one anteriorly and one posteriorly. These were approxi-mated at 2.5 to 3 cm in length. The incision was carried down through the scalp, using unipolar cautery for homeostasis. The wound was retracted using a small Weitlaner, and the soft tissue was cleared from the periosteum. Using the perforator, 2 burr holes were made, again one anteriorly and one posteriorly. The bony edges were waxed for homeostasis. The discoloration through the dura was visible, consistent with the subdural hematoma. We first opened the anterior burr hole, opening the dura. The dura was coagulated using bipolar cautery and a 15-blade knife. From here there was a flow of straw-colored fluid consistent with a chronic subdural hematoma. We irrigated from one burr hole to the other until the fluid cleared. Once the fluid was cleared, we then left a 1-French drain in the subdural space. The drain was brought out through a separate trocar incision. The burr holes were covered with Gelfoam, and then the wound was closed by reapproximating the galea with 2-0 Vicryl and staples in the skin. Postoperatively a full head dressing was applied. The patient tolerated the procedure well and remained hemodynamically stable throughout the case.

Answer the following questions, and code the case above.

Process 1: CPT

1. What is the procedure?

2. Locate the main term in the index.

3. What additional questions or set of questions can be determined?

4. Upon review of all the code choices identified in the index, what additional questions can be determined?

5. Based on the documentation, what is the correct code for this case?
   a. 61312   **c.** 61314
   b. 61150   **d.** 61154

Process 2: ICD

ICD-9-CM

1. Based on the operative report header, what is the preoperative diagnosis?

2. Is the postoperative diagnosis the same as or different from the preoperative diagnosis?

3. Is the postoperative diagnosis supported?

4. What is the main term for this condition?

5. Based on the subterm choices, what question(s) can be developed for this condition?

6. Is any sign, symptom, or additional condition documented?

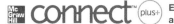 **Enhance your learning** by completing these exercises and more at mcgrawhillconnect.com

7. Is the additional condition, sign, or symptom an integral part of the primary (or other) condition coded?

8. Does the additional condition require or affect patient care, treatment, or management?

9. Based on the documentation, what is the correct ICD-9-CM code for this case?
   a. 432.1   c. 852.20
   b. 432.10   d. 432.0

ICD-10-CM

1. Based on the operative report header, what is the preoperative diagnosis?

2. Is the postoperative diagnosis the same as or different from the preoperative diagnosis?

3. Is the postoperative diagnosis supported?

4. What is the main term for this condition?

5. Based on the subterm choices, what question(s) can be developed for this condition?

6. Based on the information in the Tabular List, is additional information needed to determine the appropriate diagnosis code?

7. Is any sign, symptom, or additional condition documented?

8. Is the additional condition, sign, or symptom an integral part of the primary (or other) condition coded?

9. Does the additional condition require or affect patient care, treatment, or management?

10. Based on the documentation, what is (are) the correct ICD-10-CM code(s) for this case?
    a. I61.4   c. I62.01
    b. S06.5X0A   d. I62.01, I62.03

Process 3: Modifiers

1. Was the procedure performed different from that described by the nomenclature of the code?

2. Was the procedure performed at an anatomical site that has laterality?

3. Was the procedure performed in the global period of another procedure?

4. Were additional procedures performed during the operative session, and does the documentation support them?

5. Did the surgeon have help from another surgeon or another appropriate person?

6. Did a physician different from the surgeon provide the preoperative or postoperative portion of the procedure?

7. What modifier should be appended to the CPT code for this case?
   a. LT   c. 22
   b. 50   d. None

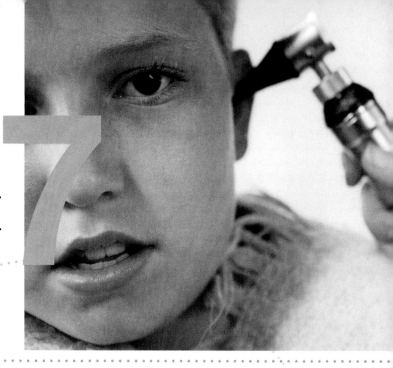

Surgery Section: Eyes, Ears, and Endocrine System

Key Terms

Audiometry
Auris dextra (AD)
Auris sinistra (AS)
Auris unitas (AU)
Cataracts
Cushing's syndrome
Glaucoma
Glucose tolerance test
  (GTT)

Graves' disease
Hypermetropia
Hypotony
Impacted cerumen
Intraocular lens (IOL)
Myopia
Oculus dexter (OD)
Oculus sinister (OS)
Oculus uterque (OU)

Otitis externa
Pineal gland
Pituitary gland
Presbyopia
Sclera
Thymus
Thyroid gland
Thyroid-stimulating
  hormone (TSH)

Thyroid storm
Tinnitus
Tympanic membrane

Learning Outcomes

After completing this chapter, you will be able to:

17.1 Review the anatomy of the eyes, ears, and endocrine system.

17.2 Understand the chapter-specific ICD guidelines and format for the eyes.

17.3 Comprehend the chapter-specific ICD guidelines and format for the ears.

17.4 Identify the guidelines and format of the eyes and ocular adnexa sections of CPT.

17.5 Recognize the guidelines and format of the ears and endocrine sections of CPT.

17.6 Apply the modifiers most commonly used with codes in the eyes, ears, and endocrine sections of CPT.

17.7 Examine the common medical and procedural terms used in operative reports.

Introduction

The eyes, ears, and endocrine system are included in the Nervous System section of the CPT manual. The endocrine system has a separate chapter in the ICD, and the guidelines for this chapter were discussed in Chapter 4 of this book. The eyes and ears are included in the Nervous System chapter of ICD-9-CM, and in ICD-10-CM they have been given separate chapters. To assign the appropriate codes for the eyes, ears, and endocrine system, a coder must be aware of the medical terminology, anatomy, and functions of each.

17.1 Anatomy of the Eyes, Ears, and Endocrine System

Eyes

The functions of the eyes are to receive and reflect light rays, which generate nerve impulses that are then transmitted to the brain via the optic nerve to become images or sight.

The structures of the eye and their functions are detailed in Table 17.1.

Path of Light

Cornea
↓
Aqueous humor of anterior chamber
↓
Pupil
↓
Vitreous humor of posterior chamber
↓
Retina
↓
Electrical signal or impulse
↓
Optic nerve
↓
Brain
↓
Image

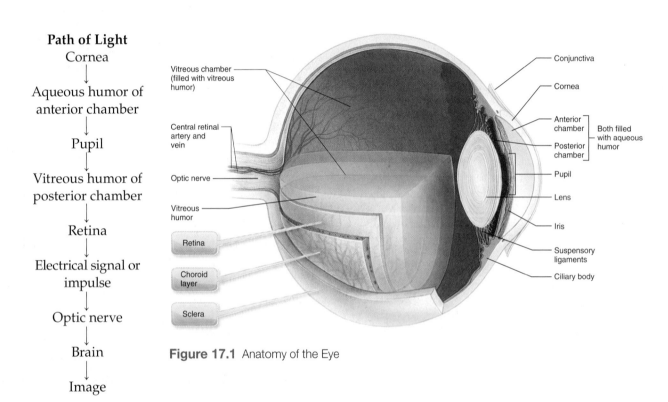

Figure 17.1 Anatomy of the Eye

sclera Structure that forms the visible white of the eye and surrounds the optic nerve.

Table 17.1 Structures of the Eye

STRUCTURE	DEFINITION/FUNCTION
Outer layer: **Sclera**	Forms the visible white of the eye and surrounds the optic nerve • Maintains the shape of the eyeball • Provides protection, since this is the hard surface of the eyeball
Cornea	Clear part of the eye that covers the pupil and iris. • Provides protection, acting as a shield for the iris and lens • Controls and focuses light entering the eye • Filters ultraviolet light
Conjunctiva	Mucous membrane lining the supporting structures of the eye and inner eyelids

Table 17.1 Structures of the Eye (*concluded*)

STRUCTURE	DEFINITION/FUNCTION
Middle layer:	
Choroid	Layer of blood vessels between the sclera and the retina • Provides nourishment to posterior areas of the eye
Iris	Colored portion of the eye between the cornea and the lens, forming the pupil
Pupil	Aperture that widens or narrows, controlling the amount of light that enters the eye
Lens	Located directly behind the cornea • Focuses light rays onto the retina
Ciliary body	Located between the iris and the choroid • Accommodates light • Produces the aqueous humor • Holds the lens in place
Inner layer:	
Retina	Sensory membrane lining the inner layer of the eye
Nerve cells	• Receive images • Convert images into signals sent through the optic nerve
Optic disc	Also known as the *optic nerve head*, junction of optic nerve and retina
Chambers:	
Anterior	Portion of the eye between the cornea and the lens and iris
Posterior	Portion of the eye between the iris and the lens

Ears

The main functions of the ears are to channel and convert sound into nerve impulses and maintain equilibrium, or balance.

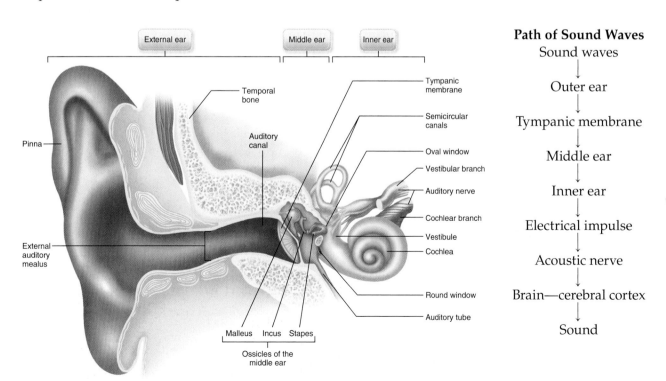

Path of Sound Waves

Sound waves
↓
Outer ear
↓
Tympanic membrane
↓
Middle ear
↓
Inner ear
↓
Electrical impulse
↓
Acoustic nerve
↓
Brain—cerebral cortex
↓
Sound

Figure 17.2 Anatomy of the Ear

Table 17.2 Structures of the Ear

STRUCTURE	DEFINITION/FUNCTION
External ear:	Focuses and directs sound to the inner auditory structures
Auricle	Also known as *pinna,* a funnel-like structure
	• Directs sound
External auditory canal	Also known as *external acoustic meatus*
	• Collects and transmits sound
Middle ear:	Begins the process of transmitting vibration to the inner ear
Tympanic membrane	Also known as *eardrum;* divides the external and middle ears
	• Converts sound to vibration
Ossicles	Amplify sound vibration from the tympanic membrane and relay it to the inner ear
	Include:
	• Malleus
	• Incus
	• Stapes
Eustachian tubes	Connect the middle ear to the nasopharynx
	• Equalize pressure
	• Drain mucus from the middle ear
Oval window	Transmits vibration from the stapes to the cochlea
	• Divides the middle and inner ears
Inner ear:	Transmits sound waves to the brain and maintains balance
Vestibule	Made up of three parts: the semicircular canals, utricle, and saccule
	• Maintains balance
	• Maintains equilibrium
Cochlea	Contains hairlike structures and lymphatic fluid (endolymph and perilymph), which aid in transforming sound vibrations to the auditory nerve

tympanic membrane Structure that divides the external and middle ears and converts sound to vibration Also called *eardrum.*

The main structures of the ear and their functions are detailed in Table 17.2.

Endocrine System

The main function of the endocrine system is to release hormones (chemicals) into the body through the bloodstream. The pancreas, testes, and ovaries also function in the endocrine system and have been discussed in earlier chapters.

The main structures of the endocrine system and their functions are detailed in Table 17.3.

Table 17.3 Structures of the Endocrine System

STRUCTURE	DEFINITION/FUNCTION
Pituitary gland	Also known as the *master gland* as it directs other endocrine glands; located near the brainstem
	• Produces growth hormone
	• Produces hormones that act upon muscles, kidneys, or other endocrine glands
	• Regulates endocrine function
	• Stores hormones produced by the hypothalamus

Table 17.3 Structures of the Endocrine System (*concluded*)

STRUCTURE	DEFINITION/FUNCTION
Pituitary gland	Hormones produced by this gland include: • Prolactin • Adrenocorticotropic hormone (ACTH) • Growth hormone (GH) • Thyroid-stimulating hormone (TSH) • Follicle-stimulating hormone (FSH) • Luteinizing hormone (LH) • Antidiuretic hormone (ADH) • Oxytocin
Pineal gland	Located near the brainstem; involved in body functions: • Influences sleep rhythms • Regulates endocrine functions • Converts nervous system signals to endocrine signals • Influences sexual development Hormones produced by this gland include: • Melatonin
Thyroid gland	Butterfly-shaped gland located low on the anterior side of the trachea • Regulates metabolism • Affects growth and development • Regulates body temperature • Influences brain development in childhood Hormones produced by this gland include: • Thyroxine (T_4) • Triiodothyronine (T_3) • Calcitonin
Parathyroid gland	Located near the thyroid gland • Controls blood levels of calcium Hormone produced by this gland: • Parathyroid hormone (PTH)
Thymus	Located in the mediastinum just behind the upper portion of the sternum • Produces and develops T cells Hormones produced by this gland include: • Thymosin • Thymopoietin • Serum thymic factor

pituitary gland Gland that is located near the brainstem and directs other endocrine glands. Also called *master gland*.

pineal gland Gland that is located near the brainstem and is involved in regulation of body functions (e.g., sleep rhythms and endocrine functions).

thyroid gland Butterfly-shaped gland, located low on the anterior side of the trachea, that influences growth and development, body temperature, and metabolism.

thymus Gland that is located in the mediastinum, just behind the upper portion of the sternum, and produces and develops T cells.

1. Explain the pathway of light.
2. Explain the path of sound waves.
3. List the structures of the endocrine system.
4. Identify the location of the tympanic membrane, and explain its function.
5. Which endocrine gland produces the hormone melatonin?

EXERCISE 17.1

Also available in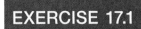

Table 17.4 Eyes Subsection Format *(Data from ICD-9-CM and ICD-10-CM, Centers for Medicare and Medicaid Services and the National Center for Health Statistics.)*

ICD-9-CM		ICD-10-CM	
SUBHEADING	**CODE RANGE**	**SUBHEADING**	**CODE RANGE**
Disorders of the Eye and Adnexa	360–379	Disorders of Eyelid, Lacrimal System, and Orbit	H00–H05
		Disorders of Conjunctiva	H10–H11
		Disorders of Sclera, Cornea, Iris, and Ciliary Body	H15–H22
		Disorders of Choroid and Retina	H30–H36
		Glaucoma	H40–H42
		Disorders of Vitreous Body and Globe	H43–H44
		Disorders of Optic Nerve and Visual Pathways	H46–H47
		Disorders of Ocular Muscles, Binocular Movement, Accommodation, and Refraction	H49–H52
		Visual Disturbances and Blindness	H53–H54
		Intraoperative and Postprocedural Complications and Disorders of Eye and Adnexa, Not Elsewhere Classified	H59

17.2 Chapter-Specific ICD Guidelines and Format for the Eyes

ICD-9-CM codes for conditions related to the eye and its supporting structures are listed in only one section in the Diseases of the Nervous System and Sense Organ chapter. This large section has become a separate chapter in ICD-10-CM. Table 17.4 lists the relevant subheadings and their code ranges.

Disorders of the Eye and Adnexa (360–379), ICD-9-CM
Diseases of the Eye and Adnexa (H00–H59), ICD-10-CM

Conditions related to disorders of the globe, category 360, include disorders and diseases that affect multiple structures of the eye. Conditions listed in this category include:

- Purulent and other endophthalmitis, 360.00–360.19 (H44.00–H44.19, ICD-10-CM)
- Degeneration of the globe, 360.20–360.29 (H44.20–H44.399, ICD-10-CM)
- **Hypotony** of the eye (low intraocular pressure), 360.30–360.34 (H44.40–H44.44, ICD-10-CM)
- Various degenerated conditions of the globe, 360.40–360.44 (H44.50–H44.539, ICD-10-CM)
- Magnetic and nonmagnetic retained foreign bodies, 360.50–360.69 (H44.60–H44.799, ICD-10-CM)
- Luxation of the eye, 360.81 (H44.821–H44.829, ICD-10-CM)

Retinal detachments and retinal defects are classified to category 361 (H33–H34, ICD-10-CM). Retinal detachment conditions are divided by the nature or type of detachment, such as with retinal defects, retinoschisis and retinal cysts, and serous. The codes are further defined by age of the detachment, partial or total, and number or type of defect.

Category 362 (H35, ICD-10-CM), "Other retinal disorders," includes retinopathy due to underlying conditions such as hypertension, 362.11, and diabetes, 362.0- (H35.2-, ICD-10-CM). Diabetic retinopathy is further defined as

hypotony Low intraocular pressure.

proliferative or nonproliferative, and the severity of nonproliferative diabetic retinopathy is defined as mild, moderate, or severe.

Other conditions included in category 362 are:

- Retinal vascular occlusion, 362.3- (H34, ICD-10-CM)
- Separation of retinal layers, 362.4- (H35.7-, ICD-10-CM)
- Degeneration of macula and posterior pole, 362.5 (H35.3-, ICD-10-CM)
- Peripheral retinal degenerations, 362.6- (H35.4-, ICD-10-CM)
- Hereditary retinal dystrophies, 362.7- (H35.5-, ICD-10-CM)

Disorders of the iris and ciliary body are listed under category 364 (H20, ICD-10-CM). Iridocyclitis is primarily divided based on acuity as either acute/subacute, 364.0- (H20.0-, ICD-10-CM), or chronic, 364.1- (H20.1-, ICD-10-CM). Acute/subacute iridocyclitis is subclassified based on the type of iridocyclitis: primary, recurrent, secondary due to infection, or not due to infection.

Other conditions listed in this category include:

- Specified types of iridocyclitis, 364.2- (H20.8-, ICD-10-CM)
- Vascular disorder of the iris and ciliary body, 364.4- (H21.1-, ICD-10-CM)
- Degeneration of the iris and ciliary body, 364.5- (H21.2-, ICD-10-CM)
- Cysts of the iris, ciliary body, and anterior chamber, 364.6- (H21.3-, ICD-10-CM)
- Adhesions and disruptions of the iris and ciliary body, 364.7- (H21.5-, ICD-10-CM)

The various types of glaucoma are category 365 (H40–H42, ICD-10-CM). This category is subcategorized based on the type or underlying cause of the condition. Codes are further defined within each subcategory by anatomical disorder, acuity or severity of the condition, stage, or associated anomalies or disorders.

Cataracts are a clouding of the lens of the eye or the lens capsule that envelopes the lens. Coded to category 366 (H25, ICD-10-CM) are several different types of cataracts that may occur as early as infancy but are predominantly conditions found in the elderly. Cataract conditions are divided by the type or underlying cause of the condition: presenile, senile, traumatic, secondary or complicated (due to underlying disease or radiation therapy), and after-cataract (cataract of posterior capsule). Codes are further defined within each category based on the location, or zone, of the cataract within the lens: anterior, posterior, or nuclear.

cataracts A clouding of the lens of the eye or the lens capsule, which envelopes the lens.

glaucoma Condition that develops when pressure builds within the eye due to an increase in fluid and leads to damage of the optic nerve.

SPOTLIGHT on Condition

Open-angle glaucoma Fluid does not flow through the trabecular meshwork properly.

Closed-angle glaucoma The angle between the iris and the cornea is too narrow, or the iris dilates too widely, closing the angle. This may be documented as *narrow-angle glaucoma*.

SPOTLIGHT on Condition

The types of cataracts include:

Congenital Occurs at or prior to birth and may or may not affect vision significantly enough to require surgery.

Age-related, or senile Typically occurs in patients over 70 years of age, but may develop as early as 40 or 50 years of age.

Secondary May develop after surgical procedures on the eye or due to an underlying condition such as diabetes or the prolonged use of medications such as steroids.

Traumatic Develops due to a direct injury to the eye, typically from blunt trauma or exposure to certain chemicals.

Category 367 identifies disorders of refraction and accommodation—the eyes' inability to focus on an object due to a disorder of the lens. This category lists codes for conditions such as **hypermetropia, also known as hyperopia** (farsightedness), 367.0 (H52.0-, ICD-10-CM), **myopia** (nearsightedness), 367.1 (H52.1-, ICD-10-CM), and **presbyopia** (errors in ability to focus due to age), 367.4 (H52.4, ICD-10-CM).

Visual disturbances such as amblyopia (lazy eye), 368.0- (H53.0, ICD-10-CM), diplopia (double vision), 368.2 (H53.2, ICD-10-CM), and color vision deficiencies (color blindness), 368.5- (H53.5-, ICD-10-CM), are included in category 368. A common condition included in this category is visual discomfort, which includes eye strain, 368.13 (H53.10, ICD-10-CM).

The various forms of blindness and visual impairment are included in category 369. The conditions listed within this category are primarily divided based on the level of impairment and whether one or both eyes are affected. Codes within each subcategory are further defined by the degree of impairment for each eye within a specific level of impairment.

FOR EXAMPLE A patient has 20/600 vision (profound impairment) of the right eye and 20/1100 vision (near-total) impairment of the left eye. This condition is assigned code 369.07 (H54.1, ICD-10-CM). ▪

ICD provides a table that breaks down the levels of impairment based on the patient's visual acuity. Note that visual acuity in this table is measured by the patient's best achievable acuity with correction. The visual acuity table includes seven levels of visual acuity, and although five levels of impairment are listed on the table, only three are included as a subcategory breakdown: Profound, moderate, and severe with near-total and total impairment are included at the code level with each of these subcategories. When coding from this category, first identify the level of visual acuity and/or impairment for each eye, and then select the code that meets the level of acuity for each eye. If both eyes are impaired at any level, use subcategories 369.0, 369.1, and 369.2 to code the condition. If one of the eyes is at normal or near-normal acuity, use codes from subcategory 369.6 or 369.7.

Categories 370 and 371 list conditions and disorders related to the cornea. Category 370 includes conditions involving inflammation of the cornea and is primarily divided as keratitis with or without conjunctivitis. Each subcategory is further defined based on the specific type of keratitis.

MENTOR
Coding Tip

Add the right-side column of Table 17.5 to the ICD manual visual acuity table to aid in selecting the correct subcategory before coding the condition.

Table 17.5 Visual Impairment Subcategories *(Data from ICD-9-CM and ICD-10-CM, Centers for Medicare and Medicaid Services and the National Center for Health Statistics.)*

LEVELS OF VISUAL IMPAIRMENT	ICD SUBCATEGORY
Moderate	369.1, one eye of lesser acuity
Severe	369.2, both eyes at this level of acuity
Profound	369.7, one eye of better visual acuity
Near-total	369.0, both eyes at this level of acuity or one at a lesser visual acuity
	369.6, one eye with better visual acuity
Total	369.00 Blindness based upon WHO definition

Conditions that affect the cornea's ability to refract light onto the lens are categorized to 371 and are defined by the nature of the condition affecting the cornea, such as corneal scars, 371.0- (H17.8-, ICD-10-CM), corneal edema, 371.2- (H18.2-, ICD-10-CM), and degeneration of the cornea 371.4- (H18.4-, ICD-10-CM). This category is primarily defined by the cause of the corneal disorder. Each code further defines the condition within the subcategory or the portion of the cornea affected by the specific condition.

FOR EXAMPLE Subcategory 371.1, corneal pigmentations and deposits, is subdivided by the location of the deposits on the cornea. ■

Acute conjunctivitis may be due to bacteria, viruses, chlamydiae, or atopic allergies and is coded to subcategory 372.0. Chronic conjunctivitis, coded to subcategory 372.1, involves persistent inflammation of the conjunctiva with acute exacerbations. Other types of conjunctivitis coded to category 372 include pterygium, 372.4- (H11.00-, ICD-10-CM), conjunctival degenerations and deposits, 372.5- (H11.1-, ICD-10-CM), conjunctival scars, 372.6- (H11.2, ICD-10-CM), and conjunctival vascular disorders and cysts, 372.7- (H11.4-, ICD-10-CM).

Disorders of the eyelid are coded to category 373, while category 374 includes other disorders such as entropion, 374.0- (H02.0-, ICD-10-CM), ectropion, 374.1- (H02.1-, ICD-10-CM), and ptosis, 374.3- (H02.4-, ICD-10-CM).

Noncongenital disorders, inflammation, and changes of the lacrimal system are found in category 375. Common conditions included in this category are dacryoadenitis, acute and chronic, 375.0- (H04.0-, ICD-10-CM), and stenosis of the lacrimal passages, 375.5- (H04.5-, ICD-10-CM).

"Disorders of the orbit," category 376, list conditions affecting the orbits, the supporting structures of the eye. The conditions within this category are primarily divided based on the nature of the condition affecting the orbit. Each condition is then further classified based on the location of the condition in the orbit or the underlying cause of the condition.

Category 377 classifies disorders affecting the optic nerve and visual pathways. The conditions within category 377 are first divided based on the condition leading to the optic nerve disorder, and they include papilledema, 377.0- (H47.1-, ICD-10-CM), atrophy, 377.1 (H47.20-, ICD-10-CM), optic disc disorders, 377.2- (H47.3-, ICD-10-CM), and neuritis 377.3-. Disorders of the optic nerve pathway are divided by location along the neural pathway: optic chiasm, 377.5 (H47.4-, ICD-10-CM), and visual cortex, 377.7 (H47.6-, ICD-10-CM).

Strabismus is a condition of the muscles of the eye that affects the ability of both eyes to point in the same direction, thus affecting the person's depth perception. (See Figure 17.3) The codes are classified based on whether one (mono) or both eyes are deviating from the axis and on the pattern of deviation. The various forms of strabismus are coded to category 378 (H50.-, ICD-10-CM).

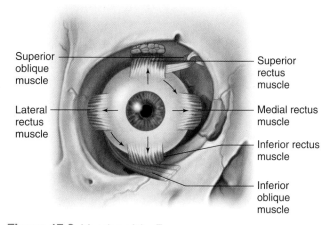

Figure 17.3 Muscles of the Eye

Strabismus is defined by the direction of the eye deviating off the axis:

Hypertropia Eye turns upward.

Hypotropia Eye turns downward.

Esotropia Eye turns inward.

Exotropia Eye turns outward.

The last category of conditions related to the eye includes various conditions not included in the other categories, such as:

- Scleritis, 379.0- (H15.00-, ICD-10-CM)
- Scleral disorders, 379.1- (H15.8-, ICD-10-CM)
- Vitreous fluid disorders, 379.2 (H43.81-, ICD-10-CM)
- Displacement of the lens, 379.3 (H27.0-, ICD-10-CM)
- Nystagmus 379.5- (H55.00-, ICD-10-CM)

EXERCISE 17.2

1. List the types of cataracts.
2. Define the two main types of glaucoma.
3. What is the subclassification for acute/subacute iridocyclitis based on?

Also available in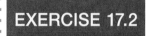

17.3 Chapter-Specific ICD Guidelines and Format for the Ears

Categories within this section are subdivided by the anatomical sites of the ear, beginning with the external ear and ending with the hearing loss due to sensorineural or conductive disorders. Table 17.6 lists the relevant subheadings and their code ranges.

Table 17.6 Ears Subsection Format *(Data from ICD-9-CM and ICD-10-CM, Centers for Medicare and Medicaid Services and the National Center for Health Statistics.)*

ICD-9-CM		ICD-10-CM	
SUBHEADING	CODE RANGE	SUBHEADING	CODE RANGE
Diseases of the Ear and Mastoid Process	380–389	Diseases of the External Ear	H60–H62
		Diseases of the Middle Ear and Mastoid	H65–H75
		Diseases of the Inner Ear	H80–H83
		Intraoperative and Postprocedural Complications and Disorders of Ear and Mastoid Process, Not Elsewhere Classified	H95

Diseases of the Ear (380–389), ICD-9-CM
Diseases of the Ear (H60–H95), ICD-10-CM

Category 380 begins conditions of the ear with perichondritis of the pinna, 380.0- (H61.0-, ICD-10-CM) and is further divided based on acuity of the condition as acute or chronic. Chondritis of the pinna, inflammation of the cartilage of the outer shell of the ear, is coded to one classification within this subcategory, 380.03 (H61.0-, ICD-10-CM).

Another condition listed in this category is **otitis externa,** 380.1–380.2 (H62.4-, ICD-10-CM). Otitis externa is an infection or inflammation that extends into the cartilage of the ear, and ICD subcategories are primarily divided into infectious and noninfectious forms of otitis externa. Conditions included in each of these subcategories are classified by the underlying cause or nature of the condition.

Otitis media is coded to categories 381 and 382 (H65–H66, ICD-10-CM). ICD categorizes otitis media as nonsuppurative, 381(H65, ICD-10-CM), and suppurative, 382 (H66, ICD-10-CM). Each of these categories is further divided based on acuity of the condition as acute or chronic. Nonsuppurative conditions are further classified based on the type: serous, mucoid, or sanguinous. Suppurative conditions are classified as acute or chronic. Acute suppurative codes are further defined based on a rupture of the eardrum, and chronic suppurative codes are further defined based on the structures affected or the location of the condition in relation to the tympanic membrane.

otitis externa Inflammation of the external ear canal. Also called *swimmer's ear.*

FOR EXAMPLE

Chronic infection of the tympanic cavity and auditory tube, 382.1 ▣

Infections, inflammations, and complications of mastoidectomy are grouped in category 383. Infections and inflammations of the mastoid are primarily divided as acute and chronic conditions. Complications following mastoidectomy are classified by the nature of the complication, such as mucosal cyst, 383.31 (H95.13-, ICD-10-CM), cholesteatoma, 383.32 (H95.0-, ICD-10-CM), and granulations, 383.33 (H95.12-, ICD-10-CM).

Disorders of the tympanic membrane not related or due to otitis media are listed in category 384 and include conditions such as acute and chronic myringitis, 384.0 and 384.1 (H73-, ICD-10-CM), and atrophy, both flaccid, 384.81 (H73.81-, ICD-10-CM), and nonflaccid, 384.82 (H73.82-, ICD-10-CM). Also listed in this category are residual conditions due to perforation injuries of the tympanic membrane, 384.2- (H72-, ICD-10-CM).

Category 385 lists various other conditions of the middle ear that are not classified elsewhere in this section. It includes conditions such as sclerosis of the tympanic membrane, 385.0- (H74.0, ICD-10-CM), adhesions, 385.1- (H74.1-, ICD-10-CM), abnormalities of the bones of the middle ear (ossicles), 385.2- (H74.3-, ICD-10-CM), and cholesteatomas, 385.3- (H71.0-, ICD-10-CM).

Disorders, diseases, and syndromes affecting the areas of the ear responsible for balance are grouped in category 386. This category includes subcategories for Ménière's disease, 386.0 (H81.0-, ICD-10-CM), labyrinthitis, 386.3 (H83.0, ICD-10-CM), labyrinthine fistulas, 386.4- (H83.1-, ICD-10-CM), and labyrinthine dysfunctions, 386.5- (H83.2-, ICD-10-CM).

Other common disorders of the ear include **tinnitus** (abnormal noises in the ear), which may be subjective, 388.31 (H93.1-, ICD-10-CM), or objective, 388.32 (H93.19, ICD-10-CM); disorders of the acoustic nerve, 388.5 (H93.3-, ICD-10-CM); and ear pain or otalgia, 388.7- (H92.0-, ICD-10-CM).

tinnitus A sensation of ringing in the ears.

Tinnitus may produce ringing, clicking, or a buzzing sound, which may be objective or subjective:

Subjective tinnitus Abnormal sounds within the ear are audible only to the patient.

Objective tinnitus Abnormal sounds within the ear are audible to others as well as the patient.

Hearing loss is coded to category 389. The conditions of hearing loss are subdivided based on the type of loss: conductive, 389.0 (H90.-, ICD-10-CM), sensorineural, 389.1- (H90.3-, ICD-10-CM), or a combination of sensorineural and conductive, 389.2 (H90.6-, ICD-10-CM). Conductive hearing loss is further classified by the location of the dysfunction leading to the loss. Sensorineural hearing loss is further defined based on laterality of the loss.

EXERCISE 17.3

1. Identify the further differentiations of nonsuppurative and suppurative conditions of otitis media.
2. Hearing loss is coded to category 389. Define the further subclassifications of hearing loss.
3. Further define the subcategories used to assign codes for otitis externa.

Also available in **connect** (plus+)

17.4 Guidelines and Format of the Eyes and Ocular Adnexa Subsections of CPT

Eyes and Ocular Adnexa Subsection General Heading Code Range (65091–68899)

The general headings and code ranges are listed in Table 17.7.

Eyeball (65091–65290)

Removal of Eye: 65091–65114

Removal of the eyeball is coded based on how much of the eyeball and orbital structures is removed with the eye. Understanding the terms used to describe each of the procedures is needed to select the correct procedure code.

Table 17.7 Eyes and Ocular Adnexa General Headings and Code Ranges *(Data from CPT 2013. © 2013 American Medical Association. All rights reserved.)*

HEADING	CODE RANGE
Eyeball	65091–65290
Anterior Segment	65400–66999
Posterior Segment	67005–67299
Ocular Adnexa	67311–67999
Conjunctiva	68020–68899

Evisceration Removal of the contents within the eye, leaving the scleral shell intact.

Enucleation Removal of the eyeball in total by cutting it free of the extraocular muscles and the optic nerve.

Exenteration Removal of the eyeball and orbital support structure, with or with orbital bone.

The codes for both evisceration and enucleation of the eye are based on the use of an implant during the removal procedure (primary). Codes for enucleation with primary ocular implants are further clarified by the attachment of the implant to the extraocular muscles (65105).

CPT divides the codes for exenteration of the orbit by the extent of the procedure: contents only, with necessary removal of bone (65112) and removal of muscle (65114).

Secondary Implant(s) Procedures: 65125–65175

A secondary ocular implant is defined as an implant placed at a later time than the removal of the eyeball. CPT provides four primary choices for this procedure: modification of an existing implant (65125), insertion either within the scleral shell or with or without muscles attachment (65130–65140), reinsertion with or without graft or reinforcement/attachment (65150–65155), and removal of a previously placed implant (65175).

Removal of Foreign Body: 65205–65265

Removals of foreign bodies of the eye are divided based on the location of the foreign body: external/conjunctival (65205–65210), corneal with or without slit lamp (65220–65222), and anterior or posterior intraocular (65235–65265). CPT further divides the codes for removal of a foreign body of the posterior segment by the material of the foreign body: magnetic (65260) or nonmagnetic (65265).

Repair of Laceration: 65270–65290

Under the subheading for laceration repairs of the eyeball, the codes are first divided based on the anatomical site of the laceration. The sites include the conjunctiva, cornea, and extraocular muscle, tendon, or Tenon's capsule. Conjunctival laceration repair codes are further defined by type of repair and hospitalization of the patient (65270–65273).

Anterior Segment (65400–66999)

Cornea: 65400–65782

Procedures performed on the cornea include excision or biopsy (65400–65426), mechanical (scraping) or chemical removal of the cornea (65430–65436), and destruction of corneal lesions (65450).

Keratoplasty, also known as a *corneal transplant,* is divided by CPT based on the thickness of the donor graft or the portion of the cornea grafted to the donor's eye, such as the endothelial disc (65756). Penetrating keratoplasties are further specified by CPT by the presence of a natural lens (65730), the absence of a lens (65750), and an artificial lens (65755).

Other procedures performed on the cornea include those to alter its shape to change its refraction and improve visual acuity (65760–65771), correct surgically induced astigmatism (65772–65775), and repair and reconstruction of the ocular surface (65778–65782).

Anterior Chamber: 65800–66030; Anterior Sclera: 66130–66250; Iris, Ciliary Body: 66500–66770

Many of the procedures performed to reduce intraocular pressure or improve the flow of vitreous fluid within the eye are listed under the subheadings Anterior Chamber, Anterior Sclera, or Iris, Ciliary Body.

Included under the Anterior Chamber subheading is monotony (65820), which may also be documented as a *divinities* or *barman's operation* and involves the use of a gonio-knife to open the angle of the trabecular meshwork. Other procedures that improve intraocular pressure by altering the trabecular meshwork include trabeculotomy ab externo (65850) and trabeculoplasty (65885).

Intraocular pressure may also be reduced through the sclera by placement or revision of an aqueous shunt (66180–66185) or trabeculectomy ab externo performed through the anterior portion of the sclera (66170–66172).

Improving vitreous flow to treat glaucoma may be done by excisional iridectomy (66625–66630), laser iridotomy/iridectomy (66761), or photocoagulation of the iris (66762).

Lens: 66820–66940

The most common procedure performed on the lens of the human eye is a cataract extraction. The catacerous lens is removed and a prosthesis inserted in its place, either at the time of the extraction or at a later time.

CPT provides separate subheadings for removal of the lens: alone (66840–66940) or with concurrent intraocular lens (IOL) prosthesis insertion during lens extraction (66982–66984).

Secondary cataracts, also known as *secondary membranous cataracts,* are corrected by creating an opening in the posterior lens capsule, allowing the image and light captured by the lens to be refracted onto the posterior segment of the eye. Creating this opening can be completed by incision (66820), by laser (66821), or with corneoscleral section (66830).

Intraocular Lens Procedures: 66982–66986

Codes for cataract lens procedures are further divided based on the method of lens removal and the complexity. A complex cataract removal as described in CPT 66982 requires additional work or devices to open the iris, such as expansion devices or sutures to enlarge and maintain the pupil's opening during the procedure.

Posterior Segment (67005–67255)

Procedures performed on the posterior segment include procedures for treatment of vitreous fluid conditions (67005–67043). Also included under this heading are procedures performed on the retina or choroid, primarily procedures for the correction of retinal detachment. The codes for repairs of retinal detachments are divided based on the method of repair and the complexity of the condition. Methods include photocoagulation (67101–67105), scleral buckling (67107–67112), and multiple-session cryotherapy or diathermy (67141) or photocoagulation (67145).

Ocular Adnexa (67311–67999)

Extraocular Muscles: 67311–67346

Strabismus surgery is performed to correct alignment of the eye muscles. CPT divides strabismus surgery by the extraocular muscle (horizontal, vertical, or oblique) altered and the number altered (67311–67318). Add-on codes are provided to identify instances in which the procedure performed is slightly altered from the norm or the patient's condition or previous surgery complicate the primary procedure.

Orbit: 67400–67599

Procedures performed on the orbit are grouped into two primary categories; those completed without a bone flap (67400–67414) and those requiring a bone flap (67420–67450). Procedures listed within each of these groupings include drainage, removal of a foreign body, decompression, and removal of a lesion.

Eyelids: 67700–67999

Blepharotomy for drainage of an abscess is assigned a code within the Incision subheading.

If the removal of a lesion involved mainly the skin of the eyelid, the coder is directed by an instructional note in the excision and destruction code range to assign codes from the Integumentary section of CPT.

To assign the accurate code from the excision and destruction code range, the coder needs to be able to identify the following information from the medical record:

- Single lesion
- Multiple lesions, same lid; multiple lesions, different lids
- General anesthesia requiring hospitalization

FOR EXAMPLE CPT code 67808 is reported for excision of a chalazion (small cyst in the eyelid caused by blockage of a small oil gland) under general anesthesia and/or requiring hospitalization, single or multiple. ■

Destruction of a lesion of the eyelid margin is also coded in this code range. An instructional note included with the destruction code directs the use of codes 17311to 17315 if Mohs micrographic surgery is performed.

CPT code range 67900–67999 contains codes assigned for various repair procedures. To assign the appropriate code from this range, a coder must answer the following questions:

- What was done (repair, reduction, or correction)?
- What condition was repaired, reduced, or corrected (brow ptosis, blepharoptosis, ectropion, or entropion)?

Conjunctiva: 68020–68899

Drainage of a cyst and expression of follicles are examples of procedures assigned codes under the Incision subheading.

Biopsy, excision, and destruction procedures involving the conjunctiva are within code range 68100–68135. The excision codes are dependent on the size of the lesion and whether the adjacent sclera was involved.

MENTOR
Coding Tip

Highlight the instructional note at the beginning of this subsection that directs the use of CPT code 65205 if a foreign body is removed.

Codes within the range 68320–68340 are used to report various conjunctivo-plasty procedures and are grouped first based on the location of the repair: buccal mucous membrane, cul-de-sac, and symblepharon. The codes within each of these groupings are then defined by the extent of the repair and the type of graft used to complete the repair.

Incision, excision, and repair procedures involving the lacrimal system are assigned codes from CPT code range 68400–68770.

EXERCISE 17.4

1. Removal of the eyeball is coded based on how much of the eyeball and orbital structures is removed with the eye. Define the terms *evisceration, enucleation,* and *exenteration.*

2. Under the subheading for laceration repairs of the eyeball, the codes are first divided based on the anatomical site of the lacerations. What are these anatomical sites, and how are the laceration repair codes further defined?

3. To accurately code a keratoplasty, what must the coder be able to determine from the medical record?

4. Describe a monotony. How else might it be described in a provider's documentation?

Also available in **connect** (plus+)

17.5 Guidelines and Format of the Ears and Endocrine Subsections of CPT

Auditory System Subsection General Heading Code Ranges (69000–69979)

The general headings and code ranges are listed in Table 17.8.

External Ear (69000–69399)

Abscess drainage and ear piercing are procedures assigned codes under the Incision subheading.

Excision: 69100–69155

Biopsies of either the external ear or the auditory canal have codes under this subheading.

Excisions of either the external ear or the auditory canal are included in this code range and are further defined by whether they are with or without neck dissection and are partial or complete amputations.

Table 17.8 Ears General Headings and Code Ranges *(Data from CPT 2013. © 2013 American Medical Association. All rights reserved.)*

HEADING	CODE RANGE
External Ear	69000–69399
Middle Ear	69400–69799
Inner Ear	69801–69949
Temporal Bone, Middle Fossa Approach	69950–69979

An excision of the external ear with complete amputation is assigned CPT code 69120. ▪

Removal: 69200–69222

Removal of a foreign body from the external auditory canal is included under this subheading. To accurately assign the code, a coder must know whether the procedure was performed with or without general anesthesia. There is a separate code for removal of **impacted cerumen** (earwax lodged within the auditory canal), CPT code 69210.

impacted cerumen An accumulation of earwax.

Repair: 69300–69320

At the beginning of this code range, there is an instructional note guiding the coder to codes in the Integumentary System section, 12011 and 14302, if the repair is a suture of a wound of the external ear.

Middle Ear (69400–69799)

The middle-ear anatomy is shown in Figure 17.4.

Introduction: 69400–69405

Introduction of the eustachian tube is within this code range and is further defined by the type of approach, such as transnasal or transtympanic, and with or without catheterization.

Incision: 69420–69450

Included in this code range is performance of a myringotomy, a procedure in which an incision is made into the tympanic membrane to gain access to the middle ear, thereby allowing middle ear fluid to be aspirated.

Often a ventilation tube is placed to allow draining of the middle-ear fluid. The codes in this section for this procedure are further defined as to the use of general anesthesia.

A myringotomy including aspiration and/or eustachian tube inflation requiring general anesthesia is assigned CPT code 69421. ▪

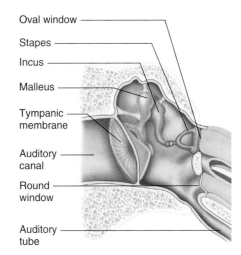

Oval window
Stapes
Incus
Malleus
Tympanic membrane
Auditory canal
Round window
Auditory tube

Figure 17.4 Anatomy of Middle Ear

A tympanostomy (see Figure 17.5) requiring the insertion of ventilating tubes is also coded using codes from this range. The coder will need to know whether local, or topical, anesthesia or general anesthesia was used for the procedure.

Excision: 69501–69554

A mastoidectomy is performed to remove infections or growths in the mastoid bone located behind the ear. Indications for this procedure could be mastoiditis, usually not responding to treatment with antibiotics, or cholesteatoma. The mastoidectomy codes, 69502–69511, are further defined as complete, modified radical (some middle-ear bones are left in place and the eardrum is rebuilt), or radical (most of the bone is removed).

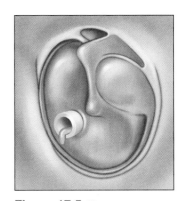

Figure 17.5 Tympanostomy

Repair: 69601–69676

Revision of a mastoidectomy is assigned codes under this subheading and is further defined by whether the revision results in complete, modified radical, or radical mastoidectomy or in tympanoplasty.

FOR EXAMPLE A revision of a mastoidectomy that results in tympanoplasty is assigned CPT code 69604. ■

Repair procedures of the stapes and oval window are also reported using codes from this subheading.

Inner Ear (69801–69949)

Incision and/or Destruction: 69801–69840

Labyrinthotomy is reported as code 69801 and with mastoidectomy as code 69802. If a labyrinthectomy is performed, code 69905 is reported.

Introduction: 69930

A cochlear device implant with or without mastoidectomy is assigned code 69930.

Operating Microscope (69990)

The description for this code is "microsurgical technique requiring use of operating microscope." This code is an add-on code, as designated by the + sign in front of the code, and must be reported in addition to the primary procedure. Many of the surgical codes have the use of an operating microscope as part of the code description, and therefore the use of 69990 as a separate code would not be appropriate.

MENTOR Coding Tip

Many coders find it useful to highlight the list of codes and code ranges located beneath CPT code 69990 as a reminder of the codes that include the use of an operating microscope in their description.

Endocrine System Subsection General Heading Code Ranges (60000–60281)

The headings and code ranges are listed in Table 17.9.

Thyroid Gland (60000–60699)

Incision/Excision: 60000–60281

Incision and drainage (I&D) of an infected thyroglossal duct cyst, code 60000, is included in this code range. This is the only incision code for the thyroid gland.

Table 17.9 Endocrine System General Headings and Code Ranges *(Data from CPT 2013. © 2013 American Medical Association. All rights reserved.)*

HEADING	CODE RANGE
Thyroid Gland	60000–60300
Parathyroid Gland, Thymus, Adrenal Glands, Pancreas, and Carotid Body	60500–60699

An instructional note below this code directs the coder to use codes from the General section (located just before the Integumentary section) if a fine-needle aspiration was performed. The notes also states the codes to be reported if imaging guidance is performed.

Also included in this range are several excision codes, 60100 to 60281. The thyroidectomy codes are further defined by the following:

- Partial or total thyroid lobectomy, with or without isthmusectomy.
- Thyroidectomy for malignancy with limited neck dissection or with radical neck dissection.
- Thyroidectomy with removal of all remaining thyroid tissue following a previous removal of a portion of the thyroid.
- Thyroidectomy, transthoracic or cervical approach. See Figure 17.6.

To assign the accurate code from this code range, coders must be able to read the operative report and decide from the documentation exactly what procedure was accomplished, what the approach was, and why the procedure was performed.

Parathyroid, Thymus, Adrenal Glands, Pancreas, and Carotid Body (60500–60699)
Excision: 60500–60605

The codes under this subheading all encompass excision. Some of the codes are further defined as exploration or reexploration. The excision codes for a thymectomy or an adrenalectomy are defined as partial or complete. If an adrenalectomy is done by a laparoscopic approach, the appropriate code is 60650. See Figure 17.7.

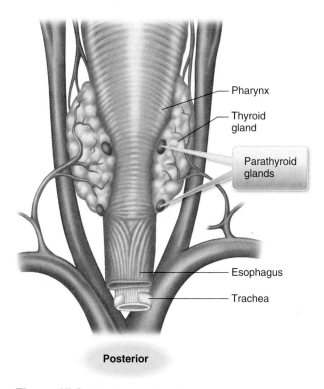

Figure 17.6 Thyroid and Parathyroids

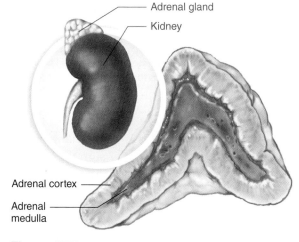

Figure 17.7 Adrenal Cortex and Adrenal Medulla

1. Would it be appropriate to append modifier 50 to CPT code 69210 when impacted cerumen is removed from both ears?
2. What must a coder be able to determine from the provider documentation in order to assign the correct code for a thyroidectomy?
3. Explain the difference between a modified radical mastoidectomy and a radical mastoidectomy.

Also available in McGraw Hill **connect** (plus+)

17.6 Modifiers Most Commonly Used with Codes in the Eyes, Ears, and Endocrine Subsections of CPT

As with all sections of the CPT manual, modifiers are used in the Eyes, Ears, and Endocrine sections to continue or modify the story of the patient's encounter. Some of the more common modifiers used within these sections are 50, bilateral procedure; 51, multiple procedures; and 62, two surgeons. There are several instructional notes throughout these sections directing the use of modifier 50 if the procedure described was performed bilaterally. (See Table 17.10.)

The appropriate use of modifiers with the codes from the relevant subsection helps to tell the patient's full story.

Table 17.10 Eyes, Ears, and Endocrine Section Modifiers *(Data from CPT 2013. © 2013 American Medical Association. All rights reserved.)*

MODIFIER	DEFINITION	EXAMPLE OF USE
50	Bilateral procedure	A tympanostomy (requiring insertion of a ventilating tube), with local or topical anesthesia, that is performed on both ears is assigned code 69433 with modifier 50 appended.
		If probing of a nasolacrimal duct, with or without irrigation, is performed bilaterally, it is assigned code 68810 with modifier 50 appended.
51	Multiple procedures	If the surgeon performs a tonsilectomy and places ventilation tubes in the tympanic membranes during the same operative session, modifier 51 would be appended to the second-procedure code, in this case the placement of the tubes.
62	Two surgeons	When two surgeons perform distinct parts of a procedure on the eye or ear each surgeon would report his or her distinct portion of the procedure, appending modifier 62 to the appropriate procedure code.
63	Procedures performed on infants less than 4 kg <<	This modifier may *not* be appended to code 65820 Goniotomy, also known as a DeVincintus or Barken's operation

1. Debridement, mastoidectomy cavity, complex, is performed bilaterally. Assign the appropriate CPT code with the appropriate modifier appended.
2. To append modifier 62, what must both surgeons document?
3. Which modifier is not to be used with CPT code 65820?

Also available in McGraw Hill **connect** (plus+)

17.7 Common Medical and Procedural Terms Used in Operative Reports

As with all sections of CPT, the Eyes, Ears, and Endocrine sections include medical terms and procedural terms that are specific to the organ or system involved. Tables 17.11 through 17.13 list some of these terms and identify some key terms that could appear in a provider's documentation concerning the eyes, ears, and endocrine system.

Table 17.11 Terms for Eyes

TERM	DEFINITION	DOCUMENTATION KEYS
Blepharoptosis	Drooping eyelid	Blepharo = eyelid; ptosis = drooping
Extra capsular cataract extraction (ECCE)	Diseased lens of the eye is removed, leaving part of the capsule covering the lens to allow implantation of an intraocular lens	*ECCE* often used in cataract procedure operative reports
Intraocular lens (IOL)	Artificial lens permanently implanted in the eye	*IOL* often used in cataract procedure operative reports
Oculus dexter (OD) **Oculus sinister (OS)** **Oculus uterque (OU)**	Right eye Left eye Each eye	Use of these modifiers defines laterality of the procedure performed and aides in payment of second procedure within a global period of the first eye procedure.

intraocular lens (IOL) Artificial lens permanently implanted in the eye.

oculus dexter (OD) Right eye.

oculus sinister (OS) Left eye.

oculus uterque (OU) Each eye.

Table 17.12 Terms for Ears

TERM	DEFINITION	DOCUMENTATION KEYS
Audiometry	Measurement of sound	Audiogram (a recording of this measurement)
Otitis externa	Inflammation of the external ear canal	Swimmer's ear
Rinne test	Test used for bone air conduction of sound waves	Vibrating tuning fork
Weber test	Test used to determine hearing deficit as conductive or sensorineural	Auditory acuity
Auris dextra (AD) **Auris sinistra (AS)** **Auris unitas (AU)**	Right ear Left ear Each ear	Use of these modifiers defines laterality of the procedure performed and aides in payment of second procedure within a global period of the first ear procedure.

audiometry Measurement of the level of hearing.

auris dextra (AD) Right ear.

auris sinistra (AS) Left ear.

auris unitas (AU) Each ear.

Table 17.13 Terms for Endocrine System

TERM	DEFINITION	DOCUMENTATION KEYS
Cushing's syndrome	Disorder in which the body is exposed to high levels of the hormone cortisol over an extended period of time. The use of oral corticosteriod medication is one of the most common causes of Cushing's.	Hypercortisolism
Graves' disease	Excessive secretion of thyroid hormone.	Hyperthyroidism, toxic diffuse goiter
Glucose tolerance test (GTT)	Determines the body's ability to breakdown glucose.	Laboratory test
Thyroid-stimulating hormone (TSH)	A test that measures the amount of TSH produced by the pituitary gland in the blood	Laboratory test
Thyroid storm	Condition that occurs in uncontrolled hyperthyroidism	Thyroid crisis

Cushing's syndrome Disorder in which the body is exposed to high levels of the hormone cortisol over an extended period of time; most commonly caused by use of oral corticosteriod medication.

Graves' disease Hyperthyroidism, or toxic diffuse goiter.

glucose tolerance test (GTT) Determines the body's ability to breakdown glucose.

thyroid-stimulating hormone (TSH) A test that measures the amount of TSH produced by the pituitary gland in the blood.

thyroid storm Condition that occurs in uncontrolled hyperthyroidism. Also called *thyroid crisis*.

EXERCISE 17.7

1. What is the difference between a Rinne test and a Weber test?
2. List the two abbreviations most commonly seen in cataract operative reports.
3. How might an excessive secretion of thyroid hormone be described in a medical record?

Also available in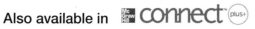

Chapter Seventeen Summary

Learning Outcome	Key Concepts/Examples
17.1 Review the anatomy of the eyes, ears, and endocrine system.	**Eyes** The functions of the eyes are to receive and reflect light rays, which generate nerve impulses that are then transmitted to the brain to become images or sight. *Path of light:* cornea → aqueous humor of anterior chamber → pupil → vitreous humor of posterior chamber → retina → electrical signal or impulse → optic nerve → brain **Ears** The main functions of the ear are balance and hearing. *Path of sound waves:* sound waves → outer ear → tympanic membrane → middle ear → inner ear → electrical impulse → acoustic nerve → brain → cerebral cortex → sound **Endocrine system** The main function of the endocrine system is to release hormones (chemicals) into the body through the bloodstream. The structures of the endocrine system are the: • Pituitary gland • Pineal gland • Thyroid gland • Parathyroid gland • Thymus
17.2 Understand the chapter-specific ICD guidelines and format for the eyes.	ICD-9-CM codes for conditions related to the eye and its supporting structures are listed in only one section in the Diseases of the Nervous System and Sense Organ Chapter. This large section has become a separate chapter in ICD-10-CM. *ICD-9-CM:* Disorders of the Eye and Adnexa, 360–379 *ICD-10-CM:* Diseases of the Eye and Adnexa, H00–H59
17.3 Comprehend the chapter-specific ICD guidelines and format for the ears.	Categories within this section are subdivided by the anatomical sites of the ear, beginning with the external ear and ending with the hearing loss due to sensorineural or conductive disorders. *ICD-9-CM:* Diseases of the Ear, 380–389 *ICD-10-CM:* Diseases of the Ear, H60–H95
17.4 Identify the guidelines and format of the eyes and ocular adnexa sections of CPT.	The codes in these sections are defined by the following general headings: • Eyeball • Anterior Segment • Posterior Segment • Ocular Adnexa • Conjunctiva These general headings are then further defined by the following subclassifications: • Incision • Excision • Removal • Repair • Destruction

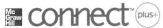 Enhance your learning by completing these exercises and more at mcgrawhillconnect.com

Learning Outcome	Key Concepts/Examples
17.5 Recognize the guidelines and format of the ears and endocrine sections of CPT.	The codes in the ear section are defined by the following general headings: • External Ear • Inner Ear • Middle Ear • Temporal Bone, Middle Fossa The codes in the endocrine section are defined by the following general headings: • Thyroid Gland • Parathyroid Gland, Thymus, Adrenal Glands, Pancreas, and Carotid Body These general headings can then be further defined by the following subclassifications: • Incision • Excision • Removal • Repair • Destruction
17.6 Apply the modifiers most commonly used with codes in the eyes, ears, and endocrine sections of CPT.	Modifiers are used in the Eyes, Ears, and Endocrine sections to continue or modify the story of the patient's encounter. Some of the more common modifiers used in these sections are: • Bilateral services, 50 • Multiple procedures, 51 • Two surgeons, 62 Several instructional notes throughout these sections direct the use of modifier 50 if the procedure described was performed bilaterally.
17.7 Examine the common medical and procedural terms used in operative reports.	The Eyes, Ears, and Endocrine sections include medical terms and procedural terms that are specific to the systems involved. Tables 17.11 through 17.13 list some of these terms and identify some key terms that could appear in a provider's documentation concerning the eyes, ears, and endocrine system.

Chapter Seventeen Review

Using Terminology

Match each key term to the appropriate definition.

_____ 1. [LO17.6] AU
_____ 2. [LO17.6] Audiometry
_____ 3. [LO17.6] Cushing's syndrome
_____ 4. [LO17.6] Graves' disease
_____ 5. [LO17.2] Hyperopia
_____ 6. [LO17.2] Hypotony
_____ 7. [LO17.6] Impacted cerumen
_____ 8. [LO17.2] Myopia

A. Gland whose functions are the production and development of T cells
B. Nearsightedness
C. Structure that forms the visible white of the eye and surrounds the optic nerve
D. Low intraocular pressure
E. Errors in focus due to age
F. Structure that divides the middle and inner ear; also known as *eardrum*
G. Farsightedness
H. Measurement of level of hearing

_____ 9. [LO17.6] Otitis externa
_____ 10. [LO17.2] Presbyopia
_____ 11. [LO17.1] Sclera
_____ 12. [LO17.1] Thymus
_____ 13. [LO17.6] Thyroid storm
_____ 14. [LO17.2] Tinnitus
_____ 15. [LO17.1] Tympanic
       membrane

I. Ringing sensation in the ears
J. Accumulation of earwax
K. Swimmer's ear
L. Abbreviation for "each ear"
M. Hyperthyroidism or toxic diffuse goiter
N. Disease that is most commonly caused by the use of oral corticosteroid medication
O. Thyroid crisis

Checking Your Understanding

Choose the most appropriate answer for each of the following questions.

1. [LO17.3] A 25-year-old patient has been diagnosed with noise-induced hearing loss due to exposure to continuous loud music. Select the appropriate ICD-9-CM code:

a. 388.12
b. 389.14
c. 389.8
d. 388.11

2. [LO17.2] A 23-year-old female presents to the ophthalmologist with type 2 diabetes mellitus with a cataract on her left eye. The patient also has been diagnosed with benign essential hypertension. Select the appropriate ICD-9-CM codes:

a. 366.9, 250.00, 401.0
b. 250.00, 366.9, 401.1
c. 250.50, 366.41, 401.1
d. 250.00, 366.41, 401.9

3. [LO17.1] The clear part of the eye that covers the pupil and iris and controls and focuses light entering the eye is the:

a. Cornea
b. Conjunctiva
c. Sclera
d. Lens

4. [LO17.4] The patient presented for removal of a foreign object from the cornea. This was performed without a slip lamp. Choose the appropriate CPT code for this procedure:

a. 65222
b. 65210
c. 65220
d. 65235

5. [LO 17.4] A patient who had previous eye surgery that did not involve the extraocular muscle presented for strabismus surgery on two horizontal muscles. Select the appropriate CPT code(s):

a. 67311
b. 67311, 67331
c. 67331, 67311
d. 67316, 67331

6. [LO 17.6] A tympanostomy (requiring insertion of a ventilating tube), with local or topical anesthesia, that is performed on both ears is assigned CPT code:

a. 69436-50
b. 69433
c. 69450
d. 69433-50

7. [LO 17.7] A procedure was performed on the oculus sinister. Which of the following modifiers should be appended to the code?

a. OD
b. OS
c. OU
d. AS

8. [LO17. 7] A 20-year-old female patient presented to the office for a test to determine whether her hearing deficit is conductive or sensorineural. This type of test is called:

a. the Rinne test
b. Audiometry
c. the Weber test
d. None of these

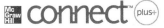

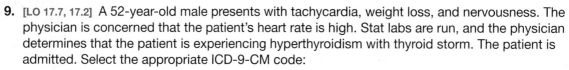

9. [LO 17.7, 17.2] A 52-year-old male presents with tachycardia, weight loss, and nervousness. The physician is concerned that the patient's heart rate is high. Stat labs are run, and the physician determines that the patient is experiencing hyperthyroidism with thyroid storm. The patient is admitted. Select the appropriate ICD-9-CM code:

a. 244.9   **c.** 242.90

b. 242.91   **d.** 242.01

10. [LO 17. 3] Robert, a 64-year-old male, presents to the office with early stage of low-tension glaucoma. Select the appropriate ICD-9-CM code(s):

a. 365.12, 365.71   **c.** 365.12

b. 365.71, 365.12   **d.** 365.12, 365.72

Applying your Knowledge

Answer the following questions and code the following case study. Be sure to follow the process steps as illustrated in Chapter 8.

Case Studies [LO 17.1–17.7] Case 1

Procedure performed: Bilateral tympanostomy

Preoperative diagnosis: Bilateral recurrent otitis media with effusion

Postoperative diagnosis: Left recurrent otitis media with effusion

Procedure: The patient was placed in the supine position and under the adequate general anesthesia; the patient was prepped and draped in the usual manner. Using the operating microscope, the left tympanic membrane was visualized. The canal was cleaned of cerumen and a radial incision was made in the anteroinferior quadrant of the membrane. A 0.40 tube was placed in the previously created myringotomy. Suspension drops were instilled, and a cotton ball was placed at the meatus.

Process 1: CPT

1. What is the procedure?

2. Locate the main term in the index.

3. What additional questions or set of questions can be determined?

4. Upon review of all the code choices identified in the index, what additional questions can be determined?

5. Based on the documentation, what is the correct code for this case?

a. 69421   **c.** 69433

b. 69436   **d.** 69424

Process 2: ICD

ICD-9-CM

1. Based on the operative report header, what is the preoperative diagnosis?

2. Is the postoperative diagnosis the same as or different from the preoperative diagnosis?

3. Is the postoperative diagnosis supported?

4. What is the main term for this condition?

5. Based on the subterm choices, what question(s) can be developed for this condition?

6. Is any sign, symptom, or additional condition documented?

7. Is the additional condition, sign, or symptom an integral part of the primary (or other) condition coded?

8. Does the additional condition require or affect patient care, treatment, or management?

9. Based on the documentation, what is the correct ICD-9-CM code for this case?
   a. 381.00　　　　　　　　　c. 382.00
   b. 381.3　　　　　　　　　　d. 381.4

ICD-10-CM

1. Based on the operative report header, what is the preoperative diagnosis?

2. Is the postoperative diagnosis the same as or different from the preoperative diagnosis?

3. Is the postoperative diagnosis supported?

4. What is the main term for this condition?

5. Based on the subterm choices, what question(s) can be developed for this condition?

6. Based on the information in the Tabular List, is additional information needed to determine the appropriate diagnosis code?

7. Is any sign, symptom, or additional condition documented?

8. Is the additional condition, sign, or symptom an integral part of the primary (or other) condition coded?

9. Does the additional condition require or affect patient care, treatment, or management?

10. Based on the documentation, what is the correct ICD-10-CM code for this case?
    a. H65.196　　　　　　　　c. H65.493
    b. H65.193　　　　　　　　d. H65.19

Process 3: Modifiers

1. Was the procedure performed different from that described by the nomenclature of the code?

2. Was the procedure performed at an anatomical site that has laterality?

3. Was the procedure performed in the global period of another procedure?

4. Were additional procedures performed during the operative session, and does the documentation support them?

5. Did the surgeon have help from another surgeon or another appropriate person?

6. Did a physician different from the surgeon provide the preoperative or postoperative portion of the procedure?

7. What modifier should be appended to the CPT code for this case?
   a. 50
   b. 51
   c. 22
   d. None

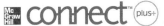

Enhance your learning by completing these exercises
and more at mcgrawhillconnect.com

Procedure performed: Extracapsular cataract extraction with intraocular lens insertion, right eye. Ophthalmic microscope was used.

Preoperative diagnosis: Senile subcapsular polar cataract, posterior

Postoperative diagnosis: Senile subcapsular polar cataract, posterior

Local anesthesia was administered with lidocaine 2 percent with epinephrine for a lid block. Retrobulbar anesthesia was administered using marcaine 0.75 percent with epinephrine and lidocaine 4 percent. Patient was prepped and draped in the usual sterile ophthalmic fashion.

The eye was stabilized with a 4-0 black silk superior rectus traction suture and was subsequently deflected downward. A scleral incision was made 2 mm superior to the superior limbus and approximately 12 mm in length. The dissection was then carried posteriorly from the base of the incision into clear cornea. A stab wound was made into clear cornea at 1 o'clock to provide an access, and a keratome was utilized to enter the anterior chamber through the base of the corneoscleral wound at 10 o'clock.

Healon was injected into the anterior chamber through a cystitome needle. The needle was subsequently used to create an anterior capsulotomy, and capsule forceps were utilized to affect a circular tear capsulorrhexis capsulotomy. Balanced salt solution was injected underneath the capsule to dissect the nucleus free from the capsule.

Using a lens loop and Colibri forceps, the nucleus was expressed through the wound. Two interrupted 10-0 nylon sutures were then inserted through the corneoscleral wound, dividing the wound into equal thirds.

Lens cortical material was irrigated and aspirated from the wound. Following this, the posterior capsule was noted to be intact, and Healon was injected into the anterior chamber.

The previously selected intraocular lens was soaked in balanced salt solution. The lens was flushed with fresh balanced salt solution and coated with Healon. Angled forceps were then used to insert the lens through the scleral incision, with the inferior foot of the haptic passing beneath the anterior capsule at 6 o'clock. Long-angled tying forceps were then used to place the superior foot of the haptic through the pupil behind the anterior capsule at 12 o'clock. The lens was rotated to ensure stability.

10-0 nylon interrupted sutures were placed to close the corneoscleral wound.

Answer the following questions, and code the case above. Be sure to follow the process steps as illustrated in Chapter 8.

Process 1: CPT

1. What is the procedure?

2. Locate the main term in the index.

3. What additional questions or set of questions can be determined?

4. Upon review of all the code choices identified in the index, what additional questions can be determined?

5. Based on the documentation, what is the correct code for this case?
   a. 66982
   b. 66984
   c. 66983
   d. 66985

Process 2: ICD
ICD-9-CM

1. Based on the operative report header, what is the preoperative diagnosis?

2. Is the postoperative diagnosis the same as or different from the preoperative diagnosis?

3. Is the postoperative diagnosis supported?

4. What is the main term for this condition?

5. Based on the subterm choices, what question(s) can be developed for this condition?

6. Is any sign, symptom, or additional condition documented?

7. Is the additional condition, sign, or symptom an integral part of the primary (or other) condition coded?

8. Does the additional condition require or affect patient care, treatment, or management?

9. Based on the documentation, what is the correct ICD-9-CM code for this case?
   a. 743.31
   b. 366.17
   c. 366.13
   d. 366.14

ICD-10-CM

1. Based on the operative report header, what is the preoperative diagnosis?

2. Is the postoperative diagnosis the same as or different from the preoperative diagnosis?

3. Is the postoperative diagnosis supported?

4. What is the main term for this condition?

5. Based on the subterm choices, what question(s) can be developed for this condition?

6. Based on the information in the Tabular List, is additional information needed to determine the appropriate diagnosis code?

7. Is any sign, symptom, or additional condition documented?

8. Is the additional condition, sign, or symptom an integral part of the primary (or other) condition coded?

9. Does the additional condition require or affect patient care, treatment, or management?

10. Based on the documentation, what is the correct ICD-10-CM code for this case?
    a. H25.039
    b. H25.041
    c. H25.049
    d. H26.051

Process 3: Modifiers

1. Was the procedure performed different from that described by the nomenclature of the code?

2. Was the procedure performed at an anatomical site that has laterality?

3. Was the procedure performed in the global period of another procedure?

4. Were additional procedures performed during the operative session, and does the documentation support them?

5. Did the surgeon have help from another surgeon or another appropriate person?

6. Did a physician different from the surgeon provide the preoperative or postoperative portion of the procedure?

7. What modifier should be appended to the CPT code for this case?
   a. 50
   b. RT
   c. OD
   d. None

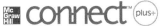

Unit 4 Exam

The questions in this exam cover material in **Chapters 13 through 17** of this book.

Choose the most appropriate answer for each question below.

1. [LO13.2, 13.3] A patient is seen in the outpatient clinic for a colonoscopy due to a family history of colon cancer. The patient has no personal history of gastrointestinal disease and is currently without signs and symptoms. The colonoscopy revealed a colonic polyp that was removed by hot biopsy forceps. What should the CPT and diagnosis codes for this case be?

   a. 45384, 211.3, V76.51, V16.0

   b. G0105, 211.3, V76.51, V16.0

   c. 45384, V76.51, V16.0, 211.3

   d. G0105, V76.51, V16.0, 211.3

2. [LO13.2] Wendy, a 23-year-old patient, is seen by Dr. Johnson for a cough with wheezing and green-colored mucus for the past four days, as well as four days of external bleeding hemorrhoids and diarrhea. Dr. Johnson gives Wendy Augmentin for acute viral bronchitis, instructions on the care of external hemorrhoids, and a diet plan to assist with the diarrhea. What diagnoses should Dr. Johnson use for this encounter?

   a. 466.0, 455.5, 787.91

   b. 787.91, 466.11, 455.5

   c. 466.11, 787.91, 455.2

   d. 466.0, 455.8, 787.91

3. [LO13.2, 13.3] A 35-year-old patient is brought to the operating room for an outpatient surgery for a hiatal hernia repair. The surgeon is able to repair the hernia laparoscopically by placing sutures in the crus diaphragmatic muscles below the esophagus and bringing them together to close the hiatal hernia. The anterior and posterior walls of the fundus are wrapped and stitched around the esophagus to complete the procedure. Select the appropriate CPT and ICD-9-CM codes for this procedure:

   a. 43281, 553.3

   b. 43279, 551.3, 551.2

   c. 43281, 750.6

   d. 43280, 553.3

4. [LO13.2, 13.3] **Operative Report**

   Preoperative diagnosis: Internal hemorrhoids

   Postoperative diagnosis: Internal hemorrhoids, anal fistula

   Procedure performed: Hemorroidectomy and repair of anal fistula

   Operative note: The patient presented today for an inpatient procedure to repair an anal fistula and remove internal hemorrhoids. The patient was put under general anesthesia, prepped, and draped. The physician entered the anus using an endoscope to determine placement of internal hemorrhoids and, upon entering, identified an intersphincteric anal fistula that had occurred since the last visit by the patient. The procedure was initiated, and removal of two columns of internal hemorrhoids was performed using rubber band ligation. Once that procedure was performed, an endoscopic repair of the anal fistula took place, using fibrin glue to seal the fistula. With this accomplished, the patient was woken up from anesthesia and taken to an inpatient room for an overnight stay.

   Select the appropriate CPT and ICD-9-CM codes:

   a. 46255, 455.3, 751.5

   b. 46258, 455.0, 751.5

   c. 46221, 46706-59, 455.0, 565.1

   d. 46262, 455.0, 565.1

5. [LO13.2, 13.3, 13.5] **Preoperative diagnosis:** (1) Cholelithiasis, (2) acute cholecystitis

Postoperative diagnosis: (1) Cholelithiasis, (2) acute cholecystitis

Name of operation: Laparoscopic cholecystectomy

Anesthesia: General

Findings: The gallbladder was thickened and showed evidence of chronic cholecystitis. There was a great deal of inflammatory reaction around the cystic duct. The cystic duct was slightly larger. There were nine stones impacted in the cystic duct. The gallbladder contained numerous stones, which were small. With the stones impacted in the cystic duct, it was felt that probably none were within the common duct. Other than rather marked obesity, no other significant findings were noted on limited exploration of the abdomen.

Procedure: Under general anesthesia after routine prepping and draping, the abdomen was insufflated with the Veress needle and the standard four trocars were inserted uneventfully. Inspection was made for any entry problems, and none were encountered.

After limited exploration, the gallbladder was then retracted superiorly and laterally, and the cystic duct was dissected out. This was done with some difficulty due to the fibrosis around the cystic duct, but care was taken to avoid injury to the duct and to the common duct. In this manner, the cystic duct and cystic artery were dissected out. Care was taken to be sure that the duct that was identified went into the gallbladder and was the cystic duct. The cystic duct and cystic artery were then doubly clipped and divided, taking care to avoid injury to the common duct. The gallbladder was then dissected free from the gallbladder bed. Again, the gallbladder was somewhat adherent to the gallbladder bed due to previous inflammatory reaction. The gallbladder was dissected free from the gallbladder bed utilizing the endo shears and the cautery to control bleeding. The gallbladder was extracted through the operating trocar site, and the trocar was reinserted. Inspection was made of the gallbladder bed. One or two bleeding areas were fulgurated, and bleeding was well controlled.

Select the appropriate CPT and ICD-9-CM codes:

a. 47562, 574.00

b. 47564, 574.21, 575.10

c. 47570, 574.21, 575.0

d. 47600, 574.21, 574.51

6. [LO13.4] An endoscopy procedure was started on a patient who was scheduled and prepped for a total colonoscopy. The physician was unable to advance the scope beyond the splenic flexure due to unforeseen circumstances. Which of the following modifiers is appended to the colonoscopy code:

a. 52

b. None; the procedure would be billed without a modifier.

c. 53

d. None; the procedure would not be billed.

7. [LO13.5] Which of the following terms refers to an abnormal accumulation of fluid in the peritoneal cavity that is often a complication of a malignancy?

a. Peritonitis

b. Crohn's disease

c. Ascites

d. Volvulus

8. [LO14.3, 14.5] A 55-year-old male patient is coming to the hospital for an outpatient service for a prostate biopsy. The patient has a family history of prostate cancer, had recent blood work showing elevated PSA levels, and has problems urinating. The patient presents and is placed under anesthesia and prepped and draped. Ultrasonic guidance is used for needle placement, and a needle biopsy is taken. The biopsy is sent to pathology, and the patient is awaiting the results. Select the appropriate CPT and ICD-9-CM codes:

a. 55706, 790.93

b. 55705, 76942, V10.46, 790.93

c. 55706, V16.42, 790.93

d. 55700, 76942, V16.42, 790.93

9. **[LO14.5]** The patient is a female transgender patient who has undergone hormonal therapy, along with other services, to prepare her for her sex change to a male. The patient is counseled on the adverse effects of surgery, as well as complications that may occur. The patient signs the consent for surgery and is taken to the operating room, prepped for surgery, and placed under general anesthesia. The patient successfully comes through surgery. Select the appropriate CPT code:

    a. 55970

    b. 55920

    c. 55980

    d. 55899

10. **[LO14.3,14.4]** **Preoperative diagnosis:** Bladder tumor, 3.4 cm

    Postoperative diagnosis: Bladder tumor, 4.2 cm

    Procedure: The patient was placed in the lithotomy position after receiving IV sedation. He was prepped and draped. A 21-French cystoscope was passed into the bladder; a previous CT scan of the bladder indicated a tumor of approximately 3.4 cm. After inspection of the bladder with the cystoscope, the findings were consistent with a bladder tumor but the size was inconsistent; the actual finding was a size of 4.2 cm. A biopsy was taken, and laser surgery was performed with fulguration on the removal of the tumor. The patient tolerated the procedure well.

Code only the procedure:

    a. 52235

    b. 52000

    c. 52341

    d. 52334

11. **[LO14.3, 14.4, 14.6]** An elderly gentleman has worsening bilateral hydronephrosis. He did not have much of a postvoid residual on bladder scan. He is taken to the OR to have a bilateral cystoscopy and retrograde pyelogram. The results come back as gross prostatic hyperplasia. Select the appropriate CPT and ICD-9-CM codes:

    a. 52005, 600.3   **c.** 52005-50, 600.91, 591

    b. 52000, 591, 600.9   **d.** 52000-50, 591, 600.9

12. **[LO14.3, 14.5]** A 25-year-old male patient presents for outpatient surgery today on penile genital warts that previously were treated with medication and have not subsided. The patient is having the genital warts removed using a cryosurgery technique. What are the correct CPT and ICD-9-CM codes?

    a. 54050, 078.19

    b. 54056, 078.11

    c. 54055, 078.10

    d. 54060, 078.11

13. **[LO15.2,15.3]** **Postoperative diagnosis:** Ovarian cyst, right

    Anesthesia: General

    Name of operation: Open drainage of cyst

    Procedure: The patient was taken to the operating room and prepped and draped in the usual manner, and adequate anesthesia was induced. An infraumbilical incision was made, and abdominal entrance was made. Gas was entered into the abdomen at 2 liters. The abdomen was visualized. The cyst was noted on the right, a 4-cm ovarian cyst. This was needled, and a hole was cut in it with the scissors. Hemostasis was intact. The instruments were removed. The patient was awakened and taken to the recovery room in good condition.

Select the appropriate CPT and ICD-9-CM codes:

    a. 58800, 620.2   **c.** 58820, 620.2

    b. 58805, 620.2   **d.** 58822, 620.2

14. **[LO17.5]** **Preoperative diagnosis:** Right eustachian tube dysfunction

Postoperative diagnosis: Right eustachian tube dysfunction

Anesthesia: General mask

Name of operation: Eustachian tube catheterization

Procedure: The patient was taken to the operating room and placed in the supine position. After general anesthesia was given, the operating microscope was brought in for full use throughout the case. The right tympanic membrane was approached using a transnasal approach. An anterior-inferior radial incision was made in the right tympanic membrane. Suction revealed a substantial amount of mucopurulent drainage. A Sheehy pressure equalization tube was placed in the site. Floxin drops were added. The patient tolerated the procedure well and returned to the recovery room awake and in stable condition.

Select the appropriate CPT and ICD-9-CM codes:

    a. 69400, 381.81

    b. 69405, 381.81

    c. 69420, 381.81

    d. 69401, 382.9, 719.41

15. **[LO15.2, 15.3]** **Operation:** LEEP procedure

Diagnosis: Cervical polyp

Procedure: With the patient in the supine position, general anesthesia was administered. The patient was put in the dorsal lithotomy position and prepped and draped for dilation and curettage in a routine fashion.

An insulated posterior weighted retractor was put in. Using the LEEP tenaculum, we were able to grasp the anterior lip of the cervix with a large wire loop at 35 cutting, 30 coagulation. The cervical polyp on the posterior lip of the cervix was excised.

Then changing to a 40 of coagulation and 4 cutting, the base of the polyp was electrocoagulated, which controlled all the bleeding. The wire loop was attached, and the pigmented raised nevus on the inner thigh was excised with the wire loop. Cautery of the base was done, and then it was closed with figure-of-eight 3-0 Vicryl sutures. A Band-Aid was applied over this.

Rechecking the cervix, no bleeding was noted. The patient was laid flat on the table, awakened, and moved to the recovery room bed and sent to the recovery room in satisfactory condition.

Select the appropriate CPT and ICD-9-CM codes:

    a. 57452, 622.3   **c.** 57455, 622.3

    b. 57461, 622.7   **d.** 57460, 622.7

16. **[LO15.2, 15.3]** The patient is a 35-year-old female who has been having prolonged and heavy bleeding during menstruation. After other testing, the patient opted to have an elective uterine ablation using NovaSure.

Procedure: After the patient was put under general anesthesia, the patient was placed in the dorsolithotomy position, after which the perineum and the vagina were prepped, the bladder was straight catheterized, and the patient was draped. After a bimanual exam was performed, a speculum was placed and the cavity integrity assessment performed. The NovaSure system uses a small amount of CO_2 to verify cavity integrity prior to performing the procedure. The NovaSure thermal endometrial ablation procedure then delivered radiofrequency energy until tissue impedance reached 50 ohms; the electrode array was retracted for easy removal, leaving the uterine lining desiccated down to the superficial myometrium. The patient was awakened from anesthesia and sent home to recover.

Select the appropriate CPT and ICD-9-CM codes:

    a. 58541, 626.2, 626.0   **c.** 58353, 626.2

    b. 58356, 626.0   **d.** 58356, 626.2

17. **[LO15.2, 15.3]** A 39-year-old female presents with an ectopic pregnancy. Due to previous abdominal surgeries, the surgeon is unable to perform a laparoscopic fallopian tube removal and must use an open procedure to successfully perform the removal. The physician elects to surgically treat this patient by using an open approach to her abdomen to remove her left fallopian tube and ovary, along with the products of conception. Select the appropriate CPT and ICD-9-CM codes:

    a. 59150, 633.90

    b. 59121-LT, 633.80

    c. 59120-LT, 633.90

    d. 59120, 633.80

18. **[LO15.2]** A patient who is 32 weeks' pregnant was admitted because of an HIV-related illness. The patient spent 3 days in the hospital and was sent home in stable condition. The baby was not delivered during this hospital stay. Select the correct ICD-9-CM codes:

    a. 042, 647.60

    b. 042, 647.63

    c. 647.83, 042

    d. 647.63, 042

19. **[LO16.5]** The medical term that can be used for pain in the head is:

    a. Agraphia

    b. Cephalgia

    c. Neuralgia

    d. Paraplegia

20. **[LO15.5]** The term *salpingo-oophorectomy* refers to:

    a. The removal of the fallopian tube

    b. The removal of a fertilized egg

    c. Cutting into the fallopian tube and ovary for a surgical procedure

    d. The removal of the fallopian tube and the ovary

21. **[LO17.1]** Which of the following is the gland that secretes a factor that causes T cells to mature and is larger in infants?

    a. Spleen

    b. Lymph

    c. Thymus

    d. Adrenal

22. **[LO17.5]** Select the appropriate CPT and ICD-9-CM codes to report the removal of 35 percent of the left thyroid lobe through an isthmusectomy. The patient's diagnosis is benign thyroid neoplasm.

    a. 60025, 226, 239.7

    b. 60212, 239.7

    c. 60240, 226

    d. 60210, 225

23. **[LO17.2]** There are two main types of glaucoma. Which type of glaucoma describes when fluid does not flow through the orbicular meshwork properly?

    a. Open angle

    b. Congential

    c. Closed angle

    d. Traumatic

24. **[LO16.1]** The nervous system is divided into two major systems. Which system includes the brain and the spinal cord?

    a. Peripheral nervous system

    b. Somatic nervous system

    c. Autonomic nervous system

    d. Central nervous system

25. **[LO16.3]** To accurately identify that a procedure was performed on the second lumbar vertebra, which of the following would be documented in the operative report?

    a. L2

    b. C2

    c. L2–3

    d. C2–3

26. **[LO16.3]** When multiple surgeons perform the complete skull base procedure (approach procedure, definitive procedure, reconstruction/repair), each surgeon reports only the code for the specific procedure each performed. If one surgeon performs all of the procedures, then all the applicable codes are reported and a modifier is added to the secondary procedure code(s). Which modifier is added?

    a. 59

    b. 62

    c. 51

    d. No modifier is needed.

Coding for Radiology, Pathology/Laboratory, General Medicine, HCPCS Category II and III, and Practice Management

5

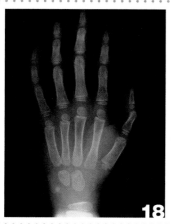

18

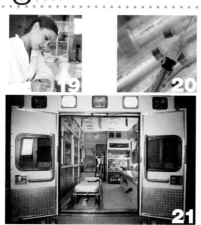

19

20

21

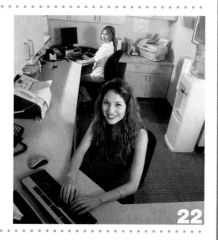

22

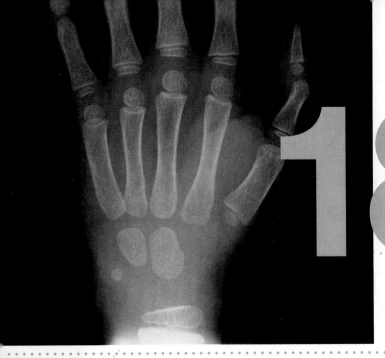

18

Radiology

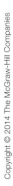

CHAPTER EIGHTEEN

Key Terms

Axial plane
Brachytherapy
Clinical treatment planning
Computed tomography (CT)
Contrast material

Coronal plane
Diagnostic nuclear medicine study
Dual-energy x-ray absorptiometry (DXA)
Extension
Flexion

Fluoroscopy
Magnetic resonance imaging (MRI)
Nuclear medicine
Pronation
Radiopharmaceutical
Sagittal plane

Simulation-aided field setting
Supination
Therapeutic nuclear medicine study
Ultrasound

Learning Outcomes

After completing this chapter, you will be able to:

18.1 Review the general ICD and CPT guidelines for radiology coding.

18.2 Identify the CPT guidelines and format of the Diagnostic Imaging subsection of CPT.

18.3 Understand the CPT guidelines and format of the Diagnostic Ultrasound and Breast, Mammography subsections of CPT.

18.4 Apply the CPT guidelines and format of the Bone/Joint Studies and Radiation Oncology subsections of CPT.

18.5 Recognize the CPT guidelines and format of the Nuclear Medicine subsection of CPT.

18.6 Evaluate the modifiers most commonly used with codes in the Radiology section of CPT.

18.7 Examine the common medical and procedural terms used in operative reports.

Introduction

Radiology involves establishing diagnoses and treating diseases and injuries. Several different methods are used to arrive at a diagnosis or to treat a condition. X-rays, computed tomography (CT), magnetic resonance imaging (MRI), ultrasound, positron emission tomography (PET), and interventional procedures are the most common methods used to perform these functions.

When coding for radiology services, coders may use codes from most sections of ICD and CPT. Therefore, coders must be very familiar with both manuals and the various "languages" used to describe radiological services and procedures.

18.1 Format and General ICD and CPT Guidelines for Radiology Coding

The general headings used in the Radiology section of the CPT manual are listed in Table 18.1. The subheadings are further divided by anatomical site.

ICD Guidelines

Signs and Symptoms

When a diagnosis has not been confirmed or the radiology report is documented as normal, signs and symptoms should be reported.

FOR EXAMPLE The indication on the radiology report is cough. The dictated chest x-ray report states "normal examination, no indication of pneumonia." The ICD diagnosis that should be reported is cough. ■

MENTOR Coding Tip

To locate a definitive or confirmed diagnosis within the provider documentation, coders should look for terms such as *impression, finding, reported as,* and *conclusion.*

Abnormal Findings

ICD abnormal-findings codes may be used when additional testing is required and the test results are negative.

FOR EXAMPLE The plain film x-ray has an inconclusive finding and therefore a CT scan is ordered. The CT scan is negative. The abnormal finding on the earlier test would be used as the diagnosis for the CT scan. ■

Encounter for Radiation Therapy

If the encounter is solely for radiation therapy, the ICD chapter-specific guidelines direct the coder to use V58.11 (ICD-9-CM) or Z51.11 (ICD-10-CM) as the first-listed diagnosis. Any side effects of the treatment, such as dehydration, and the malignancy being treated would be reported as additional codes.

Table 18.1 CPT Radiology Section Format *(Data from CPT 2013. © 2013 American Medical Association. All rights reserved.)*

GENERAL HEADING	CODE RANGE
Diagnostic Radiology (Diagnostic Imaging)	70010–76499
Diagnostic Ultrasound	76506–76999
Radiologic Guidance	77001–77032
Breast, Mammography	77051–77059
Bone/Joint Studies	77071–77084
Radiation Oncology	77261–77799
Nuclear Medicine	78012–79999

If the patient encounter is to determine the extent of a malignancy, the malignancy is the primary diagnosis and any radiation therapy during the encounter is reported as an additional code.

Fractures

Multiple fractures are sequenced in the order of severity, with the most severe first.

There is a differentiation between a traumatic fracture and a pathologic fracture.

FOR EXAMPLE The x-ray finding states that there is a fracture of the humerus due to the patient's osteoporosis. The appropriate code to report is 733.11, pathologic fracture of the humerus (ICD-9-CM), or category M80 (ICD-10-CM). ■

Other Common ICD Categories Used to Report Radiology CPT Codes

History of (personal or family): The use of a history-of code can add to the medical necessity for a diagnostic test.

Screening: Screening is performed for early detection for a patient who presents with no symptoms, and the appropriate screening code would be assigned.

If the testing is to rule out or confirm a suspected diagnosis and the patient presents with signs and symptoms, this is a diagnostic examination and not a screening examination and the signs and/or symptoms would be the primary diagnosis.

The ICD chapter-specific guidelines state that if a condition is discovered in a screening exam, the screening code remains the primary diagnosis and the condition is reported as an additional code.

Aftercare: According to the chapter-specific guidelines, aftercare codes are used for encounters after the patient has finished active treatment for the fracture and is receiving care during healing or recovery.

CPT Guidelines

Contrast Material

contrast material A dye or another substance that is used to enhance the image of an organ or tissue being examined.

Many radiological procedures require the use of **contrast material** in order to enhance the image of the organ or tissue being examined. *With contrast* is defined as contrast administered intravascularly, intraparticularly, or intrathecally. Injection of the contrast is part of the with-contrast element.

Oral and/or rectal contact is not with contrast. A combination code exists for without contrast followed by with contrast.

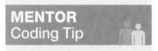

MENTOR
Coding Tip

Highlight this guideline at the beginning of the Radiology section in your CPT manual.

FOR EXAMPLE The CT study of the head states that the procedure was performed without contrast followed by IV contrast. The appropriate code to assign is 70470 since the code description is "computed tomography, head or brain; without contrast material, followed by contrast material(s) and further sections." This procedure would not be coded with separate codes for without contrast and with contrast since a combination code exists to tell the story of the use of contrast material. ■

Number of Views

Many of the code descriptions within the Radiology subsection specify a minimum number of views

FOR EXAMPLE   71020 Chest x-ray, two views ■

Fluoroscopy

Fluoroscopy creates real-time or moving images that are useful for diagnostic procedures and for guidance in interventional procedures. Fluoroscopy is inherent in many radiological procedures. Unless specifically instructed otherwise, fluoroscopy used to complete a procedure and obtain a permanent record is included in the code description and is not reported separately.

fluoroscopy A study that creates real-time or moving images that are useful for diagnostic procedures and for guidance in interventional procedures.

Component Coding

A radiologist may perform both the surgical component (CPT codes from the Surgery section) and the supervision and interpretation component (CPT codes from the Radiology section). If both components are performed by the same physician, the physician (radiologist) would report the surgical component as well as the radiology component.

There are several questions a coder needs to ask when reading an operative report and coding a procedure from the Radiology section. The following questions will help the coder, when reading through the report, to understand what actually was done and how the procedure should be translated and coded:

- At which anatomical site was the procedure performed?
- Was the procedure for diagnostic or therapeutic purposes?
- What was the approach (e.g., transvaginal or transabdominal)?
- What type of exam was done (e.g., plain film, CT, MRI, ultrasound)?
- What was the number of views?
- Was oral or IV contrast used?

1. The documentation states that the patient ingested the contrast material before the CT study was performed. Would this CT study be reported as with or without contrast?

EXERCISE 18.1

2. List some of the common procedures that are assigned codes from the Radiology section of CPT.

3. Why is it important that the medical documentation state the number of views?

4. A patient with a diagnosis of lung cancer presents today for radiation therapy and experiences severe nausea and vomiting during the encounter. Code this encounter in the appropriate sequence.

5. When the findings on a chest x-ray are normal, what should the coder look for in the report to use as the diagnosis for ICD coding?

Also available in

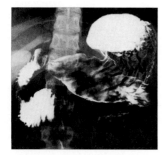

Figure 18.1 X-Ray of Stomach

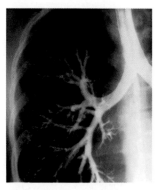

Figure 18.2 X-Ray of Lung

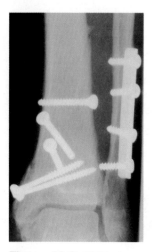

Figure 18.3 ORIF of Ankle Fracture

18.2 Guidelines and Format of the Diagnostic Imaging Subsection of the Radiology Section of CPT

Codes assigned to this subsection are further divided by anatomical site. Also included in this code range are vascular imaging procedures.

Diagnostic Imaging (70010–76499)

Diagnostic imaging is performed to identify or confirm a condition or illness. Figures 18.1 to 18.3 show diagnostic images taken of the stomach, lung, and ankle.

Codes under this subheading are further defined by the following anatomical sites:

- Head and neck, 70010–70559
- Chest, 71010–71555
- Spine and pelvis, 72010–72295
- Upper extremities, 73000–73225
- Lower extremities, 73500–73725
- Abdomen, 74000–74190
- Gastrointestinal tract, 74210–74363
- Urinary tract, 74400–74485
- Gynecological and Obstetrical, 74710–74775
- Heart, 75557–75574
- Vascular Procedures, 75600–75989
- Other Procedures, 76000–76499

Within these anatomical site code ranges, the codes are further defined by the factors discussed below.

Number of Views/Type of View

The provider documentation must be specific as to the number of views and the type of view provided in order for the coder to select the most specific CPT code.

> **FOR EXAMPLE**
>
> Radiological examination, facial bones; less than three views, 70140
>
> Radiological examination, facial bones; complete, minimum of three views, 70150
>
> Radiological examination, chest, special views (e.g., lateral, decubitus, Bucky studies), 71035
>
> Radiological examination, spine, lumbosacral; complete including bending views, minimum of six views, 72114
>
> Radiological examination, abdomen; complete acute abdomen series, including supine, erect, and/or decubitus views, single view chest, 74022
>
> Radiological examination, gastrointestinal tract, upper; with or without delayed, films, with KUB, 74241 ∎

Computed Tomography or Computed Tomography Angiography

Computed tomography (CT) and computed tomography angiography (CTA) are radiology imaging modalities used to study structures or vessels in a body plane. The scans produce computerized cross-section images.

Codes for CT or CTA exams are further defined by the following:

Specific anatomical area: The provider documentation must be specific as to the specific anatomic site being imaged in order for the coder to select the accurate CPT code.

FOR EXAMPLE

Computed tomography, head or brain, 70450–70470

Computed tomography angiography, head, 70496

Computed tomography, thorax, 71250–71270 (An instructional note below this code range directs the coder to code range 75571–75574 for cardiac CT of the heart.)

Computed tomography angiography, chest, noncoronary, 71275 ▪

Computed tomography of the abdomen and pelvis at the same encounter are reported with a combination code.

FOR EXAMPLE

Computed tomography, abdomen and pelvis, 74176–74178 ▪

SPOTLIGHT on a Guideline

Instructional notes below the CT code ranges for each anatomical site direct the coder to codes 76376 and 76377 to report 3-D rendering (reconstruction). The provider documentation must be clear that there was concurrent physician supervision of the image postprocessing and must state whether or not the image postprocessing was done at an independent workstation.

With, without, or without contrast followed by contrast (with and without): Refer to CPT guidelines in Section 18.1 concerning contrast material guidelines.

Magnetic Resonance Imaging or Magnetic Resonance Angiography

Magnetic resonance imaging (MRI) and magnetic resonance angiography (MRA) are radiology imaging modalities in which a magnetic field and radio waves produce images of organs, tissues, or vessels.

MENTOR Coding Tip

MRI scans are used to visualize and study the structure of organs, whereas MRA is used to visualize and study the vessels (arteries and veins).

---

computed tomography (CT) A radiology imaging modality used to study structures in a body plane; produces computerized cross-section views.

MENTOR Coding Tip

KUB stands for "kidney, ureters, and bladder." It is reported with code 74000 and is often included in the code descriptions for codes within the abdomen and gastrointestinal tract subsections.

MENTOR Coding Tip

CT scans are used to visualize and study the structure of organs, whereas CTA is used to visualize and study the vessels (arteries and veins).

magnetic resonance imaging (MRI) A radiology imaging modality that uses a magnetic field and radio waves to produce images of organs and tissues.

Codes for MRI or MRA exams, as with CT and CTA, are further defined by the following:

Specific anatomical area: The provider documentation must be specific as to the specific anatomic site being imaged in order for the coder to select the accurate MRI code.

FOR EXAMPLE

Magnetic resonance imaging of the abdomen, 74181–74183

Magnetic resonance angiography, lower extremity, 73725 ■

With, without, or without contrast followed by contrast (with and without): Refer to CPT guidelines in Section 18.1 concerning contrast material guidelines.

Also included in the diagnostic imaging code range are the supervision and interpretation codes for vascular procedures (75600–75989).

SPOTLIGHT on a Guideline

Nonselective and selective procedures, along with first-, second-, and third-order coding of vascular families, are discussed in the Cardiology chapter of this book. The specific guidelines for the reporting of diagnostic angiography and venography supervision and interpretation codes are located at the beginning of the specific code ranges and should be reviewed and understood by the coder before assigning these codes.

EXERCISE 18.2

1. What is the difference between a CT scan and a CTA?
2. Define *KUB*.
3. What range of codes is appropriate for cardiac computed tomography of the heart?
4. What specifically needs to be in the provider documentation to justify the use of the 3-D rendering codes, 76376 and 76377?

Also available in 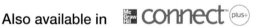 connect (plus+)

18.3 Guidelines and Format of the Diagnostic Ultrasound and Breast, Mammography Subsections of the Radiology Section of CPT

Diagnostic Ultrasound (76506–76999)

ultrasound A noninvasive test that uses high-frequency sound waves to produce images that are captured in real time and show structure, movement, and the flow of blood through blood vessels. Also called *sonography*.

Ultrasound imaging, also called *sonography*, is a noninvasive test that uses high-frequency sound waves to produce images that are captured in real time and show structure, movement, and the flow of blood through blood vessels.

Ultrasound procedures are defined as A-mode, M-mode, B-scan, and real-time scan. The definitions are located in the guidelines before the code ranges for this subsection.

The code ranges in this subsection are divided by anatomical site.

Head and Neck: 76506–76536 Chest: 76604–76645

Codes assigned to the these two subheadings are further defined by A-mode, B-scan, or real-time.

Abdomen and Retroperitoneum: 76700–76776

Codes under this subheading are further defined as to whether the abdominal or retroperitoneal area is being imaged and whether the exam is complete or limited:

- A *complete abdominal ultrasound,* code 76700, must include images of the liver, gallbladder, common bile duct, pancreas, spleen, kidneys, and upper abdominal aorta and inferior vena cava.
- A *limited abdominal ultrasound,* code 76705, is reported when a single organ or quadrant is imaged or when less than the definition of a complete abdominal ultrasound is documented.
- A *complete retroperitoneal ultrasound,* code 76770, must include images of the kidneys, abdominal aorta, common iliac artery origins, and inferior vena cava.
- A *limited retroperitoneal ultrasound,* code 76775, is assigned when less than the definition of a complete retroperitoneal ultrasound is documented.

Pelvis: 76801–76857

Codes within this range are further defined as obstetrical and nonobstetrical:

- **Obstetrical, 76801–76828:** The codes within this range are further defined by the trimester, number of gestational sacs, approach, inclusion of a detailed fetal anatomical examination, and limited or follow-up examination.

FOR EXAMPLE Ultrasound, pregnant uterus, real time with image documentation, fetal and maternal evaluation plus detailed fetal anatomical examination, transabdominal approach, single for first gestation, is assigned CPT code 76811. ■

- **Nonobstetrical, 76830–76857:** Transvaginal nonobstetric ultrasound is assigned a code within this range, 76830, while a transvaginal obstetric ultrasound is assigned code 76817. Codes within this range are also further defined as complete or limited, and the guidelines before the code range clarify the definitions.

Extremities: 76881–76886

The guidelines before this code range define a complete ultrasound of an extremity and a limited ultrasound of an extremity.

MENTOR
Coding Tip

The definitions for complete and limited ultrasounds would be good definitions to highlight in your CPT manual.

Ultrasonic Guidance: 76930–76965

Ultrasound guidance codes are assigned to this code range, while fluoroscopic, computed tomography, and magnetic resonance guidance codes are assigned to code range 77001–77032.

Breast, Mammography (77051–77059)

Diagnostic and screening mammograms are assigned codes under this subheading. Computer-aided detection (CAD) analysis should be reported as an additional code if it is performed with the mammogram.

EXERCISE 18.3

1. What is the definition of a real-time scan?
2. The radiology report documents that a patient with gallstones received an ultrasound scan, real time, with image documentation of the gallbladder only. Which CPT code would be appropriate to assign?
3. How does the CPT manual define a complete ultrasound of an extremity?
4. A bilateral diagnostic mammogram with a diagnostic computer-aided detection analysis was documented. What code(s) would be reported?
5. What is the appropriate code for an MRI of both breasts with contrast?

Also available in  connect plus+

18.4 Guidelines and Format of the Bone/Joint Studies and Radiation Oncology Subsections of the Radiology Section of CPT

Bone/Joint Studies (77071-77084)

Bone age studies, bone length studies (also known as *orthoroentgenograms* or *scan grams*), and dual-energy x-ray absorptiometry (DXA) studies are assigned codes under this subheading. Figure 18.4 shows a bone study showing osteoporosis.

Bone age studies, CPT code 77072, are used to estimate the stage of development of a child. The x-ray is usually taken of the nondominant hand and wrist and then compared to the child's chronological age standards.

Dual-energy x-ray absorptiometry (DXA) scans (codes 77080–77082) are performed to measure bone mass density, usually for patients with osteoporosis. Code 77080 is used for the axial skeleton (hips, pelvis, or spine) and code 77081 is for the appendicular skeleton (radius, wrist, or heel).

Radiation Oncology (77261-77799)

Radiation oncology codes describe therapeutic treatment that is often performed in addition to surgery and chemotherapy.

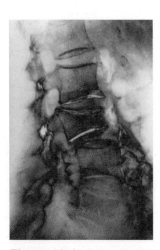

Figure 18.4 Osteoporosis

The codes under this subheading are further divided into the categories discussed below.

Clinical Treatment Planning and Simulation-Aided Field Setting: 77261–77299

Clinical treatment planning is the developing of a plan for the course of radiation therapy. It involves developing the best method of treatments by determining the number of areas of malignancy and the number of treatment ports (the sites where the beam enters the skin) and calculating the time and dosage.

Simulation-aided field setting is done before the radiation therapy course of treatment begins. This simulation visualizes and defines the exact treatment area and helps decide the size and location of the ports.

The procedures coded in this range are further defined as simple, intermediate, or complex, and the CPT manual defines these terms for the specific code ranges.

clinical treatment planning The development of a plan for the course of radiation therapy.

simulation-aided field setting Setting that is done before a radiation therapy course of treatment begins; visualizes and defines the exact treatment area and helps decide the size and location of the ports.

Radiation Treatment Delivery: 77401–77425
Radiation Treatment Management: 77427–77499

The codes in these ranges are reported in units of five fractions, or treatment sessions, which do not have to be on consecutive days. According to the CPT guidelines, these codes require and include a minimum of one examination of the patient by the physician for each reporting of the radiation treatment management service.

CPT code 77469 is for intraoperative radiation treatment management.

Proton Beam Treatment Delivery: 77520–77525

Procedures coded within this range are further defined as simple, intermediate, or complex, and the guidelines in the CPT manual before this range of codes clarify the definitions.

Clinical Brachytherapy: 77750–77799

The codes in this range are assigned for **brachytherapy,** which is the application of radioactive isotopes for internal radiation. The hospital admission and subsequent visits are included in the code description and are not coded separately.

brachytherapy The application of radioactive isotopes for internal radiation.

---

1. A dual-energy x-ray absorptiometry (DXA) scan is documented as being performed on the hips and spine. Which skeleton is being examined, and what is the appropriate code?

2. What instruction does the subheading guideline for Clinical Brachytherapy give the coder about the reporting of hospital admission and daily visits with codes in this section?

3. What is the appropriate CPT code for intraoperative radiation treatment management?

Also available in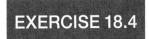

EXERCISE 18.4

18.5 Guidelines and Format of the Nuclear Medicine Subsection of the Radiology Section of CPT

nuclear medicine A field of studies that involves diagnostic and therapeutic use of radioactive materials.

The Nuclear Medicine subsection spans the code range 78012–79999. **Nuclear medicine** studies involve the diagnostic and therapeutic use of radioactive materials. Examples of radioactive materials used to perform these studies are Xenon, DTP, technetium, iodine, cardiolite, and thallium. These materials are administered by ingestion, injection, or inhalation.

> **MENTOR** Coding Tip
>
> There are terms used in provider documentation that are specific to nuclear medicine studies. *Radionuclide, radiopharmaceutical, millicures,* and *microcuries* are the most common. Being aware of these terms helps coders to identify services as nuclear medicine.

Diagnostic (78012–78999)

diagnostic nuclear medicine The use of imaging studies using radioactive materials to diagnose a condition.

Diagnostic nuclear medicine studies establish or confirm a diagnosis. Some examples of diagnostic nuclear medicine studies are bone scans, lung scans, thyroid scans and uptakes, renal imaging, SPECT, and PET studies.

Endocrine System: 78012–78099

Thyroid studies typically are uptakes or imaging scans, and they are reported using codes from this code range. These studies can include a vascular flow study. Scans produce an image of the thyroid, while an uptake study produces a value or percentage. There are codes for thyroid uptake (78012), thyroid imaging (78013), and thyroid imaging with uptake (78014).

Thyroid uptake studies are coded with one code for either single or multiple determinations (measurements) and thyroid imaging is reported with one code including vascular flow if performed. Patients swallow a radioactive capsule and return after a period of time, often 2, 3, or 6 hours. An uptake probe is used to measure the radioactive material that has accumulated in the thyroid, and this calculation is measured against a known value. In a single-determination study, the patient returns only once and only one calculation is made. In a multiple-determination study, the patient returns more than once and more than one calculation is made. In some patients, after the uptake calculation is made, a scan is taken that creates an image of the thyroid.

Gastrointestinal System: 78201–78299

Liver scans, liver-spleen scans, gallbladder scans (described as hepatobiliary system imaging in CPT) , and vitamin B_{12} absorption studies (Schilling tests) are some of the procedures included in this code range. Some of the code descriptions include static images only, while others include vascular flow.

FOR EXAMPLE

Liver imaging; static only, 78201

Liver imaging; with vascular flow, 78202 ∎

Musculoskeletal System: 78300–78399

Bone scans are assigned codes from this range. They are often done to diagnose malignancies or inflammatory diseases such as osteomyelitis or cellulitis. These procedures are further defined by:

- Limited area or localized area, such as the knee, 78300
- Multiple areas defined as two or more anatomical sites, 78305
- Whole body, defined as from the head to as least the level of the knees, 78306
- Three-phase study, which consists of initial vascular flow, blood pool images, and delayed static images, 78315

Cardiovascular System: 78414–78499

Myocardial perfusion studies, single-photon emission computed tomography (SPECT) scans and planar views, and MUGA (multigated acquisition) scans are some of the procedures assigned codes in this range. Several of these procedures are performed at rest and/or during stress.

Respiratory System: 78579–78599

Pulmonary ventilation and perfusion imaging are included in this code range.

Therapeutic (79005–79999)

Therapeutic nuclear medicine studies provide relief by the use of a radioactive material. Two examples are radioactive iodine for patients with hyperthyroidism (Graves' disease) and strontium (Metastron) for cancer patients.

The more familiar coders become with the CPT format and guidelines, the better prepared they are for selecting the appropriate code to be linked to the medically necessary diagnosis for the patient encounter.

therapeutic nuclear medicine studies The use of radioactive materials to treat a condition or disease.

---

1. How can radioactive materials be administered to a patient?
2. What is included in a nuclear medicine three-phase bone scan, code 78315?
3. Explain the difference between diagnostic and therapeutic nuclear medicine studies.

EXERCISE 18.5

Also available in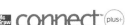

18.6 Modifiers Most Commonly Used with Codes in the Radiology Section of CPT

As with all sections of the CPT manual, modifiers are used in the Radiology section to continue or modify the story of the patient's encounter. The modifiers most commonly used in this section are 26, professional component; 52, reduced service; 59, distinct procedure; 76, repeat procedure or service by the same physician or other qualified healthcare professional; and 77, repeat procedure or service by another physician or another qualified healthcare professional. (See Table 18.2.)

Table 18.2 Radiology Section Modifiers *(Data from CPT 2013. © 2013 American Medical Association. All rights reserved.)*

MODIFIER	DEFINITION	EXAMPLE OF USE
26	Professional component	Only the professional component or supervision and interpretation is being reported.
52	Reduced service	Less than the minimum number of views was performed. For example, a single-view x-ray of the femur after a closed fracture manipulation to check for proper alignment is assigned code 73550-52.
59	Distinct procedure	A diagnostic angiography is performed at the same session as an interventional procedure when a prior study is available but the medical record documents that the patient's condition has changed since the prior study in regard to the clinical indication. The angiography is reported as a distinct procedure.
76	Repeat procedure or service by the same physician or other qualified healthcare professional	A two-view chest x-ray (71020) is interpreted by physician A at 8 a.m., and another two-view chest x-ray (71020) is interpreted by the same physician later the same day.
77	Repeat procedure or service by another physician or another qualified healthcare professional	A two-view chest x-ray (71020) is interpreted by physician A at 8 a.m., and another two-view chest x-ray (71020) is interpreted by physician B later the same day.

The appropriate use of modifiers with the codes from the Radiology section helps to tell the patient's full story.

EXERCISE 18.6

1. What is the appropriate modifier to use when less than the minimum number of views is taken and a specific code does not exist for the lower number of views?

2. If a scenario on the CPC exam instructs the test taker to code for the professional component only, which modifier would be attached to the appropriate radiology code?

3. If a one-view chest x-ray, CPT code 71010, is performed twice on the same day by the same physician, which modifier would be attached to the second x-ray?

Also available in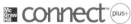

18.7 Common Medical and Procedural Terms Used in Operative Reports

As with all sections of CPT, the Radiology section includes medical terms and procedural terms that are specific to the system involved. Tables 18.3 to 18.5 list some of these terms and identify some key terms that could appear in a provider's documentation.

Body Planes

Body planes are imaginary vertical and horizontal lines used to divide the body into sections for descriptive purposes. (See Figure 18.5 and Table 18.3.)

Figure 18.6 shows the body cavities; Figures 18.7 to 18.9 show body motions.

Body Directions

Body directions are used in radiology reports to describe the locations of different parts. (See Table 18.4.)

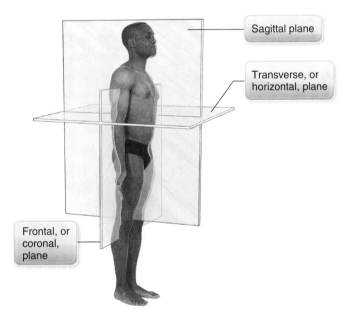

Figure 18.5 Anatomical Planes

Table 18.3 Terms for Body Planes

BODY PLANE	DEFINITION
Coronal plane (frontal plane)	Vertical plane running from side to side that divides the body into anterior and posterior portions
Sagittal plane (lateral plane)	Vertical plane running from front to back that divides the body into right and left sides
Axial plane (transverse plane)	Horizontal plane that divides the body into upper and lower portions
Median plane	Sagittal plane through the middle of the body that divides the body into right and left halves

coronal plane Vertical plane running from side to side that divides the body into anterior and posterior portions. Also called *frontal plane.*

sagittal plane Vertical plane running from front to back that divides the body into right and left sides. Also called *lateral plane* or *midline.*

axial plane Horizontal plane that divides the body into upper and lower portions. Also called *transverse plane.*

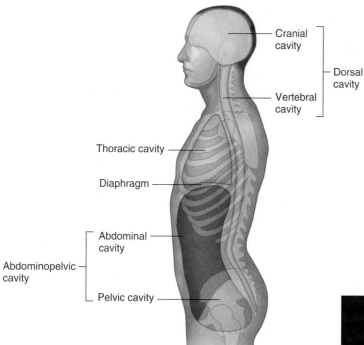

Figure 18.6 Body Cavities

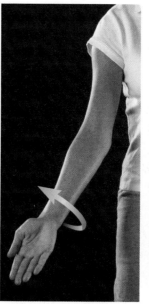

Figure 18.7 Flexion and Extension

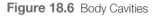

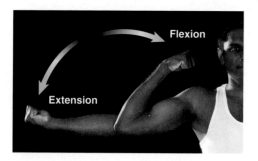

Figure 18.8 Dorsiflexion and Plantar Flexion

Figure 18.9 Supination and Pronation

Table 18.4 Terms for Body Directions

BODY DIRECTION	DEFINITION
Anterior	To the front of the body or front of an organ
Posterior	To the back of the body or back of an organ
Superior/cephalic	Above another body part or toward the head
Inferior/caudal	Below another body part or toward the feet
Proximal	Body part closest to the part of reference, midpoint, or beginning (E.g., the elbow is proximal to the wrist.)
Distal	Body part farthest from the point of reference, midpoint, or beginning (E.g., the elbow is distal to the shoulder joint.)

Additional terms used in radiology reports are defined in Table 18.5.

Table 18.5 Terms for Radiology

TERM	DEFINITION	DOCUMENTATION KEYS
Ascites	An accumulation of excess fluid in the peritoneal cavity	Centesis procedure performed to drain excess fluid.
Dual-energy x-ray absorptiometry (DXA)	A study performed to measure bone mass density, usually for patients with osteoporosis	Axial skeleton (hips, pelvis, or spine) imaged. Appendicular skeleton (radius, wrist, or heel) imaged.
Extension	Straightening movement	Increases the angle at the joint
Flexion	Bending movement	Decreases the angle at the joint
Pronation	Body motion of bending forward or downward	Rotation of the forearm with the palm facing down
Radiopharmaceutical	Radioactive drug used for therapeutic or diagnostic purposes in nuclear medicine studies	Radioactive material, MDP, Xenon, DTPA
Single-photon emission computed tomography (SPECT)	Nuclear medicine study in which images are produced in multiple dimensions in order to diagnose an abnormality within the area	CT scan performed using a radioactive tracer which lets the physician see the blood flow to tissues and organs
Supination	Body motion of bending upward	Rotation of the forearm with the palm facing up

dual-energy x-ray absorptiometry (DXA) Radiological study performed to measure bone density, usually in patients with osteoporosis.

extension A straightening movement that increases the angle at the joint.

flexion A bending movement that decreases the angle at the joint.

pronation Body motion of bending forward or downward

radiopharmaceutical Radioactive drug used for therapeutic or diagnostic purposes in nuclear medicine studies.

supination Body motion of bending upward

---

1. The radiology report finding states that there is an excess of fluid in the peritoneal cavity. What term would the coder look for in the Alphabetic Index of ICD?

2. Define *axial plane,* which is also called *transverse plane.*

3. Describe a SPECT study.

EXERCISE 18.7

Also available in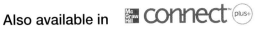

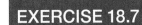

Chapter Eighteen Summary

Learning Outcome	Key Concepts/Examples
18.1 Review the general ICD and CPT guidelines for radiology coding.	**ICD Guidelines** • When a diagnosis has not been confirmed or the radiology report is documented as normal, signs and symptoms should be reported. • ICD abnormal-findings codes may be used when additional testing is required and the test results are negative. • A patient encounter for radiation therapy has definite sequencing guidelines. • Multiple fractures are sequenced in the order of severity, with the most severe first. • There is a differentiation between a traumatic fracture and a pathologic fracture. **CPT guidelines** • *Contrast material: With contrast* means that contrast is administered intravascularly, intraparticularly, or intrathecally. Oral and/or rectal contact is not with contrast. • *Number of views:* Many of the code descriptions within the Radiology subsection specify a minimum number of views. • *Fluoroscopy:* Fluoroscopy is inherent in many radiological procedures. Unless specifically instructed otherwise, fluoroscopy used to complete a procedure and obtain a permanent record is included in the code description and is not reported separately.
18.2 Identify the CPT guidelines and format of the Diagnostic Imaging subsection of CPT.	Codes under this subheading are further defined by the following: • Anatomical site • Number of views/type of view • Computed tomography (CT) or computed tomography angiography (CTA) • Magnetic resonance imaging (MRI) or magnetic resonance angiography (MRA), with or without contrast
18.3 Understand the CPT guidelines and format of the Diagnostic Ultrasound and Breast, Mammography subsections of CPT.	*Diagnostic Ultrasound:* Ultrasound imaging, or sonography, is a noninvasive test that uses high-frequency sound waves to produce images that are captured in real time and show structure, movement, and the flow of blood through blood vessels. The code ranges in this subsection are divided by anatomical site, complete or limited, and obstetrical or nonobstetrical for pelvic ultrasounds. *Breast, Mammography:* Diagnostic and screening mammograms are assigned codes within this subsection. Computer-aided detection (CAD) analysis should be reported as an additional code if it is performed with the mammogram.
18.4 Apply the CPT guidelines and format of the Bone/Joint Studies and Radiation Oncology subsections of CPT.	*Bone/Joint Studies:* Bone age studies, bone length studies (orthoroentgenograms or scan grams), and dual-energy x-ray absorptiometry (DEXA) studies are assigned codes under this subheading. Bone age studies (77072) are used to estimate the stage of development of a child. DXA scans (77080–77082) are performed to measure bone mass density. *Radiation Oncology:* Codes under this subheading describe therapeutic treatment that is often performed in addition to surgery and chemotherapy. These codes are further defined by the following subheadings: • Clinical Treatment Planning and Simulation-Aided Field Setting • Radiation Treatment Delivery • Radiation Treatment Management • Proton Beam Treatment Delivery • Clinical Brachytherapy

Learning Outcome	Key Concepts/Examples
18.5 Recognize the CPT guidelines and format of the Nuclear Medicine subsection of CPT.	Nuclear medicine studies involve the diagnostic and therapeutic use of radioactive materials. *Thyroid studies* typically are uptakes or imaging scans, and they are reported using codes from this subsection. These studies can include a vascular flow study. Scans produce an image of the thyroid, while an uptake study produces a value or percentage. *Bone scans* are often done to diagnose malignancies or inflammatory diseases such as osteomyelitis or cellulitis. These codes are further defined by: • Limited area or localized area, such as the knee • Multiple areas, defined as two or more anatomical sites • Whole body, defined as from the head to as least the level of the knees • Three-phase study, which consists of initial vascular flow, blood pool images, and delayed static images
18.6 Evaluate the modifiers most commonly used with codes in the Radiology section of CPT.	In the Radiology section the modifiers most commonly used are 26, professional component; 52, reduced service; 59, distinct procedure; 76, repeat procedure or service by the same physician or other qualified healthcare professional; and 77, repeat procedure or service by another physician or another qualified healthcare professional.
18.7 Examine the common medical and procedural terms used in operative reports.	*Body planes:* coronal, axial, sagittal, medial *Body directions:* anterior/posterior, ventral/dorsal, superior/inferior, proximal/distal

Chapter Eighteen Review

Using Terminology

Match each key term to the appropriate definition.

_____ 1. [LO18.2] Computed tomography

_____ 2. [LO18.1] Contrast material

_____ 3. [LO18.5] Diagnostic study

_____ 4. [LO18.7] Dual-energy x-ray absorptiometry

_____ 5. [LO18.7] Extension

_____ 6. [LO18.7] Flexion

_____ 7. [LO18.1] Fluoroscopy

_____ 8. [LO18.2] Magnetic resonance imaging

_____ 9. [LO18.5] Nuclear medicine

_____ 10. [LO18.7] Pronation

_____ 11. [LO18.7] Radiopharmaceutical

_____ 12. [LO18.7] Sagittal plane

_____ 13. [LO18.7] Supination

_____ 14. [LO18.3] Ultrasound

A. A radiology imaging modality used to study structures in a body plane; produces computerized cross-section images

B. Study that creates real-time or moving images that are useful for diagnostic procedures and for guidance in interventional procedures

C. Substance that is administered intravascularly, intraparticularly, or intrathecally

D. A radiology imaging modality that uses a magnetic field and radio waves to produce images of organs, tissues

E. Studies that involve the diagnostic and therapeutic use of radioactive materials

F. Vertical plane running from front to back that divides the body into right and left sides

G. Study performed to establish or confirm a diagnosis

H. A noninvasive test that uses high-frequency sound waves to produce images that are captured in real time and show structure; also called *sonography*

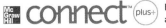

Enhance your learning by completing these exercises and more at mcgrawhillconnect.com

I. Radioactive drug for therapeutic or diagnostic use in nuclear medicine studies

I. Radioactive drug for therapeutic or diagnostic use in nuclear medicine studies
J. Rotation of the forearm with the palm facing up
K. Straightening movement that increases the angle at the joint
L. Study performed to measure bone mass density, usually for patients with osteoporosis
M. Rotation of the forearm with the palm facing down
N. Bending movement that decreases the angle at the joint

Checking Your Understanding

Choose the most appropriate answer for each of the following questions.

1. [LO18.4] George Smith was admitted for 3 days for interstitial application of six radioelement solution ribbons into his prostate for treatment of his prostate cancer by the therapeutic radiologist, who also saw the patient each day of his admission. Select the appropriate CPT and ICD-9-CM codes:

   a. 77778, 99223, 99233 x2, 186
   b. 77777, 99233 x3
   c. 77778, 186
   d. 77777, 186

2. [LO18.5] Amanda Jones presented to the ED with acute GI bleeding from the rectum as a result of her diverticulitis. The physician ordered a nuclear medicine study of the abdomen to determine the rate of blood loss and the status of her current disease. Select the appropriate ICD-9-CM and CPT codes:

   a. 78290, 562.10
   b. 78278, 562.11
   c. 74176, 562.11
   d. 74178, 562.11

3. [LO18.3] Betty presented for needle placement via ultrasonic guidance for biopsy of two breast masses. Select the appropriate supervision and interpretation codes:

   a. 76942, 611.72
   b. 76950, 611.72
   c. 76942, 19290, 19291, 174.9
   d. 76942, 19290, 611.72

4. [LO18.4] Jose is undergoing radiation therapy treatment to his larynx and salivary gland area. He is receiving EBRT 13 mev to both areas. This is the fifth day of treatment this week. Select the appropriate CPT code for the five days of treatment:

   a. 77409
   b. 77404 x5
   c. 77409 x5
   d. 77404

5. [LO18. 2] A morbidly obese male, age 46, is seen for increasing pain in his knees, which is affecting his mobility. The physician orders a bilateral x-ray of the knees, with the patient standing as part of the workup. The x-ray report indicates bilateral osteoarthritis. Select the appropriate ICD-9-CM and CPT codes:

   a. 73564-50, 715.86, 278.01
   b. 73562-50, 719.46
   c. 73560-50, 715.86, 278.01
   d. 73565, 715.36

6. [LO18.5] A 45-year-old female presents with a significant history of cardiovascular disease. The physician orders a study to determine the right ventricular ejection fraction by the first-pass technique at rest. Select the appropriate CPT code(s) for this procedure:

   a. 78742
   b. 78496
   c. 78472, 78496
   d. 78494

7. [LO18.3] An ultrasound of a pregnant uterus, real time with image documentation, fetal and maternal evaluation, second trimester, in a female carrying twins was performed. Select the appropriate code(s) for this procedure:

   a. 76801
   b. 76801, 76802
   c. 76805, 76810
   d. 76805

8. **[LO18.2]** John, a 20-year-old male, presented to his physician for evaluation of nonpainful masses on the left side of the neck. As part of the workup, the physician ordered a CT of the neck with and without contrast to aid in the diagnosis. Select the appropriate code(s):

   a. 70490, 70492

   b. 70492

   c. 70491

   d. 70490, 70491

9. **[LO18.2]** A 30-year-old male presents with flank pain and gross hematuria. The physician orders a CT of the abdomen and pelvis without contrast followed by contrast in the pelvis. Select the appropriate CPT code for the radiologist's supervision and interpretation:

   a. 72194

   b. 74177-26

   c. 74178-26

   d. 72193

10. **[LO 18.1, 18.2]** An 18-year-old patient presents today for an x-ray of his right knee and an MRI to rule out a torn ACL of the knee due to an injury sustained when checked into boards during a hockey game. After the testing is complete, the interpretation and report verify a torn ACL ligament, right knee complete. Select the appropriate CPT and ICD-9-CM codes:

   a. 73720, 73564-RT, 844.2, E886.0

   b. 73721, 73564-RT, 844.2, E886.0

   c. 73564-RT, 73720, 717.8, E886.0

   d. 73721, 73562-RT, 717.83, E886.0

Applying Your Knowledge

Answer the following questions and code the following case study. Be sure to follow the process steps as illustrated in Chapter 8.

Case Study

Indication: Right upper-quadrant abdominal pain

Procedure: Gallbladder ultrasound

There is a cyst in the left hepatic lobe. The liver is otherwise unremarkable. There is no biliary ductal dilation. There is no abdominal ascites. There are multiple gallstones noted within the gallbladder. There are no abnormalities in the visualized portions of the abdominal aorta or pancreas. The spleen does not appear enlarged. The right kidney contains a 4-cm cyst. The left kidney appears normal.

Impression:

1. Hepatic cyst

2. 4-cm kidney cyst

3. Cholelithiasis

Process 1: CPT

1. What is the procedure?

2. Locate the main term in the index.

3. What additional questions or set of questions can be determined?

4. Upon review of all the code choices identified in the index, what additional questions can be determined?

5. Based on the documentation, what is the correct code for this case?

   a. 76700-26

   b. 76705-26

   c. 76770-26

   d. 76775-26

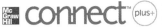

Process 2: ICD

ICD-9-CM

1. Based on the operative report header, what is the indication/diagnosis?

2. Is the postexamination diagnosis the same as or different from the preexamination diagnosis?

3. Is the postexamination diagnosis supported?

4. What is the main term for this condition?

5. Based on the subterm choices, what question(s) can be developed for this condition?

6. Is any sign, symptom, or additional condition documented?

7. Is the additional condition, sign, or symptom an integral part of the primary (or other) condition coded?

8. Does the additional condition require or affect patient care, treatment, or management?

9. Based on the documentation, what are the correct ICD-9-CM codes for this case?
   - **a.** 573.3, 753.11, 574.10
   - **b.** 573.9, 593.3, 574.00
   - **c.** 573.8, 593.2, 574.20
   - **d.** 572.0, 591, 575.0

ICD-10-CM

1. Based on the operative report header, what is the preexamination indication/diagnosis?

2. Is the postexamination diagnosis the same as or different from the preexamination diagnosis?

3. Is the postexamination diagnosis supported?

4. What is the main term for this condition?

5. Based on the subterm choices, what question(s) can be developed for this condition?

6. Based on the information in the Tabular List, is additional information needed to determine the appropriate diagnosis code?

7. Is any sign, symptom, or additional condition documented?

8. Is the additional condition, sign, or symptom an integral part of the primary (or other) condition coded?

9. Does the additional condition require or affect patient care, treatment, or management?

10. Based on the documentation, what are the correct ICD-10-CM codes for this case?
    - **a.** K75.9, Q61.01, K80.10
    - **b.** K76.9, N13.5, K80.00
    - **c.** K76.89, N28.1, K80.20
    - **d.** K75.0, N13.30, K81.0

Process 3: Modifiers

1. Was the procedure performed different from that described by the nomenclature of the code?

2. Was the procedure performed at an anatomical site that has laterality?

3. Was the procedure performed in the global period of another procedure?

4. Were additional procedures performed during the examination, and does the documentation support them?

5. Did the surgeon have help from another surgeon or another appropriate person?

6. Did a physician different from the surgeon provide the preexamination or postexamination portion of the procedure?

7. What modifier should be appended to the CPT code for this case?
   - **a.** −57
   - **b.** −26
   - **c.** −22
   - **d.** None

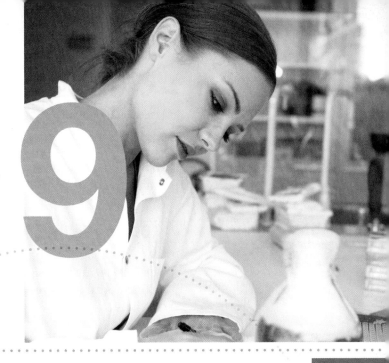

Pathology/Laboratory

Key Terms

Block
Chromatography
Coagulation
Cytogenic studies

Cytopathology
Hematology
Immunology
Ionized calcium

Molecular pathology
Mutations
Organ panel
Qualitative analysis

Quantitative analysis
Specimen

Learning Outcomes

After completing this chapter, you will be able to:

19.1 Review the general ICD and CPT guidelines for pathology/laboratory coding.

19.2 Identify the CPT guidelines and format of the Organ or Disease-Oriented Panels, Drug Testing, Therapeutic Drug Assays, Evocative/Suppression Testing, Consultations, and Urinalysis subsections of CPT.

19.3 Understand the CPT guidelines and format of the Molecular Pathology, Chemistry, Hematology, Immunology, Transfusion Medicine, and Microbiology subsections of CPT.

19.4 Apply the CPT guidelines and format of the Anatomic Pathology, Cytopathology, Cytogenic Studies, Surgical Pathology, Other Procedures, and Reproductive Medicine Procedures subsections of CPT.

19.5 Evaluate the modifiers most commonly used with codes in the Pathology/Laboratory section of CPT.

19.6 Examine the common medical and procedural terms used in operative reports.

Introduction
Pathology and laboratory CPT codes reflect services provided to give additional diagnostic and treatment management information to the treating physician. These services include the examination and evaluation of specimens obtained from patients, such as body fluids and cytological or tissue specimens.

19.1 Format and General ICD and CPT Guidelines for Pathology/Laboratory Coding

The general headings used in the Pathology/Laboratory section of the CPT manual are listed in Table 19.1.

ICD Guidelines

When a diagnosis has not been confirmed or the pathology report is documented as normal, signs and symptoms should be reported.

Abnormal test results are acceptable diagnoses when further tests are negative.

Neoplasms

The Alphabetic Index of ICD and the neoplasm table enable coders to select the appropriate neoplasm code based on the type of neoplasm and the site. The neoplasm table is divided into four sections:

- Malignant
  - Primary
  - Secondary
  - Carcinoma in situ
- Benign
- Uncertain Behavior
- Unspecified Behavior

Table 19.1 CPT Pathology/Laboratory Section Format *(Data from CPT 2013. © 2013 American Medical Association. All rights reserved.)*

GENERAL HEADING	CODE RANGE
Organ or Disease-Oriented Panels	80047–80076
Drug Testing	80100–80104
Therapeutic Drug Assays	80150–80299
Evocative/Suppression Testing	80400–80440
Consultations (Clinical Pathology)	80500–80502
Urinalysis	81000–81099
Molecular Pathology	81200–81479
Chemistry	82000–84999
Hematology and Coagulation	85002–85999
Immunology	86000–86849
Transfusion Medicine	86850–86999
Microbiology	87001–87999
Anatomic Pathology	88000–88099
Cytopathology	88104–88199
Cytogenic studies	88230–88299
Surgical Pathology	88300–88399
In Vivo	88720–88749
Other Procedures	89049–89240
Reproductive Medicine Procedures	89250–89398

CPT Guidelines

Additional Testing

After a pathology/laboratory test is performed and it is felt that additional related procedures are necessary to verify the results, these tests are considered part of the ordered test and are reported as one unit of service. An example is an automated test after a manual test to confirm the results. However, with some laboratory tests, if a positive result occurs, an additional test is then done as a follow-up. These tests are called *indicators* and allow for additional tests without the written order of a physician. This additional testing is reported separately since the initial results need additional testing to add to the clinical value of the results.

There are several questions a coder needs to ask when reading an operative report and coding a procedure from the Pathology/Laboratory section of the CPT. The following questions will help the coder, when reading through the report, to understand what actually was done and how the procedure should be translated and coded:

- At which anatomical site was the study performed (if applicable)?
- Was the study qualitative or quantitative?
- What are all of the laboratory studies that were performed during the present encounter (e.g., organ panel, surgical pathology)?
- What type of equipment was used (e.g., automated, nonautomated, microscope)?
- Which type of consultation was involved: clinical pathology or surgical pathology?
- How many tests were performed?

EXERCISE 19.1

1. What are the four sections of the neoplasm table?
2. What are some key words to look for in provider documentation to help identify a definitive diagnosis?
3. What is an indicator?

Also available in

19.2 Guidelines and Format of the Organ or Disease-Oriented Panels, Drug Testing, Therapeutic Drug Assays, Evocative/Suppression Testing, Consultations, and Urinalysis Subsections of the Pathology/Laboratory Section of CPT (80047–81099)

Organ or Disease-Oriented Panels (80047–80076)

The codes within this range are assigned to **organ panels,** or disease-oriented panels, which consist of a series of specific tests ordered to assist in the

organ panel A series of specific tests ordered to assist in the determination of a diagnosis.

determination of a diagnosis. All of the tests listed within the code description must be performed in order to assign the code.

FOR EXAMPLE CPT code 80047, basic metabolic panel (calcium, ionized), must include the following:

Calcium, ionized, 82330
Carbon dioxide, 82374
Chloride, 82435
Creatinine, 82565
Glucose, 82947
Potassium, 84132
Sodium, 84295
Urea nitrogen, 84520

If one of these tests, such as the potassium, was not performed, the panel code 80047 would not be assigned and all of the tests that were performed would be coded separately.

If all of the tests described in the panel code were performed and an additional test not listed in the series was also performed, the panel code plus the additional-test code would be reported.

FOR EXAMPLE An electrolyte panel (code 80051) was performed along with a glucose test (code 82947). This would be coded as 80051 and 82947 since the glucose is not a test listed in the description of the electrolyte panel code. ■

MENTOR Coding Tip

Highlight in your CPT manual that codes 80047 and 80048 are alike except for the calcium test: 80047 is described as "calcium, ionized," whereas 80048 is described as "calcium, total." Total calcium tests both **ionized calcium** (which is free-flowing calcium, not attached to proteins) and calcium attached to proteins.

---

ionized calcium Free-flowing calcium, not attached to proteins.

A guideline at the beginning of this code range in the CPT manual states: If a group of tests overlaps two or more panels, report the panel that incorporates the greater number of tests to fulfill the code definition and report the remaining tests using individual test codes.

Drug Testing (80100–80104)

The codes assigned to this code range are used to report drug screening, drug confirmation, and tissue preparation services. These codes are used to identify the presence of a drug, which is a **qualitative analysis.** The confirmation test, code 80102, is performed as a double check on a positive result (presence of a drug) of a drug screening test (codes 80100, 80101, 80104).

qualitative analysis Laboratory procedure that identifies the presence of a drug.

Guidelines tell coders to use 80100 for each multiple-drug-class chromatographic procedure.

Chromatography is a combination of stationary and mobile phases used to analyze the drug class or classes. The CPT guidelines direct the coder that each combination of stationary and mobile phases is to be counted as one unit. For example: Multiple drugs can be detected using one stationary phase with one mobile phase, and code 80100 would be reported once.

chromatography A combination of stationary and mobile phases used to analyze a drug class or classes.

Therapeutic Drug Assays (80150–80299)

Often, drugs used for therapeutic reasons need to be analyzed for impurities or toxicities that could lead to negative side effects for the patient, depending on the levels. Codes in this code range are used to report the tests performed to monitor and evaluate the levels of these drugs in the body. Material may be used from any source, but blood, urine, and sputum are the most common sources. This is a **quantitative analysis** to measure the amount of drug present.

The drugs are listed by generic names. The drug is measured at peaks (after the drug is given and at intervals) and troughs (before the drug is given).

MENTOR Coding Tip

Code the number of procedures, not the number of drugs tested.

quantitative analysis Laboratory procedure that measures the amount of a drug present.

Evocative/Suppression Testing (80400–80440)

The codes in this range are described as panels, and each code describes the number of times the test is performed for the particular agent. The panels involve the administration of evocative or suppressive agents and then the measurement of the effect.

The codes in this range are used for the laboratory portions of the testing.

The CPT guidelines at the beginning of the code range direct the coder to use codes 96365–96368; 96372–96376 for physician administration of the evocative or suppressive agents.

Consultations (Clinical Pathology) (80500–80502)

CPT (2013) defines a clinical pathology consultation as "a service, including a written report, rendered by the pathologist in response to a request from an attending physician in relation to a test result(s) requiring additional medical interpretive judgment."

The codes are further defined as to the level:

The reporting of only the test results is not enough to justify the use of a clinical pathology code.

- **Limited:** without review of the patient's history and medical record, 80500
- **Comprehensive:** complex diagnostic problem with review of history and medical record, 80502

An instructional note below these codes directs the coder to code range 99241–99255 for consultation involving the examination and evaluation of the patient.

Urinalysis (81000–81099)

This code range is used to report tests on urine. The codes are further defined by:

- The method of testing—reagent or dipstick.
- The constituents being tested.

- The equipment used—automated or nonautomated, with or without microscope.

Urinalysis, by dipstick or tablet reagent, for bilirubin, glucose, hemoglobin, ketones, leukocytes, nitrites, pH, protein, specific gravity, urobilinogen, or any number of these constituents, nonautomated, with microscopy is assigned CPT code 81000. ▪

- The reason for the test.

A urine pregnancy test by visual color comparison methods is assigned CPT code 81025. ▪

- The number of tests performed.

EXERCISE 19.2

1. Explain the difference between qualitative and quantitative analyses.
2. How are the codes in the urinalysis subheading further defined?
3. What is the difference between a limited clinical pathology consultation and a comprehensive one?
4. Identify the appropriate CPT code to be reported when a qualitative analysis of tissue is performed.

Also available in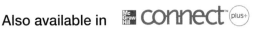

19.3 Guidelines and Format of the Molecular Pathology, Chemistry, Hematology, Immunology, Transfusion Medicine, and Microbiology Subsections of the Pathology/Laboratory Section of CPT (81200–87999)

Molecular Pathology (81200–81479)

molecular pathology Laboratory testing involving genes.

Codes under the **molecular pathology** subheading are used to report laboratory testing involving genes. The appropriate code selected is based on the specific gene or genes being analyzed. The gene name may be described in the code description as an abbreviation followed by the gene name. The gene names are based on Human Genome Organization (HUGO) approved names. The code description can also contain the protein or disease commonly associated with the gene. Figure 19.1 gives an example of the human gene structure (DNA). CPT 2013 has expanded and revised this subsection to accommodate the rapid expansion in the field of molecular diagnostics. Detailed guidelines, including examples, for use of the codes listed are included in the subsection guidelines.

81242   FANCC (Fanconi anemia, complementation group C)

This code is reported for Fanconi anemia, type C. ■

The molecular pathology codes include all analytical services performed in the test, such as cell lysis, nucleic acid stabilization, and amplification.

The analyses in this code range are qualitative (checking for a presence) unless otherwise indicated.

Several editions of the CPT manual have a section in the guidelines before this code range that lists definitions that apply to this category. Coders will find it helpful to read over this section and highlight any definitions that are new to them.

The codes in this range are further defined as:

- **Tier 1:** gene-specific and genomic procedures, 81200–81383
- **Tier 2:** procedures not listed in Tier I that are generally lower in volume than Tier 1 procedures, 81400–81479

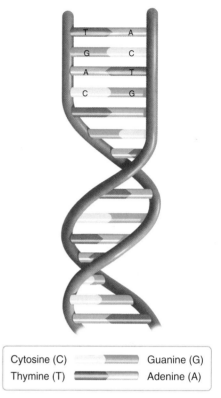

| Cytosine (C) | | Guanine (G) |
| Thymine (T) | | Adenine (A) |

Figure 19.1 DNA Structure

Chemistry (82000–84999)

Specific tests on any bodily substances such as urine, blood, breath, and feces are reported using codes from this subheading. Samples from different sources may be reported separately.

The tests are qualitative in nature unless otherwise indicated.

82379   Carnitine (total and free), quantitative, each specimen ■

Hematology and Coagulation (85002–85999)

Hematology is the study of disorders of the blood while **coagulation** is the process of blood clotting. Studies under this subheading include blood counts and are differentiated as to the following:

- Complete blood count (CBC)
- Red blood cell (RBC) count
- White blood cell (WBC) count
- Automated or manual
- Microscopic examination

See Figure 19.2 for a diagram of blood cells and platelets.

Immunology (86000–86849)

Immunology is the study of the immune system. Codes within this code range report tests used to identify immune system conditions

hematology The study of disorders of the blood.

coagulation A process of blood clotting.

immunology The study of the immune system.

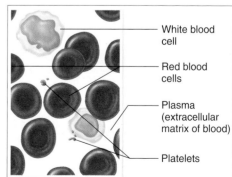

Figure 19.2 Blood Cells and Platelets

caused by antibodies and antigens. An antigen is a foreign substance that produces antibodies that fight infection and disease. The tests in this section are mostly quantitative or semiquantitative unless otherwise indicated.

86003   Allergen specific lgE: quantitative or semiquantitative, each allergen

An instructional note below this code directs the use of 82785 for total quantitative lgE. ■

Codes used to report blood banking, 86077–86079, are found under the Immunology subheading.

Transfusion Medicine (86850–86999)

Codes within this range are used for tests performed on blood or blood products. The codes are further defined by blood typing or identification, screening, and preparation or collection.

Microbiology (87001–87999)

The codes within this subheading are further differentiated by the type of study, such as bacteriology (bacteria), mycology (fungi), parasitology (parasites), and virology (viruses). The code descriptions also include the method of identification, described by CPT as:

Presumptive: identification of a microorganism by colony morphology growth on selective media, Gram stains, or up to three tests such as catalase, oxidase, indole, or urease.

Definitive: identification to the genus or species level that requires additional tests such as biochemical panels or slide cultures.

Culture, fungi (mold or yeast) isolation, with presumptive identification of isolates; skin hair or nail, 87101

or

Culture, fungi, definitive identification, each organism; yeast, 87106 ■

EXERCISE 19.3

1. Which code range and subheading include codes for reporting blood banking?
2. Identify how the codes under the Microbiology subheading are further differentiated.
3. Which type of laboratory tests is reported with codes from the range 86000–86849?
4. What are the gene names in the code descriptions in the Molecular Pathology section based on?

Also available in **connect** plus+

19.4 Guidelines and Format of the Anatomic Pathology, Cytopathology, Cytogenic Studies, Surgical Pathology, Other Procedures, and Reproductive Medicine Procedures Subsections of the Pathology/Laboratory Section of CPT (88000–89398)

Anatomic Pathology (88000–88099)

An instructional note with this range of codes states that these codes represent physician services only. It also instructs the use of modifier 90 for outside laboratory services.

These codes are for reporting postmortem examinations, that is, necropsies (autopsies). They are further divided as to:

- The extent and type of exam: gross versus gross and microscopic.
- Whether the examination is without the CNS, with the brain, or with the brain and spinal cord.

If the exam is a forensic examination, it is used for legal evidence.

MENTOR
Coding Tip

Gross examination means that the specimen is examined with the naked eye and is not prepared for examination by microscope.

Cytopathology (88104–88199)

Cytopathology is the study of cells. The codes under this subheading are used to report laboratory tests performed to identify cellular changes. The codes are divided by type of procedure and technique.

Pap smears are the most common test reported with codes in this subheading.

cytopathology The study of cells.

SPOTLIGHT on a Guideline

CPT codes 88150 to 88154 are used to report Pap smears using non-Bethesda reporting. Codes 88164 to 88167 are used to report Pap smears using the Bethesda system of reporting.

Cytogenic Studies (88230–88299)

Cytogenic studies are concerned with cellular abnormalities and pathologic conditions related to genetics.

cytogenic studies Studies concerned with cellular abnormalities and pathologic conditions related to genetics.

Surgical Pathology (88300–88399)

The codes in range 88300–88309 are defined by the following:

- Number of specimens (each specimen is a unit)
- Anatomical site and/or reason for submission
- Gross examination only
- Gross and microscopic examination (see Figure 19.3)

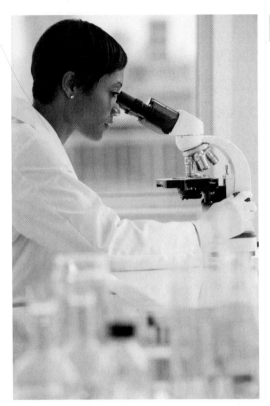

Figure 19.3 Microscopic Exam

 FOR EXAMPLE When the documentation states gross examination only, code 88300 is reported.

When the documentation indicates gross and microscopic examination on a specific anatomical site, a code from range 88302–88309 is reported. ■

MENTOR Coding Tip

The same anatomical site may be found within several codes (levels), so it is important to read the documentation and the code description carefully. For example:

Joint, loose body 88304 (level III)

Joint, resection 88305 (level IV)

These codes include accession (numbers are assigned recording the order of tissue acquisition), examination of tissue, and reporting.

Codes within this range, 88312–88319, are also used to report special stains when appropriate.

Intraoperative consultation codes, 88329 to 88334, are included in this code range and are further defined as to first tissue block with frozen section(s), each additional tissue block with frozen section(s), and cytologic examination, initial site and each additional site.

An instructional note below these codes directs the coder to use both 88331 and 88334 when an intraoperative consultation on a specimen requires both frozen section and cytologic evaluation.

MENTOR Coding Tip

A specimen is the unit submitted for evaluation, the block is a piece cut from the specimen to be frozen, and a section is a further division of the block.

EXERCISE 19.4

1. Codes within the anatomic pathology range are used to report postmortem examinations, that is, necropsies (autopsies). How are they further defined?

2. What is the difference between cytopathology studies and cytogenic studies?

3. Gross and microscopic evaluation of a pituitary tumor with first tissue block, frozen tissue, is documented. What would be the appropriate code(s)?

Also available in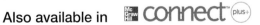

19.5 Modifiers Most Commonly Used with Codes in the Pathology/Laboratory Section of CPT

As with all sections of the CPT manual, modifiers are used in the Pathology/Laboratory section to continue or modify the story of the patient's encounter. Table 19.2 lists the modifiers that are most commonly used in this section to modify or alter the story being relayed about the patient encounter.

The appropriate use of modifiers with the codes from the Pathology/Laboratory section helps to tell the patient's full story.

Table 19.2 Pathology/Laboratory Section Modifiers *(Data from CPT 2013. © 2013 American Medical Association. All rights reserved.)*

MODIFIER	DEFINITION	EXAMPLE OF USE
26	Professional component.	When only the interpretation and report are performed, such as for a molecular pathology test, modifier 26 is reported with the appropriate molecular pathology code.
90	Outside laboratory.	This modifier is used when a lab test is performed at an outside lab and the outside lab bills the physician office and the office, in turn, bills the insurer.
91	Repeat clinical diagnostic laboratory test.	If the patient has two total bilirubin tests performed on the same day, one in the morning and one in the afternoon, the tests would be reported as 82247 and 82247-91.
QW	Service provided is a CLIA-waived test.	Simple lab test perfomed in the office or clinic such as: strep test, UA, finger stick glucose, and pregnancy.

EXERCISE 19.5

1. The patient has two tests on the same day that were ordered by the physician and not performed because of equipment malfunction. Which modifier would be appropriate to use?

2. When only the interpretation and report are performed, which modifier should be reported with the appropriate pathology/laboratory code?

Also available in 📘 **connect** (plus+)

19.6 Common Medical and Procedural Terms Used in Operative Reports

As with all sections of CPT, the Pathology/Laboratory section includes medical terms and procedural terms that are specific to the system involved. Table 19.3 lists some of these terms and identifies some key terms that could appear in a provider's documentation.

Table 19.3 Terms for Pathology/Laboratory

TERM	DEFINITION	DOCUMENTATION KEYS
Block	Portion of a tissue obtained from a specimen	Frozen piece of a specimen.
Chromatography	A combination of methods or phases used to analyze a drug class or classes	Stationary phase, mobile phase.
Cytogenic	Genetic and chromosomal studies	Harvesting, banding or culturing of cells from blood, bone marrow, amniotic fluid or solid tissue.
Cytopathology	Study of cells; used to identify cellular changes	Pap smears are the most common test reported with codes under this subheading.
Drug assay	Quantitative analysis	Amount of drug present.
Mutations	Variants associated with altered gene function that lead to functional deficits or disease	Definition is located in the molecular pathology guidelines in most editions of the CPT manual.
Necropsy	Postmortem examination	Autopsy.
Somatics	Term that refers to genetic code alterations that develop after birth (e.g., occurring in neoplastic cells); synonymous with *acquired conditions.*	Definition is located in the molecular pathology guidelines in most editions of the CPT manual.
Surgical pathology	Tissue removed during surgery for analysis	Gross examination, microscopic examination, frozen section.
Specimen	A unit submitted for evaluation, such as chemical, pathologic, or hematological	Body fluid, tissue, cytological, unit of service.

block A portion of tissue obtained from a specimen.

mutations Variants associated with altered gene function that lead to functional deficits or disease.

specimen A unit submitted for evaluation, such as chemical, pathologic or hematological.

EXERCISE 19.6

1. Define specimen, block, and section.
2. In the Pathology/Laboratory section of most editions of the CPT manual, where can definitions of terms such as *mutations, somatics, variants,* and *breakpoints* be found?
3. Pap smears are the most common test reported with codes under what subheading?

Also available in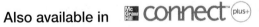

Chapter Nineteen Summary

Learning Outcome	Summary
19.1 Review the general ICD and CPT guidelines for pathology/laboratory coding.	**ICD guidelines** • When a diagnosis has not been confirmed or the pathology is documented as normal, signs and symptoms should be reported. • ICD abnormal-findings codes may be used when additional testing is required and the test results are negative. • *Neoplasms:* The Alphabetic Index of ICD and the neoplasm table enable the coder to select the appropriate neoplasm code based on the type of neoplasm and the site. **CPT guidelines** The following questions will help a coder, when reading through an operative report, to understand what actually was done and how the procedure should be translated and coded: • At which anatomical site was the study performed (if applicable)? • Was the study qualitative or quantitative? • What are all of the laboratory studies that were performed during the present encounter (e.g., organ panel, surgical pathology)? • What type of equipment was used (e.g., automated, nonautomated, microscope)? • Which type of consultation was involved: clinical pathology or surgical pathology? • How many tests were performed?
19.2 Identify the CPT guidelines and format of the Organ or Disease-Oriented Panels, Drug Testing, Therapeutic Drug Assays, Evocative/ Suppression Testing, Consultations, and Urinalysis subsections of CPT.	*Organ or Disease-Oriented Panels (80047–80076):* All of the tests listed within the code description must be performed in order to assign the code. *Drug Testing (80100–80104):* The codes in this code range are used to report drug screening, drug confirmation, and tissue preparation services. These codes are used to identify the presence of a drug, which is a qualitative analysis. *Therapeutic Drug Assays (80150–80299), Evocative/Suppression Testing (80400–80440):* The administration of pharmaceutical agents is used to measure a patient's response to those agents. The codes within this range are used for the laboratory portions of the testing. *Consultations (Clinical Pathology) (80500–80502):* The codes are further defined as to the level: limited—without review of the patient's history and medical record; comprehensive—complex diagnostic problem with review of history and medical record. *Urinalysis (81000–81099):* This code range is used to report tests on urine.
19.3 Understand the CPT guidelines and format of the Molecular Pathology, Chemistry, Hematology, Immunology, Transfusion Medicine, and Microbiology subsections of CPT.	*Molecular Pathology (81200–81099):* Codes in this range are used to report laboratory testing involving genes. The appropriate code is based on the specific gene or genes being analyzed. *Chemistry (82000–84999):* Specific tests on any bodily substance, such as urine, blood, breath, and feces, are reported using codes under this subheading. Samples from different sources may be reported separately. *Hematology and Coagulation (85002–85999):* Hematology is the study of disorders of the blood, while coagulation is the process of blood clotting. Studies under this subheading include blood counts and are differentiated as to the following: CBC, RBC, WBC, automated or manual, microscopic.

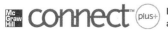

Enhance your learning by completing these exercises and more at mcgrawhillconnect.com

Learning Outcome	Summary
19.3 (continued)	*Immunology (86000–86849):* Immunology is the study of the immune study. Codes within this code range report tests used to identify immune system conditions caused by antibodies and antigens. *Microbiology (87001–87999):* The codes under this subheading are further differentiated by the type of study.
19.4 Apply the CPT guidelines and format of the Anatomic Pathology, Cytopathology, Cytogenic Studies, Surgical Pathology, Other Procedures, and Reproductive Medicine Procedures subsections of CPT.	*Anatomic Pathology (88000–88099):* An instructional note with this range of codes states that these codes represent physician services only. It also instructs the use of modifier 90 for outside laboratory services. These codes are for reporting postmortem examinations, that is, necropsies (autopsies). *Cytopathology (88104–88199):* Cytopathology is the study of cells, and the codes under this subheading are used to report laboratory tests performed to identify cellular changes. The codes are divided by type of procedure and technique. *Surgical Pathology (88300–88399):* The codes in this range are defined by the following: • Number of specimens (each specimen is a unit) • Anatomical site • Gross examination only • Gross and microscopic examination
19.5 Evaluate the modifiers most commonly used with codes in the Pathology/Laboratory section of CPT.	Modifiers commonly used include: • *26, professional component:* When only the interpretation and report are performed, such as for a molecular pathology test, modifier 26 is reported with the appropriate molecular pathology code. • *90, outside laboratory:* This modifier is used when a lab test is performed at an outside lab and the outside lab bills the physician office and the office, in turn, bills the insurer. • *91, repeat clinical diagnostic lab test:* If a patient has two total bilirubin tests performed on the same day, one in the morning and one in the afternoon, the tests would be reported as 82247 and 82247-91. • *QW:* This modifier is used when the service provided is a CLIA-waived test.
19.6 Examine the common medical and procedural terms used in operative reports.	*Chromatography:* combination of methods or phases used to analyze a drug class or classes *Cytopathology:* study of cells; used to identify cellular changes *Mutations:* variants associated with altered gene function that lead to functional deficits or disease *Necropsy (autopsy):* a postmortem exam

Chapter Nineteeen Review

Using Terminology

Match each key term to the appropriate definition.

_____ 1. **[LO19.6]** Block
_____ 2. **[LO19.6]** Chromatography
_____ 3. **[LO19.3]** Coagulation
_____ 4. **[LO19.6]** Cytogenic
_____ 5. **[LO19.4]** Cytopathology

A. Laboratory procedure that measures the presence of a drug
B. Portion of a tissue obtained from a specimen
C. Process of blood clotting
D. Series of specific tests ordered to assist in the determination of a diagnosis

_____ 6. **[LO19.3]** Hematology

_____ 7. **[LO19.3]** Immunology

_____ 8. **[LO19.1]** Ionized calcium

_____ 9. **[LO19.3]** Molecular pathology

_____ 10. **[LO19.6]** Mutations

_____ 11. **[LO19.2]** Organ panel

_____ 12. **[LO19.2]** Quantitative

_____ 13. **[LO19.2]** Qualitative

_____ 14. **[LO19.6]** Specimen

E. Laboratory procedure that measures the amount of a drug present

F. The study of cells; also, the CPT subheading for codes used to report laboratory tests performed to identify cellular changes

G. Free flowing, not attached to proteins

H. Study of disorders of the blood

I. A unit submitted for evaluation, such as chemical, pathologic, or hematological

J. Study of immune disorders

K. Genetic and chromosomal studies

L. CPT subheading for codes used to report laboratory testing involving genes

M. A combination of methods or phases, such as stationary or mobile, that is used to analyze a drug class or classes

N. Variants associated with altered gene function that lead to functional deficits or disease

Checking Your understanding

Choose the most appropriate answer for each of the following questions.

1. **[LO19.2]** A 14-year-old boy has been suspended from school for allegations that he is using marijuana and performing poorly in school as a result. The physician orders a urine drug screen to determine whether the boy has used marijuana on this occasion. Select the appropriate CPT code:

   a. 80100   **c.** 80102

   b. 80101   **d.** 80104

2. **[LO19.4]** A lump is discovered in the breast of a young woman during a routine physical examination. A breast biopsy is performed and submitted for surgical pathology and microscopic pathology and microscopic evaluation of the surgical margins. A pathologic report is completed after a comprehensive examination of the breast specimen. Select the appropriate CPT code for the pathology procedure:

   a. 88307   **c.** 88305

   b. 88309   **d.** 88302

3. **[LO19.4]**

Clinical information: Cysts, right neck and chest

Specimen submitted:

   1. Cyst, right neck
   2. Cyst, right chest

Gross description:

   1. Received, labeled with the patient's name and "right neck cyst," is a skin ellipse measuring 2.8 × 1.0 × 1.4 cm. The epithelial surface appears relatively unremarkable. A subepidermal soft white nodule is identified and sampled in one cassette.

   2. Received, labeled with the patient's name and "right chest cyst," is an ellipse of skin and subcutaneous tissue measuring 2.8 × 1.8 × 1.5 cm. On cut section, there is subepidermal white nodular cystic structure present.

Microscopic and final diagnosis:

   1. Cyst, right neck, excision. Epidermoid cyst.

   2. Cyst, right chest, excision. Epidermoid cyst.

Select the appropriate CPT codes:

   a. 88304, 216.3, 216.4   **c.** 88302, 706.2

   b. 88304 x 2, 706.2   **d.** 88305 x 2, 705.89

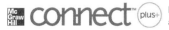 plus+   Enhance your learning by completing these exercises and more at mcgrawhillconnect.com

4. **[LO19.2]** Mrs. Jones underwent a modified mastectomy. The pathologist was unable to make a definitive diagnosis, and the oncologist requested a pathologic consultation of the slides as well as a review of the history and medical records. Select the appropriate CPT code for the consulting pathologist:

   a. 80500 **c.** 80502
   b. 88305 **d.** 88309

5. **[LO19. 2]** Sally had her first prenatal visit yesterday and presents at the laboratory today with an order for a CBC w/differential, blood typing, RH typing, antibody screen, syphilis, rubella antibody, hepatitis B surface antigen, alphafetoprotein, and urinalysis.

   Select the appropriate CPT code(s):

   a. 85027, 85007, 86901, 86850, 86592, 86762, 87370, 82105, 81000
   b. 80055
   c. 80055, 82105, 81000
   d. 80055, 81000

6. **[LO19.2]** Mrs. Thomas went to her physician with symptoms of chronic and worsening fatigue, muscle weakness, loss of appetite, and weight loss, as well as hyperpigmentation. Her physician ordered an ACTH stimulation panel and a cortisol (performed twice) to confirm a diagnosis of adrenal insufficiency. Select the appropriate CPT code(s):

   a. 80408
   b. 80400, 82533, 96372
   c. 80408, 82355 x 2, 96372
   d. 80400

7. **[LO19.4]** Mr. Green was DOA of unknown causes in the ED. A complete autopsy, including brain and spinal cord, was performed, followed by the appropriate microscopic examinations of the tissue to determine his cause of death. Select the appropriate CPT code:

   a. 88007 **c.** 88045
   b. 88027 **d.** 88025

8. **[LO19.4]** Susie Smith underwent a fine-needle aspiration of a breast mass, which was sent to the laboratory for cytology review for pathology with interpretation and report. Select the appropriate CPT code(s):

   a. 88172 **c.** 88177
   b. 88173, 88177 **d.** 88173

9. **[LO19.2, 19.3]** The patient presented in the ED complaining of nausea, vomiting, and diarrhea and is now demonstrating epigastric pain and dehydration. The ED physician ordered the following tests: basic metabolic panel with ionized calcium, CBC with automated differential, and urinalysis. Select the appropriate ICD-9-CM and CPT codes for this encounter:

   a. 80047, 85025, 81000, 787.01, 787.91, 789.06, 276.51
   b. 80047, 85027, 81000, 787.02, 787.03, 787.91, 789.05, 276.51
   c. 80048, 85025, 81000, 787.01, 787.91, 789.06, 276.51
   d. 80050, 85025, 81000, 787.01, 787.91, 789.06, 276.51

10. **[LO19.4]** A 35-year-old female underwent cystoscopy for hematuria, polyuria, and burning as well as abdominal pain. The physician found multiple papillary tumors in the trigone and sent them for gross and microscopic examination. Results of the examination revealed stage II transitional cell carcinoma. Select the appropriate codes:

    a. 88309, 188.0
    b. 88304, 188.1
    c. 88305, 188.1
    d. 88305, 188.0

Applying Your Knowledge

Case Study

Specimen: Cervix, uterus, bilateral tubes, and ovaries

Gross: The specimen received consists of a pear-shaped uterus, attached ovaries, and fallopian tubes. The uterus weighs 130 g and measures 9 × 5 × 4.2 cm. The external surface is smooth. There is a small nodule protruding through the serosal surface. On cut section, the ectocervix is smooth. The endocervical canal is patent. The endometrial cavity is pyramidal in shape and lined by 0.4-cm endometrium. Serial sectioning shows four additional nodules ranging in diameter from 0.2 to 0.3 cm.

Specimen:

A. Cervix
B. Endomyometrium and nodules
C. Right ovary, measuring 5 × 1.7 × 1.3 cm. Several subcapsular cysts are present. Adjacent fallopian tube measures 7 cm in length by 0.5 cm in diameter. Sections of the fallopian tube are unremarkable.
D. Left ovary, measuring 5.2 × 2.1 × 2 cm. There are also several small cysts present in the left ovary. The adjacent fallopian tube measures 8.2 cm in length and 0.6 in diameter. The section is unremarkable.

Microscopic: Chronic inflammation of the uterine cervix revealed in specimen A. Endometrium of proliferative histology revealed in sections of specimen B. Sections of specimens C and D show sections of ovaries with follicular cysts and serosal adhesions. Sections of fallopian tubes are unremarkable.

Diagnoses: Endometrium of proliferative histology. Follicular cysts and serosal adhesions of ovaries. Fallopian tubes, unremarkable. Chronic cervicitis.

Answer the following questions, and code the case above. Be sure to follow the process steps as illustrated in Chapter 8.

Process 1: CPT

1. What is the procedure?

2. Locate the main term in the index.

3. What additional questions or set of questions can be determined?

4. Upon review of all the code choices identified in the index, what additional questions can be determined?

5. Based on the documentation, what is (are) the correct code(s) for this case?
   a. 88305
   b. 88305, 88307
   c. 88307
   d. 88309

Process 2: ICD
ICD-9-CM

1. Based on the report header, what is the preexamination indication/diagnosis?

2. Is the postexamination diagnosis the same as or different from the preexamination diagnosis?

3. Is the postexamination diagnosis supported?

4. What is the main term for this condition?

5. Based on the subterm choices, what question(s) can be developed for this condition?

6. Is any sign, symptom, or additional condition documented?

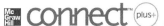
Enhance your learning by completing these exercises and more at mcgrawhillconnect.com

7. Is the additional condition, sign, or symptom an integral part of the primary (or other) condition coded?

8. Does the additional condition require or affect patient care, treatment, or management?

9. Based on the documentation, what are the correct ICD-9-CM codes for this case?
   a. 616.0, 620.0, 617.0
   b. 616.0, 620.0
   c. 616.0, 617.0
   d. 617.0, 620.0

ICD-10-CM

1. Based on the report header, what is the preexamination indication/diagnosis?

2. Is the postexamination diagnosis the same as or different from the preexamination diagnosis?

3. Is the postexamination diagnosis supported?

4. What is the main term for this condition?

5. Based on the subterm choices, what question(s) can be developed for this condition?

6. Based on the information in the Tabular List, is additional information needed to determine the appropriate diagnosis code?

7. Is any sign, symptom, or additional condition documented?

8. Is the additional condition, sign, or symptom an integral part of the primary (or other) condition coded?

9. Does the additional condition require or affect patient care, treatment, or management?

10. Based on the documentation, what are the correct ICD-10-CM codes for this case?
    a. N72, N83.0, N80.0
    b. N72, N83.0
    c. N72, N80.0
    d. N80.0, N72

Process 3: Modifiers

1. Was the procedure performed different from that described by the nomenclature of the code?

2. Was the procedure performed at an anatomical site that has laterality?

3. Was the procedure performed in the global period of another procedure?

4. Were additional procedures performed during the examination, and does the documentation support them?

5. Did the surgeon have help from another surgeon or another appropriate person?

6. Did a physician different from the surgeon provide the preexamination or postexamination portion of the procedure?

7. What modifier should be appended to the CPT code for this case?
   a. 26
   b. 58
   c. 51
   d. None

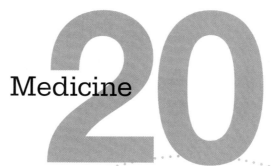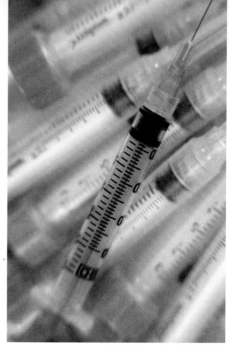

Medicine 20

Key Terms

Allergen immunotherapy
Aphakia
Biofeedback
Duplex scan
Hemodialysis
Hemofiltration
Interactive complexity

Intracutaneous
Isopter
Measles, mumps, rubella, and varicella (MMRV)
Minimally invasive procedure
Modalities

Motor studies
Nerve conduction studies
Noninvasive procedure
Nonselective debridement
Peritoneal dialysis

Photodynamic therapy (PDT)
Polysomnography
Selective debridement
Sensory nerve studies
Spirometry

Learning Outcomes

After completing this chapter, you will be able to:

20.1 Identify the chapter-specific CPT guidelines and format of the Immunization Administration for Vaccines/Toxoids, Vaccines/Toxoids, Psychiatry, Dialysis, and End-Stage Renal Disease subsections of CPT.

20.2 Understand the chapter-specific CPT guidelines and format of the Gastroenterology, Ophthalmology, Special Otorhinolaryngologic Services, Cardiovascular Services, and Noninvasive Vascular Diagnostic Studies subsections of CPT.

20.3 Apply the chapter-specific CPT guidelines and format of the Pulmonary, Allergy and Clinical Immunology, and Neurology and Neuromuscular subsections of CPT.

20.4 Recognize the CPT guidelines and format of the Hydration/Chemotherapy and Physical Medicine and Rehabilitation subsections of CPT.

20.5 Apply the modifiers most commonly used with codes in the Medicine section of CPT.

20.6 Examine the common medical and procedural terms used in operative reports.

Introduction The Medicine section consists of subsections and subheadings that contain codes to be assigned to accurately report services performed to evaluate, diagnose, and treat patients. Many of the procedures listed in this section are **noninvasive procedures,** in which surgical incision or excision is not required,

noninvasive procedure A procedure that does not require a surgical incision or excision.

minimally invasive procedure A procedure such as an injection or infusion.

or **minimally invasive procedures,** such as an injection or infusion. Codes for osteopathic manipulation treatment (OMT) and chiropractic manipulation treatment (CMT) are included in the Medicine section.

Table 20.1 identifies the general headings and code ranges for the Medicine section.

Table 20.1 CPT Medicine Section Format *(Data from CPT 2013. © 2013 American Medical Association. All rights reserved.)*

GENERAL HEADING	CODE RANGE
Immune Globulins, Serum, or Recombinant Products	90281–90399
Immunization Administration for Vaccines/Toxoids	90460–90474
Vaccines/Toxoids	90476–90749
Psychiatry	90785–90899
Biofeedback	90901–90911
Dialysis	90935–90999
Gastroenterology	91010–91299
Ophthalmology	92002–92499
Special Otorhinolaryngologic Services	92502–92700
Cardiovascular Services	92920–93779
Noninvasive Vascular Diagnostic Studies	93880–93998
Pulmonary	94002–94799
Allergy and Clinical Immunology	95004–95199
Endocrinology	95250–95251
Neurology and Neuromuscular Procedures	95782–96020
Medical Genetics and Genetic Counseling	96040
Central Nervous System Assessments/Tests	96101–96125
Health and Behavior Assessment/Intervention	96150–96155
Hydration, Therapeutic, Prophylactic, Diagnostic Injections and Infusions, and Chemotherapy and Other Highly Complex Drug or Highly Complex Biologic Agent Administration	96360–96549
Photodynamic Therapy	96567–96571
Special Dermatological Procedures	96900–96999
Physical Medicine and Rehabilitation	97001–97799
Medical Nutrition Therapy	97802–97804
Acupuncture	97810–97814
Osteopathic Manipulative Treatment	98925–98929
Chiropractic Manipulative Treatment	98940–98943
Education and Training for Patient Self-Management	98960–98962
Non-Face-to-Face Nonphysician Services	98966–98969
Special Services, Procedures, and Reports	99000–99091
Qualifying Circumstances for Anesthesia	99100–99140
Moderate (Conscious) Sedation	99143–99150
Other Services and Procedures	99170–99199
Home Health Procedures/Services	99500–99602
Medication Therapy Management Services	99605–99607

20.1 Guidelines and Format of the Immunization Administration for Vaccines/Toxoids, Vaccines/Toxoids, Psychiatry, Dialysis, and End-Stage Renal Disease Subsections of the Medicine Section of CPT

The immunization codes (90460–90474) are reported along with the vaccine and toxoid codes (90476–90749).

Immunization Administration for Vaccines/Toxoids (90460–90474)

CPT codes 90460 and 90461 include in their descriptions counseling by a physician or another qualified healthcare professional and should be assigned only when counseling of the patient and/or family is provided along with the administration of a vaccine. These codes are also to be used for ages up to 18. If the counseling and age requirements are not met, then code range 90471–90474 should be assigned.

Vaccines, Toxoids (90476–90749)

The descriptions for codes in this range apply to the vaccine product only, and these codes are to be reported in addition to the administration codes.

It is inappropriate to code each component of a combination vaccine.

FOR EXAMPLE CPT code 90710—**measles, mumps, rubella, and varicella (MMRV)** vaccine, live, for subcutaneous use—is used to code for the combination vaccine instead of coding each vaccine separately. ▪

Some codes within this range are further divided as to whether the vaccine is administered intramuscularly or subcutaneously.

SPOTLIGHT on a Guideline

Several codes under the Vaccines, Toxoids subheading have the lightning bolt symbol in front of the code. This symbol means that the code has been published prior to the drug being approved by the federal food and drug administration. The symbol will be removed once there is approval. The guidelines in many editions of the CPT manual indicate a website that can be referenced to get updates on these approvals.

Psychiatry (90785–90899)

The Psychiatry guidelines now instruct that codes within the Psychiatry subsection include diagnostic services, psychotherapy, and other services which are provided to an individual, family, or group. The services can be provided by a physician or other qualified healthcare professional in all settings (e.g. outpatient, inpatient).

SPOTLIGHT on a Guideline

The guidelines before this code range instruct the coder to not use modifier 51 when reporting both the immunization administration code and the vaccine/toxoid code.

measles, mumps, rubella, and varicella (MMRV) A combination vaccine.

Interactive Complexity: 90785

This code is to be used for **interactive complexity.** There is an instructional note with this code instructing the use of code 90785 along with codes for diagnostic psychiatric evaluation (90791, 90792), psychotherapy (90832, 90834, 90837), psychotherapy when performed with an evaluation and management service (90833, 90836, 90838, 99201–99255, 99304–99337, 99341–99350) and group psychotherapy (90853). There is a second instructional note showing code 90785 is not to be reported along with codes 90839, 90840 or with an E/M service when no psychotherapy service is also reported.

interactive complexity
Specific communication factors that complicate delivery of a psychiatric procedure. Common factors include difficult communication with emotional family members, engagement of young and verbally undeveloped patients.

Psychiatric Diagnostic Procedures: 90791–90792

The codes within this range may be reported with the interactive complexity code (90795) and the guidelines for the use of these codes is defined in the subheading guidelines for code 90785 in the CPT manual.

The guidelines for this subheading instruct the coder to use codes 90791 and 90792 for diagnostic assessment or reassessment and they do not include psychotherapeutic services.

Psychotherapy: 90832–90838

The codes within this range include ongoing assessment and adjustment of psychotherapeutic interventions. There may be involvement of family members. These are face-to-face services and the coder must know the amount of time spent with the patient. The codes are not reported for psychotherapy of less than sixteen minutes.

There are separate codes for psychotherapy services provided to a patient in a crisis state (90839 and 90840) and may not be reported in addition to codes 90832–90838.

Other Psychotherapy: 90839–90853

Psychotherapy for Crisis codes 90839 and 90840 are included in this code range and they are time based. These codes represent an urgent assessment and history of a crisis state, mental status exam, and a disposition. The guidelines in this subheading instruct the coder that typically the presenting problem is life threatening or complex requiring immediate attention.

Codes used to report psychoanalysis (90845) and family psychotherapy (90846 and 90847) are also found in this section.

Dialysis (90935–90947)

Dialysis procedures used to treat kidney failure include the following:

hemodialysis Dialysis procedure in which a man-made membrane is used to filter waste and toxins, remove and maintain fluid, and balance electrolytes by mechanically circulating the blood through a machine and transfusing it back to the body.

Hemodialysis uses a man-made membrane to filter waste and toxins, remove and maintain fluid, and balance electrolytes by mechanically circulating the blood through a machine and transfusing it back to the body. (See Figure 20.1.)

Peritoneal dialysis uses the lining of the abdominal cavity, where a solution is introduced to remove waste and excessive fluid.

Hemofiltration is similar to hemodialysis. Large amounts of blood are passed through filters that remove waste and excess fluid.

Hemodialysis: 90935–90940

The codes within this range are assigned when hemodialysis is the dialysis procedure performed.

Miscellaneous Dialysis Procedures: 90945–90947

The codes within this code range are assigned when peritoneal dialysis, hemofiltration, or other continuous renal replacement therapies are provided. As with the hemodialysis procedures, all evaluation and management services provided on the same day as the dialysis procedure related to the renal disease are included in the code description.

End-Stage Renal Disease Services (90951–90970)

To accurately code from this subheading, coders must find answers in the medical record to the following questions:

- What is the age of the patient?
- What is the number of face-to-face visits per month?
- Were the services provided in the home?
- Were the services less than a full month of services?

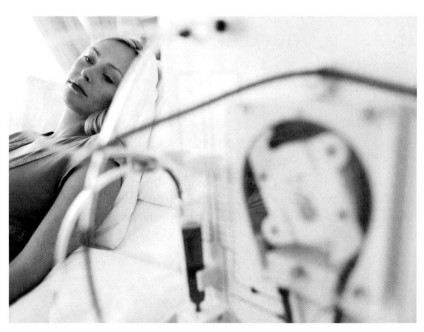

Figure 20.1 Hemodialysis Device

peritoneal dialysis Dialysis procedure in which a solution is introduced into the lining of the abdominal cavity to remove waste and excessive fluid from the body.

hemofiltration Dialysis procedure, similar to hemodialysis, in which large amounts of blood are passed through filters that remove waste and excess fluid.

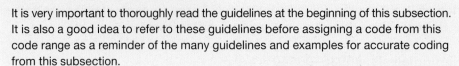
FOR EXAMPLE The CPT guidelines instruct that when the patient has had a complete assessment visit during the month and services are provided over a period of less than a month, 90951–90962 is the appropriate code range according to the number of visits performed. ■

EXERCISE 20.1

1. In the Vaccine, Toxoid subsection, what does the lightning bolt symbol before a code indicate to the coder?

2. How are codes in the Psychiatry subsection grouped and further classified?

3. To accurately code for end-stage renal disease services, what questions must coders find answers to in the medical record?

Also available in **connect** (plus+)

20.2 Guidelines and Format of the Gastroenterology, Ophthalmology, Special Otorhinolaryngologic Services, Cardiovascular Services, and Noninvasive Vascular Diagnostic Studies Subsections of the Medicine Section of CPT

Gastroenterology (91010–91299)

Codes within this subsection are assigned to motility studies of the esophagus, stomach, duodenum, and colon. Esophageal acid reflux test, code 91034, as well as esophageal function tests are coded within this code range. The code for gastrointestinal transit and pressure measurement, stomach through colon, wireless capsule, with interpretation and report, code 91112, is included in this section.

Ophthalmology (92002–92499)

General Ophthalmological Services: 92002–92014

Code selection within this subsection is determined by the status of the patient as new or established and by whether the examination was intermediate or comprehensive. An intermediate exam is typically a more limited exam focusing on a particular condition or problem, such as an acute condition that does not require a complete examination of the visual system. A comprehensive exam includes a general examination of the complete visual system.

Special Ophthalmological Services: 92015–92140

Additional services may be provided during comprehensive or intermediate exams that are not a normal part of these exams. These services include examination under anesthesia, gonioscopy (glaucoma), fitting of contact lens for treatment of disease (keratoconus, ocular surface diseases), retinal and optic nerve scans, retinal imaging and mapping, and angioscopy.

Visual field examinations are also coded to this subheading and are divided into three levels of exam: limited, intermediate, and extended. Each of these examinations is defined by the type of examination and the number of isopters plotted (92081–92083).

An **isopter** is the outer edge of a visual field; points, or isopters, are plotted around the macula lutea of the eye to aid in determining blind spots in a visual field.

isopter Outer edge of a visual field.

Spectacle Services: 92340–92371

CPT provides codes to report services for fitting of spectacles (glasses) when the service is provided by a physician. These codes report only the fitting; determining the type and strength of the lens needed is a distinct service coded elsewhere in CPT (92015). Fitting of spectacles is divided by CPT into three main categories: with **aphakia (**the absence of a lens), without aphakia, and low vision. Each code is further defined by the type of lens for which the spectacles are being fitted.

aphakia The absence of a lens.

Special Otorhinolaryngologic Services (92502–92700)

Included within this subsection are codes used to report vestibular function tests, with or without recording (92531–92548).

Audiologic Function Tests (92550–92597)

According to the CPT manual, to assign a code from this subsection, coders must verify that the medical record documents the use of calibrated electronic equipment, the recording of results, and a report with interpretation.

Evaluative and Therapeutic Services (92601–92700)

Included within this subsection are codes reported for diagnostic evaluation of cochlear implants, 92601–92604. Also included are codes to report evaluation and therapeutic services for non-speech and speech generating devices, codes 92605–92609. Codes 92611-92617 are used to report procedures for evaluating swallowing.

Cardiovascular Services (92920–93799)

Both diagnostic and therapeutic procedures are assigned codes within this subsection. For many of these procedures, the code descriptions include such services as access, monitoring, and injections, and thus these services are not reported separately.

Codes 92920–92944 and codes 92973–92979 are out of numerical sequence within this subsection.

Other Therapeutic Services and Procedures: 92950–92998

Therapeutic services assigned to this code range include:

- Cardiopulmonary resuscitation (CPR) (92950)
- Cardioversion, external or internal (92960, 92961)
- Circulatory assist, external or internal (92970, 92971)
- Percutaneous balloon valvuloplasty (92986–92990)
- Percutaneous transluminal pulmonary artery balloon angioplasty (92997–92998)

Coronary Therapeutic Services and Procedures: 92920–92978

There are extensive guidelines attached to this subheading, and they should be read thoroughly before assigning codes from this subsection.

Therapeutic services assigned to this code range include:

- Percutaneous transluminal coronary angioplasty (PTCA) (92920–92921)
- Percutaneous transluminal coronary atherectomy (92924–92925)
- Transcatheter placement of intracoronary stent(s) (92928–92929)
- Percutaneous transluminal coronary athrectomy with intracoronary stent, with coronary angioplasty (92933–92934)
- Percutanous transluminal revascularization (92937–92944)
- Percutaneous transluminal coronary thrombectomy (92973)
- Thrombolysis, intracoronary or intravenous infusion (92975, 92977)

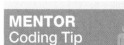

MENTOR
Coding Tip

Be aware of the difference between a PTCA and a PTA. A PTA is a percutaneous transluminal angioplasty, which would be of a noncoronary vessel.

MENTOR Coding Tip

An instructional note directs the use of CPT codes 37211 to 37214 and/or thrombolysis of other than a coronary vessel. Cerebral thrombolysis is reported with code 37195. Intravascular ultrasound (coronary vessel or graft) during diagnostic evaluation and/or therapeutic intervention is reported with 92978.

Cardiography: 93000–93042

Electrocardiograms (ECGs) are used to record the heart's electrical activity and are assigned codes under this subheading. These codes are further defined as:

93000- Electrocardiogram, routine ECG with at least 12 leads; with interpretation and report

93005- Electrocardiogram, routine ECG with at least 12 leads; tracing only, without interpretation and report

93010- Electrocardiogram, routine ECG with at least 12 leads; interpretation and report only

Cardiovascular stress testing codes are included under this subheading and are also defined by tracing only, with or without interpretation report, or with physician supervision.

Cardiovascular Monitoring Services: 93224–93278

The codes within this range are used for diagnostic services provided in person or remotely to evaluate cardiovascular rhythm. These codes are further divided by hours of continuous recording, scanning analysis with report, physician review and interpretation or scanning analysis with report only, or physician review and interpretation only.

Echocardiography: 93303–93352

Diagnostic ultrasound procedures of the heart and coronary vessels are assigned codes within this range. Code 93306 is used for a complete transthoracic echocardiography, including spectral Doppler and color-flow Doppler. Transesophageal echocardiography (TEE) is reported with codes from this subsection and is further defined by congenital cardiac anomalies. The coder needs to know whether the service provided was the probe placement, image acquisition, and interpretation and report; the placement of the probe only; or image acquisition and interpretation and report only.

Cardiac Catheterization: 93451–93533

According to the coding guidelines at the beginning of the Cardiac Catheterization subsection (CPT manual), the introduction, positioning and repositioning of catheters within the vascular system, the recording of intracardiac and intravascular pressure, and the evaluation and report are included in the code descriptions for cardiac catheterization. These guidelines also specify what is included in a right heart catheterization and a left heart catheterization.

Cardiac catheterization codes (93451–93453), other than those for congenital conditions, describe the placement of the catheter and now include the injection of the contrast and the imaging interpretation and report. If an injection procedure is performed to complete a right-ventricular, right-atrial, aortic, or pulmonary angiography during a cardiac catheterization, the injection procedure codes (93566–93568) may be reported separately.

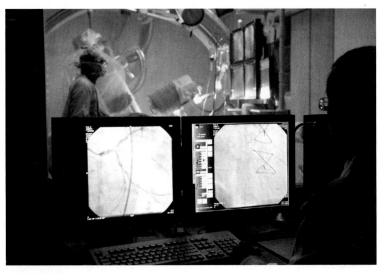

Figure 20.2 Cardiac Catheterization

Many editions of the CPT manual include a grid that can be used to determine the catheter placement-type code and any add-on procedures that can be coded separately.

CPT codes 93454 to 93461 are assigned for catheter placement in one or more coronary arteries for coronary angiography and are further defined by whether the placement is for bypass graft angiography and/or right or left or right and left heart catheterization.

FOR EXAMPLE Catheter placement in a coronary artery for coronary angiography is assigned CPT codes 93454 (catheter placement for coronary angiography) and 93567 (injection procedure). Catheter placement in a coronary artery for coronary angiography with catheter placement in a bypass graft for bypass graft angiography is assigned codes 93455 and 93567. ■

Code ranges 93530–93533 and 93563–93568 are assigned for cardiac catheterization and injection procedures during cardiac catheterization for patients with cardiac congenital anomalies.

Noninvasive Vascular Diagnostic Studies (93880–93998)

As noted at the beginning of this chapter, noninvasive procedures are procedures in which surgical incision or excision is not required.

duplex scan Ultrasound test used to evaluate the flow of blood within arteries and veins.

Duplex scans (93880, 93882) are included in this subsection. Duplex scans are performed to evaluate the direction of blood flow in the arteries or veins.

The guidelines at the beginning of this subsection explain what must be documented for limited and complete studies for lower- and upper-extremity exams.

EXERCISE 20.2

1. During comprehensive or intermediate ophthalmologic exams, additional services may be provided that are not a normal part of these exams. Identify some of these services.

2. To assign a code from the subheading Audiologic Function Tests, what does the coder need to find documented in the patient's medical record?

3. What is included in the cardiac catheterization codes that should not be reported separately?

Also available in Mc Graw Hill **connect** (plus+)

20.3 Guidelines and Format of the Pulmonary, Allergy and Clinical Immunology, and Neurology and Neuromuscular Subsections of the Medicine Section of CPT

Pulmonary (94002–94799)

Ventilator Management: 94002–94005

CPT divides the services of ventilator management primarily by the location of the patient or site of the services: hospital, nursing facility, or patient's home. The codes are further defined for each location by time. For ventilator management services reported in the hospital, CPT makes a distinction between the initial day of management (94002) and the subsequent day (94003). Ventilator management provided in a nursing facility is reported by day (94004) and in the home setting is reported once per month if 30 minutes or more of management has been provided.

Pulmonary Diagnostic Testing and Therapies: 94010–94799

Codes within this subsection identify tests and studies that measure lung volume and capacity, expiratory flow, respiratory obstructions, and pulmonary stress during exercise.

Spirometry is the measurement of breathing or breath and is used to measure both the flow (speed) of inhalation/exhalation and the amount, or volume, of air that is inhaled/exhaled (Figure 20.3). CPT divides spirometry testing based on what component of breathing is being tested and the method of testing. Codes may be further defined based on the age of the patient (94011–94013), use of an agent or gas to provoke a bronchial response (94060–94070 and 94400–94450), or use of stress to determine the location of breathing problems (94620–94621). Also included in this subsection are services to aid the patient with respiration difficulties due to disease or lung disorder (94640–94662) and noninvasive determination of blood oxygen saturation (94760–94762).

Allergy and Clinical Immunology (95004–95199)

CPT divides services listed under this subheading into two categories: testing and immunotherapy.

Allergy Testing: 95004–95071

Allergy testing may be done percutaneously, by scratching the skin; **intracutaneously,** by injecting a small amount of the allergen just below the skin or placing the agent directly on the skin or mucous membrane; or by inhalation. CPT primarily groups allergy testing by the method of the test. Codes within the two most commonly performed testing methods, percutaneous and intracutaneous, are further defined based on the type and number of allergens, venoms, drugs, or other agents tested.

At the beginning of this subsection, CPT provides definitions of many of the procedures described for pulmonary diagnostic testing. Read through the definitions, and map the terms to the codes within this subsection.

spirometry The measurement of breathing or breath; used to measure both the flow (speed) of inhalation or exhalation and the amount, or volume, of air inhaled or exhaled.

intracutaneous Within the skin.

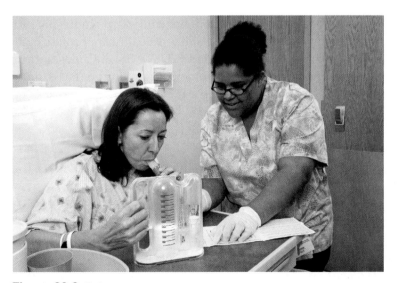

Figure 20.3 Spirometry

Ingestion Challenge Testing: 95076–95079

The codes within this range are used to report testing to confirm a significant reaction to food, drug, or other substances when a medical history suggests an allergy to one of these. Code 95076 is to be reported for the initial 120 minutes of testing and 95079 is the add-on code to report each additional 60 minutes of testing.

Allergen Immunotherapy: 95115–95199

Allergen immunotherapy involves injecting small doses of what the patient is allergic to and increasing the amount of the dose over time to gradually desensitize the patient to the substance. CPT divides codes for such services into two groups. The first group involves administration of the allergen (95115–95134). This group is further divided based on who is providing the service: the prescribing physician (typically the allergist/immunologist) or another physician (such as the primary care provider). Codes within each of these subgroups indicate the number of injections, with specific codes provided for insect venoms.

The second group under this subheading involves the preparation and provision of the antigens given for immunotherapy (95144–95170). CPT divides this category by the type of antigen prepared: stinging-insect venom and/or other antigens.

At times it may be appropriate to report codes from both the administration and the provision groups.

> **FOR EXAMPLE** A patient returns to her allergist for therapy for her allergy to dust, mold, and grass. The allergist prepares the antigens and administers the first dose in one injection in the office. The patient remains in the office for observation for 30 minutes. These services are reported with codes 95165 and 95120. ■

Neurology and Neuromuscular Procedures (95782–96020)

Sleep Medicine Testing: 95782–95811

CPT divides the services for sleep medicine and sleep studies into those that are unattended by a technologist or qualified healthcare professional (95800–95801) and those that must be attended (95782–95811). Codes within each of these groups are then defined by what is being monitored and/or measured during the study.

> **FOR EXAMPLE** Actigraphy testing monitors and records the patient's sleep-wake cycles over a 3-day period (95803), while latency studies measure the length of time it takes the patient to fall asleep. ■

Attended studies are divided by whether the service is a study (95807) or a recorded test, polysomnography (95782–95811). The codes for polysomnography are further defined by the number of parameters studied.

Parameters that may be studied during sleep medicine testing include:

Frontal, central, and occipital lobes by EEG, submental EMG, and bilateral EOG.

Electrocardiogram.

Airflow, nasal and/or oral.

Goniometry.

Bilateral anterior tibia by EMG.

Muscle activity.

Vital signs.

Snoring.

Routine Electroencephalography: 95812–95830

CPT divides electroencephalography (EEG) by the length of time of testing and the state of the patient at the time of the testing, such as awake and asleep, asleep or in coma, or during surgery. Timing of the test indicated within the codes may be defined by time of day, as all night (95827), or by a specific length of time: 41 to 60 minutes or greater than 1 hour (95812–95813).

Electromyography: 95860–95887

Electromyography testing is divided according to the nerve or branch of nerves innervating a body area. CPT divides the codes for these services by body area, number of extremities, and extent of the study (95862–95872). CPT provides add-on codes to identify instances in which EMG testing is performed at the same session as conduction studies (see "Nerve Conduction Test," below). These add-on codes (95885–95887) define whether an extremity or a nonextremity is being examined. Codes 95885 and 95886 are reported once for each extremity tested and are further divided as limited or complete based on the number of muscles and nerves studied.

Nerve Conduction Test: 95905–95913

Nerve conduction studies measure the time required for a signal to traverse the nerve pathway to and from the muscle. CPT divides these tests based on what conduction is being studied: motor nerves (with or without F waves) or sensory:

Motor studies are studies of efferent impulses, nerve signals going from the spinal cord to the muscles. If the nerve conduction is studied in the distal segment of the nerve only, it is considered a motor study without F wave. A study with F waves measures conduction in the proximal portion of the nerve, between the spinal cord and the muscle as well as the distal segment of the nerve.

Sensory nerve studies are studies of afferent impulses, nerve signals traveling to the spinal cord. Sensory nerve studies test only the sensory portion of the nerve. H-reflex studies are also afferent nerve impulse studies.

CPT divides these codes by the number of studies performed: 1-2 studies (95907), 3-4 studies (95908), 5-6 studies (95909), 7-8 studies (95910), 9-10 studies (95911), 11-12 studies (95912), and 13 or more studies (95913). These tests are coded by the number of studies performed and not the number of nerves studied.

MENTOR
Coding Tip

CPT provides direction for reporting routine EEGs (those of less than 41 minutes duration). Locate and highlight this directional note at the beginning of the subsection.

nerve conduction studies Studies that measure the time required for a signal to traverse the nerve pathway to and from a muscle.

motor studies Studies of efferent impulses, nerve signals going from the spinal cord to the muscles.

sensory nerve studies Studies of afferent impulses, nerve signals traveling to the spinal cord.

FOR EXAMPLE Motor and sensory study of the left ulnar nerve and motor study with F-wave and sensory of right ulnar nerve would equate to 4 studies: 95908. ∎

Neurostimulators, Analysis-Programming: 95970–95982

CPT divides analysis and programming of neurostimulators first based on whether the analysis is performed without programming (95970 and 95981) or with programming. The codes are further defined by the anatomical site in which the neurostimulator is implanted (spinal cord; brain; peripheral, cranial, or sacral nerve) and the type of neurostimulator (simple or complex).

EXERCISE 20.3

1. Explain what nerve conduction studies measure.
2. List the parameters that may be studied during sleep medicine testing.
3. Define *allergen immunotherapy*.

Also available in **connect** (plus+)

20.4 Guidelines and Format of the Hydration/Chemotherapy and Physical Medicine and Rehabilitation Subsections of the Medicine Section of CPT

Hydration, Therapeutic, Prophylactic, Diagnostic Injections and Infusions, and Chemotherapy and Other Highly Complex Drug or Highly Complex Biologic Agent Administration (96360–96549)

There are very detailed guidelines at the beginning of this subsection. They should be reviewed very carefully before assigning codes from this subsection. Some of the guidelines are listed below:

- The following services are included with infusion and injection procedures:
  - Use of local anesthesia.
  - IV start.
  - Access to indwelling IV/subcutaneous catheter or port.
  - Flush at conclusion of infusion.
  - Standard tubing, syringes, and supplies.
- When multiple infusions, injections, or combinations are administered, only one initial code is reported per day unless protocol requires two separate IV sites.
- The first IV push given subsequent to an initial 1-hour infusion is reported using a subsequent IV-push code.

- *Initial infusion* is defined as the key, or primary, reason for the encounter, regardless of the order in which the infusions or injections are administered.
- *Sequential infusion* is defined as an infusion or IV push of a new substance or drug following a primary or initial service.
- *Concurrent infusion* is defined as an infusion of a new substance or drug at the same time as the infusion of another substance or drug. This type of infusion is not time-based and is reported only once per day.

Hydration: 96360–96361

Codes within this subsection are used for infusions, under direct physician supervision, of a hydration solution (prepackaged such as saline and electrolytes). These codes are not to be used for infusion of substances other than for hydration. These codes are further defined by time (31 minutes to 1 hour and each additional hour).

Therapeutic, Prophylactic, and Diagnostic Injections and Infusions: 96365–96379

The codes within this range are reported for injections and infusions for reasons other than hydration. When fluids are used to aid in the administration of the drugs, this is considered incidental and hydration codes are not reported separately. These codes are further defined by time and by initial, subsequent, or concurrent infusion.

Chemotherapy and Other Highly Complex Drug or Highly Complex Biologic Agent Administration: 96401–96549

These codes require direct physician supervision. The guidelines instruct that the word *chemotherapy*, in regard to codes in this subheading, includes other highly complex drugs or highly complex biologic agents. The codes are further defined by time, intralesional or intravenous technique, and, if intralesional, the number of lesions.

Physical Medicine and Rehabilitation (97001–97799)

Within this subsection, CPT divides evaluations and reevaluations for therapy into three groups: physical (97001–97002), occupational (97003–97004), and athletic training (97005–97006).

Modalities: 97010–97039

Modalities are the application of an agent or device used to change tissues and include heat, sound, light, and mechanical or electrical energy. CPT groups modalities as those that are watched as needed but not constantly (97010–97028) and those that are monitored by the therapist from initiation to completion of the therapy (97032–97039).

Modalities indicated as supervised are further described by the specific modality or therapy applied and include thermal, traction, electrical (e-stim), whirlpool, and light therapies. Codes indicating constant attendance differ from supervised modalities in two distinct ways: the type of modality and the time for each modality. As the description of modalities within CPT range 97032–97039 states, modalities within this range may be listed in 15-minute units when performed.

modalities The application of an agent or device used to change tissues; include heat, sound, light, and mechanical or electrical energy.

> **FOR EXAMPLE** If the patient received a total of 35 minutes of contrast bath, the service is reported as 97034 at 2 units. ∎

MENTOR Coding Tip

Payers establish how many additional minutes are needed over the 15 minutes indicated by each code before an additional unit is billable. For the purposes of the CPC exam, an additional 8 minutes or more must be provided to report an additional unit of modality.

Therapeutic Procedures: 97110–97546

CPT guidelines clarify that these procedures require direct face-to-face contact with the provider or the therapist and must be provided or performed to affect change in a body area. Therapeutic procedures may be performed as a team with both the provider and the therapist working together to move or reeducate a body part, either in a group setting or one on one.

Active Wound Care Management: 97597–97606

selective debridement Procedure in which instruments or devices are used to cut away only dead (necrotic) or devitalized tissue.

nonselective debridement Procedure in which devitalized tissue is removed with healthy tissue by scrubbing the wound and using wet-to-dry dressings or enzymes. Also called *mechanical debridement.*

Three distinct methods of wound care are included under this subheading: selective debridement (97597–97598), nonselective debridement (97602), and negative pressure wound therapy (97605–97606).

   Selective debridement is performed using instruments or devices to *cut* away only dead (necrotic) or devitalized tissue. In **nonselective debridement,** devitalized tissue is removed with healthy tissue by scrubbing the wound and using wet-to-dry dressings or enzymes. Nonselective debridement may also be documented as mechanical debridement.

EXERCISE 20.4

1. Define *modality* as used in physical medicine and rehabilitation.
2. What are the three distinct methods of active wound care?
3. What services are included with infusion and injection procedures?

Also available in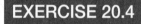

20.5 Modifiers Most Commonly Used with Codes in the Medicine Section of CPT

As with all sections of the CPT manual, modifiers are used in the Medicine Section to continue or modify the story of the patient's encounter. Some of the more common modifiers used within this section are 25, significant, separately identifiable evaluation and management service by the same physician on the same day of the procedure or other service; 26, professional services; 52, reduced services; and 59, distinct procedural service. (See Table 20.2.)

Table 20.2 Medicine Section Modifiers *(Data from CPT 2013. © 2013 American Medical Association. All rights reserved.)*

MODIFIER	DEFINITION	EXAMPLE OF USE
25	Significant, separately identifiable evaluation and management service by the same physician on the same day of the procedure or other service	Separate evaluation and management service is provided on the same day as the administration of a vaccine.
26	Professional services	For interpretation and report only for code 93278, signal-averaged electrocardiography, with or without ECG, append modifier 26 to the code.
52	Reduced services	When assigning code 93224, external electrocardiographic recording up to 48 hours by continuous rhythm recording and storage (which includes recording, scanning analysis with report, physician review and interpretation), and less than 12 hours of continuous recording is documented, append modifier 52 to the code.
59	Distinct procedural service	For code 93922, limited bilateral noninvasive physiologic studies of upper- or lower-extremity arteries, modifier 59 would be appended when both the upper and lower extremities are evaluated in the same setting.
LC RC LD	Left circumflex artery Right coronary artery Left descending artery	These modifiers are used instead of modifier 59 when procedures are performed in separate arteries.

The appropriate use of modifiers with the codes from the Medicine section helps to tell the patient's full story.

EXERCISE 20.5

1. A limited bilateral noninvasive physiologic study of both the upper- and lower-extremity arteries during the same encounter was performed. Since both the upper and lower extremities were studied, which modifier would need to be appended?

2. Which modifiers are used instead of modifier 59 to show that separate coronary arteries were involved?

3. The patient was seen in the office for a vaccination and a separate evaluation and management service. Which modifier should be appended to the evaluation and management code?

Also available in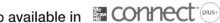

20.6 Common Medical and Procedural Terms Used in Operative Reports

As with all sections of CPT, the Medical section includes medical terms and procedural terms that are specific to the procedures involved. Table 20.3 lists some of these terms and identifies some key terms that could appear in a provider's documentation.

Table 20.3 Terms for Medicine

biofeedback Training in which the patient is taught how certain responses to thought processes, stimuli, and actions can affect physical responses.

TERM	DEFINITION	DOCUMENTATION KEYS
Biofeedback	Training in which the patient is taught how certain responses to thought processes, stimuli, and actions can affect physical responses	Physical therapists use biofeedback to help stroke victims regain movement in paralyzed muscles. Psychologists use it to help tense and anxious clients learn to relax. Specialists in many different fields use biofeedback to help their patients cope with pain.
Chiropractic manipulative treatment (CMT)	Manipulation of the vertebrae by a chiropractor in order to increase range of motion, reduce nerve irritability, or improve function	Spinal adjustment
Diphtheria and tetanus (DT)	Vaccine	This vaccine is often abbreviated as DT in provider documentation
Diphtheria, tetanus, and pertussis (DTP)	Vaccine	This vaccine is often abbreviated as DTP in provider documentation
Duplex scan	Ultrasound test used to evaluate the flow of blood within arteries and veins	Combination of real-time and Doppler studies
Photodynamic therapy (PDT)	Therapy in which a photosensitizing agent is applied to a lesion, such as an actinic keratosis, and the patient returns for light treatment, which activates the chemical agent in order to destroy the lesion.	This type of therapy is often abbreviated PDT in provider documentation
Polysomnography	Test performed to measure sleep cycles and sleep stages, REM and NREM.	Sleep study

photodynamic therapy (PDT) Therapy in which a photosensitizing agent is applied to a lesion (e.g., an actinic keratosis) and the patient returns for light treatment, which activates the chemical agent to destroy the lesion.

polysomnography A test performed to measure sleep cycles and sleep stages, REM and NREM.

EXERCISE 20.6

1. What type of ultrasound study is often performed to check for blockage of blood flow in an extremity?

2. What type of study could be abbreviated *REM* or *NREM* in the medical documentation?

3. Explain photodynamic therapy.

Also available in McGraw Hill **connect**™ (plus+)

Chapter Twenty Summary

Learning Outcome	Key Concepts/Examples
20.1 Identify the chapter-specific CPT guidelines and format of the Immunization Administration for Vaccines/Toxoids, Vaccines/Toxoids, Psychiatry, Dialysis, and End-Stage Renal Disease subsections of CPT.	*Immunization Administration and Vaccines/Toxoids:* The immunization codes (90460–90474) are reported along with the vaccine and toxoid codes (90476–90749). *Psychiatry:* The Psychiatry guidelines now instruct that codes within the Psychiatry subsection include diagnostic services, psychotherapy, and other services which are provided to an individual, family, or group. The services can be provided by a physician or other qualified healthcare professional in all settings (e.g. outpatient, inpatient). *Dialysis and End-Stage Renal Disease:* *Hemodialysis:* The codes within this range are assigned when hemodialysis is the dialysis procedure performed, and they include the evaluation and management services provided to the patient on the day of the hemodialysis procedure involving the renal disease. *End-Stage Renal Disease:* To accurately code from this subheading, coders must find answers in the medical record to the following questions: • What is the age of the patient? • What is the number of face-to-face visits per month? • Were the services provided in the home? • Were the services less than a full month of services?
20.2 Understand the chapter-specific CPT guidelines and format of the Gastroenterology, Ophthalmology, Special Otorhinolaryngologic Services, Cardiovascular Services, and Noninvasive Vascular Diagnostic Studies subsections of CPT.	*Gastroenterology:* Codes within this subsection are assigned to motility studies of the esophagus, stomach, duodenum, and colon. *Ophthalmology:* Code selection within this subsection is determined by the status of the patient as new or established and by whether the examination was intermediate or comprehensive. *Special Otorhinolaryngologic Services:* Included within this subsection are codes used to report vestibular function tests with or without recording. *Audiologic Function Tests:* To assign a code from this subsection, coders must verify that the medical record documents the use of calibrated electronic equipment, the recording of results, and a report with interpretation. *Cardiovascular Services:* Both diagnostic and therapeutic procedures are assigned codes within this subsection. For many of these procedures, the code descriptions include such services as access, monitoring, and injections, and thus these services are not reported separately. *Noninvasive Vascular Diagnostic Studies:* Duplex scans (93880 and 93882) are included in this subsection. Duplex scans are performed to evaluate the direction of blood flow in the arteries or veins.
20.3 Apply the chapter-specific CPT guidelines and format of the Pulmonary, Allergy and Clinical Immunology, and Neurology and Neuromuscular Subsections of CPT.	*Pulmonary:* *Ventilator Management:* CPT divides the services of ventilator management primarily by the location of the patient or site of the services: hospital, nursing facility, or patient's home. The codes are further defined for each location by time. *Pulmonary Diagnostic Testing and Therapies:* Codes within this subsection identify tests and studies that measure lung volume and capacity.

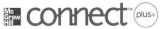 Enhance your learning by completing these exercises and more at mcgrawhillconnect.com

Learning Outcome	Key Concepts/Examples
20.3 *(concluded)*	*Allergy and Clinical Immunology:* *Allergy Testing:* This testing may be done percutaneously, by scratching the skin; intracutaneously, by injecting a small amount of antigen just below the skin or by placing the agent directly on the skin or mucous membrane; or by inhalation. *Allergen Immunotherapy:* CPT divides codes in this subsection into two groups. The first group involves administration of the allergen. This group is further divided based on who is providing the service: the prescribing physician (typically the allergist/immunologist) or another physician (such as the primary care provider). The second group involves the preparation and provision of the antigens given for immunotherapy. *Sleep Medicine Testing:* CPT divides the services for sleep medicine and sleep studies by attended and not attended by a technologist or qualified healthcare professional. The codes are further divided by the parameters monitored and/or measured during the study. *Routine electroencephalography:* Codes are divided by time of testing and patient's state of consciousness at the time of the testing. *Electromyography:* Codes are divided by nerve or nerve branch innervating a body area and the body area, number of extremities, and extent of the study. Add-on codes are used to report EMG testing performed with conduction studies. *Nerve Conduction Test:* Codes are divide by the number of studies performed, not the number of nerves studied.
20.4 Recognize the CPT guidelines and format of the Hydration/Chemotherapy and Physical Medicine and Rehabilitation subsections of CPT.	*Hydration:* There are very detailed guidelines at the beginning of this subsection. They should be reviewed very carefully before assigning codes from this subsection. When multiple infusions, injections, or combinations are administered, only one initial code is reported per day unless protocol requires two separate IV sites. *Therapeutic Injections/Infusions:* The codes in this subsection are reported for injections and infusions for reasons other than hydration. When fluids are used to aid in the administration of the drugs, this is considered incidental and hydration codes are not reported separately. *Physical Medicine and Rehabilitation:* Within this subsection, CPT divides evaluations and reevaluations for therapy into three groups: physical (97001–97002), occupational (97003–97004), and athletic training (97005–97006).
20.5 Apply the modifiers most commonly used with codes in the Medicine section of CPT.	Some of the more common modifiers used within this section are 25, significant, separately identifiable evaluation and management service by the same physician on the same day of the procedure or other service; 26, professional services; and 52, reduced services.
20.6 Examine the common medical and procedural terms used in operative reports.	*Biofeedback:* Training in which the patient is taught how certain responses to thought processes, stimuli, and actions can affect physical responses *Duplex scan:* Ultrasound test used to evaluate the flow of blood within arteries and veins *Photodynamic therapy (PDT):* Therapy in which a photosensitizing agent is applied to a lesion, such as an actinic keratosis, and the patient returns for light treatment, which activates the chemical agent in order to destroy the lesion

Chapter Twenty Review

Using Terminology

Match each key term to the appropriate definition.

_____ 1. [LO20.3] Allergen immunotherapy

_____ 2. [LO20.2] Aphakia

_____ 3. [LO20.1] Hemodialysis

_____ 4. [LO20.1] Hemofiltration

_____ 5. [LO20.2] Sensory nerve studies

_____ 6. [LO20.1] Interactive complexity

_____ 7. [LO20.3] Intracutaneous

_____ 8. [LO20.2] Isopter

_____ 9. [LO20.1] Minimally invasive

_____ 10. [LO20.2] MMRV

_____ 11. [LO20.4] Modalities

_____ 12. [LO20.1] Noninvasive

_____ 13. [LO20.1] Peritoneal dialysis

_____ 14. [LO20.3] Spirometry

A. Procedure in which surgical incision or excision is not required

B. Measurement of breathing or breath; used to measure both the flow (speed) of inhalation/exhalation and the amount, or volume, of air that is inhaled/exhaled

C. The application of an agent or device used to change tissues; include heat, sound, light, and mechanical or electrical energy

D. Procedure such as injection or infusion

E. Treatment that involves injecting small doses of the substance the patient is allergic to and increasing the amount of the dose over time to gradually desensitize the patient to the substance

F. Injection of an agent just below the skin for allergy testing

G. Outer edge of a visual field

H. The absence of a lens

I. Measles, mumps, rubella, and varicella

J. Dialysis procedure that uses a man-made membrane to filter waste and toxins, remove and maintain fluid, and balance electrolytes by mechanically circulating the blood through a machine and transfusing it back to the body

K. Studies of afferent impulses, nerve signals traveling to the spinal cord

L. This dialysis procedure uses the lining of the abdominal cavity, where a solution is introduced to remove waste and excessive fluid

M. Specific communication factors that complicate delivery of a psychiatric procedure; verbal communications to achieve therapeutic interaction

N. Procedure in which large amounts of blood are passed through filters that remove waste and excess fluid

Checking Your Understanding

Choose the most appropriate answer for each of the following questions.

1. [LO20.2] The patient undergoes an initial 2-D echocardiogram, including spectral Doppler and color flow, to confirm a diagnosis of mitral valve stenosis with aortic insufficiency. Select the appropriate ICD-9-CM and CPT codes:

   a. 93306, 396.1

   b. 93308, 394.25

   c. 93307, 394.25, 395.2

   d. 93308, 396.1

2. [LO20.1] Misty, an 18-year-old female, was seen today and received hepatitis A and hepatitis B vaccines, adult dose, with counseling by her physician about the risks and advantages. Select the appropriate CPT codes for this encounter:

   a. 90636, 90460

   b. 90636, 90472, 90473

   c. 90636, 90460, 90461

   d. 96036, 90472

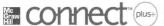 plus+ Enhance your learning by completing these exercises and more at mcgrawhillconnect.com

507

Copyright ©2014 The McGraw-Hill Companies   CPT only © 2013 American Medical Association. All rights reserved.

3. **[LO20.1]** A 35-year-old female patient presented for a psychiatric diagnostic evaluation which included a history, mental status exam, and recommendations. The evaluation and treatment plan were communicated to the family as the patient has requested their involvement in her care. Select the appropriate CPT code:

   a. 90792, 90785   **c.** 90791

   b. 90791, 90785   **d.** 90832

4. **[LO20.2]** A patient undergoes a left heart catheterization, with coronary angiography and catheter placement in the bypass graft, and a bypass graft angiography. Select the appropriate code(s) for the procedure:

   a. 93459   **c.** 93454, 93459

   b. 93452, 93454   **d.** 93452, 93459

5. **[LO20.2]** Barry has been diagnosed with intracranial stenosis within the arteries, and the physician has ordered a complete bilateral transcranial Doppler study to determine the flow of blood of the right and left circulation territories of the brain. Select the appropriate CPT code:

   a. 93880   **c.** 93890

   b. 93888   **d.** 93886

6. **[LO20.3]** Keegan presented to the office today for allergy testing as a result of chronic sinusitis. He received intracutaneous testing with allergenic extracts for airborne allergens. Interpretation of the tests revealed an allergy to dust and dust mites. Select the appropriate CPT code(s):

   a. 95024, 99213–25

   b. 95004

   c. 95004

   d. 95027, 99213–25

7. **[LO20.3]** A 60-year-old patient was in a car accident and arrived at the ED in a coma. Based on the injuries, it was determined that his condition was terminal. An EEG was ordered for cerebral death evaluation. Select the appropriate CPT code for this procedure:

   a. 95822   **c.** 95824

   b. 95829   **d.** 95812

8. **[LO20.4]** Phil has been having problems with a previous bucket-handle injury to the medial meniscus of his left knee. He presents today for initial physical therapy evaluation followed by these modalities: isotonic massage to his knee and active and passive range-of-motion exercises to develop strength and endurance. Select the appropriate CPT codes:

   a. 97001, 97010, 97110

   b. 97002, 97010, 97110 × 2

   c. 97001, 97110 × 2

   d. 97002, 97110 × 2

9. **[LO20.4]** Beth, a 46-year-old female with breast cancer, presents today for her chemotherapy treatment. An IV line was started, and an antiemetic was administered over 35 minutes; then the patient received Cytoxan via IV infusion over 60 minutes, followed by a 1-hour infusion of Adriamycin. Select the appropriate CPT codes for this encounter:

   a. 96360, 96413, 96417

   b. 96360, 96416

   c. 96360, 96415, 96417

   d. 96413, 96417

Applying Your Knowledge

Answer the following questions and code the following case study. Be sure to follow the process steps as illustrated in Chapter 8.

Case Studies [LO 20.1–20.6] Case 1

Preoperative diagnosis: Coronary artery disease

Postoperative diagnosis: Two-vessel coronary disease with ejection fraction of 60 to 65 percent

Procedures performed: Left heart catheterization, left ventriculogram, and coronary angiography via the left femoral artery

Indications: This is an elderly male with palpitations with no significant chest discomfort and no previous cardiac history. Echocardiogram showed cardiomyopathy, ejection fraction of 60 percent, with slow heart movement globally. A cardiac catheterization was recommended to determine the cause of his cardiomyopathy. Risks and benefits were explained, and informed consent was obtained.

Procedure: The patient was prepped and draped in a sterile manner, and the left groin was anesthetized with 1 percent plain lidocaine. Entry into the right femoral artery was accomplished by means of a single-wall puncture. A guidewire was inserted into the left femoral artery, and a hemostatic sheath with its dilator was advanced over the guidewire into the left femoral artery. The guidewire and dilator were removed, and the hemostatic sheath was flushed with normal saline. A pigtail catheter was inserted with its guidewire and passed into the left ventricular chamber. The pigtail catheter was connected to the injection system, and left ventricular pressures were obtained.

Left ventriculogram was obtained. The catheter was removed, leaving the guidewire in place. The left coronary catheter was advanced over the guidewire to the aortic root and left main coronary artery; the guidewire was removed and the catheter connected to the injection system, and multiple injections of the left coronary system were completed.

At this time the injection system was disengaged from the catheter, and the left coronary catheter was removed, leaving the guidewire in place; a right coronary catheter was then advanced over the guidewire up to the aortic root and attached to the injection system. The catheter was then placed into the right coronary artery, and views were obtained.

The injection system was then disconnected from the catheter, and the catheters were removed.

Findings:

The left heart systemic blood pressure was 128/72 and left ventricular end-diastolic pressure 20 mmHg.

Left ventriculogram demonstrated mild global hypokinesis with ejection fraction 60 to 65 percent. There was no significant mitral regurgitation, and the aortic valve appeared normal.

The left anterior descending had 20 to 25 percent distal narrowing. The remainder of the left anterior descending was free of focal stenosis. The left circumflex was found to have 30 percent smooth, discrete narrowing in the proximal portion. The right coronary artery was found to be free of narrowing or focal stenosis.

Answer the following questions, and code the case above. Be sure to follow the process steps as illustrated in Chapter 8.

Process 1: CPT

1. What is the procedure?

2. Locate the main term in the index.

3. What additional questions or set of questions can be determined?

4. Upon review of all the code choices identified in the index, what additional questions can be determined?

5. Based on the documentation, what is (are) the correct code(s) for this case?

   a. 93452, 93454

   b. 93458, 93563

   c. 93458

   d. 93458, 93462

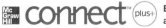
Enhance your learning by completing these exercises and more at mcgrawhillconnect.com

Process 2: ICD

ICD-9-CM

1. Based on the operative report header, what is the preoperative diagnosis?

2. Is the postoperative diagnosis the same as or different from the preoperative diagnosis?

3. Is the postoperative diagnosis supported?

4. What is the main term for this condition?

5. Based on the subterm choices, what question(s) can be developed for this condition?

6. Is any sign, symptom, or additional condition documented?

7. Is the additional condition, sign, or symptom an integral part of the primary (or other) condition coded?

8. Does the additional condition require or affect patient care, treatment, or management?

9. Based on the documentation, what is (are) the correct ICD-9-CM code(s) for this case?
   - **a.** 414.00
   - **b.** 414.01
   - **c.** 414.00, 414.8
   - **d.** 414.01, 414.8

ICD-10-CM

1. Based on the operative report header, what is the preoperative diagnosis?

2. Is the postoperative diagnosis the same as or different from the preoperative diagnosis?

3. Is the postoperative diagnosis supported?

4. What is the main term for this condition?

5. Based on the subterm choices, what question(s) can be developed for this condition?

6. Based on the information in the Tabular List, is additional information needed to determine the appropriate diagnosis code?

7. Is any sign, symptom, or additional condition documented?

8. Is the additional condition, sign, or symptom an integral part of the primary (or other) condition coded?

9. Does the additional condition require or affect patient care, treatment, or management?

10. Based on the documentation, what is (are) the correct ICD-10-CM code(s) for this case?
    - **a.** I25.10
    - **b.** I25.720
    - **c.** I25.111
    - **d.** I25.10, I25.5

Process 3: Modifiers

1. Was the procedure performed different from that described by the nomenclature of the code?

2. Was the procedure performed at an anatomical site that has laterality?

3. Was the procedure performed in the global period of another procedure?

4. Were additional procedures performed during the operative session, and does the documentation support them?

5. Did the surgeon have help from another surgeon or another appropriate person?

6. Did a physician different from the surgeon provide the preoperative or postoperative portion of the procedure?

7. What modifier(s) should be appended to the CPT code for this case?
   - **a.** 59
   - **b.** 51
   - **c.** LD, LC, and RC
   - **d.** None

The patient returns for a follow-up ocular examination 1 year after cataract surgery of the left eye.

The exam shows best acuity of 20/400 secondary to macular degenerative changes. Her pupils are normal; her pressures are 10. There is a small hemorrhage just inferior to the fovea in the left macula. The remainder of the ocular exam is unremarkable.

Diagnosis: No new ocular changes or disease of note apart from a right lower-lid marginal chalazion.

The patient was instructed to use a warm compress on the right lower-lid chalazion. There are no other ocular concerns at present. Unfortunately, no treatment is available that would restore her acuity given her current retinal findings. She should continue to be examined periodically to make sure no other ocular disease develops.

Process 1: CPT

1. What is the procedure or service?

2. Locate the main term in the index.

3. What additional questions or set of questions can be determined?

4. Upon review of all the code choices identified in the index, what additional questions can be determined?

5. Based on the documentation, what is the correct code for this case?
   a. 92002
   b. 92004
   c. 92012
   d. 92014

Process 2: ICD

ICD-9-CM

1. Based on the documentation, what is the diagnosis or reason(s) for the encounter?

2. What is the main term for this condition?

3. Based on the subterm choices, what question(s) can be developed for this condition?

4. Is any sign, symptom, or additional condition documented?

5. Is the additional condition, sign, or symptom an integral part of the primary (or other) condition coded?

6. Does the additional condition require or affect patient care, treatment, or management?

7. Based on the documentation, what is (are) the correct ICD-9-CM code(s) for this case?
   a. V72.0, 362.50, 373.2
   b. V72.0
   c. V43.1, 362.50, 373.2
   d. 362.50, 373.2, V43.1

ICD-10-CM

1. Based on the documentation, what is the diagnosis or reason(s) for the encounter?

2. What is the main term for this condition?

3. Based on the subterm choices, what question(s) can be developed for this condition?

4. Based on the information in the Tabular List, is additional information needed to determine the appropriate diagnosis code?

5. Is any sign, symptom, or additional condition documented?

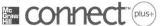 **plus+**   Enhance your learning by completing these exercises and more at mcgrawhillconnect.com

6. Is the additional condition, sign, or symptom an integral part of the primary (or other) condition coded?

7. Does the additional condition require or affect patient care, treatment, or management?

8. Based on the documentation, what is (are) the correct ICD-10-CM code(s) for this case?
   a. Z96.1, H35.3, H00.19
   b. Z01.00
   c. Z96.1, H35.3, H00.12
   d. H35.3, H00.12, Z96.1

Process 3: Modifiers

1. Was the service performed different from that described by the nomenclature of the code?

2. Was the service performed at an anatomical site that has laterality?

3. Was the service performed in the global period of another procedure?

4. Were additional procedures performed during the encounter, and does the documentation support them?

5. Did the surgeon have help from another surgeon or another appropriate person?

6. Did a physician different from the surgeon provide the preoperative or postoperative portion of the procedure?

7. What modifier should be appended to the CPT code for this case?
   a. 52
   b. E4
   c. LT
   d. None

HCPCS Level II: Category II and Category III Codes

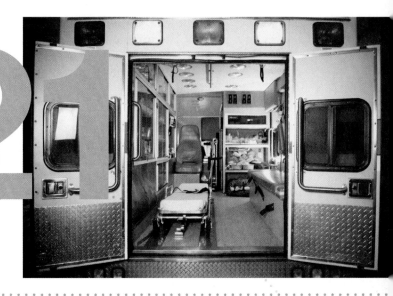

CHAPTER TWENTY ONE

Key Terms

Advanced life support (ALS)

Basic life support (BLS)

Durable medical equipment (DME)

Enteral therapy

Intra-arterial (IA)

Intramuscular (IM)

Intrathecal (IT)

Intravenous (IV)

Orthotic procedures and devices

Outpatient Prospective Payment System (OPPS)

Parenteral therapy

Route of administration

Learning Outcomes

After completing this chapter, you will be able to:

21.1 Identify the general HCPCS II guidelines and format.

21.2 Recognize the chapter-specific HCPCS Level II guidelines and format.

21.3 Review the most commonly used HCPCS modifier codes.

21.4 Examine the common abbreviations and acronyms used in HCPCS Level II.

21.5 Understand the chapter-specific CPT guidelines and format of the category II and category III codes.

Introduction

The Healthcare Common Procedure Coding System, which is more commonly termed *HCPCS*, consists of two levels. Level I comprises the Current Procedural Terminology (CPT) codes, and Level II comprises the national codes. This chapter focuses on HCPCS Level II codes as HCPCS Level I (CPT) codes have been discussed in previous chapters.

HCPCS Level II is maintained by the Center for Medicare and Medicaid Services (CMS). Multiple healthcare providers can use HCPCS Level II codes to continue telling the accurate stories of patient encounters.

These providers include physicians, nurse practitioners, physician assistants, ambulance providers, dentists, and durable medical equipment suppliers. Home health providers, therapists, and outpatient departments also need to be familiar with HCPCS Level II code guidelines and the appropriate use of these codes.

21.1 HCPCS Level II General Guidelines and Format

HCPCS Level II codes, like CPT Level I codes, are made of up five characters. HCPCS Level II codes always begin with an alphabetic letter that is followed by four numeric digits.

FOR EXAMPLE A0422 ∎

Guidelines exist in the front of many editions of the HCPCS Level II manual, and additional guidelines are included before each subsection range of codes.

The index for this manual is used in the same manner as the indexes for ICD and CPT. A coder must determine the main term, which can be a medical or surgical supply, service, orthotic, prosthetic, or drug, and locate this main term in the index. After identifying a possible code, the coder locates the code(s) under the appropriate subheading and checks the selected code(s) for any instructional notes or indicators such as age. The coder should review the appendix for any specific coverage guidelines that may be listed. Then the coder determines whether any modifiers are needed and assigns the code. As a review, here are the steps used to locate an appropriate HCPCS Level II code:

1. Identify the main term.
2. Locate the main term in the index, including the table of drugs.
3. Locate the code(s) identified in the index in the appropriate subsection (such as B Codes).
4. Look for any instructional notes, indicators, and so on, and review the appendix coverage guides. (Not all editions have this appendix, so a coder needs to be familiar with other resources for obtaining these coverage guidelines.)
5. Determine whether a modifier is needed.
6. Assign the code(s).

To determine whether it is appropriate to use a HCPCS Level I or Level II code, coders need to determine certain factors or criteria and follow these rules:

- If a Level I (CPT) code description and a Level II code description are identical, the CPT code should be used unless otherwise indicated by Medicare or another payer.
- If the Level I and Level II codes are not identical and the Level II code is more specific, the Level II code is to be reported.

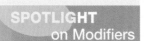

SPOTLIGHT on Modifiers

The table of drugs lists brand and generic names and also includes the amount (dose) and route of administration (i.e., IV, IM, IA).

MENTOR Coding Tip

It is very important to know the different abbreviations and acronyms used in the HCPCS Level II manual. This helps in selecting both the appropriate code and the most correct answer on the CPC exam. Many of the manuals include an abbreviation list.

Table 21.1 HCPCS Format *(Data from CPT 2013. © 2013 American Medical Association. All rights reserved.)*

GENERAL HEADING	CODE RANGE
Transportation Services, Including Ambulance	A0021–A0999
Medical and Surgical Supplies	A4206–A9999
Enteral and Parenteral Therapy	B4034–B9999
Outpatient and Prospective Payment System	C1300–C9899
Durable Medical Equipment (DME)	E0100–E9999
Procedures/Professional Services (Temporary)	G0008–G9156
Alcohol and Drug Abuse Treatment Services	H0001–H2037
Drugs Administered Other than by Oral Method	J0120–J8499
Temporary (Durable Medical Equipment)	K0000–K9999
Orthotic Procedures and Devices	L0000–L4199
Medical Services	M0000–M0301
Pathology and Laboratory Services	P0000–P9999
Temporary (Miscellaneous Services)	Q0035–Q9968
Diagnostic Radiology Services	R0000–R5999
Temporary National Codes (Non-Medicare)	S0000–S9999
National T Codes	T1000–T9999
Vision Services	V5000–V5999

Table 21.1 references the general headings and the code ranges for HCPCS Level II codes.

21.2 Chapter-Specific HCPCS Level II Guidelines and Format

There are often guidelines before each subheading that give specific instructions for the codes within the subheading range. Before selecting the appropriate code, be sure to read these guidelines and look for any additional coverage guidelines that may be included in the HCPCS Level II manual.

A Codes

Transportation Services, Including Ambulance: A0021–A0999

Codes within this subheading are further defined by the following criteria:

- Ground or air ambulance services:
  - Basic life support (BLS).
  - Advanced life support (ALS).

- Emergency or nonemergency status.
- Number of miles.
- Ambulance waiting time.

Generally, the definition of **basic life support** concerning ambulance services includes the following: basic CPR, trauma care such as splinting and control of bleeding, basic airway management, and use of pulse oximetry equipment. **Advanced life support** services can include the above procedures for BLS and the following: establishment of an IV, drawing of blood, use of a cardiac monitor, intubation, tracheotomy, use of continuous positive airway pressure (CPAP), and nasogastric tube placement.

- Nonemergency transportation:
  - Type of transportation, such as taxi, bus, automobile, wheelchair, or van.
  - Number of miles (several codes are per mile).
  - Provider of the vehicle, such as individual, family member, or volunteer.

Modifiers must be reported with ambulance service codes. Origin and destination modifiers are used to identify the site where the patient was picked up and the site the patient was transported to. They are two-digit modifiers; the first digit represents the origin site, and the second digit represents the destination site. See Table 21.2 for a list of these modifiers.

FOR EXAMPLE If the patient is picked up at his or her residence and transported to the physician's office, the appropriate modifier would be RP. ■

Medical and Surgical Supplies: A4206–A9999

Some subheadings included in this code range cover:

- Miscellaneous supplies (includes codes for syringes, infusion sets, replacement batteries for home blood glucose monitoring kits, and breast pump supplies).
- Vascular catheters.
- Incontinence appliances and care supplies.

Table 21.2 HCPCS Ambulance Services Modifiers *(Data from CPT 2013. © 2013 American Medical Association. All rights reserved.)*

MODIFIER	DEFINITION
D	Diagnostic or therapeutic site other than "P" or "H" when either is used as the origin code
G	Hospital-based ESRD facility
H	Hospital
I	Site of transfer (e.g., airport or helicopter pad) between modes of ambulance transport
J	Free-standing ESRD facility
N	Skilled nursing facility (SNF)
P	Physician office
R	Residence
S	Scene of accident or acute event
X	Intermediate stop at a physician's office on the way to the hospital (destination code only)

An instructional note states that these supplies are covered by Medicare when the medical record indicates incontinence is permanent or of long and indefinite duration.

- Ostomy supplies.
- Supplies for oxygen and related respiratory equipment such as nasal cannula, tubing, and mouthpiece.
- Dialysis supplies.
- Diabetic shoes, fillings, and modifications.

A guideline note informs coders that Medicare requires documentation from the prescribing physician showing that one of the following criteria has been met: peripheral neuropathy with callus formation, history of preulcerative calluses, history of ulceration, foot deformity, previous amputation, or poor circulation.

- Dressings (codes are defined by type of dressing and size of dressing).

FOR EXAMPLE

Foam dressing, wound cover, sterile, pad size 16 sq in or less, without adhesive border

Each dressing is assigned HCPCS code A6209. ▪

Nonprescription drugs, noncovered items and services, and radiopharmaceuticals are assigned codes from this subheading. For radiopharmaceuticals, the specific agent the code is describing is often listed below the code choice.

FOR EXAMPLE
Code A9500—technetium Tc-99m sestamibi, diagnostic, per study dose, up to 40 millicuries—is used for Cardiolite. ▪

B Codes

Enteral and Parenteral Therapy: B4034–B9999

Enteral therapy and **parenteral therapy** are forms of routes of administration. A **route of administration** is the method or path used for the entrance of a drug or another substance into the body. Enteral therapy is administered within the intestine, and this is often accomplished through the gastrointestinal tract via a gastric feeding tube or gastrostomy. In parenteral therapy, the patient receives the nutritional material in ways other than through the intestine, such as subcutaneously, intravenously, or intramuscularly. Included in the code choices for this subheading are the enteral formulae and medical supplies, such as gastrostomy tubes. Parenteral solutions and infusion pumps are also assigned codes within this subsection.

enteral therapy Therapy administered within the intestine; often accomplished through the gastrointestinal tract via a gastric feeding tube or gastrostomy.

parenteral therapy Therapy in which the patient receives the nutritional material subcutaneously, intravenously, or intramuscularly.

route of administration The method or path used for the entrance of a drug or other substance into the body.

MENTOR Coding Tip

Some routes of administration and their abbreviations are shown in Table 21.3.

intra-arterial (IA) Route of administration through the arterial system.

intravenous (IV) Route of administration through the venous system.

intramuscular (IM) Route of administration through the muscular system.

intrathecal (IT) Route of administration within the sheath through the membrane.

Table 21.3 Routes of Administration

ROUTE	ABBREVIATION
Intra-arterial (through the arterial system)	IA
Intravenous (through the venous system)	IV
Intramuscular (through the muscular system)	IM
Intrathecal (within the sheath through the membrane)	IT
Subcutaneous	SC
Inhalation	INH

C Codes

Outpatient PPS: C1300–C9899

The **Outpatient Prospective Payment System (OPPS)** is Medicare's system for payment to outpatient departments of hospitals and other outpatient facilities.

Outpatient Prospective Payment System (OPPS) Medicare's system for payment to outpatient departments of hospitals and other outpatient facilities.

This code range includes drug, biological, and device codes that must be used by OPPS hospitals. These codes can be reported only for facility or technical services.

Some of the items and services reported with codes in this subsection include:

- Brachytherapy sources
- Cardioverter-defibrillator, single- or dual-chamber pacemaker
- Catheters
- Leads for pacemakers and cardioverter-defibrillators
- Magnetic resonance imaging (MRI)
- Transesophageal echocardiography (TEE)

FOR EXAMPLE C1750 is assigned for catheter, hemodialysis/peritoneal, long term. ■

E Codes

Durable Medical Equipment E0100–E9999

durable medical equipment (DME) Equipment that can withstand extended use and is often prescribed for patients' home use.

Durable medical equipment (DME) is equipment that can withstand extended use and is often prescribed for patients' home use. Some equipment generally defined as DME includes canes, wheelchairs, crutches, hospital beds, oxygen equipment, and safety equipment (see Figure 21.1). Codes within this subsection can be very specific, and therefore both the code description and the documentation must be reviewed carefully.

FOR EXAMPLE Codes for walkers, range E0130–E0147, are defined as rigid, folding, enclosed, heavy duty, and with or without wheels. ■

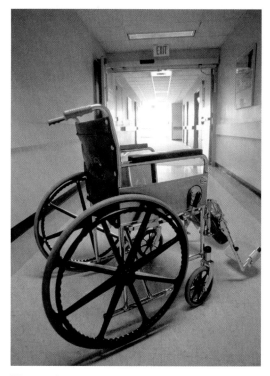

Figure 21.1 Durable Medical Equipment

G Codes

Procedures/Professional Services (Temporary): G0008–G9156

Codes in this subsection are commonly used for Medicare patients but may be used by all payers. These codes describe services for which there is no appropriate code description in HCPCS Level I (CPT).

Some frequently used G codes are listed below:

- G0102, prostate cancer screening, digital rectal examination.
- G0104, colorectal cancer screening, flexible sigmoidoscopy.
- G0121, colorectal cancer screening, colonoscopy on an individual not meeting the criteria for high risk.
- G0402, initial preventive physical examination, face-to-face visit, services limited to a new beneficiary during the first 12 months of Medicare enrollment.
- G0403, electrocardiogram, routine ECG with 12 leads, performed as a screening for the initial preventive physical examination with interpretation and report.

H Codes

Alcohol and Drug Abuse Treatment Services: H0001–H2037

The codes under this subheading are generally used by Medicaid agencies to identify mental health services that include services for drug and alcohol treatment.

J Codes

Drugs Administered Other than Oral Method: J0120–J8499

Codes in this code range are commonly used for drugs that cannot be self-administered, such as chemotherapy drugs, immunosuppressive drugs, and

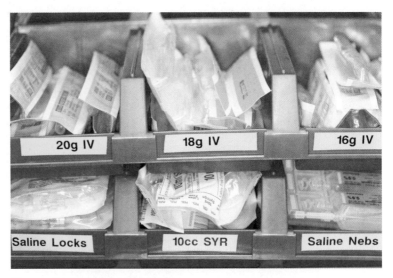

Figure 21.2 Drugs and Supplies

inhalation solutions. To assign the accurate code, a coder needs to know the following (see Figure 21.2):

- What drug was administered?
- How was the drug administered—injection, infusion, or inhalation?
- How much of the drug was administered, and how was it measured (e.g., units, cubic centimeters, grams, milligrams, or milliliters)?

L Codes

Orthotic Procedures and Devices: L0000–L4199

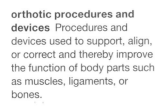

orthotic procedures and devices Procedures and devices used to support, align, or correct and thereby improve the function of body parts such as muscles, ligaments, or bones.

Orthotic procedures and devices are used to support, align, or correct and thereby improve the function of body parts such as muscles, ligaments, or bones. Some devices covered in this subsection are braces, slings, shoes, and prosthetic devices (see Figure 21.3). Codes within this subsection are further classified by the following subheadings:

- Orthotic Devices—Spinal
- Cervical
- Thoracic
- Cervical-Thoracic-Lumbar-Sacral
- Halo Procedure
- Orthotic Devices
- Scoliosis Procedures
- Lower Limb (further defined by knee, hip, ankle, foot)
- Upper Limb (further defined by shoulder, elbow, wrist-hand-finger)
- Orthopedic Shoes (further defined by inserts, arch support, lifts, wedges, heels)

Prosthetic Procedures: L5000–L9999

Multiple codes may be used from this subsection. Several of the codes are "base" codes, and additional codes from the Additions subheadings may be used.

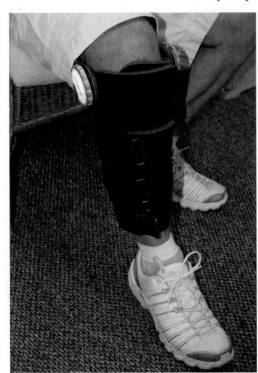

Figure 21.3 Orthotics

FOR EXAMPLE Code L5595—preparatory, hip disarticulation/ hemipelvectomy, pylon, no cover, SACH foot, laminated socket, molded to patient model—could have L5626—addition to lower extremity, test socket, hip disarticulation—as an additional code. ∎

Codes within this subheading are further classified by the following:

- Lower limb.
- Upper limb (hooks, hands, and gloves).
- Prosthetic implants (artificial larynx, ocular implants, cochlear implants).

Q Codes

Temporary Miscellaneous Services Q0035–Q9968

Codes within this subsection are mainly temporary codes for casting supplies. Codes Q4001 to Q4051 are used to report casting and splint materials supplied by the physician.

S Codes

Temporary National Codes (Non-Medicare): S0000–S9999

Codes in this subsection are used to report codes to non-Medicare payers, such as Blue Cross/Blue Shield and other commercial payers. These codes are used by Medicaid but not Medicare. The codes in this subsection are used to report drugs, services, and supplies that do not have codes in HCPCS Level I (CPT) or elsewhere in the HCPCS Level II manual.

V Codes

Vision Services: V0000–V2999

Codes included in this subsection are reported for vision-related supplies such as spectacles, contact lenses, intraocular lenses, and prosthetic eyes.

Hearing Services: V5000–V5999

Codes included in this subsection are reported for hearing-related supplies such as hearing aids and assistive hearing devices. Also included are codes for hearing tests, speech-language pathology screening tests, and repairs of augmentative communication systems.

EXERCISE 21.2

1. Assign the appropriate modifier to report a patient's origin site as an SNF and destination site as the hospital.
2. Using your HCPCS Level II manual, assign the appropriate code for a body-worn hearing aid, monaural, for bone conduction loss.
3. Using your HCPCS Level II manual, assign the appropriate code(s) for trimming of five dystrophic nails, and indicate where you would look in the index to locate the code(s).
4. What criteria does Medicare require for the use of codes under the subheading Diabetic Shoes?

Also available in Connect (plus+)

Table 21.4 HCPCS Level II Modifiers *(Data from CPT 2013. © 2013 American Medical Association. All rights reserved.)*

MODIFIER	DEFINITION
AD	Medical supervision by a physician: more than four concurrent anesthesia procedures
AQ	Physician providing a service in an unlisted health professional shortage area (HPSA)
BO	Orally administered nutrition, not by feeding tube
GS	ESRD patient for whom less than 6 dialysis sessions have been provided in a month
GA	Waiver-of-liability statement on file (This is the modifier used with an ABN.)
GH	Diagnostic mammogram converted from screening mammogram on the same day, same patient
GW	Service not related to the hospice patient's terminal condition
NU	New equipment
Q3	Live kidney donor surgery and related services
SH	Second concurrently administered infusion therapy

21.3 Most Commonly Used HCPCS Modifiers

Modifiers are used to continue or modify the story of the patient's encounter. Some of the HCPCS Level II modifiers are listed inside the front cover of many editions of the HCPCS Level I CPT manual. The HCPCS Level II modifiers are listed in an appendix of many editions of the Level II manual. If the modifiers are not listed in an appendix, they are located somewhere else within the manual. Some of the more common Level II modifiers are identified in Table 21.4.

The appropriate use of modifiers with the codes from Level II helps to tell the patient's full story.

EXERCISE 21.3

For the following exercises, use both HCPCS Level I and Level II manuals as resources.

1. Identify the appropriate HCPCS Level II modifiers for the following:
   a. Right foot, great toe
   b. Left hand, fourth digit
   c. Upper-left eyelid
2. Identify the appropriate HCPCS Level II modifiers for the following:
   a. Ambulance service provided under arrangement by a provider or service.
   b. Ambulance service furnished directly by a provider of service.
3. Identify the appropriate HCPCS Level II modifier for the following:
   a. Performance and payment of a screening mammogram and diagnostic mammogram on the same patient, same day.

Also available in McGraw Hill **connect** (plus+)

Table 21.5 HCPCS Level II Symbols, Abbreviations, and Acronyms *(Data from CPT 2013. © 2013 American Medical Association. All rights reserved.)*

SYMBOL, ABBREVIATION, OR ACRONYM	DEFINITION	USE IN HCPCS II	ABBREVIATION OR ACRONYM	DEFINITION	USE IN HCPCS II
<	Less than	A codes	LAUP	Laser-assisted uvulopalato plasty	S codes
≤	Less than or equal to	A codes	NG	Nasogastric	B codes
>	Greater than	A codes	PTK	Phototherapeutic keratectomy	S codes
AKA	Above-the-knee amputation	L codes			
FPD	Fixed partial denture	D codes	SACH	Solid ankle cushion heel	L codes
HKAFO	Hip-knee-ankle-foot orthosis	L codes	SGD	Speech-generating device	E codes
LVEF	Left-ventricular ejection fraction	G codes	TENS	Transcutaneous electrical nerve stimulation	E codes B codes
			TPN	Total parenteral nutrition	

21.4 Common Medical and Procedural Terms Used in Operative Reports

There are medical terms and procedural terms that are specific to HCPCS Level II. Table 21.5 lists some of the abbreviations, acronyms, and symbols most commonly used in the HCPCS Level II manual. Many editions of this manual include an appendix that lists many of the abbreviations and acronyms. It is extremely important that coders have an understanding of these terms and their use in HCPCS Level II coding.

1. Give an example in which *less than or equal to* is a factor in a code in the A-code range.
2. The abbreviation *TENS* stands for transcutaneous electrical nerve stimulation and is located in the E codes. Give an example of a code that has this abbreviation in the code description.
3. The abbreviation *TPN* is used for total parenteral nutrition. Give an example of a code that has this abbreviation in the code description.

Also available in 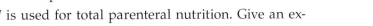 connect plus+

21.5 Chapter-Specific CPT Guidelines and Format of Category II and III Codes

Category II Codes

The codes within category II (F codes) are supplemental tracking codes used for performance measurement. Modifiers (1P, 2P, and 3P) attached to these codes indicate that a specified service was considered but not performed due to medical, patient, or system reasons. These category II modifiers are to be reported only with category II codes. These codes are optional.

The subheadings in this subsection are divided as follows:

- Composite Codes (very similar to panel codes in CPT category I)
- Patient Management
- Patient History
- Physical Examination
- Diagnostic/Screening Processes or Results
- Therapeutic, Preventive, or Other Interventions
- Follow-Up or Other Outcomes
- Patient Safety

Category III Codes

The codes within this subsection are T codes, which are temporary codes used for emerging technology services and procedures when an appropriate code in CPT category I does not exist. The guidelines at the beginning of this subsection contain much information about this code set and should be reviewed carefully. These guidelines instruct the use of a category III code instead of a category I unlisted code if there is an appropriate category III code. The codes in this subsection are five characters: four numeric digits followed by an alphabetic letter.

FOR EXAMPLE

0099T Implantation of intrastromal corneal ring segments ■

The codes in the category III subsection are updated semiannually on the AMA/CPT website and published annually in the CPT manual.

Some of the subheadings include the following:

- Remote Real-Time Interactive Videoconferenced Critical Care Services
- Atherectomy (Open or Percutaneous) for Supra-Inguinal Arteries
- Acoustic Cardiography
- Implantantion
- Injection

As with category I codes, there are several instructional notes within the code ranges directing the use of modifiers, and in some cases category I codes are listed that can be used in conjunction with category III codes.

FOR EXAMPLE

0213T Injection(s), diagnostic or therapeutic agent, paravertebral facet joint (or nerves innervating that joint) with ultrasound guidance, cervical or thoracic, single level

To report a bilateral procedure, use 0213T with modifier 50. ■

MENTOR
Coding Tip

There are several guidelines at the beginning of this subheading, and before selecting a code from this code range, the coder should review these guidelines. Codes such as the critical care codes in category I are time-based.

EXERCISE 21.5

1. Which category I codes do category III codes supersede?
2. Which set of codes includes codes that are optional and are used to track performance measurement of services and procedures?
3. How often are category III codes updated?

Also available in Mc Graw Hill connect plus+

Chapter Twenty-One Summary

Learning Outcome	Key Concepts/Examples
21.1 Identify the general HCPCS Level II guidelines and format.	HCPCS Level II codes are made of up five characters beginning with an alphabetic letter that is followed by four numeric digits. Steps used to locate the appropriate HCPCS Level II code are: 1. Identify the main term. 2. Locate the main term in the index, including the table of drugs. 3. Locate the code(s) identified in the index in the appropriate subsection. 4. Look for any instructional notes, indicators, and so on, and review the appendix coverage guides. 5. Determine whether a modifier is needed. 6. Assign the code(s).
21.2 Recognize the chapter-specific HCPCS Level II guidelines and format.	There are often guidelines before each subheading that give specific instructions for the codes within the specific range. Before selecting the appropriate code, be sure to read these guidelines and look for any coverage guidelines that may be included in the HCPCS Level II manual. *Outpatient Prospective Payment System (OPPS):* This is Medicare's system for payment to outpatient departments of hospitals and other outpatient facilities. The OPPS code range includes drug, biological, and device codes that must be used by OPPS hospitals. These codes can be reported only for facility or technical services. *Dental Procedures:* The codes within this subsection are maintained by the American Dental Association.
21.3 Review the most commonly used HCPCS modifier codes.	Modifiers are used to continue or modify the story of the patient's encounter. Some of the HCPCS Level II modifiers are listed inside the front cover of many editions of the HCPCS Level I CPT manual. The HCPCS Level II modifiers are listed in an appendix of many editions of the Level II manual. If the modifiers are not listed in an appendix, they are located somewhere else within the manual.
21.4 Examine the common abbreviations and acronyms used in HCPCS Level II.	There are medical terms and procedural terms that are specific to HCPCS Level II. Table 21.5 lists some of the abbreviations, acronyms, and symbols most commonly used in the HCPCS Level II manual. Many editions of this manual include an appendix that lists many of the abbreviations and acronyms. It is extremely important that coders have an understanding of these terms and their use in HCPCS Level II coding.
21.5 Understand the chapter-specific CPT guidelines and format of the category II and category III codes.	*Category II:* The codes within category II (F codes) are supplemental tracking codes used for performance measurement. Modifiers (1P, 2P, and 3P) attached to these codes indicate that a specified service was considered but not performed due to medical, patient, or system reasons. These category II modifiers are to be reported only with Category II codes. These codes are optional. *Category III:* The codes within this subsection are T codes, which are temporary codes used for emerging technology services and procedures when an appropriate code in CPT category I does not exist. The guidelines at the beginning of this subsection contain much information about this code set and should be reviewed carefully. These guidelines instruct the use of a category III code instead of a category I unlisted code if there is an appropriate category III code. The codes in this subsection are five characters: four numeric digits followed by an alphabetic letter.

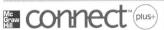

Enhance your learning by completing these exercises and more at mcgrawhillconnect.com

Chapter Twenty-One Review

Using Terminology

Match each key term to the appropriate definition.

_____ 1. [LO21.2] Advanced life support (ALS)

_____ 2. [LO21.2] Basic life support (BLS)

_____ 3. [LO21.2] Durable medical equipment (DME)

_____ 4. [LO21.2] Enteral

_____ 5. [LO21.2] Intra-arterial (IA)

_____ 6. [LO21.2] Intramuscular (IM)

_____ 7. [LO21.2] Intrathecal (IT)

_____ 8. [LO21.2] Intravenous (IV)

_____ 9. [LO21.2] Orthotic

_____ 10. [LO21.2] Outpatient Prospective Payment System (OPPS)

_____ 11. [LO21.2] Parenteral

_____ 12. [LO21.2] Route of administration

A. Route of drug administration through the arterial system

B. Administration of nutrients into the body by a route other than through the small intestine

C. Administration of nutrients into the body through the small intestine via a gastrostomy tube

D. Reusable materials such as walkers, canes, and crutches

E. Type of device used to support, align, or correct muscles, ligaments, and bones

F. Route of drug administration through the venous system

G. Type of life support certification that generally allows basic CPR, trauma care such as splinting and control of bleeding, basic airway management, and use of pulse oximetry equipment to be performed by EMT personnel in an ambulance

H. Route of drug administration through the muscular system

I. Medicare's system for payment to outpatient departments of hospitals and other outpatient facilities

J. Route of administration within a sheath

K. Type of life support certification that generally allows services including establishment of an IV, drawing of blood, use of a cardiac monitor, intubation, tracheotomy, use of continuous positive airway pressure (CPAP), and nasogastric tube placement to be performed by EMT personnel in an ambulance

L. Method or path used for the entrance of a drug or another substance into the body

Checking Your Understanding

Choose the most appropriate answer for each of the following questions.

1. [LO21.2] A 20-year-old female is seen in her OB/GYN clinic. She receives an injection of Depo-Provera, 150 mg, for family planning. Select the appropriate HCPCS Level II code:

   a. J1000

   b. L8030

   c. J1055

   d. J1056

2. [LO21.5] Which of the following best describes category III codes?

   a. Emerging technology temporary codes

   b. Optional performance measurement codes

   c. Deleted codes

   d. HCPCS codes

3. [LO21.4] HCPCS Level II modifiers may be added to:

   a. HCPCS Level II codes

   b. ICD-9-CM codes

   c. CPT HCPCS Level I codes

   d. HCPCS Level I and II codes

4. [LO21.2] A patient's family receives 30 minutes of family training and counseling. This training and counseling was done for child development purposes. Select the appropriate HCPCS Level II code:

   a. T1025

   b. T1026

   c. T1027

   d. T1027 x2

5. **[LO21.2]** HCPCS Level II dental codes (D0000 to D9999) are maintained by the:

    a. HCPCS National Panel   **c.** American Dental Association

    b. CMS   **d.** OIG

6. **[LO21.2]** The patient receives an IV injection of 5 percent dextrose with water. Select the appropriate HCPCS Level II code:

    a. J7100   **c.** J7042

    b. J7060   **d.** J1720

7. **[LO21.3]** Which of the following HCPCS modifiers is appropriate to report when a diagnostic mammogram is converted from a screening mammogram on the same day for the same patient?

    a. GS   **c.** GW

    b. GA   **d.** GH

8. **[LO21.3]** The HCPCS Level II modifier for new equipment is:

    a. NU   **c.** NQ

    b. NR   **d.** NH

9. **[LO21.2]** A patient received Level 2 advanced life support (ALS). Select the appropriate HCPCS Level II code:

    a. A0432   **c.** A0433

    b. A0428   **d.** A0429

10. **[LO21.5]** A category III code can be used in place of a(n):

    a. HCPCS Level II code   **c.** ICD-9-CM code

    b. Unlisted CPT Level I code   **d.** HCPCS Level I code (CPT)

Applying Your Knowledge

1.   **[LO21.2]** Explain C codes (Outpatient PPS, C1000–C9999).

    _____

2.   **[LO21.1]** Explain the criteria needed to determine the appropriate use of a HCPCS Level I or Level II code.

    _____

3.   **[LO 21.1]** Discuss routes of administration, and give examples of some of the abbreviations and their definitions.

    _____

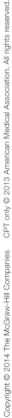

connect (plus+)   Enhance your learning by completing these exercises and more at mcgrawhillconnect.com

CHAPTER TWENTY-ONE REVIEW

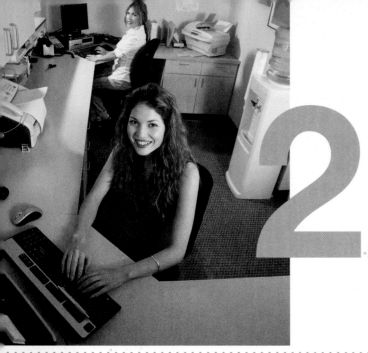

22

Practice Management

CHAPTER TWENTY-TWO

Key Terms

Advance Beneficiary
Notice (ABN)

American Recovery and
Reinvestment Act
(ARRA)

Centers for Medicare and
Medicaid Services
(CMS)

Compliance plan

Covered entity

Health Information
Technology for
Economic and Clinical
Health (HITECH) Act

Health Insurance
Portability and
Accountability Act
(HIPAA)

Hierarchical condition
categories (HCCs)

Local Coverage
Determination (LCD)

Medically unlikely edits
(MUEs)

Medicare Administrative
Contractor (MAC)

National Correct Coding
Initiative (NCCI)

National Coverage
Determinations
(NCDs)

Office of Inspector
General (OIG)

Protected health
information (PHI)

Learning Outcomes

After completing this chapter, you will be able to:

22.1 Recognize the AAPC professional code of ethics.

22.2 Understand the definitions of providers and payers, including Medicare, Medicaid, TRICARE, and managed care entities.

22.3 Identify regulations and the parties responsible for maintaining and enforcing the regulations.

Introduction

Practice management consists of many components, all of which the coder needs to be aware of in order to be most effective in a practice. One component is knowledge of government payers, such as Medicare, Medicaid, and TRICARE, and of third-party payers, including managed care entities and their reimbursement guidelines. Other significant components of practice management are compliance with regulations and awareness of the entities responsible for these regulations. Certified coders also must adhere to the professional code of ethics defined by the AAPC.

Copyright © 2014 The McGraw-Hill Companies

22.1 AAPC Professional Code of Ethics

It is vital that professional coders know the AAPC's code of ethics. Coders should refer to these ethics to remind themselves of why they were interested in the profession of medical coding in the first place and to make sure that they are complying with the code.

AAPC Code of Ethics

Commitment to ethical professional conduct is expected of every AAPC member. The specification of a Code of Ethics enables AAPC to clarify to current and future members, and to those served by members, the nature of the ethical responsibilities held in common by its members. This document establishes principles that define the ethical behavior of AAPC members. All AAPC members are required to adhere to the Code of Ethics and the Code of Ethics will serve as the basis for processing ethical complaints initiated against AAPC members.

AAPC members shall:

Maintain and enhance the dignity, status, integrity, competence, and standards of our profession.

Respect the privacy of others and honor confidentiality.

Strive to achieve the highest quality, effectiveness and dignity in both the process and products of professional work.

Advance the profession through continued professional development and education by acquiring and maintaining professional competence.

Know and respect existing federal, state and local laws, regulations, certifications and licensing requirements applicable to professional work.

Use only legal and ethical principles that reflect the profession's core values and report activity that is perceived to violate this Code of Ethics to the AAPC Ethics Committee.

Accurately represent the credential(s) earned and the status of AAPC membership.

Avoid actions and circumstances that may appear to compromise good business judgment or create a conflict between personal and professional interests.

Adherence to these standards assures public confidence in the integrity and service of medical coding, auditing, compliance and practice management professionals who are AAPC members.

Failure to adhere to these standards, as determined by AAPC's Ethics Committee, may result in the loss of credentials and membership with AAPC.

1. What does adhering to the AAPC code of ethics mean to coders and the coding profession?
2. List three of the items in the code of ethics.

EXERCISE 22.1

Also available in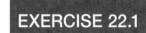

22.2 Definitions of Providers and Payers, Including Medicare, Medicaid, TRICARE, and Managed Care Entities

Providers

Over the last 20 years healthcare has expanded the role of the medical practitioner to encompass more than physicians. Today the term *provider* encompasses a wide range and level of practitioners as well as nonphysician providers (NPPs). The most common types of providers include:

Physician (MD)

Doctor of osteopathy (DO)

Nurse practitioner (NP)

Physician assistant (PA)

Payers

Medicare was established in 1965 and is administered by the **Centers for Medicare and Medicaid Services (CMS)** through **Medicare Administrative Contractors (MACs).** Medicare provides coverage for persons 65 years and older, disabled persons (after 2 years of disability), and persons with end-stage renal disease (ESRD).

The Medicare program is made up of four parts:

A. **Hospital insurance:** pays for inpatient facility care (includes hospital, skilled nursing facility, hospice, and some home healthcare services)

B. **Medical insurance:** pays for provider services, outpatient hospital and lab services, and durable medical equipment (DME).

C. **Medicare Advantage:** as an alternative to the original Medicare plan, provides managed care and private fee-for-service plan options. Reimbursement for Part C claims are impacted by the provider's management of the patient's health. Payments are adjusted based on CMS **hierarchical condition categories (HCCs),** which are a means of assessing the risk of medically managing each patient based on current conditions and comorbid conditions that are impacting care.

D. **Prescription drug plan:** provides prescription drug coverage through various Medicare plans.

> **SPOTLIGHT** on Practice Management
>
> **Claim forms:** There are typically two types of claim forms used to report healthcare services: the CMS-1500 (see Figure 22.1) and the UB-04. Provider and outpatient facility services are reported on the CMS-1500 (Medicare Part B and C services). Inpatient facility services are reported on the UB-04 (Medicare Part A services).

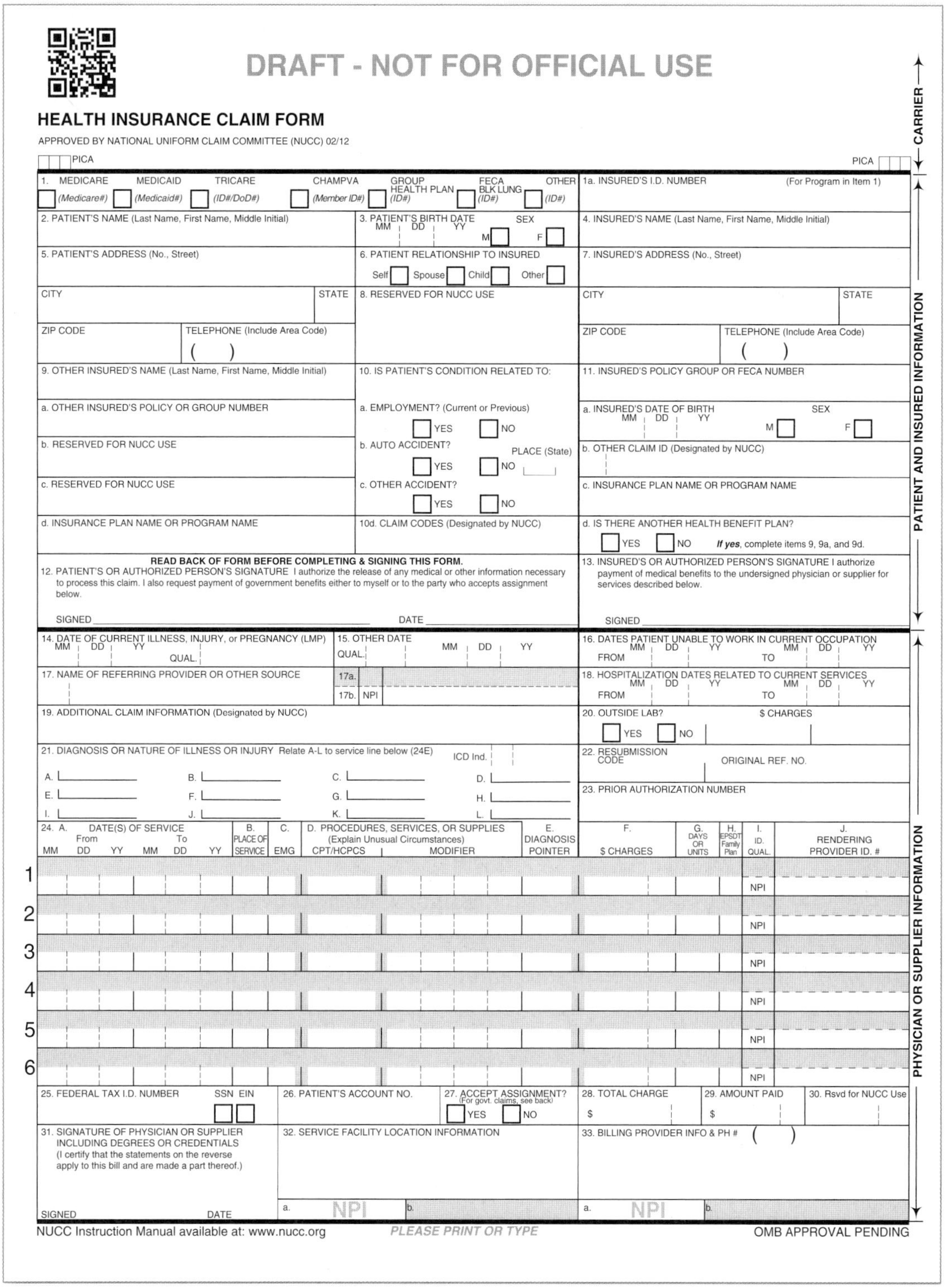
DRAFT - NOT FOR OFFICIAL USE

HEALTH INSURANCE CLAIM FORM

APPROVED BY NATIONAL UNIFORM CLAIM COMMITTEE (NUCC) 02/12

PICA PICA

CARRIER

1. MEDICARE (Medicare#) MEDICAID (Medicaid#) TRICARE (ID#/DoD#) CHAMPVA (Member ID#) GROUP HEALTH PLAN (ID#) FECA BLK LUNG (ID#) OTHER (ID#)

1a. INSURED'S I.D. NUMBER (For Program in Item 1)

2. PATIENT'S NAME (Last Name, First Name, Middle Initial)

3. PATIENT'S BIRTH DATE MM DD YY SEX M F

4. INSURED'S NAME (Last Name, First Name, Middle Initial)

5. PATIENT'S ADDRESS (No., Street)

6. PATIENT RELATIONSHIP TO INSURED Self Spouse Child Other

7. INSURED'S ADDRESS (No., Street)

CITY STATE

8. RESERVED FOR NUCC USE

CITY STATE

ZIP CODE TELEPHONE (Include Area Code) ( )

ZIP CODE TELEPHONE (Include Area Code) ( )

9. OTHER INSURED'S NAME (Last Name, First Name, Middle Initial)

10. IS PATIENT'S CONDITION RELATED TO:

11. INSURED'S POLICY GROUP OR FECA NUMBER

a. OTHER INSURED'S POLICY OR GROUP NUMBER

a. EMPLOYMENT? (Current or Previous) YES NO

a. INSURED'S DATE OF BIRTH MM DD YY SEX M F

b. RESERVED FOR NUCC USE

b. AUTO ACCIDENT? YES NO PLACE (State)

b. OTHER CLAIM ID (Designated by NUCC)

c. RESERVED FOR NUCC USE

c. OTHER ACCIDENT? YES NO

c. INSURANCE PLAN NAME OR PROGRAM NAME

d. INSURANCE PLAN NAME OR PROGRAM NAME

10d. CLAIM CODES (Designated by NUCC)

d. IS THERE ANOTHER HEALTH BENEFIT PLAN? YES NO *If yes*, complete items 9, 9a, and 9d.

READ BACK OF FORM BEFORE COMPLETING & SIGNING THIS FORM.

12. PATIENT'S OR AUTHORIZED PERSON'S SIGNATURE I authorize the release of any medical or other information necessary to process this claim. I also request payment of government benefits either to myself or to the party who accepts assignment below.

SIGNED DATE

13. INSURED'S OR AUTHORIZED PERSON'S SIGNATURE I authorize payment of medical benefits to the undersigned physician or supplier for services described below.

SIGNED

PATIENT AND INSURED INFORMATION

14. DATE OF CURRENT ILLNESS, INJURY, or PREGNANCY (LMP) MM DD YY QUAL.

15. OTHER DATE QUAL. MM DD YY

16. DATES PATIENT UNABLE TO WORK IN CURRENT OCCUPATION MM DD YY FROM TO

17. NAME OF REFERRING PROVIDER OR OTHER SOURCE 17a. 17b. NPI

18. HOSPITALIZATION DATES RELATED TO CURRENT SERVICES MM DD YY FROM TO

19. ADDITIONAL CLAIM INFORMATION (Designated by NUCC)

20. OUTSIDE LAB? YES NO $ CHARGES

21. DIAGNOSIS OR NATURE OF ILLNESS OR INJURY Relate A-L to service line below (24E) ICD Ind.

A. B. C. D.
E. F. G. H.
I. J. K. L.

22. RESUBMISSION CODE ORIGINAL REF. NO.

23. PRIOR AUTHORIZATION NUMBER

24. A. DATE(S) OF SERVICE From MM DD YY To MM DD YY | B. PLACE OF SERVICE | C. EMG | D. PROCEDURES, SERVICES, OR SUPPLIES (Explain Unusual Circumstances) CPT/HCPCS MODIFIER | E. DIAGNOSIS POINTER | F. $ CHARGES | G. DAYS OR UNITS | H. EPSDT Family Plan | I. ID. QUAL. | J. RENDERING PROVIDER ID. #

1 NPI
2 NPI
3 NPI
4 NPI
5 NPI
6 NPI

PHYSICIAN OR SUPPLIER INFORMATION

25. FEDERAL TAX I.D. NUMBER SSN EIN

26. PATIENT'S ACCOUNT NO.

27. ACCEPT ASSIGNMENT? (For govt. claims, see back) YES NO

28. TOTAL CHARGE $

29. AMOUNT PAID $

30. Rsvd for NUCC Use

31. SIGNATURE OF PHYSICIAN OR SUPPLIER INCLUDING DEGREES OR CREDENTIALS (I certify that the statements on the reverse apply to this bill and are made a part thereof.)

SIGNED DATE

32. SERVICE FACILITY LOCATION INFORMATION

a. NPI b.

33. BILLING PROVIDER INFO & PH # ( )

a. NPI b.

NUCC Instruction Manual available at: www.nucc.org PLEASE PRINT OR TYPE OMB APPROVAL PENDING

Figure 22.1 CMS-1500 Claim Form

Medicare contracted providers, also known as participating (PAR) providers, agree to accept assignment of the claim and Medicare's allowed amount as identified by the Medicare provider fee schedule (MPFS) for approved and medically necessary services. PAR providers are allowed 100 percent of the MPFS, with 80 percent paid by Medicare and 20 percent paid by the beneficiary. Another incentive for participation is faster processing of claims, resulting in more timely and direct reimbursement of services.

Nonparticipating, or non-PAR, providers are those providers who have chosen not to contract with Medicare and can decide whether or not to accept assignment for each claim. However, non-PAR providers incur more reimbursement risk as a high percentage of the total payment is the responsibility of the beneficiary. Medicare allows only 95 percent of the MPFS for non-PAR providers, of which Medicare pays 80 percent. Non-PAR providers may bill beneficiaries up to 15 percent above the MPFS in addition to the 20 percent remaining from the non-PAR Medicare payment.

SPOTLIGHT on Practice Management

Payer contracts typically require that a good-faith attempt be made to collect the patient's coinsurance, copayment, and deductible.

Coinsurance The patient-responsible portion, which is based on a percentage of the allowed charge.

Copayment The patient-responsible portion of a set amount per service or encounter.

Deductible A predetermined amount that is deemed the patient's responsibility before the payer benefits begin.

Non-PAR providers face additional restrictions:

- Fees are restricted to no more than the limiting charge.
- Claims must be filed by the provider.
- Only the deductible and/or coinsurance can be collected at the time of service.
- Surgical fees over $500 require that a Surgical Disclosure Notice be signed by the patient.
- Lab fees are paid as accept assignment only at the allowed fee schedule regardless of the providers status as PAR or Non-PAR.

Medicaid, created in 1965 and funded by both state and federal funds, provides medical care for persons falling below the national poverty level. The Medicaid program is administered by each state and monitored by CMS to keep track of funding, ensure delivery of services, check eligibility of beneficiaries, and see that quality-of-care standards are met.

TRICARE and CHAMPVA provide healthcare coverage and benefits to active or retired uniformed service members and their families. TRICARE provides coverage for active-duty and retired members who are not eligible for Medicare benefits. CHAMPVA provides coverage for retired members who are eligible for Medicare and enrolled in Part A but not enrolled in Part B.

In addition to the government healthcare coverage listed above, several other forms of insurance are available that are generally offered by third-party payers. Third-party payers employ a variety of methodologies to manage, negotiate, and contract with providers of services while keeping healthcare costs down. These methods include:

Health maintenance organizations (HMOs)

Preferred provider organizations (PPOs)

Point of service (POS)

Fee for service (FFS)

SPOTLIGHT on Practice Management

Medicaid is considered the payer of last resort as the claim must first be submitted to and adjudicated by any other health or medical entity whose coverage is available to the patient before reimbursement is sought from the Medicaid program.

SPOTLIGHT on Practice Management

Third-party payers are so named as they are the third party in the patient (first party), provider (second party), and payer relationship.

EXERCISE 22.2

1. Define *coinsurance, copayment,* and *deductible.*
2. Identify the four parts of Medicare.
3. Which type of provider agrees to accept assignment of the claim and Medicare's allowed amount as identified by the Medicare provider fee schedule for approved and medically necessary services?

Also available in connect(plus+)

22.3 Regulations and the Parties Responsible for Regulation Maintenance and Enforcement

Office of Inspector General

Within the executive branch of the federal government, the **Office of Inspector General (OIG)** investigates allegations of fraud, waste, abuse, or misconduct and assists the executive branch in identifying and correcting operational deficiencies. When federal funds are involved, the OIG's jurisdiction encompasses any relevant department or agency, state or federal, and the programs within it. Working through the Department of Health and Human Services (HHS), the OIG has jurisdiction over healthcare programs regulated and administered at the state and/or federal level, Medicaid, and TRICARE.

Within HHS, the integrity of the Centers for Medicare and Medicaid Services (CMS) is protected through OIG activities such as audits, evaluations, and, when necessary, enforcement and compliance actions. Each of these management activities may be done at either the national level, through the OIG or CMS, or the local level, through CMS Medicare Administrative Contractors. In essence, OIG is responsible for protecting the Medicare and Medicaid programs and their beneficiaries by identifying and preventing fraud, waste, and abuse; recognizing opportunities to improve the economy, effectiveness, and efficiency of the programs; and holding responsible any persons or entities that do not adhere to program requirements or that violate federal laws.

The OIG provides direction to providers in a number of ways:

- Each year the OIG publishes a work plan that identifies new and ongoing reviews and activities that the OIG will track during the next 12 months based on issues identified or brought forth during the year. The work plan is published annually, usually in October of the year preceding the calendar year for the plan.
- The OIG encourages the development and use of an effective **compliance plan** by outlining the benefits of such a plan, some of which are that it:
  - Increases accuracy of documentation, which will enhance patient care.
  - Speeds and optimizes proper payment of claims.
  - Minimizes billing mistakes.
  - Reduces chances of an audit by CMS or the OIG.
  - Avoids conflicts with the self-referral and anti-kickback statutes.
  - Shows good-faith effort to submit accurate claims.
  - May mitigate fines and penalties due to claim errors.

Office of Inspector General (OIG) Agency that investigates allegations of fraud, waste, abuse, or misconduct and assists the executive branch in identifying and correcting operational deficiencies.

Compliance plan A written plan consisting of standards and procedures designed to implement compliance and practice standards.

In October 2000, the OIG published "Compliance Program Guidance for Individual and Small Group Physician Practices," which lists seven components as the basis of developing a voluntary compliance program for a physician practice:

- Designating a compliance officer or contact(s) to monitor compliance efforts and enforce practice standards.
- Implementing compliance and practice standards through the development of written standards and procedures.
- Conducting internal monitoring and auditing through the performance of periodic audits.
- Conducting appropriate training and education on practice standards and procedures.
- Developing open lines of communication.
- Responding appropriately to detected violations through the investigation of allegations and disclosure of incidents to appropriate government entities.
- Enforcing disciplinary standards through well-publicized guidelines.

Centers for Medicare and Medicaid Services

The Centers for Medicare and Medicaid Services (CMS) operates in two parts or levels: national and local. At the national level CMS oversees and develops payment policy and integrates management of administrative contractors. At the local level Medicare Administrative Contractors (MACs) assume the responsibility of enrolling and educating providers; receiving, adjudicating, and paying claims; and detecting fraud and abuse within their jurisdictions.

In its efforts to reduce waste from improper payments, CMS developed edits and medical coverage rules identifying when payment for services will and will not be allowed. Medical coverage rules are administered at both the national level and the local level:

National Coverage Determinations (NCDs): Developed by CMS, NCDs identify payment coverage for a specific service, procedure, test, or technology based on medical necessity or frequency.

Local Coverage Determination (LCD): When there is no NCD or when clarification is needed regarding determination of payment coverage of services, procedures, tests, or technology, the MAC may create an LCD. The LCD may not be more restrictive than the CMS's NCD regarding a specific service or code and must be consistent with all statutes, rulings, regulations, and NCDs.

An **Advance Beneficiary Notice** (ABN) of Noncoverage is needed for any service that does not meet the coverage criteria established in an NCD or LCD. An ABN, also known as form CMS-R-131 (see Figure 22.2), is not intended to be used when the service provided is never covered by Medicare but when a service usually covered by Medicare may not be covered under a particular circumstance, such as diagnosis restrictions, frequency of the service or procedure, or another payment limitation.

The ABN allows the provider to collect payment from the patient for services that Medicare determines are not medically necessary based on coverage

National Coverage Determinations (NCDs) CMS national-level rules that identify payment coverage for a specific service, procedure, test, or technology based on medical necessity or frequency.

Local Coverage Determinations (LCDs) Rules developed at the local level by Medicare Administrative Contractors that identify payment coverage for a specific service, procedure, test, or technology based on medical necessity or frequency.

Advance Beneficiary Notice (ABN) A waiver needed for any service that does not meet the coverage criteria established in an NCD or LCD.

(A) Notifier(s): _____

(B) Patient Name: _____ **(C)** Identification Number: _____

Advance Beneficiary Notice of Noncoverage (ABN)

NOTE: If Medicare doesn't pay for **(D)** _____ below, you may have to pay.

Medicare does not pay for everything, even some care that you or your healthcare provider have good reason to think you need. We expect Medicare may not pay for the **(D)** below.

(D)	**(E) REASON MEDICARE MAY NOT PAY**	**(F) ESTIMATED COST**

What you need to do now:

- Read this notice, so you can make an informed decision about your care.
- Ask us any questions that you may have after you finish reading.
- Choose an option below about whether to receive the **(D)** listed above.

Note: If you choose Option 1 or 2, we may help you to use any other insurance that you might have, but Medicare cannot require us to do this.

(G) OPTIONS: Check only one box. We cannot choose a box for you.

☐ **OPTION 1.** I want the **(D)** listed above. You may ask to be paid now, but I also want Medicare billed for an official decision on payment, which is sent to me on a Medicare Summary Notice (MSN). I understand that if Medicare doesn't pay, I am responsible for payment, but **I can appeal to Medicare** by following the directions on the MSN. If Medicare does pay, you will refund any payments I made to you, less co-pays or deductibles.

☐ **OPTION 2.** I want the **(D)** _____ listed above, but do not bill Medicare. You may ask to be paid now as I am responsible for payment. **I cannot appeal if Medicare is not billed.**

☐ **OPTION 3.** I don't want the **(D)** _____ listed above. I understand with this choice I am **not** responsible for payment, and **I cannot appeal to see if Medicare would pay.**

(H) Additional Information:

This notice gives our opinion, not an official Medicare decision. If you have other questions on this notice or Medicare billing, call **1-800-MEDICARE** (1-800-633-4227/**TTY**: 1-877-486-2048).

Signing below means that you have received and understand this notice. You also receive a copy.

(I) Signature: _____ **(J)** Date: _____

According to the Paperwork Reduction Act of 1995, no persons are required to respond to a collection of information unless it displays a valid OMB control number. The valid OMB control number for this information collection is 0938-0566. The time required to complete this information collection is estimated to average 7 minutes per response, including the time to review instructions, search existing data resources, gather the data needed, and complete and review the information collection. If you have comments concerning the accuracy of the time estimate or suggestions for improving this form, please write to: CMS, 7500 Security Boulevard, Attn: PRA Reports Clearance Officer, Baltimore, Maryland 21244–1850.

Form CMS-R-131 (03/08)   Form Approved OMB No. 0938–0566

Figure 22.2 CMS Advance Beneficiary Notice

criteria. A properly executed ABN informs the patient in advance of possible additional financial responsibility. However, the patient's or legal representative's refusal to sign the ABN does not waive his or her financial responsibility should the services be provided after the patient has been informed of a potential denial of coverage for services rendered.

CMS specifies that a properly completed and executed ABN should meet the following requirements:

- The following fields must be completed:
  - Notifiers (physicians, providers, practitioners, or suppliers):
    - Include name, address, and telephone number.
    - Notifier information may be added to the ABN in the form of a label, handwritten, or preprinted.
    - For a practice using a billing agency, the notifier information may include both the provider of the ABN and the billing agency.
  - Patient name.
  - Patient identification number (optional):
    - Do *not* include the patient's Medicare or Social Security number.
  - Service, procedure, test, or supply provided or given that the provider believes may not be covered:
    - Specification of frequency should be included in certain circumstances, such as repeat procedures or tests.
  - Reason for denial:
    - Explain in language the patient can easily understand.
    - Include one valid reason for each item or service listed.
  - Estimated cost:
    - The estimate should be within $100 or 25 percent of the actual cost.
    - A statement for a cost estimate of "No more than" or "between $ and $" is also acceptable as long as this statement still meets the $100 or 25 percent requirement.
    - Multiple items can be added together to provide a single cost estimate.
    - If the cost cannot reasonably be estimated during the completion and delivery of the ABN, the notifier may indicate that no cost estimate is available.
  - Selection of one of the three options by the patient or his or her representative:
    - Preselection or selection of an option by the notifier will cause the ABN to be invalid.
  - Additional information (if needed).
- The ABN must be reviewed verbally with the patient or patient's representative far enough in advance of delivery of the service or procedure so that the patient and/or representative has time to consider options, receive answers to questions, and make an informed decision.
- The signature of an authorized representative must be obtained on the completed ABN before the service or procedure is provided. An authorized representative can be a legal representative, spouse, adult child, adult sibling, parent, or close friend.
- The date the signature is obtained must be included.
- Signature of a witness must be obtained should the patient or authorized representative refuse to sign a properly executed ABN and request the service be provided without the ABN.

A completed and signed copy of the ABN must be retained, and the claim should be filed with the appropriate modifier:

GA **Waiver of liability statement on file:** This modifier notifies the payer that the patient was informed prior to receipt of services that the services may not be covered and has accepted financial responsibility for these services. Proper use of this modifier results in reduction of payer-based requests for patient refunds and timely adjudication of claims, as needed, for submission of additional insurance claims.

GY **Item or service statutorily excluded:** This modifier informs the payer that although payment is not expected, a denial is requested. Use of this modifier allows timely filing to secondary insurance payers.

The **National Correct Coding Initiative (NCCI)** was created to encourage correct coding methodologies and control inappropriate payments due to improper coding of Part B claims. Originally there were two distinct tables of edits: column 1/column 2 edits and mutually exclusive edits. In April 2012 these two tables were combined into one table that identifies inappropriate code pairs based on the CPT manual, NCD and LCD policies, national societies' guidelines, standard medical and surgical practices, and a review of current coding practices.

FOR EXAMPLE A biopsy of a lesion of the right forearm (11100) and an 0.8-cm excision of a benign lesion of the arm (11401) reported on the same day for the same patient would produce an NCCI edit as the work to perform an excision for a biopsy is included in the excision of the lesion. ■

MENTOR
Coding Tip

Modifier 59 may be used to identify circumstances in which it is appropriate to report NCCI-identified code pairs together, such as a skin lesion biopsy of the arm and an excision of a skin lesion of the trunk performed during the same encounter.

SPOTLIGHT on Practice Management

Modifier 59 distinct procedural service: A distinct or separate procedure or service may be a different procedure, surgery, site, organ system, incision, excision, lesion, or injury. *As this modifier is under scrutiny by the OIG due to misuse, careful consideration is required prior to appending modifier 59.* If a more specific modifier is available to describe the situation in which the services were rendered, modifier 59 should not be used.

Medically unlikely edits (MUEs) are edits that identify limits for units of service for a given service or procedure completed by a single provider per patient per day.

FOR EXAMPLE Amputation of the right forearm (CPT 25900) has a limit of 1 unit of service allowed. ■

Office of Civil Rights

The Office of Civil Rights (OCR) was established to prevent discrimination due to color, race, national origin, disability, age, gender, or religion. The OCR is responsible for enforcing the rules of the **Health Insurance Portability and Accountability Act (HIPAA)** of 1996. HIPAA consist of two parts: Title I protects health insurance coverage for an employee when he or she loses or changes jobs. Title II, also known as *Administrative Simplification,* created an additional means of detecting fraud and abuse and established guidelines and procedures for the use and storage of protected health information (PHI) through the development of several rules:

- **Transactions and code sets:** HIPAA requires that all entities that transmit healthcare–related data electronically use HIPAA Electronic Data Interchange standardized code sets.

- **Unique identifiers:** Every covered entity completing electronic transactions must use a single, unique identifier. For providers this identifier is known as the National Provider Identifier (NPI).

- **Privacy:** This rule regulates the use and disclosure of protected health information. **Protected Health Information (PHI)** is any medical or financial information held or managed by a covered entity. PHI may be disclosed without the patient's permission only for the purposes of facilitating treatment, payment, or healthcare operations. The Privacy Rule also requires or allows the following:

  - A patient may request a copy of his or her PHI and the request must be completed within 30 days of receipt of the written request.

  - Patients have the right to request that a covered entity correct errors in the PHI.

  - A written request must be obtained from the patient for disclosure of PHI, and the covered entity must ensure that only the minimum necessary information is disclosed.

  - Covered entities must take reasonable steps to ensure confidentiality of communication of PHI.

  - Covered entities must track disclosures of PHI.

  - Covered entities must provide a privacy notice that describes how the covered entity may use and disclose PHI, the patient's rights regarding PHI and how the patient may exercise these rights, the covered entity's legal responsibilities regarding PHI, and whom the patient may contact to discuss the privacy policy.

- **Security:** This rule identifies security standards for Electronic Protected Health Information (EPHI) and is broken down into three parts:
  - Administrative Safeguards
  - Physical Safeguards
  - Technical Safeguards

- **Enforcement:** This rule created procedures for investigation of and hearings for violations of HIPAA rules and sets civil and monetary penalties for these violations.

SPOTLIGHT on Practice Management

A **covered entity** is any provider or organization that transmits health information electronically. Examples are healthcare providers (only if they transmit information in an HHS-adopted transaction standard), healthcare clearinghouses, and health plans (payers).

Worker's compensation and automobile and home owners insurance are not considered covered entities and thus are exempt from HIPAA rules.

American Recovery and Reinvestment Act

The **American Recovery and Reinvestment Act (ARRA)** of 2009 was enacted to promote economic recovery and growth and provide the opportunity to enhance the nation's healthcare system through investment in health information technology (HIT) and Electronic Health Records (EHRs).

To promote implementation of the meaningful use of health information technology, ARRA includes the **Health Information Technology for Economic and Clinical Health (HITECH) Act.** The HITECH Act addresses security and privacy issues related to the electronic transmission of health information. In addition to the security and privacy rules set out by HIPAA, the HITECH Act outlines rules and regulations as well as penalties for violations of these rules:

- Authorized disclosures of PHI in an electronic format must be provided at a cost equal to the cost incurred to process the request.
- Notification of a breach in PHI that affects 500 or more patients must be provided to both HHS and the media in addition to the patients.

American Recovery and Reinvestment Act (ARRA) Legislation enacted to promote economic recovery and growth and provide the opportunity to enhance the nation's healthcare system through investment in health information technology.

Health Information Technology for Economic and Clinical Health (HITECH) Act Legislation that addresses security and privacy issues related to the electronic transmission of health information; outlines rules and regulations as well as penalties for violations of the rules.

---

1. Explain the American Recovery and Reinvestment Act (ARRA).
2. Define *PHI*.
3. Describe an ABN.

Also available in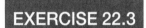

EXERCISE 22.3

Chapter Twenty-Two Summary

Learning Outcome	Key Concepts/Examples
22.1 Recognize the AAPC professional code of ethics.	"Commitment to ethical professional conduct is expected of every AAPC member. The specification of a Code of Ethics enables AAPC to clarify to current and future members, and to those served by members, the nature of the ethical responsibilities held in common by its members."
22.2 Understand the definitions of providers and payers, including Medicare, Medicaid, TRICARE, and managed care entities.	The most common providers include physicians, doctors of osteopathy, nurse practitioners, and physician assistants. *Medicare* provides coverage for persons 65 years and older, disabled persons (after 2 years of disability), and persons with end-stage renal disease (ESRD). The Medicare program is made up of four parts: A. Hospital insurance B. Medical insurance, which pays for provider services, outpatient hospital and lab services, and Durable Medical Equipment C. Medicare Advantage, which provides managed care and private fee-for-service plan options D. Prescription drug plan *Medicaid,* created in 1965 and funded by both state and federal funds, provides medical care for persons falling below the national poverty level. The Medicaid program is administered by each state and monitored by CMS. *TRICARE* and *CHAMPVA* provide healthcare coverage and benefits to active or retired uniformed service members and their families. In addition to the government healthcare coverage listed above, several other forms of insurance are available that are generally offered by third-party payers.
22.3 Identify regulations and the parties responsible for maintaining and enforcing the regulations.	*Office of Inspector General (OIG)* investigates allegations of fraud, waste, abuse, or misconduct and assists the executive branch in identifying and correcting operational deficiencies. *National Coverage Determinations (NCDs)* are developed by the CMS. NCDs identify payment coverage for a specific service, procedure, test, or technology based on medical necessity or frequency. An *Advanced Beneficiary Notice (ABN)* of Noncoverage is needed for any service that does not meet the coverage criteria established in an NCD or LCD. *National Correct Coding Initiative (NCCI)* was created to encourage correct coding methodologies and control inappropriate payments due to improper coding of Part B claims. *Office of Civil Rights (OCR)* was established to prevent discrimination due to color, race, national origin, disability, age, gender, or religion. The OCR is responsible for enforcing the rules of the Health Insurance Portability and Accountability Act (HIPAA) of 1996.

Chapter Twenty-Two Review

Using Terminology

Match each key term to the appropriate definition.

_____ 1. [LO22.3] Advance Beneficiary Notice (ABN)

_____ 2. [LO22.3] American Recovery and Reinvestment Act (ARRA)

_____ 3. [LO22.3] Covered Entity

_____ 4. [LO22.3] Health Insurance Portability and Accountability Act (HIPAA)

_____ 5. [LO22.2] Hierarchical Condition Category (HCC)

_____ 6. [LO22.3] Medically Unlikely Edits (MUEs)

_____ 7. [LO22.2] Medicare Administrative Contractor (MAC)

_____ 8. [LO22.3] National Correct Coding Initiative (NCCI)

_____ 9. [LO22.3] National Coverage Determinations (NCDs)

_____ 10. [LO22.3] Office of Inspector General (OIG)

_____ 11. [LO22.3] Protected Health Information (PHI)

A. Waiver needed for any service that does not meet the coverage criteria established in an LCD

B. Entity through which Medicare is administered by the Centers for Medicare and Medicaid Services

C. Provides a method of assessing the risk of medically managing each patient based on current conditions and comorbid conditions that are impacting care

D. Investigates allegations of fraud, waste, abuse, or misconduct and assists the executive branch in identifying and correcting operational deficiencies

E. Identify payment coverage for a specific service, procedures, test, or technology based on medical necessity or frequency at a national level

F. Created to encourage correct coding methodologies and control inappropriate payment due to improper coding of Part B claims

G. Edits that identify limits for units of service for a given service or procedure completed by a single provider per patient per day

H. Any medical or financial information held or managed by a covered entity

I. Any provider or organization that transmits health information electronically

J. Enacted to promote economic recovery and growth and provide the opportunity to enhance the nation's healthcare system through investment in health information technology (HIT)

K. Addresses security and privacy issues related to the electronic transmission of health information

Checking Your Understanding

Choose the most appropriate answer for each of the following questions.

1. [LO22.2] Which of the following statements are *not* true for a non-PAR provider? Choose all that apply.
   a. Claims must be filed by the provider.
   b. Fees are restricted to no more than the limiting charge.
   c. Payment is sent directly to the provider.
   d. Only the deductible and/or coinsurance can be collected at the time of service.

2. [LO22.2] Medicare provides coverage for:
   a. Individuals over the age of 65
   b. Patients with ESRD
   c. Disabled persons
   d. All of these

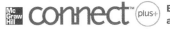 **Enhance your learning** by completing these exercises and more at mcgrawhillconnect.com

3. **[LO22.2]** The patient-responsible portion of a set amount per service or encounter is the definition of:
   a. Coinsurance
   b. Deductible
   c. Copayment
   d. Allowed amount

4. **[LO22.2]** Which type of claim form is used to report inpatient facility services?
   a. UB-04
   b. UB-92
   c. CMS-1500
   d. HCFA 1500

5. **[LO22.2]** Which service is *not* considered a Medicare Part A benefit?
   a. DME
   b. Inpatient stay
   c. Hospice
   d. Home health service

6. **[LO22.2]** Methods of reimbursement include:
   a. Capitation
   b. Point of service
   c. Fee for service
   d. All of these

7. **[LO22.3]** Which of the following statements is *not* a benefit of an effective compliance plan?
   a. Eliminates the risk of an audit
   b. Minimizes billing mistakes
   c. Speeds and optimizes proper payment of claims
   d. Increases accuracy of documentation

8. **[LO22.3]** Which modifier is under scrutiny by the OIG, making it important for coders to be knowledgeable about the correct use of this modifier?
   a. Modifier 51
   b. Modifier 59
   c. Modifier 22
   d. None of these

9. **[LO22.3]** Which of the following is responsible for enforcing the rules of HIPAA?
   a. OIG
   b. NCCI
   c. OCR
   d. NCD

10. **[LO22.3]** Which of the following is *not* considered a covered entity?
    a. Any provider or organization that transmits health information electronically
    b. Healthcare clearinghouses
    c. Health plans (payers)
    d. Worker's compensation

Applying Your Knowledge

1. **[LO22.3]** Discuss the HITECH Act and its implications to a practice.

   _____

2. **[LO22.3]** Discuss the completion of the required fields of an ABN and the appropriate modifiers needed.

   _____

3. **[LO22.1]** Discuss the AAPC code of ethics.

   _____

Unit 5 Exam

The questions in this exam cover material in Chapters 18 through 22 of this book.

Choose the most appropriate answer for each question below.

1. [LO22.2] What is the portion of payment that patients are responsible for each time they visit a physician's office?
   - **a.** Co-pay
   - **b.** Deductible
   - **c.** Premium
   - **d.** Coinsurance

2. [LO22.2] A PAR provider is a:
   - **a.** Physician assistant reporter
   - **b.** Preferred provider
   - **c.** Physician account receivables
   - **d.** Participating provider

3. [LO21.2] A 20-year-old female is seen in her OB/GYN clinic. She receives an injection of Depo-Provera, 150 mg, for family planning. Select the correct HCPCS Level II code:
   - **a.** J1000
   - **b.** L8030
   - **c.** J1055
   - **d.** J1056

4. [LO21.2] Which of the following is considered an inhalation drug?
   - **a.** Albuterol
   - **b.** Ampicillin
   - **c.** Estradiol valerate
   - **d.** Phenobarbital

5. [LO21.5] Category II codes are:
   - **a.** Emerging-technology temporary codes
   - **b.** Optional performance measurement codes
   - **c.** Deleted codes
   - **d.** HCPCS codes

6. [LO21.2] Madison, a 7-year-old patient, receives a fluoride treatment at a dentist's office. Select the correct HCPCS Level II code:
   - **a.** D1110
   - **b.** D1120
   - **c.** D1206
   - **d.** D1203

7. [LO21.2] A patient who has terminal lung cancer is admitted to the hospice unit for general inpatient care. Select the appropriate HCPCS Level II code:
   - **a.** T2042
   - **b.** T2043
   - **c.** T2044
   - **d.** T2045

8. [LO22.2] COP is an abbreviation for:
   - **a.** Coordination of procedures
   - **b.** Conditions of participation
   - **c.** Coordination of practices
   - **d.** Condition of practices

9. [LO19.2] A 78-year-old male presents to his primary care provider's office with a complaint of urinary retention. Upon examination, the PC documents a smooth enlarged prostate. The physician orders a PSA to rule out prostate cancer and documents the DX as hypertrophy of the prostate. Select the appropriate CPT and ICD-9-CM codes:
   - **a.** 84152, 600.00
   - **b.** 84154, 788.20
   - **c.** 84153, 600.01, 788.20
   - **d.** 84152, 600.01, 788.20

10. **[LO20.3]** A patient is exhibiting symptoms of dysphasia and chest pain. Evaluation to this point has ruled out cardiac origins and GERD. The physician orders a manometric study of the esophagus and gastroesophageal junction with stimulation of gastric acid to rule out achalasia. Select the appropriate CPT code(s):

   a. 91010

   b. 91010, 91013

   c. 91013, 91010

   d. 91020, 91013

11. **[LO20.3]** A patient experiencing nystagmus and dizziness is being seen for vestibular function testing and receives the following test with recording: spontaneous test for nystagmus including gaze and function, testing for nystagmus in three positions, and optokinetic testing. Select the appropriate CPT code(s):

   a. 92540

   b. 92541

   c. 92541, 92542, 92544

   d. 92545

12. **[LO20.2]** Kiera, a bright 8-year-old, has received a cochlear implant. She is here today for postoperative analysis and the fitting of this implant, as well as the connection and programming of the stimulator. Select the appropriate CPT code:

   a. 92601

   b. 92602

   c. 92604

   d. 92603

13. **[LO20.2]** Fred, age 60, has been experiencing abdominal pain and is undergoing testing for Crohn's disease. His physician orders a capsule endoscopy in order to gain visualization of the gastrointestinal tract and esophagus through the ileum with interpretation and report. Select the appropriate CPT code(s):

   a. 91111

   b. 91110, 91111

   c. 91110

   d. 91110, 91117

14. **[LO19. 3]** For coding anatomic pathology when the specimen is not viewed using a microscope, which of the following codes would be appropriate?

   a. 88302

   b. 88300

   c. 88309

   d. 88305

15. **[LO20.1]** A psychiatrist provided psychotherapy for crisis for a patient experiencing a high degree of anxiety. A history of the crisis state, a mental status exam, and a disposition were performed. The provider documented the time spent as 35 minutes. Select the appropriate CPT code(s):

   a. 90839

   b. 90832

   c. 90839, 90741

   d. 90845

16. **[LO20.1]** Frank is a 42-year-old ESRD patient. To properly manage his disease this month, as he has had several issues, he has been to his physician three times. Select the appropriate codes:

   a. 90960, 585.4

   b. 90961, 585.6

   c. 90962, 585.6

   d. 90964, 585.6

17. **[LO20.4]** A patient has been suffering from sleep apnea, and his physician orders a sleep study to measure his heart rate, O_2 saturation, respiration analysis, and sleep time. Select the appropriate code(s) for this test:

   a. 95806

   b. 95806, 93041

   c. 95800

   d. 95800, 93041

18. **[LO20.4]** A patient undergoes a left heart catheterization with catheter placement in the bypass graft, and the physicain performs a bypass graft angiography. Code this procedure:

   a. 93459

   b. 93452, 93454

   c. 93454, 93459

   d. 93452, 93459

19. **[LO19.1]** Mrs. Tent was sent to the lab following her yearly examination with Dr. Jones. Dr. Jones ordered a general health panel, WBC count, bilirubin analysis, and a qualitative urinalysis for her Urinary Tract Infection (UTI). Select the appropriate CPT and ICD-9-CM codes:

    a. 80050, 81005, V70.0, 599.0

    b. 80050, 85007, 82247, 81005, V72.6

    c. 80050, 81005, V72.6

    d. 80048, 85007, 82247, 81005, V72.6, 599.0

20. **[LO18.1]** A patient presents at his primary care provider's office with pain in the left wrist. The physician orders an x-ray to be done in the outpatient department of the local hospital. The hospital will bill the technical component of the wrist x-ray. How will the radiologist bill for his services?

    a. 73115   **c.** 73115-25

    b. 73115-26   **d.** 73115-57

21. **[LO21.5]** What is the coder instructed to do with category III codes in the CPT?

    a. Use of these codes is optional.

    b. Never use category III codes for hospital encounters.

    c. If there is a category III code available, it must be used instead of an unlisted category I code.

    d. Use a category III code along with a category I unlisted code.

22. **[LO19.2]** A patient comes in with a 2-day history of sore throat, fever, and chills. The physician performs a rapid-strep test and prescribes a 10-day course of penicillin. Code the lab test:

    a. 87081   **c.** 87899

    b. 87880   **d.** None of these

23. **[LO22.2]** Which of the following is the best description of an Advance Beneficiary Notice?

    a. A written notice given to a Medicare patient after a denial of a claim is received

    b. A written notice given to any patients who present at a physician's office which informs them that they will be responsible for all charges

    c. A written notice from Medicare given to a patient before certain services are performed which explains that Medicare may deny payment and, if so, the patient is responsible

    d. A written notice that a Medicare patient signs which states that the patient is unable to pay the 20 percent left over after Medicare pays

24. **[LO20.4]** The procedure that records the electrical impulses of the brain is called a(n):

    a. Encephalogram   **c.** Electroencephalogram

    b. Myelogram   **d.** Transcranial sonogram

25. **[LO21.3]** The patient is at his physician's office for a routine physical when he suffers cardiac arrest. The physician performs lifesaving measures and stabilizes the patient until the ambulance arrives. The ambulance team continues to administer lifesaving treatment to the patient and transports the patient to the hospital, which is 7 miles away from the physician's office. Select the appropriate HCPCS Level II codes:

    a. A0422, A0888

    b. A0433-XH, A0888 x7

    c. A0433-SH, A0888 x7

    d. A0427-PH, A0425 x7

Final Exam: ICD-9-CM

· ·

Anesthesia

1. **History:** A 62-yr-old woman (height, 1.7 m; weight, 61 kg) was scheduled for resection of a sigmoid colon carcinoma. Her medical history revealed hypothyroidism, vitamin B12 deficiency, and SPS. This syndrome started with low back pain, which rendered her unable to walk. She was experiencing stiffness, involuntary jerks, and painful cramps. Neurologic examination revealed extreme hypertonia of the body and proximal legs, with intercurrent, painful spasms. Reflexes were symmetrical without Babinski signs. Laboratory findings showed positive glutamic acid decarboxylase (GAD) and negative amphiphysin antibodies. The patient was successfully treated with baclofen and diazepam. Subsequently, prednisone as immunosuppressive therapy was started. The stiffness diminished, and the patient was able to walk unaided. The neurologic examination was unremarkable, except for a slight stiffness in the legs. Her medication at admission was prednisone 20 mg once a day, baclofen 12.5 mg twice a day (daily dose = 25 mg), diazepam 7.5 mg twice a day (daily dose = 15 mg), levothyroxine 25 µg once a day, and vitamin B_{12} injections. Her medical history included urologic and gynecologic surgery under general anesthesia before she experienced stiff person syndrome (SPS).

   Procedure: No premedication was given. Anesthesia was induced with propofol (2.5 mg/kg) and sufentanil (0.25 µg/kg). After the administration of atracurium (0.6 mg/kg), the trachea was intubated, and anesthesia was continued with isoflurane (0.6–1.0 vol %) and oxygen/air for the duration of the procedure. Cefuroxime 1,500 mg, clindamycin 600 mg, and dexamethasone 10 mg were administered IV. In the following 2 hours, additional atracurium (35 mg), sufentanil (10 µg), and morphine (8 mg) were administered. At the end of the procedure, which was uneventful, neuromuscular monitoring showed four strong twitches. Although the patient was responsive, she could not open her eyes, grasp with either hand, or generate tidal volumes beyond 200 mL. Neostigmine 2 mg (0.03 mg/kg) and glycopyrrolate 0.2 mg did not alter the clinical signs of muscle weakness.

   The patient was sedated with propofol 5 and further mechanically ventilated in the recovery room. After 1 hour, the sedation was stopped and mechanical ventilation was terminated. At that time, baclofen 12.5 mg was administered into the gastric tube. Two hours later she was in a good clinical condition, and her trachea was extubated.

   Select the appropriate CPT and ICD-9-CM codes:

   a. 00790, 153.3, 244.9, 281.1, 333.91   **c.** 00810, 153.9, 281.1, 244.9, 333.1

   b. 00800, 153.9, 281.1, 333.91   **d.** 00792, 153.3, 244.9, 281.1, 333.1

2. **History:** A 73-year-old 81-kg male with a history of non-Hodgkin's lymphoma and moderate in situ adenocarcinoma of the prostate presents for transurethral resection of the prostate (TURP). The preoperative evaluation reveals a history of smoking (60 pack-years), normal ejection fraction and heart valves, and normal chest x-ray and EKG. No other significant findings.

   Procedure: He was taken to the operating room and monitored as per routine for cystoscopy and TURP. After appropriate preoxygenation, general anesthesia was uneventfully induced with fentanyl, propofol, and rocuronium. The patient was intubated, ventilated, and placed in the lithotomy position. The operative procedure was started without difficulty. After 90 minutes, the patient's temperature had dropped from 35.9EC at the beginning of the case to 32.9EC. Blood was sent to the lab due to the length of the surgery. The patient's vital signs were stable. Shortly thereafter the following values were sent back from the laboratory to the operating room: NA 109 mEq/L, K 4.7 mEq/L, CL 83 mEq/L, glucose 83 mg/dl, Hct 34. The anesthesiologist informed the surgeon about the findings, and the surgery was then stopped. The patient was transferred to the surgical intensive care unit (SICU).

   At arrival in the SICU: The patient was still intubated and sedated. The body temperature was 33.5EC. The laboratory measurements revealed NA 107 mEq/L, K 5.7 mEq/L, CL 79 mEq/L, CO_2 109 mEq/L, ammonia level of 60 mmol/L, and serum osmolarity of 273. A radial arterial catheter and a central venous catheter were inserted, and rewarming with hot air (Bair Hugger) was initiated. EKG and chest x-ray are shown below.

Select the appropriate CPT and ICD-9-CM codes:

a. 00914-53, 99100, 233.4, 202.80

b. 00910, 201.9, 233.4

c. 00914, 99100, 233.4, 201.9

d. 00912-53, 202.8, 233.4

3. **Preprocedure diagnosis:** Lumbar radiculopathy

   Postprocedure diagnosis: Lumbar radiculopathy

   Procedure performed: Lumbar epidural steroid injection

   Anesthesia given: Local

   Indications for procedure: This 53-year-old female presents with symptoms consistent with a lumbar radiculopathy. Previous epidural steroid injections have resulted in significant improvement of her pain. This is the second in a series of three of those injections.

   Description of procedure: The patient was placed in the left lateral decubitus position. The L4–5 interspace was identified with deep palpation. Local infiltration was carried out with 3 cc of 1% lidocaine. The area was prepped and draped in the usual sterile fashion. An 18-gauge Tuohy needle was advanced to the epidural space with the loss-of-resistance technique. Then a mixture of Depo-Medrol 80 mg, normal saline 10 cc, and lidocaine 1% at 5 cc was injected. No complications were encountered, and the patient was returned to the outpatient surgery department in stable condition.

   Plan: To repeat this procedure in two weeks.

   Select the appropriate CPT and ICD-9-CM codes:

   a. 62311, 724.4

   b. 62310, 722.10

   c. 62310, 724.4

   d. 62311, 722.10

4. **Preoperative diagnosis:** Left hip pain and bilateral chest and back pain

   Postoperative diagnosis: Left hip pain and bilateral chest and back pain

   Procedures: Bilateral lumbar paravertebral sympathetic nerve block under ultrasound guidance

   Left hip greater trochanter bursa injection

   Procedure in detail: All questions were answered. His back was palpated to try to elicit areas of discomfort. This was quite difficult to do, since he said he hurt all over. Of note is that we had looked at his legs, and on his right leg he had an area of excoriation or erythema that was unusual for him, and he stated that his pain seemed to correlate with his edema and erythema of his legs. With this in mind, we turned our attention first to his left hip pain and asked him to move his left hip to where we could elicit a point of maximum tenderness. Point of maximum tenderness was elicited over what appeared to be the greater trochanter of the left hip area itself. We then injected what appeared to be the bursa of the left hip with 10 cc of 0.25% Marcaine with 20 mg of Depo-Medrol. He was then placed in a prone position with a pillow supporting his upper abdomen. In light of his symptoms down his legs, we felt that a lumbar paravertebral sympathetic nerve block was indicated at this time. We identified the spinous process of L2. The midpoint of the spinous process of L2 was marked. A line perpendicular to the spinous process of L2 was then drawn on his skin, and a point that was 1¾ inches from the midline was then marked. The skin at this point was anesthetized with 1.5% lidocaine using a 25-gauge B-bevel needle. This was then followed with a 22-gauge 3½-inch needle that was advanced under a slightly cephalic medial direction, approximately 85 degrees off midline. Under fluoroscopic guidance, the needle was advanced. On the first attempt on the left, we encountered the transverse process of L2. The needle was repositioned left of cephalic, and we were able to bypass the transverse process. The needle was advanced until we encountered the vertebral body of L2 under ultrasound guidance. We then obtained a lateral view and found that indeed we were at the level of the midbody of L2. With this needle felt to be adequately placed, we then injected 6 cc of 0.25% Marcaine with 20 mg of Depo-Medrol. The needle was left in place, and the stylet was replaced.

We then turned our attention to the right-hand side because of the excoriation on his legs and the edema that he said he experiences with increased levels of his pain. The skin was once again marked 1¾ inch from the midline at the midlevel of the spinous process of L2. The skin was anesthetized with 1.5% lidocaine. This was then followed with a 22-gauge 3½-inch spinal needle that was advanced under fluoroscopic guidance. Of note, we made three or four passes in the attempt to approximate the needle next to the vertebral body of L2. Interesting to note is that in order to obtain the maximum view of the spinous process of L2, we were approximately 5 degrees to the right in terms of off midline. Once the 22-gauge 3½-inch spinal needle was placed on the right after several attempts, he did not complain of any paresthesias at this time. We then took a lateral view and found that our needle was not as deep as it should be. We then withdrew the needle, and on ultrasound guidance, using a lateral view, the needle was advanced until it was felt that we were at the appropriate depth. An AP view was then retaken, and we were found to be not at the body of L2 in terms of next to it. The needle was then removed and repositioned in a slightly medial fashion, and it was felt that we encountered bone. We then turned to the lateral view once again and found that we were at this time at the midbody of L2. This was felt to be adequately placed after three attempts. Then 6 cc of 0.25% Marcaine with 20 mg of Depo-Medrol was injected. The needle stylet was then replaced, and we then waited approximately 4 minutes for the Marcaine to set.

We then removed the needles of both the right and the left sides, respectively, and pressure was applied at the skin to prevent any bleeding. He was then placed in the supine position and was discharged home in satisfactory condition. He was instructed to call if he had any changes in edema of his legs.

Select the appropriate CPT and ICD-9-CM codes:

a. 64520, 719.45, 786.50

b. 0213T, 714.95, 786.50, 724.5

c. 0213T-50, 719.45, 786.50, 724.5

d. 64520-50, 719.45, 786.50, 724.1

5. A 43-year-old male came into the doctor's office to have a hemorrhoidopexy by stapling. He was very uneasy since he had never had this procedure before. Dr. Hanson administered an IV of Versed, for the anxiety. The procedure is not really painful, so there was no need for a full anesthetic or painkiller. Myrtle Pape, a certified registered nurse anesthetist (CRNA), sat with the patient throughout the procedure to ensure his safety and comfort level. The procedure was complete in one stage, taking 30 minutes.

Select the appropriate CPT and ICD-9-CM codes:

a. 46947, 455.6

b. 46947, 99143 × 2, 455.6

c. 46947, 99144 × 2, 455.6

d. 46947, 99144-QX, 455.6

6. Dr. Willow is called in to administer general anesthesia to a 3-month-old female patient diagnosed with congenital tracheal stenosis. Dr. Gordon performs a surgical repair of her trachea. The patient is released to the recovery room staff in good condition. Select the appropriate CPT and ICD-9-CM codes for Dr. Willow:

a. 00320, 99100, 784.3

b. 00326, 99100, 519.19

c. 00320, 519.19

d. 00326, 748.3

7. Scott Ray, a 43-year-old male cyclist, came to see Dr. Klios for a repair of his extensor tendon in his right wrist. Dr. Klios administered a regional nerve block and then performed the repair. Select the appropriate CPT codes for Dr. Klios:

a. 25260, 64450

b. 25270, 64450

c. 25272, 64450

d. 25270-47, 64450

8. Esther Nelson, a 79-year-old female, came to see Dr. Talbot for a right total-knee arthroplasty due to acute arthritis. Dr. Clearwater administered the general anesthesia for the procedure. Esther is in otherwise good health. Select the appropriate CPT and ICD-9-CM codes for Dr. Clearwater:

   a. 01400, 99100, 719.4

   b. 01402, 99100, 719.96

   c. 01400-P1, 99100, 719.46

   d. 01402-P1, 99100, 716.96

9. Anesthesia is administered to a normal, healthy patient for a cesarean hysterectomy following neuraxial labor anesthesia. Select the appropriate CPT code(s):

   a. 01967-P1

   b. 01969-P1

   c. 01969-P1, 01967-P1

   d. 01967-P1, 01969-P1

10. Maurice Nelson, a 72-year-old businessman, undergoes a total-hip arthroplasty. Dr. Julia Hanson assesses the patient before surgery and determines that Mr. Nelson has severe systemic diseases, including diabetes, hypertension, and coronary artery disease. Mr. Nelson is taken to the operating room for the procedure, which is accomplished without complication. He is then taken to the recovery room, and care is transferred to the nursing staff. Select the appropriate CPT code(s):

   a. 01212-P3, 99100

   b. 01214-P3, 99100

   c. 01214-P3

   d. 01210-P3

Integumentary System

1. Jerry, an established patient, is seen today for evacuation of a subungual hematoma of his left index finger, sustained while hanging a picture. The physician performs a problem-focused history and problem-focused examination to evaluate the extent of the damage and determines that evacuation of the hematoma is needed. He then evacuates the subungual hematoma. Select the appropriate CPT and ICD-9-CM codes:

   a. 11740, 99212, 923.3

   b. 11740, 923.3

   c. 11740, 99212-25, 923.3

   d. 11740-25, 923.3

2. Mary underwent removal of 20 skin tags on her neck with use of ligature strangulation and cauterization. Select the appropriate CPT and ICD-9-CM codes:

   a. 11200 × 20, 701.9

   b. 11201, 701.9

   c. 11200, 11201, 701.9

   d. 11200, 11201 × 5, 701.9

3. Mrs. Jones was seen today for puncture aspiration of three cysts on the left breast and one on the right. The pathology report revealed cystic breast disease. Select the appropriate CPT and ICD-9-CM codes:

   a 19100, 610.0

   b. 19000 × 4, 610.0

   c. 19000, 19001, 610.0

   d. 19000, 19001 × 3, 610.0

4. Sally was seen today for repair of four lacerations following a fall on some broken glass. The physician evaluated and performed simple repair on the following: a 6-cm laceration on the right forearm, a 2.5-cm laceration on the right forearm, a 0.5-cm laceration on the left hand, and a 20-cm laceration on the left upper arm. Select the appropriate CPT and ICD-9-CM codes:

   a. 12004-RT, 12006-LT, 884.0, 881.00, 882.0

   b. 12002-RT, 12006-LT, 884.0

   c. 12006, 884.0, 881.00, 882.0

   d. 12006-LT, 12002-RT, 884.0, 881.00, 882.0

5. **Preoperative diagnosis:** Morbid obesity

   Postoperative diagnosis: Morbid obesity

   Procedure performed: Abdominal panniculectomy

   Estimated blood loss: Throughout the procedure, approximately 20 mL

   Anesthesia: General endotracheal anesthesia

   Indications for procedure: This is a 49-year-old female who previously underwent gastric bypass surgery and has lost 120 pounds, leaving a large lower pannus of the abdomen. This pannus needs to be resected. The nonoperative versus operative management options were discussed with the patient. The operative risks included bleeding, infection, hematoma, chance for further surgery as well as pain, and a resulting scar. The patient accepted the risks, and consented to surgery.

   Procedure in detail: The patient was placed under general endotracheal anesthesia. The patient was draped in the proper manner, and the lower abdominal pannus was identified. It was preoperatively marked prior to going to the OR. The lower incision was from the superior iliac crest with the middle being the pubic tubercle. That lower incision was then made. The pass was then elevated at the level of the anterior abdominal fascia and was elevated superiorly to the level of the inferior umbilicus. Then incisions were made on the umbilicus to the superior iliac crest, and the skin and subcutaneous pannus was passed off table as a specimen. The wound was then made hemostatic with the use of electrocautery. JP drains were placed. The abdominal skin flap was then brought to the inferior skin flap and sutured in place with 2-0 Vicryl sutures at the dermal level. The drains were then secured, and then the skin was closed with running 3-0 Monocryl suture. The skin was further dressed with Steri-strips, gauze, and abdominal binder. The patient tolerated the procedure well. All needle and instrument counts at the end of the procedure were correct, and the patient was taken to PACU in good condition.

   Select the appropriate CPT and ICD-9-CM codes:

   a. 15830, 13000, 13101, 278.01

   b. 15830, 278.1, 278.01

   c. 15830-51, 278.01

   d. 15830, 278.01

6. Joan underwent excision of a benign lesion of the right leg, 4 cm × 4 cm, with a rotation flap to repair the incision site. The flap measures 12 cm × 5.2 cm. Select the appropriate CPT and ICD-9-CM codes:

   a. 11404, 14301, 216.7

   b. 11403, 14021, 216.7

   c. 11404, 216.7

   d. 11403, 216.7

7. A patient presents to his physician today complaining of pain in the left gluteal area. The physician gathers an expanded problem-focused history and performs an expanded problem-focused examination and decision making of straightforward complexity, determining that the cause of the

pain is an infected sebaceous cyst in this area. An incision and drainage of the cyst is performed. Select the appropriate CPT and ICD-9-CM codes:

a. 10060, 99212, 685.1

b. 10080, 99213, 685.1

c. 10081, 99212-25, 706.2

d. 10060, 99213-25, 706.2

8. Jerome, a 15-year-old male, is seen by the dermatologist today for treatment of his acne vulgaris. The physician uses liquid nitrogen to destroy lesions on the left side of his face. Select the appropriate CPT and ICD-9-CM codes:

a. 17340, 706.0

b. 17340, 706.1

c. 17360, 706.1

d. 17380, 706.0

9. The Mohs micrographic technique is used for removal of complex or ill-defined skin cancers. During this procedure, the physician acts as:

a. Surgeon

b. Pathologist

c. Both surgeon and pathologist

d. Consultant

10. Mrs. Mustin undergoes insertion of a left custom breast prosthesis 3 months after a mastectomy for breast cancer. The patient needed to undergo radiation to that area prior to the insertion of the prosthesis. Select the appropriate CPT and ICD-9-CM codes:

a. 19342, 19396, V10.3

b. 19340, 19396, 175.9

c. 19340, 175.9

d. 19342, V10.3

Musculoskeletal

1. Mrs. Jones is in the operating room today for repair of a nontraumatic tear of the rotator cuff of the right shoulder. The physician performs an arthroscopy subacromial decompression with an open repair of the rotator cuff. Select the appropriate CPT and ICD-9-CM codes:

a. 29826, 727.61, 840.4

b. 23412, 29826-59, 727.61

c. 23412, 29826, 727.61

d. 29821, 727.61, 840.4

2. Tommy was climbing the tree in front of his house, fell, and sustained a greenstick fracture of the ulna of his left arm. The orthopedic surgeon performed a closed manipulation and applied a short arm cast. Select the appropriate CPT and ICD-9-CM codes:

a. 25500, 813.82

b. 25530, 29075, 813.82

c. 25505, 29075, 813.82

d. 25535, 813.82

3. A 2-year-old with osteogenesis imperfecta was brought to the OR for application of a halo with placement of seven pins. Select the appropriate CPT and ICD-9-CM codes:

a. 20661, 756.50   c. 20660, 756.51

b. 20664, 756.51   d. 20664, 756.50

4. The patient was seen for I&D of a subfascia soft tissue abscess on the left thigh. Code this procedure with the appropriate CPT and ICD-9-CM codes:

   a. 10060, 682.6
   b. 20005, 682.6
   c. 10061, 682.5
   d. 20005, 682.5

5. Mrs. Jones was brought to the OR for open reduction by posterior approach of fractures to vertebrae at L4 and L5 as a result of a car accident. Select the appropriate CPT and ICD-9-CM codes:

   a. 22327, 805.5
   b. 22325, 805.4
   c. 22327, 22328, 805.5
   d. 22325, 22328, 805.4

6. The surgeon performed a correction of hallux valgus with sesamoidectomy and tendon transplants using the Joplin procedure on the left foot to correct a bunion. Select the appropriate CPT and ICD-9-CM codes:

   a. 28294, 727.1
   b. 28290, 727.1
   c. 28292, 727.1
   d. 28296, 727.1

7. John underwent disarticulation at the knee as a result of a traumatic crushing injury to the right tibia and fibula caused by a motorcycle accident. Select the appropriate CPT and ICD-9-CM codes:

   a. 27598, 928.10
   b. 27592, 823.91
   c. 27598, 823.91
   d. 27592, 823.92

8. Mr. Dell is a farrier, and he was kicked in the sacral-coccygeal area by a horse that he was shoeing. The injury was significant enough to require an open treatment to repair the coccygeal fracture. Select the appropriate CPT and ICD-9-CM codes:

   a. 27202, 805.6
   b. 27200, 805.6
   c. 27202, 807.70
   d. 27200, 806.60

9. The patient underwent partial excision of the posterior C7 and L1 and L2 vertebrae to remove intrinsic bony lesions. Two surgeons worked simultaneously as primary surgeons to remove the lesions. Surgeon A removed the lesion at C7, and surgeon B removed the lesions at L1 and L2. Code the services of surgeon B with the appropriate CPT and ICD-9-CM codes:

   a. 22100-62, 22102-62, 22103-62, 213.2
   b. 22100-59, 22102, 22103, 213.2
   c. 22102-62, 22103-62, 213.2
   d. 22102-62, 213.2

10. Mrs. Jones, an established patient, is seen by the rheumatologist for repeated pain in her left knee due to osteoarthritis. Today she presents with pain and swelling. The rheumatologist performs an arthrocentesis of the left knee followed by injection of Dexa-Methasone sodium phosphate, 5 mg. No E/M service is performed. Select the appropriate CPT and ICD-9-CM codes:

   a. 20605, 99212-25, 715.16
   b. 20610, J1100 5u, 715.16
   c. 20605, J1100 5u, 99212-25, 715.16
   d. 20610, 99212-25, J110 5u, 715.16

Respiratory/Cardiovascular

1. Jeffrey has developed cellulitis in his tracheostomy from his surgery for adenocarcinoma of the larynx. A tracheostoma revision, simple without flap rotation, was performed. Select the appropriate CPT and ICD-9-CM codes:

   a. 31613, 519.01, 682.1

   b. 31614, 519.01, 682.1, 161.9

   c. 31600, 519.01, 682.1, 161.9

   d. 31613, 519.01, 682.1, 161.9

2. **Pre-op diagnosis:** Left lung abscess

   Post-op diagnosis: Same

   Procedure performed: Left upper lobectomy with decortication and drainage

   Indications: The patient is a 56-year-old female with evidence of a left upper-lobe abscess seen on the MRI. She was admitted with tension pneumothorax, which was treated with double-lumen intubation and a chest tube.

   Procedure: The patient was brought to the operating room and placed in the supine position, with general intubation from the double-lumen tube. The patient was rolled onto the right lateral decubitus position, with left side up. A posterior lateral thoracotomy was performed. Adhesions were taken down sharply and bluntly and with cautery. Following this a standard artery first left-upper lobectomy was carried out utilizing 0 silk and hemoclips. The left upper pulmonary vein was secured with a single application of the stapling machine. The posterior fissure was created with multiple applications of the automatic stapling machine and the bronchus secured with a single application of the bronchus stapling machine. Following this the wound was drained with three 24-French strium chest tubes and hemostasis obtained with spray Tisseel and surgical gauze. The bronchus was sealed with bio glue and the wound closed in layers. A sterile compression dressing was applied, and the patient was returned to the surgical intensive care unit after the double-lumen tube was changed to a single-lumen tube. The patient received 3 units of packed cells intraoperatively to maintain hemostasis. Sponge count and needle count correct × 2. Large abscess in the left upper lobe accounted for approximately 70% of the left upper-lobe parenchyma.

   Select the appropriate CPT and ICD-9-CM codes:

   a. 32480-LT, 513.0

   b. 32482-LT, 513.0, 512.89

   c. 32320, 32480-LT, 513.0, 512.89

   d. 32503, 512.89

3. **Procedure performed:** Fiber-optic bronchoscopy, bronchial biopsy, bronchial washings, and bronchial brushings

   Preprocedure diagnosis: Abnormal chest x-ray

   Postprocedure diagnosis: Inflammation in all lobes, pneumonia; with pleural placquing consistent with possible candidiasis

   The patient was already on a ventilator, so the bronchoscope tube was introduced through the ET tube. We saw 2.5 cm above the carina of the trachea, which was red and swollen as was the carina. The right lung: All entrances were patent, but they were all swollen and red, with increased secretions. The left lung was even more involved, with more swelling and more edema and had bloody secretions, especially at the left base. This area from the carina all the way down to the smaller airways on the left side had shown white placquing consistent with possible candidiasis. These areas were brushed, washed, and biopsied. A biopsy specimen was also sent for tissue culture, as well as two biopsy specimens sent for pathology. Sheath brushings were also performed. The patient tolerated the procedure well and was sent back to the ICU.

APPENDIX A

Select the appropriate CPT and ICD-9-CM codes:

a. 31625, 486, 112.9

b. 31625, 793.19, 486, 112.9

c. 31625, 486

d. 31625, 793.19, 486

4. Operations performed:

1. Flexible bronchoscopy.

2. Right muscle-sparing lateral thoracotomy with complete decortication of the lung with drainage of right lower-lobe lung abscess.

Description of operation: The patient was brought to the operative suite and placed in the supine position. After satisfactory induction of general endotracheal anesthesia, a flexible Olympus bronchoscope was passed through the endotracheal tube, visualizing the distal trachea, carina, right and left main stem bronchi with primary and secondary divisions. No evidence of any endobronchial tumor was noted. What I did see was some crowding involving the right middle-lobe and right lower-lobe bronchi. The scope was then withdrawn.

A double-lumen endotracheal tube was then positioned by the anesthesiologist. The patient was placed in the left lateral decubitus position and prepped and draped in the usual sterile fashion. A right muscle-sparing lateral thoracotomy was made. We entered via the fifth intercostal space. Careful exploration was carried out, and findings were as stated above. The gelatinous material present in the right pleural space was completely evacuated. Adhesiolysis was carried out, freeing up the entire right lung.

Decortication was next carried out, being careful not to injure the underlying lung parenchyma. The patient had a very thick pleural rind. While performing the decortication, I unroofed a 2- × 2-cm right lower-lobe lung abscess. The contents were evacuated. I sent cultures of the abscess cavity as well as of the empyema cavity in separate containers to microbiology for examination. All decorticated tissue was also sent to pathology for examination as well. Excellent lung expansion was noted. I irrigated the entire region using several liters of warm antibiotic saline solution until the effluent came back clear, and then I irrigated with several more liters.

Attention was then directed at closing. Two 32-French chest tubes were placed, one anteriorly and one posteriorly, and they were brought out through inferior stab wounds. The ribs were approximated using heavy Vicryl sutures. The chest wall muscles, fascia, skin, and subcutaneous tissues were approximated using the same suture material. Dressings were applied. Marcaine 0.25% was used as a paravertebral/interfacet block at the level of T2 to T9. The patient tolerated the procedure well and was sent to the intensive care unit in stable condition

Select the appropriate CPT code(s):

a. 31623

b. 31623, 32505

c. 31624

d. 32505, 31623

5. Preoperative diagnosis: Respiratory insufficiency

Postoperative diagnosis: Respiratory insufficiency

Operation: Tracheotomy with division of thyroid isthmus

Estimated blood loss: Less than 10 mL

Fluids: Crystalloid

Complications: None

Technique: The patient was brought to the operating room and placed in the supine position. He was given general anesthesia through his existing oral intubation tube. The anterior neck was prepped and draped in the usual sterile fashion. Lidocaine 1% with 1:100,000 epinephrine was infiltrated into the skin at the lower neck.

A transverse incision was made at the cricoid ring level through skin and subcutaneous fat. The platysmal layer was traversed, and then the strap muscles were separated in the midline. The thyroid isthmus was ligated and divided with #2-0 silk ligatures. An inferiorly based tracheotomy flap was created using the second and third tracheal rings and sewn into place with a #3-0 chromic stitch to the inferior dermis margin.

Hemostasis was achieved using suction cautery. At this point, the oral intubation tube was withdrawn, and a #8 Shiley low-pressure cuffed tube was passed into the newly created trach site. The trach ties were tied securely into place, and the cuff was inflated to a comfortable pressure. The patient then received further ventilation through the newly placed trach tube. The patient was then allowed to awaken from general anesthesia and was taken back to the ICU in stable condition.

Select the appropriate CPT and ICD-9-CM codes:

a. 31600, 60200, 518.82

b. 31600, 518.82

c. 31605, 518.82

d. 31605, 60200, 518.82

6. **Preoperative diagnosis:** Left perihilar mass

   Postoperative diagnosis: Left perihilar mass, mucosal abnormality in the posterior subsegment of the left upper lobe

   Procedure performed: Bronchoscopy, transbronchial lung biopsy and bronchial lung biopsy, brushing and washing

   Assistant: None

   Anesthesia: MAC

   Description of procedure: With the patient in the supine position, under monitored anesthesia care, the scope was introduced through the mouth, and the larynx and the laryngeal area were inspected. All of them were normal. The scope was then inserted through the trachea into the carina, which was sharp and clear. There was a moderate amount of thick-thin secretions that were suctioned through both right and left main bronchi. The scope was then directed into the right main bronchus, and then the right upper-lobe bronchus with its subsegments was inspected. All of them were normal. Right middle-lobe and right lower-lobe bronchi with their subsegments were also inspected and were normal. The scope was then directed into the left side, where the left main bronchus was normal. Left lower-lobe and middle-lobe bronchi with their subsegments were normal. The left upper-lobe bronchus, anterosuperior segment, showed an anterior subsegment to have a bulging in one of its sub-bronchi. Under fluoroscopy, biopsy forceps were inserted and several pieces of lung tissue were obtained from the area of the left perihilar lesion. Then brushing was done in the same area. Washing was also done in the same area. Then, in a separate container, several pieces of bronchial tissue were taken from the area that was bulging, anterosuperior subsegment of the left upper-lobe bronchus. All specimens were submitted for cytology, pathology, and/or culture. The patient tolerated the procedure well, with no apparent complications. Chest x-ray is pending.

   Select the appropriate CPT and ICD-9-CM codes:

   a. 31628, 00635, 786.6

   b. 31628, 786.6

   c. 31629, 786.6, 162.9

   d. 31628, 31620, 786.6, 162.9

7. **Coronary Artery Bypass Graft**

   Title of procedure: Coronary artery bypass graft (CABG)

   Procedure in detail: The patient was brought to the operating room and given general endotracheal anesthesia. The pulmonary artery catheter was inserted by anesthesia under sterile technique in the right internal jugular vein. The distal right saphenous vein was harvested from the medial malleolus to just above the knee using multiple small serial incisions with skin bridges. It was a good-quality vein. The leg was closed in layers with 2-0 and 3-0 Vicryl, with 3-0 Vicryl subcuticular suture in the skin.

A midline sternotomy was performed. The patient was heparinized. The ascending aorta was found to be extremely calcified after opening the pericardium. There was diffuse atherosclerosis with visible plaque emanating from the ascending aorta. The aortic arch was cannulated beyond the ascending aorta. The atrium was cannulated, and the patient was placed on bypass. A vent was inserted into the left ventricle via the right superior pulmonary vein. Coronaries were marked for bypass, including a very large posterior descending artery and a good-size posterior lateral branch just prior to its bifurcation with two smaller branches. A single-clamp technique was utilized. The aorta was cross-clamped in the least calcified place. One liter of cardioplegia was given antegrade to arrest the heart. It was packed with ice and then flushed posteriorly.

Bypasses were accomplished, first using the reverse saphenous vein in an end-to-side fashion to the PDA, which was a good-quality 2.5- to 3-mm vessel. This was done with a reverse vein and running 7-0 Prolene suture. The second bypass was to the posterolateral branch, which was smaller but easily took a 1.5-mm probe. This was done with a separate piece of vein and a running 7-0 Prolene suture. A bolus of cold cardioplegia was given, and the patient was rewarmed. With the cross clamp still in place, a single aortotomy was made in the ascending aorta. The area was thickened and calcified, but it had a decent lumen to allow suture of the proximal end of the PDA up to the ascending aorta with running 5-0 Prolene suture in an end-to-side fashion. After concluding this anastomosis, hot cardioplegia was given into the aortic root. The cross clamp was removed after a total of 30 minutes' cross-clamp time. The remaining proximal anastomosis of the posterolateral branch was brought onto the hood of the PDA graft. The PDA was isolated with bulldog clamps. Venotomy was made, and the end-to-side anastomosis of the posterior left ventricle to the PDA was accomplished using running 6-0 Prolene suture in an end-to-side fashion. The system was back bled and de-aired, and the bulldog clamps were removed. Vessels were inspected, and they were both hemostatic.

Two atrial and two ventricular pacing wires were placed and brought out through the skin. One single chest tube was placed into the mediastinum. Neither pleura was opened. The left ventricular vent was clamped and removed, and the purse string was ligated. The lungs were inflated. The patient was ventilated and weaned off bypass successfully without the aid of inotropic support. Protamine was started, and the atrial cannula was removed. Volume status was normalized, and the heparin fully reversed with protamine. The aortic cannula was removed and the site ligated and reinforced with pledgeted 4-0 Prolene stitch. The chest tube was positioned. The wound was closed using figure-of-eight 0 Ethibond to reapproximate fascia, seven sternal wires, and two layers of running 2-0 Vicryl and a running 3-0 Vicryl in the skin. The patient tolerated the procedure and was transferred to the intensive care unit in stable condition.

Select the appropriate CPT code(s):

a. 33511, 35572

b. 33511

c. 33511, 33518

d. 33534, 35572

8. **Procedure:** Permanent pacemaker implantation

Indication for the procedure: Sick sinus syndrome with decreased mentation and confusion

Description of the procedure: After a detailed description of the procedure, indications, and potential risks of permanent pacemaker implantation was given to the patient as well as the patient's daughter, informed consent was obtained. The patient was transferred to the cardiac catheterization lab. A left subclavian area was prepared and draped in the usual sterile manner, and the left subclavian vein was accessed by Seldinger technique. A guidewire was placed. The left subclavian vein was accessed, and a separate guidewire was placed.

Following this, a deep subcutaneous pacemaker pocket was created using the blunt dissection technique without any excessive bleeding.

Following this, a French-7 introducer sheath was advanced over the guidewire, and the guidewire was removed. A Medtronic bipolar endocardial lead, model #5054 and serial #LEH025605V, was advanced under fluoroscopic guidance, and the tip of the pacemaker lead was positioned in the right ventricular apex.

Following this, the French-9.5 introducer sheath was advanced over a separate guidewire under fluoroscopic guidance, and the guidewire was removed.

Through this sheath, a bipolar atrial screw-in lead by Medtronic, model #4568 , was selected. It was positioned in the right atrial appendage, and the lead was screwed in.

Following this, the stimulation thresholds were obtained for the atrial lead. The amplitude was millivolts (mv) of resistance of 549 ohms, with pulse rate of 0.5 ms.

Following the ventricular stimulation, threshold perimeters were obtained, including R-wave entry of 4.6 mv with resistance of 1,427 ohms, with a pulse wave of 0.5 ms. Minimum-stimulation threshold voltage was 0.4 volts for the ventricular lead, and minimal-stimulation voltage was 2 volts for the atrial lead.

Select the appropriate CPT and ICD-9-CM codes:

a. 33207, 427.81

b. 33210, 427.10

c. 33202, 33212, 427.81

d. 33208, 427.81

9. **Preoperative diagnosis:** Carcinoma of the lung with right neck metastasis

Postoperative diagnosis: Carcinoma of the lung with right neck metastasis

Operative procedures: Cervical esophagoscopy, microlaryngoscopy, and biopsy

Procedure and findings: With the patient under general anesthesia, the 101 14 × 23 Roberts esophagoscope was passed. It was noticed that the left piriform sinus was of normal appearance. There was edema of the free tip of the epiglottis. The scope was advanced through the left piriform sinus into the cervical esophagus, and the cervical esophagus and postcricoid area were essentially normal. Also, the upper cervical esophagus was normal. The scope was slowly withdrawn through the right piriform sinus. It was noticed that there was a tumor involving the anterior wall of the right piriform sinus, extending approximately 1 cm below the pharyngeal epiglottic fold. This tumor then also involved the lateral hypopharyngeal wall to a minor degree. The scope was removed.

The Dedo microlaryngoscope was passed. It was now noticed that the above findings were further defined. It was noticed that there was an exit through the tumor involving the vallecula on the right side going into the base of the tongue for a distance of approximately 0.5 cm. This tumor was quite exophytic, and it extended laterally above the pharyngeal epiglottic fold, extending, therefore, approximately 0.75 cm to the lateral hypopharyngeal wall. It also involved heavily the medial wall of the right piriform sinus without crossing over onto the laryngeal surface of the epiglottic fold. The vocal cords are of normal appearance. The right vocal cord is fixed in the midline. Inferiorly the tumor extends onto the medial wall of the piriform sinus just about 0.5 cm below the level of the right vocal cord. The scope was suspended. These findings were confirmed, and under 10× magnification, several biopsies were obtained. The scope was removed. The neck was carefully palpated. The endoscopy had been preceded by a tracheostomy. The patient was initially prepared with Betadine solution and draped in the usual manner. A horizontal incision was made approximately 2 cm above the sternal notch and carried through the subcutaneous tissue down to the strap muscles. The strap muscles were divided in the midline. The cricoid cartilage was identified, the trach ties were tied securely into place, and the cuff was inflated to a comfortable pressure. The patient then received further ventilation through the newly placed trach tube. The patient tolerated all procedures well.

Select the appropriate CPT and ICD-9-CM codes:

a. 43202, 198.89, 162.9

b. 43200, 31541, 198.2, 162.9

c. 31541, 43200-59, 31600-59, 198.89, 162.9

d. 31541, 43200, 198.2, 162.9

10. **Arteriogram:** Left Renal Artery Stenosis

Procedure in detail: The procedure, indications, possible complications of an abdominal aortogram, and possible renal arteriogram were discussed with the patient. The patient agreed to have the procedure done and signed the consent.

Under sterile technique with fluoroscopy control, a vascular sheath was introduced in the right common femoral artery using the Seldinger technique. Through this sheath, a 5-French pigtail catheter was introduced and placed at the proximal abdominal aorta. Flush aortogram followed, and a digital subtraction study of the abdominal aorta, by placing the catheter close to the renal artery origin, was performed.

Evidence of mild atheromatous plaque disease involving the infrarenal abdominal aorta, causing focal dilation, is seen. No significant stenosis is noted at the aortic bifurcation.

The celiac axis, including the splenic artery, gastroduodenal artery, and hepatic artery, is normal.

On the right side, the renal artery is normal in caliber, without any significant stenosis. Segmental arteries are normal. Contrast nephrogram was also uniform.

On the left side, there is segmental narrowing at the origin of the left renal artery. The narrowed segment is approximately 2 cm in length, with the narrowing more than 50% to 60% seen. No significant distal stenotic dilation of the renal artery is seen. Segmental arteries of the left renal artery are normal. Nephrogram of the left kidney is also normal.

Since the digital subtraction study was done with stenosis analysis, left renal artery stenosis is in the range of 50% to 65%. Hence, a selective renal arteriogram was not performed.

Impression: A 2-cm stenotic segment involving the origin of the left renal artery with stenosis in the range of 50% to 65% is noted. Segmental arteries of the left kidney are normal. Nephrogram of the left kidney is also normal.

Select the appropriate CPT and ICD-9-CM codes:

a. 36246-LT, 440.1

b. 36245-50, 440.1

c. 36245 × 2, 440.1-lt

d. 36252, 440.1

11. **Preoperative diagnoses:**

1. Sick sinus syndrome, status post-pacemaker insertion.
2. Infected pacemaker with exposed wires.
3. Coronary artery disease with history of coronary artery bypass graft.
4. Essential hypertension.

Postoperative diagnoses:

1. Sick sinus syndrome, status post-pacemaker insertion.
2. Infected pacemaker with exposed wires.
3. Coronary artery disease with history of coronary artery bypass graft.
4. Essential hypertension.

Operations performed:

1. Explant of pacemaker generator and two wires under fluoroscopic guidance and xenon laser.
2. Pocket revision.
3. Intraoperative transesophageal echocardiography with interpretation.

Select the appropriate CPT and ICD-9-CM codes:

a. 33233, 33222, 93318, 996.61, 427.81, V45.01, 414.0, 401.9

b. 33233, 33222, 93318, 996.61, 427.81, 414.07, V45.01, 401.9, V45.81

c. 33233, 33222, 93318, 427.81, 996.61, 414.07, 401.9

d. 33233, 33222, 93318, 427.81, V45.01, 996.61, 414.0

12. A 75-year-old patient was brought to the operating room for operative ablation of her atrial fibrillation via a combined Wolff-Parkinson-White atrio-ventricular node tissue ablation and reconstruction of

the atria using the Maze procedure. Cardiopulmonary bypass was not required. The patient tolerated the procedure well and was sent to ICU for continued monitoring.

a. 33250, 427.31

b. 33255, 33257, 427.32

c. 33258, 427.31

d. 33250, 33258, 427.31

Digestive

1. Mr. Jones is a patient with recurrent stage IV colon carcinoma of the sigmoid colon. He had previously undergone a laparoscopic low anterior resection (LAR). He was brought to the operating room today and under general anesthesia underwent a laparoscopic lysis of adhesions. The small bowel loops were found to be adherent to the anterior abdominal wall and also near the colostomy. These adhesions were lysed. There was one loop of small bowel that was adherent to the anterior abdominal wall of the RLQ, and this adhesion was not disturbed. Select the appropriate CPT and ICD-9-CM codes:

   a. 44180, 568.0, 153.3

   b. 44340, 568.0, 153.3

   c. 44180, 153.3, 568.0

   d. 44340, 44180, 153.3, 568.0

2. Jeremy presented to the ED complaining of severe odynophagia after eating chicken wings. Upon initial x-rays, no perforation of the esophagus was noted. The gastrointestinal specialist was called, and the patient was taken to the endoscopy suite. There, with the patient under moderate sedation, the gastroenterologist performed an esophagoscopy and removed a small chicken bone lodged in the esophagus above the diaphragm. Select the appropriate CPT and ICD-9-CM codes:

   a. 43247. 935.1

   b. 43200, 787.20

   c. 43215, 935.1

   d. 43215, 787.20

3. The patient underwent a hemorrhoidectomy for removal of two columns of prolapsed internal hemorrhoids and resolution of a chronic anal fissure—fissurectomy. Select the appropriate CPT and ICD-9-CM codes:

   a. 46255, 455.2, 565.0

   b. 46250, 455.2, 565.0

   c. 46260, 455.2, 565.0

   d. 46261, 455.2, 565.0

4. Mrs. Jones presented with pain in the right upper quadrant. Upon a CT of the abdomen and an ultrasound of the gallbladder a diagnosis of cholelithiasis and acute cholecystitis was confirmed, and the patient was taken to the operating room. The patient underwent a laparoscopic cholecystectomy with a normal intraoperative cholangiogram to remove the gallstones. Select the appropriate CPT and ICD-9-CM codes:

   a. 47562, 574.10

   b. 47561, 574.10

   c. 47563, 574.10

   d. 47570, 574.10

5. A 4-year-old male underwent a frenoplasty using the Z technique to correct his speech difficulty due to ankyloglossia. Select the appropriate CPT and ICD-9-CM codes:

   a. 41115, 750.0

   b. 41520, 750.0

   c. 40819, 750.0

   d. 41116, 750.0

6. A 45-year-old male with pancreatic cancer presents with a distended abdomen. The ultrasound reveals fluid in the peritoneal cavity. The patient undergoes a therapeutic paracentesis with ultrasound imaging guidance to drain the fluid. Select the appropriate CPT and ICD-9-CM codes:

   a. 49062, 157.9

   b. 49084, 157.9

   c. 49082, 157.9

   d. 49083, 157.9

7. A 1-year-old female underwent a uvulopalatopharyngoplasty to repair a congenital bilateral cleft lip and bilateral cleft hard palate. Select the appropriate CPT and ICD-9-CM codes:

   a. 42145, 749.23

   b. 42145, 749.24, 749.03

   c. 42145, 749.13, 749.03

   d. 42145, 749.25

8. Taylor was born at 36 weeks and is now 1 month old. He presented with a reducible R. inguinal hernia and hydrocele. He was taken to the OR for a repair. Select the appropriate CPT and ICD-9-CM codes:

   a. 49492, 550.90, 603.9

   b. 49495, 550.90, 603.9

   c. 49491, 550.90, 603.9

   d. 49496, 550.90, 603.9

9. A patient with morbid obesity presents for laparoscopic revision of a previous gastro-restrictive procedure. Select the appropriate CPT and ICD-9-CM codes:

   a. 43770, 278.01

   b. 43771, 278.01

   c. 43772, 278.01

   d. 43774, 278.01

10. A patient undergoes a percutaneous liver biopsy with US guidance. The pathology report reveals autoimmune hepatitis. Select the appropriate CPT and ICD-9-CM codes:

    a. 47000, 571.42

    b. 47000, 76942, 571.40

    c. 47000, 571.41

    d. 47000, 76942, 571.42

Urinary, Male/Female Reproductive Systems, Maternity/Delivery

1. **Preoperative diagnosis:** Left hydrocele

   Postopertive diagnosis: Left hydrocele

   Procedure performed: Left hydrocelectomy

   Procedure description: The initial incision was made, and the left hydrocele was delivered out of the wound and incised. The hydrocele was emptied of about 500 mL and then incised completely. About 90% of the hydrocele sac was removed with the Bovie. The hydrocele sac was involuted and sewn to itself using running 3-0 Vicryl in the manner of Jabuolay. The testicle was replaced in the left scrotum, and the patient tolerated the procedure well.

   Select the appropriate CPT and ICD-9-CM codes:

   a. 55040-LT, 603.9

   b. 55041-LT, 603.9

   c. 55000-LT, 603.9

   d. 55060-LT, 603.9

APPENDIX A

2. Sally was seen today for a percutaneous aspiration of a cyst of the left kidney with a translumbar renal cyst study. Select the appropriate CPT and ICD-9-CM codes:

a. 50391-LT, 593.2

b. 50390-LT, 593.1

c. 50391-LT, 74470, 593.1

d. 50390-LT, 74470, 593.2

3. Doug, a 45-year-old patient with ESRD, receives a unilateral cadaver kidney transplant. The surgeon performs the backbench work in addition to the transplant. Select the appropriate CPT and ICD-9-CM codes:

a. 50320, 50323, 585.6

b. 50300, 50323, V42.0, 585.6

c. 50320, V42.0

d. 50300, 585.6

4. A surgeon performs a ritualistic surgical circumcision on a 30-day-old male. Select the appropriate CPT and ICD-9-CM codes:

a. 54161, V50.2

b. 54161-63, V50.2

c. 54160-63, V50.2

d. 54160, V50.2

5. Gregory underwent a prostatomy for drainage of a complicated prostatic abscess. Select the appropriate CPT and ICD-9-CM codes:

a. 55706, 601.2

c. 55725, 601.2

b. 55720, 601.2

d. 55801, 601.2

6. Jeff has detected a mass in his right testicle and undergoes a needle biopsy of the mass. Code this encounter with the appropriate CPT and ICD-9-CM codes:

a. 10021, 608.89

c. 10020, 608.89

b. 54500, 608.89

d. 54505, 608.89

7. Sally was seen in the ED for an acute onset of lower abdominal pain. US determined the presence of bilateral twisted ovarian cysts. Sally was taken to the OR for removal of both cysts. Select the appropriate CPT and ICD-9-CM codes:

a. 58940, 620.2

c. 58925-50, 620.2

b. 58925, 620.2

d. 58940-50, 620.2

8. Ms. Jones had been seen by Dr. Stork throughout her second pregnancy, and he performed a cesarean delivery of twin girls. Select the appropriate CPT and ICD-9-CM codes:

a. 59510, V22.1, V24.2

b. 59515, V22.1, V27.2

c. 59514, V22.1, V24.2

d. 59515, 651.00, V27.2

9. The patient underwent abdominal pan-hysterectomy to remove a malignant hydatiform mole. Select the appropriate CPT and ICD-9-CM codes:

a. 58150, 236.1

b. 58200, 630

c. 58150, 630

d. 58152, 236.1

10. The patient is seen in the OB/GYN office for follow-up postpartum. She had been seen by her previous physician throughout her pregnancy but has relocated since the normal vaginal delivery of her daughter 6 weeks ago. Select the appropriate CPT and ICD-9-CM codes:

a. 59426, V24.2

b. 59400, V24.2

c. 59430, V24.2

d. 59514, V24.2

11. A 28-year-old patient was seen today for her annual physical exam by her OB/GYN. After discussion with the physician, the patient expressed her decision to have her IUD removed as she and her husband are ready to begin a family. This procedure was performed at this visit. Select the appropriate CPT and ICD-9-CM codes:

a. 99395-25, 58301, V70.0, V25.12

b. 99394-25, 58301, V70.0, V25.12

c. 99294-25, 58301, V70.0, V25.12

d. 99295-25, 58301, V70.0, V25.12

12. Mary was seen today for a surgical hysteroscopy with lysis of intrauterine adhesions. Select the appropriate CPT and ICD-9-CM codes:

a. 58558, 621.6

b. 58560, 621.8

c. 58555, 621.5

d. 58559, 621.5

Nervous System, Eyes, Ears, Endocrine

1. The patient was diagnosed with Graves' disease and underwent a total thyroidectomy. Select the appropriate CPT and ICD-9-CM codes:

a. 60271, 242.01

b. 60240, 242.01

c. 60252, 242.10

d. 60260, 242.00

2. A patient diagnosed with myasthenia gravis undergoes partial removal of the thymus gland using a transthoracic approach. Select the appropriate CPT and ICD-9-CM codes:

a. 60520, 358.00

b. 60522, 358.10

c. 60521, 358.00

d. 60521-52, 358.01

3. A patient underwent fine-needle aspiration of a thyroid cyst. Select the appropriate CPT and ICD-9-CM codes:

a. 60100, 246.2   c. 60200, 246.2

b. 10021, 246.2   d. 10022, 246.24

4. **Preoperative diagnosis:** Right subdural hematoma

Postoperative diagnosis: Right subdural hematoma

Procedure performed: Right temporoparietal craniotomy for evacuation of subdural hematoma

Anesthesia: General endotracheal

Complications: None

Condition: Stable

Indications for procedure: Mr. Green is a 45-year-old male with a known history of alcoholism. He reported falling today, with loss of consciousness for about 20 minutes. Upon arrival at the ED, he was minimally responsive, with some spontaneous movement on the right side. He was intubated and taken to CT, which demonstrated a large right temporal subdural hematoma with 2.5-cm midline shift and effacement of the right lateral ventricle.

Description of procedure: The patient was brought to the OR already intubated. General anesthesia was induced. He was given Ancef for preoperative prophylactic IV antibiotics. Lacri-Lube was placed in both eyes, which were then taped shut. A Foley was placed. The patient was positioned supine on the operating room table with the right side elevated with a gel roll. The head was secured in the three-point Mayfield head-holder with the right side up. All pressure points were inspected and padded adequately. The patient's scalp was clipped, prepped, and draped in standard sterile surgical fashion. Local anesthetic was infiltrated along the line of the planned skin incision. A right temporoparietal inverted-question-mark incision was performed with a #10 blade down to the level of the periosteum. The scalp flap, along with the muscle and periosteum, was elevated and reflected anteriorly and held in place with fishhooks. Raney clips were applied to the skin edges. Using the high-speed Midas Rex drill with the perforator bit, burr holes were placed in the temporoparietal region, and they were connected with the B1 and footplate. The bone flap was elevated from the dura and set aside. The underlying brain appeared to be tense. The dura was opened with a 15-blade, and a large amount of subdural hematoma was immediately released. The subdural space was copiously irrigated, and hemostasis was achieved.

Select the appropriate CPT and ICD-9-CM codes:

a. 61314, 853.00

b. 61314, 853.02

c. 61314, 853.04

d. 61314, 853.01

5. George presented with chronic intractable pain of unknown origin in his left leg. The neurologist used stereotaxis to create a lesion in the spinal cord in order to attempt to block the pain and provide sustainable relief. Select the appropriate CPT and ICD-9-CM codes:

   a. 63600, 338.29, 729.5

   b. 65220, 338.19, 729.5

   c. 65222, 338.29, 729.5

   d. 63621, 338.19, 729.5

6. The patient underwent a laminectomy for creation of a lumbo-subarachnoid shunt. Select the appropriate CPT code:

   a. 62190   **c.** 63740

   b. 63741   **d.** 62220

7. The patient was seen for complaints of persistent cluster headaches and blurring vision. As part of the workup, a lumbar puncture was performed, the pressure of the spinal fluid was measured, and some fluid was removed for analysis. Select the appropriate CPT and ICD-9-CM codes:

   a. 62271, 339.02

   b. 62270, 339.01

   c. 62270, 339.02

   d. 62271, 339.01

8. Sam, a welder, was seen today by the ophthalmologist for removal of a welding flash from his left eye. The flash had caused a nonperforating tear in the cornea. The ophthalmologist removed the flash and repaired the cornea. Select the appropriate CPT and ICD-9-CM codes:

   a. 65220, 65275, 930.0   **c.** 65221, 65275, 930.0

   b. 65202, 930.1   **d.** 65275, 930.0

9. Sam underwent scleral buckling for repair of a detached retina of the right eye with cryotherapy and drainage of subretinal fluid. Select the appropriate CPT and ICD-9-CM codes:

   a. 67101, 67105, 361.9

   b. 67107, 361.9

   c. 67966, 361.81

   d. 67110, 361.89

10. The patient underwent blepharoplasty of the left eyelid, including lid margin and tarsus with a full-thickness skin graft for paralytic ptosis. Select the appropriate CPT and ICD-9-CM codes:

    a. 15820, 374.33

    b. 67961, 374.31

    c. 67966, 374.30

    d. 15821, 374.31

11. Jimmy, age 4, has a history of repeated ear infections and is in the OR today for myringotomy and eustachian tube inflation to reduce the damage from chronic purulent otitis media. Select the appropriate CPT and ICD-9-CM codes:

    a. 69433, 382.3

    b. 69420, 382.3

    c. 69421, 382.3

    d. 69440, 382.3

12. A patient underwent tympanoplasty with a mastoidectomy and ossicular chain reconstruction for removal of a cholesteatoma of the right ear. Select the appropriate CPT and ICD-9-CM codes:

    a. 69641, 385.30

    b. 69643, 385.30

    c. 69637, 385.30

    d. 69642, 385.30

13. A patient underwent fenestration of the semicircular canal to improve bone conduction and decrease hearing loss due to obliterative otosclerosis involving the oval window of the left ear. Select the appropriate CPT and ICD-9-CM codes:

    a. 69805, 387.1

    b. 69840, 387.9

    c. 69840, 387.1

    d. 69820, 387.1

Radiology

1. Upon orders from Dr. Clyos, a portable x-ray machine was transported to the city nursing home for chest x-rays of a patient with possible tuberculosis. The diagnosis was nodular lesions and patchy infiltrates in the upper lobes. Select the appropriate CPT and ICD-9-CM codes:

   a. 71020, V71.2

   b. 71010, 011.90, V71.2

   c. 71010, 017.20

   d. 71010, V71.2

2. **CT Scan of the Chest and Adrenals**

   History: Left pulmonary nodule on chest x-ray

   Technique: Helical transaxial images, 7 mm, of the chest were obtained after the administration of oral and intravenous contrast.

Findings: The patient's chest x-rays from February 24 and 25 were reviewed. There is an ill-defined opacity suggested in the left midlung zones on those studies, including oblique views.

Within the left lower lobe laterally, there is an approximately 2-cm area of parenchymal density that has the appearance of interstitial changes without findings of a significant nodule or mass. This finding can relate to scarring. There is no other nodule, mass, or effusion. Within the mediastinum, there is no evidence of adenopathy seen. The heart and great vessels are normal in appearance. There is a suggestion of minimal pericardial thickening anteriorly that is not specific. Osseous structures show degenerative changes with osteophyte formation at multiple levels in the thoracic spine.

Visualized upper abdominal structures, including liver, spleen, kidneys, pancreas, aorta, and para-aortic retroperitoneum, show no specific finding. The adrenal glands are not enlarged.

Impression: There is a small focal area of increased parenchymal density that has an interstitial pattern. There is no significant nodule or mass. This is suggestive of scarring. There is no nodule, mass, effusion, or adenopathy seen. Consider chest x-ray follow-up of this lesion to assess stability.

Select the appropriate CPT and ICD-9-CM codes:

a. 71260, 518.89

b. 71250, 518.89

c. 71270, 518.89

d. 71250, 71260, 518.89

3. **CT Scan of the Abdomen and Pelvis**

   History: Malignant testicular neoplasm

   Technique: Axial CT images of the abdomen and pelvis were obtained with intravenous and oral contrast.

   Findings: Images of the lung bases are normal. Images of the abdomen show the liver, spleen, gallbladder, pancreas, and adrenal glands to be normal. No mass is seen. There is no evidence of cholelithiasis. A retroaortic left renal vein is seen. No obvious mass or enlarged lymph nodes are noted in the retroperitoneum. Mesenteric structures appear normal. A prominent inferior vena cava is seen. Gas is identified in the left inguinal structures, likely representing previous left orchidectomy and removal of the inguinal ring. No enlarged lymph node is identified in the pelvis.

   Impression: Left retroaortic renal vein is seen. No adenopathy is noted within the abdomen or pelvis. No enlarged lymph node is seen; no mass is identified.

   Select the appropriate CPT and ICD-9-CM codes:

   a. 74177, V10.47

   b. 74150, 74175, V10.47

   c. 74177 × 2, V10.47

   d. 74160, 74150, V10.47

4. **Barium Swallow**

   Technique: This study was performed in the presence of a speech pathologist. Thin, thick, and pureed barium were used in the evaluation.

   After swallowing the thick barium, the patient aspirated into the larynx. There was no reflux cough. However, voluntary cough was initiated to clear the remaining part of the contrast. Subsequent swallowing with the thin barium did not reveal any aspiration. However, there was a significant delay in the oropharyngeal transit time as seen on the videography. Significant pooling of the barium was seen in the vallecula and piriform sinuses. Since the patient demonstrated aspiration with the thick barium, solid food material was not given. Thus, the patient is still at risk for unsupervised oral feeding because of aspiration.

   Impression: Aspiration is documented for the thick barium. Oropharyngeal transit time is delayed. Significant pooling in the vallecula and piriform sinuses is still noted.

   Select the appropriate CPT code:

   a. 74220-52

   b. 74220

   c. 74230

   d. 74210

5. **KUB:** No radiopaque density is noted below the renal region. No radiopaque density is noted along the course of the ureters. A few faint calcific densities are noted in both sides on the bony pelvis. One of them could be in the ureter, but it most certainly looks like they are calcified phleboliths.

Impression: No calcific densities are noted over the renal region. If symptoms persist, repeat this urography, intravenous pyelogram.

Select the appropriate CPT code:

a. 74425

b. 74400

c. 74246

d. 74270

6. **Examination:** Gastric-emptying study

Reason for examination: This is a study of elimination for gastroparesis, abdominal cramping, and pain.

Interpretation: One millicurie of technetium-99m sulfur colloid was given through a gastrostomy tube in saline. The normal half-time of clearance of liquid material from the stomach is 12 minutes. The patient's clearance is 50 minutes, which is a fourfold increase in time and is compatible with a marked delay in gastric emptying.

Select the appropriate CPT and ICD-9-CM codes:

a. 78264, 536.6

c. 78262, 536.3, 789.07

b. 78264, 563.3, 789.07

d. 78264, 536.3

7. **Myocardial Perfusion Scan**

Persantine was positive at 5 minutes.

Technique: Following the intravenous administration of 25.5 mCi of technetium-99m MIBI following pharmacologic stress, SPECT images of the right ventricle were obtained with assessment and ejection fraction. Subsequently, following the intravenous administration of 26.1 mCi of technetium-99m MIBI at rest, the study was repeated and was correlated with prior examination.

Findings: There was no evidence of an ischemia on today's examination. There was no ventricular cavity dilation at stress. Fixed decreased uptake was noted in the inferior wall, with no normalization at rest. Findings are consistent with prior inferior infarction.

Conclusion: No evidence of stress ischemia.

Select the appropriate CPT code(s):

a. 78472, 78496

b. 78473

c. 78481, 78496

d. 78496

8. **Clinical Indication:** Carcinoma of the breast with skeletal metastases

Procedure: CT scan of l. lung shows no dominant nodules within the lung. Multiple osteolytic metastases are present in several of the ribs in the posteriolateral aspect involving 3, 4, 5, 6, and 7th ribs. Small amount of pleural reaction is noted in the l. costophrenic angle. Hilar shadows are unremarkable. Shadow for l. breast is absent.

Impression: No definite metastatic nodules in l. lung. Multiple mixed osteolytic and osteoblastic changes in several ribs in the l. chest due to metastatic neoplasm.

a. 71250, 174.9, 198.5, V10.3

b. 71260, 198.5, 174.9

c. 71260, 174.9, 198.5

d. 71250, 198.5, V10.3

9. **Clinical History:** Carcinoma of the breast, currently being treated, with skeletal metastases

   Study Performed: Total Body Bone Scan

   Impression: Abnormal total body bone scan from the head to below the knees showed abnormalities in the ribs and spine and the skull, representing the skeletal metastases.

   a. 78300, 198.5, 174.9

   b. 78305, 198.5, 174.9

   c. 78315, 198.5, V10.3

   d. 78306, 198.5, 174.9

10. An eleven-year-old boy is brought to the ED with fever, malaise, and a stiff neck. The ED physician performs a spinal tap to R/O meningitis. The patient is admitted to University Hospital to further monitor his status. Later during the evening, the boy complains of a severe headache along with a "runny nose." The physician orders a nuclear medicine study to detect CSW fluid leakage and localization. Code the correct CPT and ICD-9-CM codes.

    a. 78645, 322.9

    b. 78630, 036.0, 320.9

    c. 78650, 349.0, 349.81

    d. 78650, 784.0, 478.19

Pathology

1. **Laboratory data:** Complete blood cell count on admission 9,700. White blood cell count 9,200. Sodium 140, potassium 4.2, chloride 101, CO_2 30, BUN 14, creatinine 1.2, glucose 103, calcium 9.2, total bilirubin 0.7, and total protein 8.1. AST 195, ALT 116, alkaline phosphatase 120, albumin 4.1. Urinalysis shows trace protein, 1+ occult blood, negative nitrites, negative leukocyte esterase, 5–10 red blood cells and less than 2 WBCs, trace bacteria, trace mucus, and rare epithelial cells. Valproic acid level is 61.6.

   Select the appropriate CPT codes:

   a. 80050, 85025, 81005

   b. 80050, 81005

   c. 80053, 85025, 81003

   d. 80069, 85025, 82247, 84155, 81003

2. **Postoperative diagnosis:** Carcinoma of bladder, R/O scalene node metastasis

   Procedure preformed: Bx of bladder and left scalene node

   Gross description: The specimen is received in two parts. They are labeled 1, biopsy bladder tumor, and 2, scalene node left. Part 1 consists of multiple fragments of gray-brown tissue that appear slightly hemorrhagic. They are submitted in their entirety for processing. Part 2 consists of multiple fragments of fatty yellow tissue that range in size from 0.2 cm to 1.0 cm in diameter. They are submitted in their entirety for processing.

   Microscopic: Section of bladder contains areas of transitional cell carcinoma. No area of invasion can be identified. A marked acute and chronic inflammatory reaction with eosinophils automated count is noted together with some necrosis. Sections are examined at six levels. Section of lymph node contains normal node with reactive germinal centers

   Diagnoses:

   1. Papillary transitional cell carcinoma, grade II bladder, biopsy.

   2. Acute and chronic inflammation, most consistent with recent biopsy procedure.

   3. Scalene lymph node, left, no pathologic diagnosis.

Select the correct CPT and ICD-9-CM codes

ICD-9-CM

a. 88305, 88305, 188.9, 196.2   **c.** 88306, 88307, 188.9, 196.2

b. 88305 × 2, 188.9   **d.** 88307, 88305, 188.9, 196.2

3. **Section:** Kidney (left): Adenocarcinoma

MACROSCOPIC

Specimen type: Radical nephrectomy

Laterality: Left

Tumor site: Upper pole

Focality: Unifocal

Tumor size: Greatest dimension is 7.2 cm.

Macroscopic extent of tumor: Tumor extends into major veins.

MICROSCOPIC

Histologic type: Clear cell (conventional) renal carcinoma

Histologic grade: Furhman Nuclear Grade 2

PATHOLOGIC STAGING (pTN)

Primary tumor (pT): pT3

Regional lymph nodes (pN): N×

Number of lymph nodes examined: 0

Number of lymph nodes involved: 0

Margins: Renal vein margin positive

Adrenal gland: Unevolved

Venous (large vessel) invasion (V) (excluding renal vein and inferior vena cava): Negative

Lymphatic (small vessel) invasion (L): Present

Additional pathologic findings: Chronic glomerulonephritis present in noninvolved renal parenchyma

Clinical history: A 76-year-old male with a left renal mass in the upper pole; hematuria

Gross description section: Received in formalin, labeled "left kidney," is a 12.2- × 7.1- × 2.5-cm kidney with unremarkable perirenal fat present at the upper pole (suture oriented, per requisition). A 2.3 cm in length segment of ureter exits from the hilum. The renal vein appears occluded. The cut sections demonstrate a 7.2- × 1.5- × 1.5-cm brown-orange circumscribed tumor with sharp borders present in the upper pole. Gerota's fascia appears uninvolved. The tumor extends into the renal vein; the venous margin appears positive for tumor.

Microscopic section: Microscopic examination was performed.

Select the appropriate CPT and ICD-9-CM codes:

a. 88307-LT, 189.0, 582.81

b. 88307-LT, 189.0

c. 88307, 189

d. 88307, 189.0, 582.9

3. **History:** The patient is a 79-year-old male with dyspepsia and weight loss. A recent supraclavicular lymph node biopsy revealed signet-ring cell adenocarcinoma.

Specimen site: Stomach

Gross description: Received in formalin is a 10.0- × 6.5- × 3.2-cm segment of stomach, with a palpable firm 4.0 × 2.2 cm mass on the designated lesser curvature. The external surface of the specimen is unremarkable and inked black. The cut surfaces demonstrate the mass and adjacent firm areas of nodularity. The remainder of the gastric mucosa is unremarkable. Six lymph node candidates and representative sections of the stomach are submitted.

Microscopic description: Microscopic examination was performed. See synoptic report. The uninvolved stomach shows chronic inactive gastritis with intestinal metaplasia.

Diagnosis: Stomach (proximal): Invasive adenocarcinoma

Comment: Signet-ring cell carcinomas are not typically graded but are high-grade and would correspond to grade 3.

Select the appropriate CPT and ICD-9-CM codes:

a. 88309, 151.9, 536.8, 783.21

b. 88309, 88307, 151.9

c. 88309, 88307 × 6, 151.9

d. 88309 × 2, 151.9, 536.8

4. **Specimen site:** Cervical biopsy

Preoperative Diagnosis: Severe squamous dysplasia, consistent with CIN III (high-grade dysplasia)

Gross description: Cervical biopsy: One fragment of gray-white tissue, measuring 0.5 centimeters in diameter. Totally submitted with a request for levels. Submitted request for stains.

Microscopic description: Sections of the cervical biopsy show high-grade dysplasia, consistent with CIN III. No evidence of invasive malignancy is present.

Select the appropriate CPT and ICD-9-CM codes:

a. 88305, 88312, 622.11

b. 88305, 622.11

c. 88305, 233.1

d. 88305, 88312, 622.10

5. **Specimen site:** Right medial cheek

Specimen site: Left dorsal hand

Gross description: Right medial cheek: The specimen is one gray-white fragment measuring 0.3 × 0.2 cm. Totally submitted in one cassette with a request for levels labeled "A."

Left dorsal hand: The specimen is one gray-white fragment measuring 0.3 × 0.3 cm. Totally submitted in one cassette with a request for levels labeled "B."

Microscopic description: The right medial cheek shows atypical keratinocytes within the entire thickness of the epidermis extending to the stratum corneum. The lesion appears to have been excised. The dermis shows elastosis.

The dorsal hand shows hyperkeratosis. The epidermis is mildly acanthotic. There is extensive dermal elastosis.

Final diagnoses:

1. Right medial cheek, biopsy:

—Squamous cell carcinoma in-situ (See comment.).

2. Left dorsal hand, biopsy:

—Dermal elastosis.

—No malignant changes seen.

Comment: The lesion from the cheek appears to reside within the confines of the histologic section. The skin lesion shows no invasive malignancy.

Select the appropriate CPT and ICD-9-CM codes:

a. 88305, 173.3, 701.1

c. 88304 × 2, 173.3, 701.9

b. 88305 × 2, 232.3, 701.1

d. 88305, 88305 173.3, 701.8

6. **Specimen site:** Gastric biopsy

Gross description: Gastric biopsy: Received in formalin, the specimen consists of two fragments of gray-brown mucosa, each measuring approximately 0.3 centimeter in diameter. Totally submitted for routine and special stains and additional levels.

Microscopic description: Sections show benign-appearing gastric mucosa with acute and chronic inflammatory cells within the lamina propria. The surface and pit-lining epithelium are also infiltrated with neutrophils. There is no dysplasia or malignancy. Special stains for *H. pylori* are positive.

Final diagnosis:

Gastric biopsy:

Chronic active gastritis.

—Warthin-Starry stain positive for *H. pylori.*

—Negative for intestinal metaplasia, dysplasia, or malignancy.

Select the appropriate CPT and ICD-9-CM codes:

a. 88305 × 2, 88312 × 22, 535.1, 041.86

b. 88305 × 2, 535.10, 041.86

c. 88305, 88312, 535.10, 041.86

d. 88305, 535.1, 041.86

7. **Microscopy**

Cytology:

Gross: 50 cc of slightly cloudy yellow fluid in a urocyte container. ThinPrep and residual fluid submitted for FISH testing.

Microscopic: Review of the ThinPrep prepared from this urine for FISH testing shows scattered atypical urothelial cells with increased nuclear cytoplasmic ratios and features suggesting advanced dysplasia suspicious for malignancy.

FISH: Review of the FISH reaction on cytology from this urine specimen shows increased numbers of mutations associated with transitional and urothelial cell malignancy. The combination of increased numbers of nuclear mutations as well as the cytology is consistent with a malignant diagnosis.

Diagnosis:

1. Urine for cytology, ThinPrep:

—Atypical urothelial cells suspicious for malignancy.

2. FISH testing:

—Increased mutations associated with urothelial malignancy, consistent with neoplastic transformation.

Select the appropriate CPT codes:

a. 88112, 88108

c. 88112, 88108, 88271

b. 88112, 88271

d. 88108, 88271

8. **History:** 76-year-old female with colonic mass

Diagnosis: Invasive adenocarcinoma, 3.4 × 3.0 cm, involving muscularis propria

All margins negative.

No lymphatic invasion.

No metastatic tumor identified.

Gross description: Received fresh is a right colon, 32 cm in length. Upon opening of the specimen, there is a 3.4- × 3.0-cm nodular mass. 36 lymph nodes were retrieved. Representative sections are submitted.

Microscopic description: Microscopic examination performed

Select the appropriate CPT and ICD-9-CM codes:

a. 88309, 153.9

b. 88309, 153.6

c. 88309, 153.8

d. 88307, 574.10

9. Mary Jane underwent cholecystectomy for acute cholecystitis. Select the appropriate CPT and ICD-9-CM codes for the gross and microscopic examination by the pathologist:

a. 88304, 574.10   c. 88309, 574.01

b. 88304, 574.00   d. 88307, 574.10

10. **Diagnosis:** Stomach (distal): Invasive adenocarcinoma

Gross description: Received in formalin two specimens, 9.0- × 5.5- × 4.3-cm and 2.0- × 1.5- × 3.4-cm segments of the stomach, with a palpable firm 3.0- × 2.5-cm mass on the designated lesser curvature of the larger specimen. The external surfaces of the specimens are unremarkable and inked black. The curved surfaces demonstrate the mass and adjacent firm areas of nodularity. The remainder of the gastric mucosa is unremarkable.

Microscopic description: Microscopic examination was performed. See synoptic report.

Select the appropriate CPT and ICD-9-CM codes:

a. 88307, 151.9   c. 88309 × 2, 151.9

b. 88307, 88309, 151.9   d. 88309, 88302, 151.9

Medicine

1. An echocardiogram was obtained for assessment of left ventricular function. The patient has been admitted with diagnosis of syncope. Overall, the study was suboptimal due to poor sonic window.

Findings:

1. Aortic root appears normal.

2. Left atrium is mildly dilated. No gross intraluminal pathology is recognized, although subtle abnormalities could not be excluded. Right atrium is of normal dimension.

3. There is echo dropout of the interatrial septum. Atrial septal defects could not be excluded.

4. Right and left ventricles are normal in internal dimension. Overall left ventricular systolic function appears to be normal. Eyeball ejection fraction is around 55%. Again, due to poor sonic window, wall motion abnormalities in the distribution of lateral and apical walls could not be excluded.

5. Aortic valve is sclerotic with normal excursion. Color-flow imaging and Doppler study demonstrate trace aortic regurgitation.

6. Mitral valve leaflets are also sclerotic with normal excursion. Color-flow imaging and Doppler study demonstrates a trace to mild degree of mitral regurgitation.

7. Tricuspid valve is delicate and opens normally. Pulmonic valve is not clearly seen. No evidence of pericardial effusion.

Conclusions:

Poor-quality study.

Eyeball ejection fraction is 55%.

Trace to mild degree of mitral regurgitation.

Trace aortic regurgitation.

Select the appropriate CPT and ICD-9-CM codes:

a. 93306, 780.2

b. 93307, 780.02

c. 93308, 780.2

d. 93307, 780.2

2. **S:** A 46-year-old male who was in a car accident presents for a prosthetic spectacle.

   O: HEENT is unremarkable. Monofocal measurements are taken, and data for the creation of an appropriate prosthesis are recorded.

   A: Aphakia, left eye.

   P: Return in 10 days for a final fitting.

   Select the appropriate CPT and ICD-9-CM codes:

   a. 92354, 379.3, E89.11

   b. 92352, 379.31

   c. 92340, 379.31

   d. 92352, 373.9, E89.11

3. Jim Jones is a 32-year-old from Maryland who was in town last week with ESRD. He was seen for four dialysis treatments this month. Select the appropriate CPT and ICD-9-CM codes:

   a. 90960, 585.6

   b. 90970-G6 $\times$ 4, 585.6

   c. 90967 $\times$ 4, 585.6

   d. 90960-G6 $\times$ 4, 585.6

4. **Office outpatient:** A Medicare patient, age 83, is seen for a therapeutic infusion of saline solution with prepackaged 5% detrose IV 500 mL for dehydration, lasting 1 hour 20 minutes. Select the appropriate CPT and ICD-9-CM codes:

   a. 96360 $\times$ 2, J7042, 276.51   **c.** 96360, 276.51

   b. 96360, 96361, J7042, 276.51   **d.** 96360, J7042, 276.51

5. **Procedure performed:** Left-sided heart catheterization, selective coronary angiography and left ventriculography

   Indication: Chest pain and abnormal Cardiolite stress test

   RESULTS

   Hemodynamics: The left ventricular pressure before the LV-gram was 117/1 with an LVEDP of 4; after the LV-gram it was 111/4 with an LVEDP of 10. The aortic pressure on pullback was 111/17.

   Left ventriculography: The left ventriculography showed that the left ventricle was of normal size. There were no significant segmental wall motion abnormalities. The overall left ventricular systolic function was normal, with an ejection fraction of better than 60%.

   Selective coronary angiography:

   a. Right coronary artery: The right coronary artery is a medium- to large-size dominant artery that has about 80% to 90% proximal/mid eccentric stenosis. The rest of the artery has only mild surface irregularities.

   b. Left main coronary artery: The left main has mild distal narrowing.

   c. Left circumflex artery: The left circumflex artery is a medium-size, nondominant artery. It gives rise to a very high first obtuse marginal/intermedius, which is a bifurcation medium-size artery that has only mild surface irregularities. The second obtuse marginal is also a medium-size artery that has about 20% to 25% proximal narrowing. After that second obtuse marginal, the circumflex artery is a small-size artery that has about 20% to 30% narrowing, a small aneurismal segment.

   d. Left anterior descending coronary artery: The left anterior descending artery is a medium-size artery that is mildly calcified. It gives rise to a very tiny first diagonal that has mild diffuse atherosclerotic disease. Right at the origin on the second diagonal, the LAD has about 30% narrowing. The rest of the artery is free of significant obstructive disease. The second diagonal is also a small-caliber artery that has no significant obstructive disease.

Conclusion: Severe single vessel atherosclerotic heart disease

Select the appropriate CPT and ICD-9-CM codes:
a. 93454, 78635, 786.50, 794.30
b. 93458, 414.01
c. 93455, 794.30, 414.01
d. 93454, 78635, 786.50, 794.39

6. **Bilateral Doppler Study:** Carotid Arteries

Indications: Status post-carotid endarterectomy imaging. The patient states that he was told that the right carotid artery is blocked. The right internal carotid artery is not identified, probably completely blocked.

Velocity measurements on the right side:

Common carotid artery: 58.9 cm/sec

Right external carotid: 142 cm/sec

Right vertebral: 44 cm/sec and showing antegrade flow

Velocity measurements on the left side:

Common carotid artery: 35 cm/sec

Carotid bulb: 60 cm/sec

Internal carotid: 52 cm/sec

External carotid: 236 cm/sec

Left vertebral: 55 cm/sec

Status postendarterectomy changes are noted in the left internal carotid and the bulb. There is evidence of ectasia. On the right, the common carotid artery shows ectasia.

Judging from the velocity measurements, the right internal carotid artery has a stenosis in the range of 50% to 79%.

The left internal carotid artery has a stenosis in the range of 16% to 49%. The left external carotid artery is in the range of 50% to 79%.

Impression: The right internal carotid artery is completely occluded. Status postendarterectomy change in the left internal carotid and the bulb is noted. No significant occlusive disease is seen in the left internal carotid artery. Both vertebral arteries are showing antegrade flow.

Select the appropriate CPT and ICD-9-CM codes:
a. 0126T, 433.10, V45.89
b. 93880, 433.10, V45.89
c. 93882, V67.00
d. 93880, V67.00

7. **Holter Monitor Report**

History: This is a 36-year-old male referred for evaluation of syncope episodes and dizziness. He also has a history of depression and anxiety.

A Holter monitor was placed on April 2 for 24 hours. Recording revealed sinus rhythm with three VPCs and three isolated APCs. There were no SVTs, no VTs, and no pauses. The patient had multiple complaints of dizziness, anxiety, panic, and feeling near syncopal. Rhythms at these times documented normal sinus rhythm at rates between 80 and 104 beats per minute. No significant arrhythmias.

Impression: Normal Holter

Select the appropriate CPT and ICD-9-CM codes:

a. 93225, 780.02

b. 93226, 780.2

c. 93227, 780.2, 780.4

d. 93224, 780.02, 780.4

8. Gary Grimm is admitted today for his chemotherapy, which consists of an antineoplastic drug 500-mg IV infusion over 3 hours. Dr. Michele Rosenberger is in attendance during Gary's treatment. Select the appropriate CPT code:

a. 93405

b. 96413, 96415, 96415

c. 96413 × 3

d. 96416, 96415 × 2

9. A 55-year-old female was having a problem with menopause. Because of the reported concerns about hormone replacement therapy, she decided to try acupuncture. After discussing her symptoms and discussing a treatment plan, Dr. Kind inserted several needles; the needles were removed 20 minutes later. Dr. Kind reviewed the follow-up plan and made an appointment for the patient's next visit. Dr. Kind spent 30 minutes in total face-to-face with Charlene. Select the appropriate CPT and ICD-9-CM codes:

a. 97810, 97813, 97814 × 2, 672.2

b. 97810, 97811, 627.2

c. 97810, 97811 × 3, 672.2

d. 97810, 97811 × 2, 627.2

10. This is a new 35–year-old male who is experiencing a piercing ringing sound in his left ear that began 6 months ago. The ringing interferes with his daily life, and he has problems sleeping. The patient is taken to a testing suite for a bilateral tinnitus assessment; pitch frequency matching loudness and masking procedures are included. The findings of the testing indicate a positive determination of tinnitus, acute tinnitus. Follow-up masking therapy. Select the appropriate CPT and ICD-9-CM codes:

a. 92625, 92562, 388.30

b. 92625, 388.30

c. 92625-52, 388.32

d. 92558, 388.32

11. A 36–year-old female who was the driver in a car accident presents with whiplash for chiropractic manipulative treatment of her cervical spine. The chiropractor provided a complete history and examination prior to the treatment plan of one visit a week for 2 months, at which point her status will be reevaluated. Today the first manipulation was performed. Select the appropriate CPT and ICD-9-CM codes:

a. 99213, 98940, 847.00, E811.0

b. 99213, 98940, 847.00

c. 98940, 847.0, E811.0

d. 98940, 847.0

12. A 75–year-old female recently underwent a stroke assessment of her aphasia. The following assessments were performed using Boston diagnostic aphasia examination: expressive and receptive speech, language function, language comprehensive, speed production ability, reading, spelling, and writing skills. Total time 60 minutes. Select the appropriate CPT and ICD-9-CM codes:

a. 92502, 784.3

b. 92506, 438.11

c. 92507, 784.3

d. 92511, 438.11

13. A child is being seen for immunizations. The first immunization is a subcutaneous injection of live varicella virus, and the other is an oral administration of live poliovirus. Select the appropriate CPT and ICD-9-CM codes:

a. 90716, 90471, 90712, 90474, V05.4, V04.0

b. 90716 × 2, 90471 × 2, V05.04, V05.09

c. 90716, 90712, 90471 × 2 V06.8

d. 90716, 90716, 90471, 90474, V05.4, V04.0

Medical Terminology

1. The patient underwent an examination of the esophagus, stomach, and duodenum. Which of the following terms describes this procedure?
   a. Esophagogastroduodenoscopy
   b. Duodenoscopy
   c. Esophagoscopy
   d. Upper GI

2. The patient presented with jaundiced skin. The color of jaundiced skin is:
   a. Red
   b. Blue
   c. White
   d. Yellow

3. The coiled tubules on top of the testicles that hold the testicles in place are called:
   a. Vas deferens
   b. Epididymis
   c. Spermatic cord
   d. None of these

4. The jellylike substance found inside the eye is called the:
   a. Aqueous humor
   b. Bilious humor
   c. Vitreous humor
   d. Lacrimal humor

5. A disease caused by overproduction of the growth hormone after puberty is:
   a. Gigantism
   b. Dwarfism
   c. Cushing's syndrome
   d. Acromegaly

6. The rapid discharge of menstrual blood between periods is called:
   a. Menorrhagia
   b. Menometrorrhagia
   c. Metrorrhagia
   d. Dysmenorrhea

7. The term meaning "many pregnancies" is:
   a. Multigravida
   b. Nulligravida
   c. Primigravida
   d. Multipara

8. Which of the following terms best describes presbycusis?
   a. Hardening of the stapes
   b. Inflammation of the outer ear
   c. Sense of revolving of the body or the environment
   d. Hearing impairment of old age

9. The patient was taken to the OR for draining of the pus from the middle ear. The surgeon accomplished this with an incision in the tympanic membrane. Which of the following terms best describes this procedure?
   a. Labyrinthectomy
   b. Stapedectomy
   c. Myringotomy
   d. Mastoidectomy

10. An abnormal hump caused by increased convexity of the thoracic spine is called:
    a. Kyphosis
    b. Lordosis
    c. Scoliosis
    d. Osteopenia

APPENDIX A

11. Which of the following terms pertains to the muscle tissue of the heart?
    a. Peritoneal
    b. Presbyopia
    c. Myocardium
    d. Carditis

12. A wall dividing two cavities is the definition of:
    a. Striated muscle
    b. Septum
    c. Bundle of His
    d. Pleural cavity

13. The area between the lungs that contains the heart, aorta, venae cavae, esophagus, and trachea is called the:
    a. Thoracic cavity
    b. Mediastinum
    c. Pleural cavity
    d. Upper abdominal

14. Which of the following is the medical term for difficulty breathing?
    a. Dyspnea
    b. Respiratory failure
    c. Shortness of breath
    d. Emphysema

15. Which of the following is one of the largest veins in the body?
    a. Vena cava
    b. Renal artery
    c. Biliary duct
    d. Carotid artery

16. Which of the following terms means "air in the pleural cavity"?
    a. Pneumothorax
    b. Visceral pleuritis
    c. Hemothorax
    d. Pneumoperitoneum

17. Which of the following terms refers to an examination of the interior of the tracheobronchial tree with an endoscope?
    a. Laryngoscopy
    b. Tracheostomy
    c. Bronchoscopy
    d. Laparoscopy

18. Which of the following tests involves delineation of deep structures using sound waves?
    a. Lithotripsy
    b. Audiometric testing
    c. Ultrasonography
    d. Mediastinoscope

19. Spread of a disease from one part of the body to another is called:
    a. Metastasis
    b. Adenocarcinoma
    c. Carcinogenesis
    d. Necrosis

20. Which of the following procedures is surgical removal of a lobe of the lung?
    a. Lobectomy
    b. Lobotomy
    c. Labiectomy
    d. Lobular excision

Evaluation and Management

1. Mr. Jones, a new patient with a history of prostate cancer 6 years ago, presented today with pain in his lower back and weakness in his extremities. He brought films from x-rays taken earlier in the week and his previous records from his internal medicine physician. The physician takes a comprehensive PMFSH and ROS and performs a comprehensive examination. Based on review of the records and his findings, the physician's diagnosis is metastatic prostate cancer to the sacral vertebrae. The physician discussed treatment options with the patient, including risks and benefits. Select the appropriate CPT and ICD-9-CM codes:
    a. 99204, 186, 198.5
    b. 99204, V10.46
    c. 99205, 186, 198.5
    d. 99205, 198.5, V10.46

2. Jeremy is seen at the clinic today by his regular physician for a rash on his arm that developed while camping in the woods this past weekend. After the problem-focused history and examination the physician determines that the problem was caused by poison oak, and Jeremy is diagnosed with allergic contact dermatitis and prescribed corticosteroid skin cream to reduce the inflammation. Select the appropriate CPT and ICD-9-CM codes:

   a. 99212, 692.6

   b. 99212, 692.0

   c. 99211, 692.6

   d. 99211, 692.3

3. An 80-year-old female with NIDDM was brought to the ED after she fell at home. She complains of pain in her left hip and is unable to stand. The physician obtains a detailed history and performs a detailed examination. X-rays reveal a closed midcervical fracture of the left femur, and arrangements for surgical and endocrine consultations are initiated. Select the appropriate CPT and ICD-9-CM codes:

   a. 99285, 820.03, 250.00

   b. 99284, 820.03, 250.00

   c. 99284, 820.13, 250.00

   d. 99285, 820.13, 250.00

4. Dr. Green works for a house call physician service. She was called to evaluate a new patient, an 88-year-old bedridden patient, who has developed a painful rash on her posterior left side of the trunk, extending from C6 to C7 around the right side and ending midline on the anterior trunk just below the sternum. The physician performs a detailed history and a detailed examination and diagnoses the patient with shingles. Select the appropriate CPT and ICD-9-CM codes:

   a. 99342, 053.9

   b. 99343, 053.9

   c. 99203, 053.9

   d. 99204, 053.9

5. Dr. Black, a cardiologist, is seeing Mrs. Smythe, a 72-year-old Medicare patient, today at the request of her internist regarding her atrial fibrillation. After a comprehensive history, comprehensive cardiology, specific examination, and decision making of moderate complexity, Dr. Black prescribes some adjustments to her medications and sends a letter to her internist with his findings and suggested follow-up. Select the appropriate CPT and ICD-9-CM codes:

   a. 99245, 427.31

   b. 99205, 427.31

   c. 99204, 427.31

   d. 99244, 427.32

6. **Patient Infant Male Crowley**

   I was present at the delivery at 5:07 p.m. of a male infant, 29 weeks' gestation with a spontaneous cry. At the 1 minute mark the Apgar was 5; the decreases were in tone, grimace, and color. An Apgar of 8 was reached at the 5 minute mark, with decreases continued in grimace and tone. The infant was taken to NICU for further management. Upon examination, decreased breath sounds and increased work to breathe was noted. The infant was intubated with difficulty. The patient did tolerate this well.

   An umbilical artery catheter was placed without difficulty, and labs were ordered. A chest x-ray and abdominal films were done. Both UAC and the endotracheal tube are in proper placement. The OG has been advanced; the lung fields do show significant granularity. Blood gas is 8.32, PCO_2 of 50, PO_2 of 102 on a setting of 22/4 rate of 60, and 80% FiO_2.

   PE: Patient currently is intubated. His weight is 1,706 kg; OFC is 30.5; length is 39.6 cm. Heart rate is in the 120s to 130s. Respiratory rate is 60 on the ventilator; O_2 saturation is in the mid-90s. Blood pressure in right arm is 67/34, with a mean of 46, and in right leg is 67/32, with a mean of 44.

Plan: Observation for sepsis

Maternal hypermagnesemia.

Admission to the NICU, continued mechanical ventilation.

Select the appropriate CPT and ICD-9-CM codes:

a. 99464, 99468, 769, 765.17, 765.25, 775.5, V29.0, V30.01

b. 99468, 769, 765.17, 765.24, 775.4, V29.0, V30.02

c. 99468, 769, 765.17, 775.5, V29.0, V30.02

d. 99468, 99464, 769, 765.17, 765.24, 775.4, V29.0, V30.02

7. Dr. Klinger, a cardiologist, has been asked by Dr. Swartz to see a 74-year-old female inpatient for a second time. Last week, the patient suffered an anterior wall myocardial infarction. Despite following the medical management suggested by Dr. Klinger, she continued to have angina and ventricular tachycardia. Dr. Klinger closely examined all of the documentation and test results that had been generated in the past week and performed a complete ROS with an extended HPI including the detailed interval history. The detailed physical examination performed was a complete cardiovascular system examination. Based on the subjective and objective findings, Dr. Klinger concluded that more aggressive medical management was in order. Given the patient's multiple problems, coupled with the new threat of cardiorespiratory failure, the patient was immediately transferred to the ICU. Select the appropriate CPT and ICD-9-CM codes:

a. 99233, 410.11

b. 99253, 410.01

c. 99233, 410.51

d. 99234, 410.81

8. Dr. Mathis has been called to the ICU to provide care for a 37-year-old male patient who has received second-degree burns of 50% of his body. Dr. Mathis provides support from 1 p.m. to 3 p.m. After leaving the unit to do his rounds, Dr.Mathis is called back around 5 p.m., and he provides critical care support to the patient until 6 p.m. Select the appropriate CPT and ICD-9-CM codes:

a. 99291, 99292 × 5, 948.50

b. 99291 × 3, 948.50

c. 99291, 99292 × 4, 948.50

d. 99291 × 2, 99292, 948.50

9. A 76-year-old female is admitted for IV antibiotic therapy to treat pneumonia due to pseudomonas bacteria and a level 3 initial inpatient visit was provided. On days 2 and 3, the patient had not yet responded to treatment as noted after an expanded problem-focused exam and history. On day 4, the patient showed significant improvement and the physician recorded a problem-focused history and exam. On day 5, the patient was discharged to home and the physician spent 30 minutes in discharge day management. Select the appropriate CPT and ICD-9-CM codes of the physician visits from the admit to the discharge.

a. 99222, 99232, 99231, 99238, 482.1

b. 99223, 99232, 99232, 99231, 99238, 482.1

c. 99223, 99232, 99231, 99231, 99238, 486

d. 99223, 99232, 99232, 99231, 99238, 486

10. **Chief complaint:** Cardiopulmonary arrest

History of present illness: The patient is a 53-year-old male with a history of aortic valve replacement and severe cardiomyopathy, chronic left bundle-branch block, and diabetes who presents after being found with agonal respirations by his wife. The patient was in his usual state of good health until last night at 3, when he apparently awoke from sleep with nonspecific complaints. The patient returned to sleep. At 4 a.m., the patient's wife noted him having agonal breathing and tried to wake him up. She immediately called 911 and began giving the patient ventilations. The patient's wife reports that the rescue squad arrived within 5 minutes and initiated CPR. Upon arrival, initial rhythm was a wide complex tachycardia, which most likely was ventricular tachycardia. The patient was cardioverted multiple times, probably eight. Subsequent rhythm appeared to be sinus tachycardia with a left bundle-branch block. The patient presented unconscious and has not regained consciousness. There were no preceding complaints other than left-shoulder cramping, which was short-lived. The patient has been compliant with medications apparently. The patient had no history of prior significant arrhythmic events. He does have a history of aortic valve replacement approximately 10 years ago. He has had subsequent decrease in left ventricular function since that time and has had episodes of congestive heart failure. He had a cardiac catheterization at the time of the aortic valve replacement, which showed normal coronary vessels.

Past medical history:

1. Positive for AVR.

2. Cardiomyopathy.

3. Diabetes.

4. Negative for hypertension, lung, liver, or kidney disease.

Medications on admission: Coumadin, Lasix, potassium, Zestril, Lanoxin

Social history: The patient does not smoke.

Family history: Positive for coronary artery disease. There is no premature coronary disease noted, however.

Review of systems: Otherwise unobtainable at present.

Physical examination: Blood pressure is currently 110/70. Initial blood pressure was approximately 80 systolic. Pulse is 110 and respirations are 14 on ventilator. The patient is afebrile.

HEENT: The pupils are 3 to 4 mm and reactive; doll's eyes are normal. Neck is supple. Carotids have diminished upstroke without bruits. Lungs are clear. Anteriorly heart is tachycardiac and distant, without murmur. There is a prosthetic S2. The abdomen is soft and nontender, without masses. Extremities have trace edema. Distal pulses are present.

Neurologic exam: The patient is unresponsive. He appears to decorticate with ventilatory respirations. He has spontaneous respirations. Pupils are reactive as noted above. Doll's eyes are normal.

EKG shows sinus tachycardia with left bundle-branch block. Labs are significant for initial potassium of 2.8. Initial blood gas pH of 7.29, CO_2 30, O_2 321 on the ventilator. Initial ABG prior to this showed a pH of 7.077 with a PCO_2 of 64. White count is currently normal. CPK is elevated at 600. Glucose is elevated at 411. BUN is 22. Creatinine is 1.8. Digoxin dose is noted to be 0.3.

Impression:

Cardiopulmonary arrest. The patient most likely had a primary arrhythmic event and was noted to have wide-complex tachycardia. He has a severe cardiomyopathy that is long-standing and a chronic left bundle-branch block. His initial potassium was low at 2.8. Currently the patient's rhythm is stable after having magnesium and calcium partially repleted, which is ongoing. The patient initially was treated with pressors; both these have been able to be weaned off partially with fairly stable blood pressure.

Status post-aortic valve replacement: The patient has had subsequent worsening of left ventricular function and now has a cardiomyopathy with a left ventricular ejection fraction of approximately 20%. This is controlled by bedside electrocardiogram.

Chronic left bundle-branch block is likely secondary to cardiomyopathy. Initial EKG suggested possibility of acute ischemic event. However, this most likely is spurious due to left bundle-branch block and possibly metabolic abnormalities.

Diabetes.

Neurologic: The patient currently has signs of a midbrain function; however, he has evidence for significant cortical dysfunction at present. It is unclear how long the patient was down prior to the wife attempting to wake him and finding him with agonal respirations.

Plan:

Admit to ICU.

Rule out MI.

Pressor support as necessary.

Neurologic evaluation.

Pulmonary evaluation

Replete potassium.

Check echocardiogram.

I have discussed the possibility of a cardiac catheterization with the family. This patient has a chronic cardiomyopathy and left bundle-branch pattern on EKG. I feel it is a very low likelihood that he is having an acute ischemic episode. The patient also is noted to have normal coronary arteries on previous cardiac catheterization. Cardiac catheterization at this point is felt to have a very high risk-benefit ratio and will not be attempted unless the patient shows some signs of neurologic improvement.

Select the appropriate CPT and ICD-9-CM codes:

a. 92950, 99288, 427.5

b. 99285, 92950, 99233, 427.1, 425.4, 426.3

c. 99223, 427.1, 425.4, 426.3, V42.2, 250.00

d. 99285, 427.1, 425.4, 426.3, V42.2, 250.00

HCPCS Level II

1. On May 18 a respiratory suction pump was provided to Roger Gordon, who has been diagnosed with emphysema. The first unit was found to be defective, so another unit was delivered on May 19. Select the appropriate HCPCS Level II and ICD-9-CM codes:

   a. E0600 × 2, 492.8

   b. E0600, 492.8

   c. E0600, E0600-RA, 492.8

   d. E0600, E0600-59, 492.8

2. Health and behavior intervention each 15 minutes face-to-face and/or family for a patient's morbid obesity. Select the appropriate CPT, HCPCS Level II, and ICD-9-CM codes:

   a. 96154-HR, 278.01

   b. 96155-HR, 278.00

   c. 96154, 278.01

   d. 96155, 278.01

3. A 10-year-old, who has broken the same arm in the past, now presents to the orthopedic office for a cast application. The physician puts on a long-arm fiberglass cast. Select the appropriate CPT and HCPCS Level II codes:

   a. 29065, Q4007

   b. 29065, Q4008

   c. 29065, Q4020

   d. 29065, A4590

4. A 50-year-old Medicare patient is seen in the office for a colorectal cancer screening, fecal occult blood test, and immunoassay. Select the appropriate HCPCS Level II and ICD-9-CM codes:

   a. G0107, V76.51

   b. G0328, V76.51

   c. 88270, V76.51

   d. 88272, V76.51

5. The patient is given an infusion of dextran 75 w/NaCl 1,000 mL for iron replacement for anemia. Select the appropriate CPT and ICD-9-CM codes:

   a. J7110 × 2, 280.9
   b. J7100 × 2, 280.9
   c. J7042 280.9
   d. J7030, 280.9

Practice Management

1. Medicare Part A pays for all of the following except:
   a. Hospital
   b. Hospice
   c. Nursing home—acute care
   d. Durable medical equipment

2. The purpose of the medical record includes:
   a. Source of statistics
   b. Compliance with coding and reimbursement
   c. Continuity of care
   d. All of these

3. Managed care policies include all of the following except:
   a. PPO
   b. FFS
   c. HMO
   d. EPO

4. Once the claim is processed, the insurance company sends the following to the provider:
   a. Letter of explanation
   b. Explanation of benefits
   c. No communication
   d. Remittance advice

5. Government health insurance programs include all of the following except:
   a. Blue Cross/Blue Shield
   b. Medicaid
   c. Medicare
   d. TRICARE

GLOSSARY

A

ablation Procedure that involves scarring or destroying cardiac tissue that triggers an abnormal heart rhythm.

accounts receivable (A/R) Revenue that is due to the practice or provider for services or procedures rendered to the patient; may be due from health insurance coverage, workers' compensation, liability coverage, or the patient.

acute Condition with a sudden onset, usually without warning, and of brief duration.

adjacent tissue transfer Type of tissue transfer in which the tissue remains attached to its original anatomical location.

Advance Beneficiary Notice (ABN) A waiver needed for any service that does not meet the coverage criteria established in an NCD or LCD.

advanced life support (ALS) Ambulance services that include BLS procedures as well as establishment of an IV, drawing of blood, use of a cardiac monitor, intubation, tracheotomy, use of CPAP, and nasogastric tube placement.

airway management Process of maintaining an open airway for ventilation of the lungs; methods include endotracheal, through an existing tracheotomy, or via a mask or nasal cannula.

allergen immunotherapy The injecting of small doses of an allergen and increasing the amount of the dose over time to desensitize the patient to the substance.

allograft Skin graft in which tissue from a human donor is applied to the recipient. Also called *nonautologous graft*.

alveoli Air sacs located at the end of the bronchioles through which oxygen and carbon dioxide pass

Alzheimer's disease Disease due to the destruction of subcortical white matter of the brain.

amenorrhea Lack of menstruation.

American Academy of Professional Coders (AAPC) Organization that administers the CPC exam and confers the Certified Professional Coder credential; supports its members by providing coding education, identifying job opportunities, and offering networking opportunities.

American Recovery and Reinvestment Act (ARRA) Legislation enacted to promote economic recovery and growth and provide the opportunity to enhance the nation's health care system through investment in health information technology.

and In ICD, notation meaning "and/or."

anesthesia Without sensation or loss of sensation; can be partial or complete.

aneurysm A bulge or swelling in the wall of a vessel.

angina pectoris Severe chest pain due to insufficient blood supply to the heart.

angiography X-ray exam of the arteries or veins to diagnose conditions of the blood vessels, such as blockage.

antepartum The period beginning with conception and ending at the time of delivery.

anterior Body direction that is to the front of the body or front of an organ.

anterior nasal hemorrhage control Insertion of gauze packing or anterior packing or cauterization

aorta The largest artery; carries oxygenated blood from the left ventricle to the body.

aortic valve Valve located between the left ventricle and the aorta; when open, allows the blood to exit the left ventricle and enter the aorta.

aphakia The absence of a lens.

appendicular skeleton The bones of the upper and lower extremities, which make body movement possible.

approach The means by which the provider gains access to the body to complete a service or procedure.

arrhythmia An irregular heartbeat.

ascites Abnormal accumulation of fluid in the peritoneal cavity.

audiometry Measurement of the level of hearing.

auris dextra (AD) Right ear.

auris sinistra (AS) Left ear.

auris unitas (AU) Each ear.

autograft Skin graft in which tissue harvested from a patient's own body is applied to another area of the patient's body.

autonomic nervous system System that controls the muscles of internal organs; divided into the sympathetic nervous system and the parasympathetic nervous system.

axial plane Horizontal plane that divides the body into upper and lower portions. Also called *transverse plane*.

axial skeleton The skull, spinal column, ribs, and sternum, which protect major organs of the nervous, respiratory, and circulatory systems.

B

Bartholin's glands Glands that are located next to the vaginal opening; function is to produce mucous secretions.

base units Units of value assigned by the ASA to all CPT surgical codes; the first component in the formula for assigning a cost-revenue value to an anesthesia service.

basic life support (BLS) Ambulance services that include basic CPR, trauma care, basic airway management, and use of pulse oximetry equipment.

benign Noninvasive tumor that remains localized.

benign prostatic hyperplasia (BPH) Enlargement of the prostate gland, which can interfere with urinary function.

billing language A medical coding language that includes terms such as *accounts receivable (A/R), clean claims, denials, modifiers,* and *advanced beneficiary notices (ABNs).*

biofeedback Training in which the patient is taught how certain responses to thought processes, stimuli, and actions can affect physical responses.

biopsy The removal of all or part of a lesion for pathologic examination.

block A portion of tissue obtained from a specimen.

bolus A mixture of food and digestive enzymes in the saliva.

brachytherapy The application of radioactive isotopes for internal radiation.

bronchi In the lungs, tubular structures that branch into bronchioles.

bullet (●) In CPT, the symbol that designates a new code for the current edition of the manual.

bull's-eye (◉) In CPT, the symbol designating that the use of moderate sedation is included in the code description and is not to be reported separately.

C

carcinoma in situ A neoplasm whose cells are localized in the epithelium and do not invade or metastasize into surrounding tissue.

cataracts A clouding of the lens of the eye or the lens capsule, which envelopes the lens.

cecum Pouch at the beginning of the large intestine that links to the ileum.

Centers for Medicare and Medicaid Services (CMS) Government agency that, nationally, oversees and develops payment policy and integrates management of administrative contractors and, locally, administers Medicare through the MACs.

central nervous system (CNS) System that includes the brain and spinal cord and is responsible for coordination and communication within the entire body.

cerclage The suturing of the opening of the cervix—treatment for incompetent cervix (i.e., the cervix is unable to contain the pregnant uterus).

cerebellum Brain structure that is located posterior to the brainstem and inferior to the cerebrum; responsible for fine motor coordination and movement, posture, and balance. Also called *hindbrain.*

cerebrum Brain structure that directs conscious motor functions, processes sensory input, and governs intelligence and reasoning, allowing for speech, memory, and learning.

Certified Professional Coder (CPC) An individual who has demonstrated his or her knowledge of medical coding by successfully completing the CPC exam.

Certified Professional Coder (CPC) exam Exam that tests the coder's skill in translating data from the patient's medical record accurately and completely so that the provider is reimbursed correctly and fairly and within compliance guidelines.

Certified Registered Nurse Anesthetist (CRNA) A provider of anesthesia care who may act under the direction of an anesthesiologist or may provide the service without medical direction.

cervix uteri The lower, narrow part of the uterus where it joins with the vagina. Also called *neck of the uterus.*

chief complaint The reason for the present encounter, usually in the patient's own words.

choledocholithiasis Condition in which stones form in the biliary duct and gallbladder.

cholelithiasis Gallstones.

chromatography A combination of stationary and mobile phases used to analyze a drug class or classes.

chronic Condition with a slow onset and of long duration.

cilia Hairlike projections within each fallopian tube that aid in the movement of the egg through the tube.

clean claim A CMS-1500 claim that is complete and accurate from the demographic portion to the diagnosis and procedure. If it is not, the contractual turnaround, or adjudication, timeframe does not have to be met.

clinical treatment planning The development of a plan for the course of radiation therapy.

closed fracture A fracture that is closed to the environment or does not protrude through the skin (e.g., greenstick fracture).

closed procedure Procedure that is completed without incision and is considered noninvasive in nature.

closed treatment Fracture treatment in which the fracture is not surgically opened and directly visualized.

coagulation A process of blood clotting.

code first Informs the coder that the code being referenced is sequenced second to the primary code.

colposcopy Visualization of the vagina and cervical tissue through a scope.

complex repair Repair that requires additional repair work, such as retention suturing, debridement, or placement of stents or drains.

compliance language A medical coding language that brings terms such as *unbundling, fraud, false claim,* and *abuse* into the translation of the medical record.

compliance plan A written plan consisting of standards and procedures designed to implement compliance and practice standards.

computed tomography (CT) A radiology imaging modality used to study structures in a body plane; produces computerized cross-section views.

conduction disorder A disturbance in the electrical impulse of the heart.

conscious sedation See **moderate sedation.**

consultation A visit that is requested in writing and that involves the rendering of an opinion and the compilation of a written report.

contrast material A dye or another substance that is used to enhance the image of an organ or tissue being examined.

cornea The clear part of the eye that covers the pupil and iris.

coronal plane Vertical plane running from side to side that divides the body into anterior and posterior portions. Also called *frontal plane.*

coronary artery bypass graft (CABG) A procedure used to improve blood flow to the heart by bypassing a vessel blockage with a grafted vessel.

corpectomy The removal or resection of the anterior portion of the vertebrae (spinal column).

corpus uteri The main body of the uterus; function is to protect a developing fetus.

covered entity Any provider or organization that transmits health information electronically.

Cowper's glands Pea-size structures on the sides of the urethra, below the prostate. Also called *bulbourethral glands.*

craniectomy An excision of the cranium in which a bone flap is removed and not returned to the original site.

craniotomy An incision into the cranium in which a bone flap is removed and then returned either immediately or at a later time (delayed) to the original site.

critical care Service that is provided to a patient suffering from an illness or injury that impairs one or more organ systems and has a high potential of life-threatening deterioration.

Cushing's syndrome Disorder in which the body is exposed to high levels of the hormone cortisol over an extended period of time; most commmonly caused by use of oral corticosteriod medication.

cytogenic studies Studies concerned with cellular abnormalities and pathologic conditions related to genetics.

cytopathology The study of cells.

D

debridement Removal of a foreign object or damaged tissue either by excision (surgically cutting away) or nonexcision (e.g., brushing or irrigating).

deep vein thrombosis (DVT) Inflammation of a vein with development of a thrombus in a deep vein.

default codes In ICD-10-CM, codes that are unspecified or are most often used with a condition; located directly behind the boldface main term and used only when the provider's documentation has no additional detail on the patient's condition or disease.

defibrillator An electrical device inserted into the body to shock the heart into regular rhythm through a combination of antitachycardia pacing, low-energy cardioversion, and shocks; generally used to treat ventricular tachycardia or ventricular fibrillation.

dermis The middle layer of the skin; lies below the epidermis.

destruction The destroying of tissue by means of heat, cold, or chemicals.

diagnostic nuclear medicine study A study performed to establish or confirm a diagnosis.

diaphragm Separates the thoracic and abdominal cavities.

diaphysis The shaft of a long bone.

direct laryngoscopy Visualization of the larynx by means of a rigid or fiber-optic endoscope.

dislocation Displacement of a bone from its normal location.

distal A body part that is farthest from the point of reference, midpoint, or beginning.

diverticulitis Inflammation of the diverticula.

diverticulosis A condition of the diverticula.

dual-energy x-ray absorptiometry (DXA) Radiological study performed to measure bone density, usually in patients with osteoporosis.

duodenal ulcer An ulcer in the first, or upper, section of the intestine.

duodenum The first section of the small intestine.

duplex scan Ultrasound test used to evaluate the flow of blood within arteries and veins.

durable medical equipment (DME) Equipment that can withstand extended use and is often prescribed for patients' home use.

dystocia Difficult or painful labor.

E

ectomy Suffix meaning removal by cutting all or part.

electronic health record Electronic documentation of patient's medical history.

embolus A foreign object, such as a detached blood clot, that moves through the bloodstream, lodges in a blood vessel, and occludes the vessel.

emegency condition Any condition for which a delay in treatment would lead to a significant increase in the threat to life or a body part.

emergency department (ED) A 24-hour facility that provides services to unscheduled patients who have immediate concerns.

encephalititis Inflammation of the brain tissue and spinal cord. Also called *myelitis.*

endocardium The inner layer of the heart-wall tissue.

endometrium Innermost layer of the uterus; functions as a lining.

endoscopic retrograde cholangiopancreatography (ERCP) X-ray exam of the pancreatic and biliary ducts.

endoscopy Visual examination within a cavity.

enteral therapy Therapy administered within the intestine; often accomplished through the gastrointestinal tract via a gastric feeding tube or gastrostomy.

epicardium The outer layer of the heart-wall tissue.

epidermis The outer layer of the skin; forms a protective covering.

epididymis A long, coiled tube located on the back of the testicle.

epiglottis A small flap of cartilage that closes over the trachea, preventing food from entering the larynx and thus the lungs.

epiphyses The ends of a long bone.

eponym The proper name of the person who first identified the condition or disease, the physician who first developed the treatment or procedure for the condition, or the first patient diagnosed with the condition.

erythropoiesis Production of red blood cells.

erythropoietin Hormone that stimulates erythropoiesis.

escharotomy Release of scar from underlying tissue by means of incising or cutting.

established patient A patient who *has* received services from the physician or another physician of the *exact same specialty or subspecialty* in the same group within the past 3 years.

ethmoid sinus Paranasal sinus between the nose and the eyes.

etiology The underlying cause, or origin, of a condition or disease.

eustachian tubes Structures that connect the middle ear to the nasopharynx and that equalize pressure and drain mucus from the middle ear.

excision Removal by cutting all or part. Suffix is *-ectomy.*

excludes In ICD-9-CM, a note that lists conditions, diseases, or injuries that are not included in the code being considered in the Tabular List (Volume 1).

Excludes 1 In ICD-10-CM, a note indicating that the condition, disease, or injury being coded is located elsewhere in the manual and should never be coded with the code under which it is located. Conditions identified by this note cannot be present together and therefore are never coded during the same encounter.

Excludes 2 In ICD-10-CM, a note indicating that the condition excluded is distinct from the code condition and is coded elsewhere in the manual. The condition excluded may occur with the condition represented by the code, and these two codes may be coded together during the same encounter.

expiration/exhalation Opposite of inspiration; as the diaphragm and intercostal muscles relax, air is pushed out of the lungs.

extenders In ICD-10-CM, alphabetic seventh characters used to complete the description of many codes by conveying additional information (e.g., episode of care, type of fracture, late effects, or trimester of pregnancy).

extension A straightening movement that increases the angle at the joint.

external approach Approach through the skin to the respiratory tract.

external fixation Fracture treatment in which skeletal pins are attached to an external mechanism.

extubation Removal of a flexible tube previously placed in the trachea for airway management.

F

face-to-face time The actual time the provider spends with the patient and/or family in the office or outpatient setting.

facetectomy Removal of the facet or bony overgrowth from the facet that leads to compression of the nerve root.

facing triangles (▶◀) In CPT, the symbol that designates which portion of the code text describing the procedure or text in the guideline or note has been revised for the current edition of the manual.

fascia A sheet of fibrous connective tissue that covers, supports, and separates muscle.

fimbriae Fingerlike structures at the end of each fallopian tube that capture and sweep the egg into the tube.

first listed The reason for the visit; used for provider and outpatient coding.

fissure A groove or a crack.

flexion A bending movement that decreases the angle at the joint.

fluoroscopy A study that creates real-time or moving images that are useful for diagnostic procedures and for guidance in interventional procedures.

foraminotomy Enlargement of the foramen, or hole, through which the nerve root exits the spinal canal.

full-thickness graft Skin graft that involves all layers through to the subcutaneous.

gastric ulcer An ulcer in the stomach.

gastroesophageal reflux disease (GERD) Weakness of the valve between the esophagus and stomach that can cause stomach acid to reflux.

gastrojejunal ulcer An ulcer in the stomach and jejunum (third, or last, section of the intestine).

general anesthesia Type of anesthesia in which the patient airway must be managed by an anesthesiologist or another qualified professional.

glaucoma Condition that develops when pressure builds within the eye due to an increase in fluid and leads to damage of the optic nerve.

global surgical package A prescribed period of time surrounding a surgical procedure. Also called *postoperative*, or *post-op, period.*

glomerulus A region of the kidney through which blood passes as it enters the kidney and which filters the blood, removing water and waste products.

Graves' disease Hyperthyroidism, or toxic diffuse goiter.

harvest Removal of a donor's organ, tissue, or bone for implantation into another anatomical site or patient.

Health Information Technology for Economic and Clinical Health (HITECH) Act Legislation that addresses security and privacy issues related to the electronic transmission of health information; outlines rules and regulations as well as penalties for violations of the rules.

Health Insurance Portability and Accountability Act (HIPAA) Legislation that addresses security and privacy issues related to the electronic transmission of health information.

hematology The study of disorders of the blood.

hemilaminectomy See **Laminotomy.**

hemiparesis Weakness on one side of the body.

hemiplegia Loss of the ability to move one side of the body; total paralysis.

hemodialysis Dialysis procedure in which a man-made membrane is used to filter waste and toxins, remove and maintain fluid, and balance electrolytes by mechanically circulating the blood through a machine and transfusing it back to the body.

hemofiltration Dialysis procedure, similar to hemodialysis, in which large amounts of blood are passed through filters that remove waste and excess fluid.

hernia Protrusion of an anatomical structure through the wall of the cavity in which it is normally located.

hierarchical condition categories (HCCs) A means of assessing the risk of medically managing each patient based on current conditions and comorbid conditions that are impacting care.

history of present illness (HPI) Description of the illness or injury that precipitated the present encounter.

hydrocephalus A disorder of the ventricle and/or cerebrospinal fluid that leads to increased intracranial pressure.

hypermetropia Farsightedness.

hypothalamus Structure that links the nervous system to the endocrine system, regulates hormone secretion, and is the control center for many autonomic functions of the peripheral nervous system.

hypotony Low intraocular pressure.

I

ileum The last section of the small intestine.

immunology The study of the immune system.

impacted cerumen An accumulation of earwax.

impending conditions In ICD, specific diagnostic conditions whose codes are used only when the condition was averted due to medical intervention. Also called *threatened conditions.*

impingement syndrome Condition in which inflamed and swollen tendons are caught in the narrow space between the bones within the shoulder joint.

incision Creation of an opening by surgically cutting into the skin or other tissue. Suffix is *-tomy.*

incision and drainage (I&D) Procedure in which either a needle or scalpel is used to open or access and then drain an area or site.

includes ICD instructional note that clarifies the code or category being considered by providing definitions or examples of conditions included in the code.

indirect laryngoscopy Visualization of the larynx by means of a mirror positioned at the back of the throat.

infarction The death of tissue.

infection Invasion of the body by a pathogenic organism.

inferior Body direction that is below another body part or toward the feet. Also called *caudal.*

inflammation A localized response to an injury or destruction of tissue.

inpatient An individual who has been formally admitted to a heath care facility.

insight-oriented behavior modifying and/or supportive psychotherapy Psychotherapy that involves the patient's attaining insight and understanding through the use of behavior modification and supportive interaction.

inspiration/inhalation Diaphragm and intercostal muscles contract. Air is drawn into the lungs.

interactive complexity Specific communication factors that complicate delivery of a psychiatric procedure.

interactive psychotherapy Psychotherapy that involves the use of physical aids, such as play equipment, and non-verbal communications to achieve therapeutic interaction.

intermediate repair Repair in which a wound is closed in layers, such as by suturing the subcutaneous in one layer and then the dermis in a second layer.

internal approach Approach through the respiratory system.

internal fixation Fracture treatment in which wires, pins, screws, etc., are placed through or within the fracture site to stabilize the fracture.

intra-arterial (IA) Route of administration through the arterial system.

intracerebral Within the cerebrum.

intracranial Within the skull.

intracutaneous Within the skin.

intramuscular (IM) Route of administration through the muscular system.

intraocular lens (IOL) Artificial lens permanently implanted in the eye.

intrathecal (IT) Route of administration within the sheath through the membrane.

intravenous (IV) Route of administration through the venous system.

intubation Placement of a flexible tube into the trachea to maintain an open airway.

intussusception The sliding of one part of the intestine into another.

ionized calcium Free-flowing calcium, not attached to proteins.

irreversible ischemia Condition in which heart muscle is denied adequate blood flow for an extended period of time and the muscle dies.

ischemia Condition in which heart muscle is denied adequate blood flow for an extended period of time and the muscle dies.

isopter Outer edge of a visual field.

J

jejunum The middle section of the small intestine.

L

labia majora Outermost structure of the vulva; contains sweat- and oil-secreting glands.

labia minora Structure that lies inside the labia majora; contains the vaginal and urethral openings and the clitoris.

laceration A tear, cut, or open wound.

laminectomy Removal of the lamina of a vertebral segment.

laminotomy Removal of the superior or inferior half of the lamina. Also called *hemilaminectomy.*

laparoscopy Process of inserting a scope through the wall of the abdomen for examination of the abdominal cavity.

larynx Structure that houses the vocal cords. Also called *voice box.*

late effect Used to describe a residual condition that occurs after the initial illness or injury has healed.

lesion An abnormal or pathologic change in tissue due to disease or injury.

ligament A band of fibrous tissue that connects two or more bones or cartilages.

linkage The process of supporting the medical necessity of the CPT code(s) with the ICD code(s).

Local Coverage Determinations (LCDs) Rules developed at the local level by Medicare Administrative Contractors that identify payment coverage for a specific service, procedure, test, or technology based on medical necessity or frequency.

luna Moon-shaped, whitish area located beneath the proximal end of the nail.

lymph node A collection of tissue located along the lymph vessels that acts as a filter and produces antibodies and lymphocytes.

M

magnetic resonance imaging (MRI) A radiology imaging modality that uses a magnetic field and radio waves to produce images of organs and tissues.

main term In the provider's diagnostic statement, the term that identifies the patient's condition, injury, or disease; used in locating a code in the Alphabetic Index of ICD.

male reproductive system System whose functions include production of male hormones and production and transportation of sperm.

malignant An invasive tumor that spreads beyond the tumor site.

malunion An incorrectly healing (i.e., faulty, incomplete) fracture.

manifestation The way a condition due to an underlying disease or condition presents itself.

manipulation Attempted reduction or restoration of a fracture or joint to its normal anatomical alignment by the application of manually applied force.

matrix Substance located beneath the skin of the finger at the proximal end of the nail.

measles, mumps, rubella, and varicella (MMRV) vaccine A combination vaccine.

maxillary sinus Cavity in the skull which opens into the nasal cavity located under the eyes within the maxillary bone.

medical coding The process of translating provider documentation and medical terminology into codes that illustrate the procedures and services performed by medical professionals.

medical decision making (MDM) A key component used to determine the appropriate level of an E/M code; includes the number of management options or diagnoses, data reviewed, and risk factors the physician encounters during the E/M encounter.

medical direction Physician involvement with and direction of anesthesia that is carried out by a qualified provider.

medical necessity Any diagnosis, condition, procedure, and/or service that is documented in the patient record as having been treated or medically managed.

medically managed A diagnosis which may not receive direct treatment during an encounter but which the provider has to consider when determining treatment for other conditions.

medically unlikely edits (MUE) Edits that identify limits for units of service for a given service or procedure completed by a single provider per patient per day.

Medicare Administrative Contractor (MAC) CMS contracting entities responsible for enrolling and educating providers; receiving, adjudicating, and paying claims; and detecting fraud and abuse within their jurisdictions.

meningitis Inflammation of the meninges of the brain and/or spinal cord.

metastasis Secondary site or spread of the primary malignancy.

methicillin resistant staphylococcus aureus (MRSA) septicemia Antibiotic-resistant staph infection.

micturition Urination.

minimally invasive procedure A procedure such as an injection or infusion.

mitral valve A two-flapped valve that allows blood to flow from the left atrium into the left ventricle. Also called *bicuspid valve.*

modalities The application of an agent or device used to change tissues; include heat, sound, light, and mechanical or electrical energy.

moderate sedation A level of consciousness in which the patient can still respond to verbal commands. Also called *conscious sedation.*

modifier In CPT, an addition to the code that is used to show that the service or procedure performed was altered in some way.

Mohs surgery Procedure in which the physician acts as both the surgeon and the pathologist.

molecular pathology Laboratory testing involving genes.

monitored anesthesia care (MAC) Type of anesthesia reported when the patient airway is managed by the patient or when no information is documented indicating that the airway was managed by a provider.

mononeuritis Inflammation of a single nerve; may affect the body along the entire nerve path.

motor studies Studies of efferent impulses, nerve signals going from the spinal cord to the muscles.

mutations Variants associated with altered gene function that lead to functional deficits or disease.

myelitis See **Encephalititis.**

myocardium The muscle layer of the heart-wall tissue.

myometrium Smooth muscle that forms the wall of the uterus; functions to expel the fetus and placenta and reduce blood loss during labor and delivery.

myopia Nearsightedness.

N

nasal hemorrhage Nasal bleeding, epistasis.

National Correct Coding Initiative (NCCI) Program designed to encourage correct coding methodologies and control inappropriate payments due to improper coding of Part B claims.

National Coverage Determinations (NCDs) CMS national-level rules that identify payment coverage for a specific service, procedure, test, or technology based on medical necessity or frequency.

NEC Notation meaning "not elsewhere classified"; indicates that a more specific code is not provided in the ICD manual.

nephrons Kidney cells whose functions are to filter blood and form urine.

nerve conduction studies Studies that measure the time required for a signal to traverse the nerve pathway to and from a muscle.

nerve plexus A network of intersecting nerves and blood and lymph vessels; named for the area of the body in which it is located.

neurorrhaphy Repair of transected nerves by suturing.

new patient A patient who has *not* received services from the physician or another physician of the *exact same specialty or subspecialty* in the same group within the past 3 years.

nonautologous graft See **allograft.**

noninvasive procedure A procedure that does not require a surgical incision or excision.

nonsegmental instrumentation Spinal instrumentation in which a device (rod) is attached by hooks or screws to the spine only at each end of the device.

nonselective debridement Procedure in which devitalized tissue is removed with healthy tissue by scrubbing the wound and using wet-to-dry dressings or enzymes. Also called *mechanical debridement.*

nonunion Failure of a fracture to heal.

NOS Notation meaning "not otherwise specified"; the equivalent of unspecified.

nuclear medicine A field of studies that involve diagnostic and therapeutic use of radioactive materials.

null zero (ϕ) In CPT, the symbol designating that modifier 51 is not to be used with the code.

O

oculus dexter (OD) Right eye.

oculus sinister (OS) Left eye.

oculus uterque (OU) Each eye.

Office of Inspector General Agency that investigates allegations of fraud, waste, abuse, or misconduct and assists the executive branch in identifying and correcting operational deficiencies.

open fracture A fracture that is open to the environment and protrudes outside the skin (e.g., compound and missile fractures).

open procedure Procedure that involves an incision in the skin or other membranes so that the provider has full view of the organs or structures.

open treatment Fracture treatment in which the skin is surgically opened and the fracture is visualized or the fracture site is opened remotely in order to insert an intramedullary nail across the site.

opportunistic infections (OIs) HIV-related illnesses. When an OI is documented in conjunction with HIV-positive status, convert the patient's diagnosis from HIV-positive status V08 to (AIDS) 042.

organ panel A series of specific tests ordered to assist in the determination of a diagnosis.

orthotic procedures and devices Procedures and devices used to support, align, or correct and thereby improve the function of body parts such as muscles, ligaments, or bones.

-oscopy Suffix meaning visual examination through a scope.

ossicles Small bones that amplify sound vibration from the tympanic membrane and relay it to the inner ear.

osteoarthritis Condition characterized by inflammation of the bone and joint. Also called *wear-and-tear arthritis.*

osteoporosis Condition characterized by thinning of bone tissue and loss of bone density, causing the bones to become brittle and weak.

-ostomy Suffix meaning surgical creation of an artificial opening.

otitis externa Inflammation of the external ear canal. Also called *swimmer's ear.*

-otomy Suffix meaning creation of an opening by surgically cutting into the skin or other tissue.

outpatient An individual who has not been formally admitted to a healthcare facility.

Outpatient Prospective Payment System (OPPS) Medicare's system for payment to outpatient departments of hospitals and other outpatient facilities.

ovary Small oval-shaped gland that produces the oocyte, and female hormones.

oviduct Also known as fallopian tubes. Primary function is transportation of the oocyte.

P

parenteral therapy Therapy in which the patient receives the nutritional material subcutaneously, intravenously, or intramuscularly.

parentheses Punctuation marks used in the ICD manuals to enclose supplemental terms, or nonessential modifiers.

parenthetical notes Notes that provide additional information about the code; may inform the coder that the service/procedure described by the code(s) being reviewed is a part of or included in the code for the service/procedure listed in the parenthetical note.

paring The removal of cornified epithelial layers by skinning or trimming back the overgrowth.

Parkinson's disease Disease due to the degeneration of nigral neurons, which are responsible for creating dopamine (a neurotransmitter).

past, family, and social history (PFSH) A listing of a patient's past surgeries, allergies, marital status, and family illnesses.

pathologic fracture A fracture that is caused by disease rather than trauma.

payer language Language that comprises terms such as *noncovered services, medical necessity, compliance language, and unbundling.*

percutaneous Type of surgical procedure completed through the skin that involves viewing the site indirectly (e.g., via fluoroscopy) rather than directly through an open view.

pericardium The membrane sac that encases the heart.

peripartum The period that begins 30 days prior to delivery and extends to 5 months after delivery.

peripheral nervous system (PNS) System that consists of nerves only and connects the brain and spinal cord to the body.

peritoneal dialysis Dialysis procedure in which a solution is introduced into the lining of the abdominal cavity to remove waste and excessive fluid from the body.

pharynx Structure that connects the nose and the mouth to the larynx. Also called *throat.*

photodynamic therapy Therapy in which a photosensitizing agent is applied to a lesion (e.g., an actinic keratosis) and the patient returns for light treatment, which activates the chemical agent to destroy the lesion.

physical status modifiers Modifiers used with all anesthesia procedure codes to rank the physical condition of the patient and the level of anesthesia complexity inherent in each ranking.

pineal gland Gland that is located near the brainstem and is involved in regulation of body functions (e.g., sleep rhythms and endocrine functions).

pituitary gland Gland that is located near the brainstem and directs other endocrine glands. Also called *master gland.*

placeholder character In ICD-10-CM, an "×" placed in the fourth-, fifth-, or sixth-character position when needed to enable the seventh-character extender to remain in the seventh-character position.

-plasty Suffix meaning "the reshaping or replacing of a body part by surgical means."

pleura Membrane surrounding the lung. It contains two layers; one covers the lungs and the other lines the chest cavity.

plus sign (+) In CPT, the symbol designating that a code is an additional code to be used with the primary procedure and never to be used alone.

polysomnography A test performed to measure sleep cycles and sleep stages, REM and NREM.

post-anesthesia care unit (PACU) The unit where a patient is monitored by a nurse specializing in postsedation care.

posterior A body part that is closest to the point of reference, midpoint, or beginning.

posterior nasal hemorrhage control Procedure which often requires the use of nasal stents, balloon catheters, or posterior packing.

postpartum The period of 6 weeks following delivery.

prepuce Foreskin which surrounds and protects the head of the penis.

presbyopia Condition characterized by errors in focus of the eyes due to age.

preventive care Service that is provided to a patient in order to maintain health and prevent disease.

primary neoplasm Site of origin of a malignancy.

principal diagnosis The reason for admission after study; used for facility coding.

pronation Rotation of the forearm with the palm facing down.

protected health information (PHI) Any medical or financial information held or managed by a covered entity.

provider language Medical billing and coding language that is built on medical terminology, anatomy, and pathophysiology and describes services, procedures, and their medical necessity.

puerperium The period that begins with the delivery of the placenta and extends through 6 weeks after delivery.

Q

qualifying-circumstance modifiers Modifiers used to report challenging circumstances under which anesthesia may be provided.

qualitative analysis Laboratory procedure that identifies the presence of a drug.

quantitative analysis Laboratory procedure that measures the amount of a drug present.

R

radiopharmaceutical Radioactive drug used for therapeutic or diagnostic purposes in nuclear medicine studies.

repair Restoration of diseased or damaged tissue, organ, bone, etc.; can be described in documentation as *suture, revise,* or *restore.*

revenue cycle The flow of a practice's revenue, which begins when charges for services, procedures, or supplies are incurred and continues until those charges are paid in full or adjusted off the account.

reversible ischemia The heart muscle function is below normal levels.

review of systems (ROS) A series of questions presented to the patient in order to identify any signs, symptoms, or contributing factors relevant to the present encounter.

route of administration The method or path used for the entrance of a drug or other substance into the body.

S

sagittal plane Vertical plane running from front to back that divides the body into right and left sides. Also called *lateral plane.*

sclera Structure that forms the visible white of the eye and surrounds the optic nerve.

secondary diabetes mellitus Diabetes due to an underlying condition or cause.

secondary neoplasm The spread or metastases of a malignancy.

segmental instrumentation Spinal implementation in which a device (rod) is attached by hooks or screws to the spine at each end of the device and at least one other point of the spine along the device.

selective debridement Procedure in which instruments or devices are used to cut away only dead (necrotic) or devitalized tissue.

semicolon (;) In CPT, the punctuation mark indicating that the verbiage preceding it in a stand-alone code is shared with all dependent codes that follow it, thus providing a full description of the service or procedure for each dependent code.

seminal vesicle A saclike pouch that is attached to the vas deferens and produces seminal fluid.

seminiferous tubules Coiled masses of tubes that are responsible for producing sperm cells through a process called *spermatogenesis.*

sensory nerve studies Studies of afferent impulses, nerve signals traveling to the spinal cord.

separate procedure Although it may be performed alone, a service/procedure that, when performed with a more extensive service/procedure at the same site, is considered a part of the more extensive service/procedure and therefore is not separately reportable.

sepsis A response specifically to infection.

septic shock A form of organ failure of the vascular system.

septicemia The presence of toxins or disease in the blood, such as bacteria or a fungus.

septum The wall dividing the right and left sides of the heart.

sequela The condition produced after the initial injury or condition has healed.

severe sepsis Sepsis with organ failure.

shaving A sharp removal by transverse incision or horizontal slicing.

sign An objective condition that can be measured and recorded.

simple repair Repair in which a wound is closed in one layer regardless of the wound depth.

simulation-aided field setting Setting that is done before a radiation therapy course of treatment begins; visualizes and defines the exact treatment area and helps decide the size and location of the ports.

skeletal traction Application of force to a limb through a wire, pin, screw, or clamp that is attached to a bone.

skin traction Application of force to a limb by means of felt or strapping applied directly to the skin only.

slanted brackets In ICD-9-CM, punctuation marks used to identify the mandatory sequencing of etiology/manifestation coding.

somatic nervous system System that regulates body movement through control of skeletal or voluntary muscles.

specimen A unit submitted for evaluation, such as chemical, pathologic or hematological.

spermatic cord Cord that secures the testes in the scrotum.

sphenoid sinus Paranasal sinus at the center of the skull base.

spirometry The measurement of breathing or breath; used to measure both the flow (speed) of inhalation or exhalation and the amount, or volume, of air inhaled or exhaled.

split-thickness graft A graft that involves the epidermis and part of the dermis.

sprain A joint injury that usually involves a stretched or torn ligament.

square brackets In ICD-9-CM, punctuation marks used to enclose explanatory phrases or synonyms of a condition and, when directly below the code in the Tabular List, to enclose valid fifth digits for that code. In ICD-10-CM, punctuation marks used in the Tabular List to enclose explanatory phrases or synonyms of the condition and valid fifth digits for the code; used in the Alphabetic Index to identify mandatory sequencing of etiology/manifestation coding.

status migrainous A severe migraine that lasts for 72 hours or more and may lead to hospitalization.

stenosis Narrowing of a artery or a valve.

stereotactic Medical imaging technique that creates a 3-D image of a specific anatomical site for therapeutic surgical or diagnostic interventions or localization of a tumor prior to radiation therapy.

strabismus A condition that affects the ability of both eyes to point in the same direction, thus affecting a person's depth perception.

strain An injury to the body of a muscle or the attachment of a tendon; usually associated with overuse injuries that involve a stretched or torn muscle or tendon attachment.

subcutaneous The deepest layer of the integumentary system; located below and attached to the dermis but does not extend beyond the fascia that covers the muscle.

superior Body direction that is above another body part or toward the head. Also called *cephalic.*

supination Rotation of the forearm with the palm facing up.

symptom A subjective condition that is relayed to the provider by the patient.

syringobulbia A syringomyelia that has extended into the brainstem area.

syringomyelia A cyst or syrinx of the spinal cord that may destroy the spinal cord over time, leading to numbness and dysfunction of the nerves and muscles.

systemic inflammatory response syndrome (SIRS) The body's response to septicemia, trauma, or, in some cases, cancer.

T

tendon Narrow band of nonelastic, dense, fibrous connective tissue that attaches muscle to a bone.

testes Oval organs that are located in the scrotum and produce testosterone and sperm. Also called *testicles.*

therapeutic nuclear medicine study Study that provides relief by the use of a radioactive material (e.g., radioactive iodine and strontium).

threatened conditions See **impending conditions.**

thrombus A clot in a blood vessel.

thymus Gland that is located in the mediastinum, just behind the upper portion of the sternum, and produces and develops T cells.

thyroid gland Butterfly-shaped gland, located low on the anterior side of the trachea, that influences growth and development, body temperature, and metabolism.

thyroid storm Condition that occurs in uncontrolled hyperthyroidism. Also called *thyroid crisis.*

thyroid stimulating hormone (TSH) A test that measures the amount of TSH produced by the pituitary gland in the blood.

time (anesthesia) Period that begins when the patient is being prepared for anesthesia and ends when the patient is no longer being attended by the anesthesiologist; converted into units and added to base units in the reimbursement formula.

tinnitus A sensation of ringing in the ears.

total body surface area (TBSA) Total body surface area is based on the rule of nines, which divides the patient's body into segments of 9 percent.

trachea Structure of muscular tissue that branches into the bronchi. Also called *windpipe.*

triangle (▲) In CPT, the symbol designating that a code has been revised.

tricuspid valve Valve located on the right side of the heart between the atrium and the ventricle that stops the backflow of blood between these two chambers.

tympanic membrane Structure that divides the external and middle ears and converts sound to vibration. Also called *eardrum.*

U

ultrasound A noninvasive test that uses high-frequency sound waves to produce images that are captured in real time and show structure, movement, and the flow of blood through blood vessels. Also called *sonography.*

ureters Two structures that transport urine from the kidney to the urinary bladder.

urethra Tube that carries urine from the urinary bladder to the outside of the body; in the male, also functions as a reproductive outlet.

urinary system System that consists of the kidneys, ureters, urinary bladder, and urethra, which function together to filter blood and create and maintain balance of water and chemicals.

use additional code Informs the coder that the code being referenced is sequenced as the first listed code in a pairing of codes.

V

vagina Hollow muscular tube extending from the cervix to the labia; functions are to receive sperm and provide a passageway for births.

vas deferens Tube from the epididymis to the pelvic cavity that transports mature sperm to the urethra.

vertebral interspace The nonbony area between two vertebral segments, including the intervertebral disc (nucleus pulpous, annulus fibrosus, and cartilaginous end plates).

vertebral segment One complete vertebral bone, including laminae and articulating processes.

vestibule The part of the oral cavity outside the dento-alveolar structures; it includes the mucosal and submucosal tissue of lips and cheeks.

volvulus Knotting, strangulation, torsion, or twisting of the intestine, bowel, or colon.

vulva Female external genitalia that protects internal reproductive organs and enables sperm to enter the body.

W

with In ICD-10-CM, notation indicating that a separate associated complication or comorbidity is present.

without In ICD-10-CM, notation indicating that a separate associated complication or comorbidity is not present.

X

xenograft Skin graft in which tissue procured (harvested) from another species (e.g., porcine graft) is applied to the recipient.

CREDITS

Text and Illustration Credits

CHAPTER 1

Figures 1.1–1.3: CMS 1500 form from National Uniform Claim Committee.

American Academy of Professional Coders. (2011). *Certified Professional Coder*. Retrieved October 20, 2011, from American Academy of Professional Coders website: www.aapc.com/certification/cpc.aspx

CHAPTER 2

Table 2.1: Data from ICD-9-CM, Centers for Medicare & Medicaid Services, and National Center for Health Statistics.

OptumInsight. (2011). *International Classification of Diseases, 9th Revision, Clinical Modification* (6th ed.). Salt Lake City, UT: Ingenix.

CHAPTER 3

Table 3.1: Data from ICD-10-CM, Centers for Medicare & Medicaid Services and National Center for Health Statistics.

AAPC. (2012). *International Classification of Diseases, 10th Revision, Clinical Modification* (2012 draft). Salt Lake City, UT: Contexo Media.

CHAPTER 4

Tables 4.1–4.5: Data from ICD-9-CM and ICD-10-CM, Centers for Medicare & Medicaid Services, and National Center for Health Statistics.

OptumInsight. (2011). *International Classification of Diseases, 9th Revision, Clinical Modification* (6th ed.). Salt Lake City, UT: Ingenix.

AAPC. (2012). *International Classification of Diseases, 10th Revision, Clinical Modification* (2012 draft). Salt Lake City, UT: Contexo Media.

OptumInsight. (2011). *Coders' Desk Reference 2012—Diagnoses*. Salt Lake City, UT: Ingenix.

CHAPTER 5

Figure 5.1: CMS 1500 form from National Uniform Claim Committee.

Tables 5.1–5.3: Data from CPT 2013. © 2013 American Medical Association. All rights reserved.

American Medical Association. (2012). *Current Procedural Terminology 2013—Professional Edition*. Chicago, IL: AMA Press.

OptumInsight. (2011). *Healthcare Common Procedural Coding System—2012*. Salt Lake City, UT: Ingenix.

CHAPTER 6

Tables 6.3–6.7: Data from CPT 2013. © 2013 American Medical Association. All rights reserved.

American Medical Association. (2012). *Current Procedural Terminology 2013—Professional Edition*. Chicago, IL: AMA Press.

CHAPTER 7

Tables 7.1 and 7.2: Data from CPT 2013. © 2013 American Medical Association. All rights reserved.

Tables 7.3–7.5: Data from HCPCS (Healthcare Common Procedure Coding System) Level II National Codes, Centers for Medicare & Medicaid Services.

American Medical Association. (2012). *Current Procedural Terminology 2013—Professional Edition*. Chicago, IL: AMA Press.

CHAPTER 8

Tables 8.1–8.3: Data from CPT 2013. © 2013 American Medical Association. All rights reserved.

OptumInsight. (2011). *International Classification of Diseases, 9th Revision, Clinical Modification* (6th ed.). Salt Lake City, UT: Ingenix.

AAPC. (2012). *International Classification of Diseases, 10th Revision, Clinical Modification* (2012 draft). Salt Lake City, UT: Contexo Media.

American Medical Association. (2012). *Current Procedural Terminology 2013—Professional Edition*. Chicago, IL: AMA Press.

CHAPTER 9

Figures 9.1, 9.2, and 9.4: From Rod Seeley et al., *Seeley's Anatomy & Physiology* (9th ed.). © 2011 McGraw-Hill Companies, Inc. Reprinted with permission.

Figure 9.3: Image provided by The British Association of Plastic, Reconstructive, and Aesthetic Surgeons. Reprinted with permission.

Tables 9.3 and 9.8: Data from ICD-9-CM and ICD-10-CM, Centers for Medicare & Medicaid Services, and National Center for Health Statistics.

Tables 9.4–9.7: Data from CPT 2013. © 2013 American Medical Association. All rights reserved.

American Medical Association. (2012). *Current Procedural Terminology 2013—Professional Edition*. Chicago, IL: AMA Press.

OptumInsight. (2011). *International Classification of Diseases, 9th Revision, Clinical Modification* (6th ed.). Salt Lake City, UT: Ingenix.

AAPC. (2012). *International Classification of Diseases, 10th Revision, Clinical Modification* (2012 draft). Salt Lake City, UT: Contexo Media.

OptumInsight. (2011). *Coders' Desk Reference 2012—Procedures*. Salt Lake City, UT: Ingenix.

OptumInsight. (2011). *Coders' Desk Reference 2012—Diagnoses*. Salt Lake City, UT: Ingenix.

Centers for Medicare & Medicaid Services. (2011). *National Correct Coding Initiative Policy Manual for Medicare Services*, Chapter 3. Retrieved November 2, 2011, from Centers for Medicare & Medicaid Services website: www.cms.gov/Medicare/Coding/National CorrectCodInitEd/

CHAPTER 10

Figure 10.1: From Rod Seeley et al., *Seeley's Anatomy & Physiology* (9th ed.). © 2011 McGraw-Hill Companies, Inc. Reprinted with permission.

Figures 10.2, 10.4, 10.9, and 10.10: From David Shier et al., *Hole's Human Anatomy & Physiology* (12th ed.). © 2010 McGraw-Hill Companies, Inc. Reprinted with permission.

Figures 10.5–10.7: From Christine Eckel, *Human Anatomy Laboratory Manual* (2nd ed.). © 2011 McGraw-Hill Companies, Inc. Reprinted with permission.

Figure 10.8: From Deborah Roiger, *Anatomy & Physiology: Foundations for the Health Professions* (1st ed.). © 2013 McGraw-Hill Companies, Inc. Reprinted with permission.

Table 10.3: Data from ICD-9-CM and ICD-10-CM, Centers for Medicare & Medicaid Services, and National Center for Health Statistics.

Tables 10.4–10.10: Data from CPT 2013. © 2013 American Medical Association. All rights reserved.

American Medical Association. (2012). *Current Procedural Terminology 2013—Professional Edition.* Chicago, IL: AMA Press.

OptumInsight. (2011). *International Classification of Diseases, 9th Revision, Clinical Modification* (6th ed.). Salt Lake City, UT: Ingenix.

AAPC. (2012). *International Classification of Diseases, 10th Revision, Clinical Modification* (2012 draft). Salt Lake City, UT: Contexo Media.

OptumInsight. (2011). *Coders' Desk Reference 2012—Procedures.* Salt Lake City, UT: Ingenix.

OptumInsight. (2011). *Coders' Desk Reference 2012—Diagnoses—2012.* Salt Lake City, UT: Ingenix.

Centers for Medicare & Medicaid Services. (2011). *National Correct Coding Initiative Policy Manual for Medicare Services—Chapter 4.* Retrieved November 2, 2011, from Centers for Medicare & Medicaid Services website: www.cms.gov/Medicare/Coding/National CorrectCodInitEd/

CHAPTER 11

Chapter-opening figure and Figures 11.2 and 11.5: From David Shier et al., *Hole's Human Anatomy & Physiology* (12th ed.). © 2010 McGraw-Hill Companies, Inc. Reprinted with permission.

Figure 11.1: From Deborah Roiger, *Anatomy & Physiology: Foundations for the Health Professions* (1st ed.). © 2013 McGraw-Hill Companies, Inc. Reprinted with permission.

Table 11.2: Data from ICD-9-CM and ICD-10-CM, Centers for Medicare & Medicaid Services, and National Center for Health Statistics.

Tables 11.3 and 11.4: Data from CPT 2013. © 2013 American Medical Association. All rights reserved.

American Medical Association. (2012). *Current Procedural Terminology 2013—Professional Edition.* Chicago, IL: AMA Press.

OptumInsight. (2011). *International Classification of Diseases, 9th Revision, Clinical Modification* (6th ed.). Salt Lake City, UT: Ingenix.

AAPC. (2012). *International Classification of Diseases, 10th Revision, Clinical Modification* (2012 draft). Salt Lake City, UT: Contexo Media.

OptumInsight. (2011). *Coders' Desk Reference 2012—Procedures.* Salt Lake City, UT: Ingenix.

OptumInsight. (2011). *Coders' Desk Reference 2012—Diagnoses.* Salt Lake City, UT: Ingenix.

Centers for Medicare & Medicaid Services. (2011). *National Correct Coding Initiative Policy Manual for Medicare Services,* Chapter 5. Retrieved November 2, 2011, from Centers for Medicare & Medicaid Services website: www.cms.gov/Medicare/Coding/National CorrectCodInitEd/ ●

CHAPTER 12

Chapter-opening figure and Figures 12.1–12.9: From David Shier et al., *Hole's Human Anatomy & Physiology* (12th ed.). © 2010 McGraw-Hill Companies, Inc. Reprinted with permission.

Tables 12.5 and 12.6: Data from ICD-9-CM and ICD-10-CM, Centers for Medicare & Medicaid Services, and National Center for Health Statistics.

Tables 12.7–12.9: Data from CPT 2013. © 2013 American Medical Association. All rights reserved.

American Medical Association. (2012). *Current Procedural Terminology 2013—Professional Edition.* Chicago, IL: AMA Press.

OptumInsight. (2011). *International Classification of Diseases, 9th Revision, Clinical Modification* (6th ed.). Salt Lake City, UT: Ingenix.

AAPC. (2012). *International Classification of Diseases, 10th Revision, Clinical Modification* (2012 draft). Salt Lake City, UT: Contexo Media.

OptumInsight. (2011). *Coders' Desk Reference 2012—Procedures.* Salt Lake City, UT: Ingenix.

OptumInsight. (2011). *Coders' Desk Reference 2012—Diagnoses.* Salt Lake City, UT: Ingenix.

Centers for Medicare & Medicaid Services. (2011). *National Correct Coding Initiative Policy Manual for Medicare Services,* Chapter 5. Retrieved November 2, 2011, from Centers for Medicare & Medicaid Services website: www.cms.gov/Medicare/Coding/National CorrectCodInitEd/

CHAPTER 13

Chapter-opening photo and Figure 13.2: From Rod Seeley et al., *Seeley's Anatomy & Physiology* (9th ed.). © 2011 McGraw-Hill Companies, Inc. Reprinted with permission.

Figure 13.1: From Deborah Roiger, *Anatomy & Physiology: Foundations for the Health Professions* (1st ed.). © 2013 McGraw-Hill Companies, Inc. Reprinted with permission.

Figures 13.3–13.6: From David Shier et al., *Hole's Human Anatomy & Physiology* (12th ed.). © 2010 McGraw-Hill Companies, Inc. Reprinted with permission.

Table 13.2: Data from ICD-9-CM and ICD-10-CM, Centers for Medicare & Medicaid Services, and National Center for Health Statistics.

Tables 13.4 and 13.5: Data from CPT 2013. © 2013 American Medical Association. All rights reserved.

American Medical Association. (2012). *Current Procedural Terminology 2013—Professional Edition.* Chicago, IL: AMA Press.

OptumInsight. (2011). *International Classification of Diseases, 9th Revision, Clinical Modification* (6th ed.). Salt Lake City, UT: Ingenix.

AAPC. (2012). *International Classification of Diseases, 10th Revision, Clinical Modification* (2012 draft). Salt Lake City, UT: Contexo Media.

OptumInsight. (2011). *Coders' Desk Reference 2012—Procedures.* Salt Lake City, UT: Ingenix.

OptumInsight. (2011). *Coders' Desk Reference 2012—Diagnoses.* Salt Lake City, UT: Ingenix.

Centers for Medicare & Medicaid Services. (2011). *National Correct Coding Initiative Policy Manual for Medicare Services*, Chapter 6. Retrieved November 2, 2011, from Centers for Medicare & Medicaid Services website: www.cms.gov/Medicare/Coding/National CorrectCodInitEd/

CHAPTER 14

Chapter-opening figure: From Deborah Roiger, *Anatomy & Physiology: Foundations for the Health Professions* (1st ed.). © 2013 McGraw-Hill Companies, Inc. Reprinted with permission.

Figures 14.1–14.4: From David Shier et al., *Hole's Human Anatomy & Physiology* (12th ed.). © 2010 McGraw-Hill Companies, Inc. Reprinted with permission.

Table 14.3: Data from ICD-9-CM and ICD-10-CM, Centers for Medicare & Medicaid Services, and National Center for Health Statistics.

Tables 14.4–14.6: Data from CPT 2013. © 2013 American Medical Association. All rights reserved.

American Medical Association. (2012). *Current Procedural Terminology 2013—Professional Edition*. Chicago, IL: AMA Press.

OptumInsight. (2011). *International Classification of Diseases, 9th Revision, Clinical Modification* (6th ed.). Salt Lake City, UT: Ingenix.

AAPC. (2012). *International Classification of Diseases, 10th Revision, Clinical Modification* (2012 draft). Salt Lake City, UT: Contexo Media.

OptumInsight. (2011). *Coders' Desk Reference 2012—Procedures*. Salt Lake City, UT: Ingenix.

OptumInsight. (2011). *Coders' Desk Reference 2012—Diagnoses*. Salt Lake City, UT: Ingenix.

Centers for Medicare & Medicaid Services. (2011). *National Correct Coding Initiative Policy Manual for Medicare Services*, Chapter 7. Retrieved November 2, 2011, from Centers for Medicare & Medicaid Services website: www.cms.gov/Medicare/Coding/National CorrectCodInitEd/

CHAPTER 15

Figure 15.1: From David Shier et al., *Hole's Human Anatomy & Physiology* (12th ed.). © 2010 McGraw-Hill Companies, Inc. Reprinted with permission.

Figure 15.2: From Deborah Roiger, *Anatomy & Physiology: Foundations for the Health Professions* (1st ed.). © 2013 McGraw-Hill Companies, Inc. Reprinted with permission.

Tables 15.2 and 15.3: Data from ICD-9-CM and ICD-10-CM, Centers for Medicare & Medicaid Services, and National Center for Health Statistics.

Tables 15.4–15.6: Data from CPT 2013. © 2013 American Medical Association. All rights reserved.

American Medical Association. (2012). *Current Procedural Terminology 2013—Professional Edition*. Chicago, IL: AMA Press.

OptumInsight. (2011). *International Classification of Diseases, 9th Revision, Clinical Modification* (6th ed.). Salt Lake City, UT: Ingenix.

AAPC. (2012). *International Classification of Diseases, 10th Revision, Clinical Modification* (2012 draft). Salt Lake City, UT: Contexo Media.

OptumInsight. (2011). *Coders' Desk Reference 2012—Procedures*. Salt Lake City, UT: Ingenix.

OptumInsight. (2011). *Coders' Desk Reference 2012—Diagnoses—2012*. Salt Lake City, UT: Ingenix.

Centers for Medicare & Medicaid Services. (2011). *National Correct Coding Initiative Policy Manual for Medicare Services*, Chapter 7. Retrieved November 2, 2011, from Centers for Medicare & Medicaid Services website: www.cms.gov/Medicare/Coding/National CorrectCodInitEd/

CHAPTER 16

Chapter-opening figure and Figures 16.1, 16.3, and 16.6: From David Shier et al., *Hole's Human Anatomy & Physiology* (12th ed.). © 2010 McGraw-Hill Companies, Inc. Reprinted with permission.

Figures 16.2, 16.4, and 16.5: From Deborah Roiger, *Anatomy & Physiology: Foundations for the Health Professions* (1st ed.). © 2013 McGraw-Hill Companies, Inc. Reprinted with permission.

Table 16.2: Data from ICD-9-CM and ICD-10-CM, Centers for Medicare & Medicaid Services, and National Center for Health Statistics.

Tables 16.3–16.5: Data from CPT 2013. © 2013 American Medical Association. All rights reserved.

American Medical Association. (2012). *Current Procedural Terminology 2013—Professional Edition*. Chicago, IL: AMA Press.

OptumInsight. (2011). *International Classification of Diseases, 9th Revision, Clinical Modification* (6th ed.). Salt Lake City, UT: Ingenix.

AAPC. (2012). *International Classification of Diseases, 10th Revision, Clinical Modification* (2012 draft). Salt Lake City, UT: Contexo Media.

OptumInsight. (2011). *Coders' Desk Reference 2012—Procedures*. Salt Lake City, UT: Ingenix.

OptumInsight. (2011). *Coders' Desk Reference 2012—Diagnoses—2012*. Salt Lake City, UT: Ingenix.

Centers for Medicare & Medicaid Services. (2011). *National Correct Coding Initiative Policy Manual for Medicare Services*, Chapter 8. Retrieved November 2, 2011, from Centers for Medicare & Medicaid Services website: www.cms.gov/Medicare/Coding/National CorrectCodInitEd/

CHAPTER 17

Figures 17.1, 17.2, and 17.4: From Rod Seeley et al., *Seeley's Anatomy & Physiology* (9th ed.). © 2011 McGraw-Hill Companies, Inc. Reprinted with permission.

Figures 17.3 and 17.5: From Deborah Roiger, *Anatomy & Physiology: Foundations for the Health Professions* (1st ed.). © 2013 McGraw-Hill Companies, Inc. Reprinted with permission.

Figures 17.6 and 17.7: From David Shier et al., *Hole's Human Anatomy & Physiology* (12th ed.). © 2010 McGraw-Hill Companies, Inc. Reprinted with permission.

Tables 17.4–17.6: Data from ICD-9-CM and ICD-10-CM, Centers for Medicare & Medicaid Services, and National Center for Health Statistics.

Tables 17.8–17.10: Data from CPT 2013. © 2013 American Medical Association. All rights reserved.

American Medical Association. (2012). *Current Procedural Terminology 2013—Professional Edition*. Chicago, IL: AMA Press.

OptumInsight. (2011). *International Classification of Diseases, 9th Revision, Clinical Modification* (6th ed.). Salt Lake City, UT: Ingenix.

AAPC. (2012). *International Classification of Diseases, 10th Revision, Clinical Modification* (2012 draft). Salt Lake City, UT: Contexo Media.

OptumInsight. (2011). *Coders' Desk Reference 2012—Procedures.* Salt Lake City, UT: Ingenix.

OptumInsight. (2011). *Coders' Desk Reference 2012—Diagnoses.* Salt Lake City, UT: Ingenix.

Centers for Medicare & Medicaid Services. (2011). *National Correct Coding Initiative Policy Manual for Medicare Services,* Chapter 8. Retrieved November 2, 2011, from Centers for Medicare & Medicaid Services website: www.cms.gov/ Medicare/Coding/National CorrectCodInitEd/

CHAPTER 18

Figure 18.5: From Rod Seeley et al., *Seeley's Anatomy & Physiology* (9th ed.). © 2011 McGraw-Hill Companies, Inc. Reprinted with permission.

Figure 18.6: From David Shier et al., *Hole's Human Anatomy & Physiology* (12th ed.). © 2010 McGraw-Hill Companies, Inc. Reprinted with permission.

Tables 18.1 and 18.2: Data from CPT 2013. © 2013 American Medical Association. All rights reserved.

American Medical Association. (2012). *Current Procedural Terminology 2013—Professional Edition.* Chicago, IL: AMA Press.

OptumInsight. (2011). *International Classification of Diseases, 9th Revision, Clinical Modification* (6th ed.). Salt Lake City, UT: Ingenix.

AAPC. (2012). *International Classification of Diseases, 10th Revision, Clinical Modification* (2012 draft). Salt Lake City, UT: Contexo Media.

OptumInsight. (2011). *Coders' Desk Reference 2012—Procedures.* Salt Lake City, UT: Ingenix.

OptumInsight. (2011). *Coders' Desk Reference 2012—Diagnoses.* Salt Lake City, UT: Ingenix.

Centers for Medicare & Medicaid Services. (2011). *National Correct Coding Initiative Policy Manual for Medicare Services,* Chapter 9. Retrieved November 2, 2011, from Centers for Medicare & Medicaid Services website: www.cms.gov/ Medicare/Coding/National CorrectCodInitEd/

CHAPTER 19

Figure 19.1: From Rod Seeley et al., *Seeley's Anatomy & Physiology* (9th ed.). © 2011 McGraw-Hill Companies, Inc. Reprinted with permission.

Figure 19.2: From David Shier et al., *Hole's Human Anatomy & Physiology* (12th ed.). © 2010 McGraw-Hill Companies, Inc. Reprinted with permission.

Tables 19.1 and 19.2: Data from CPT 2013. © 2013 American Medical Association. All rights reserved.

American Medical Association. (2012). *Current Procedural Terminology 2013—Professional Edition.* Chicago, IL: AMA Press.

OptumInsight. (2011). *International Classification of Diseases, 9th Revision, Clinical Modification* (6th ed.). Salt Lake City, UT: Ingenix.

AAPC. (2012). *International Classification of Diseases, 10th Revision, Clinical Modification* (2012 draft). Salt Lake City, UT: Contexo Media.

OptumInsight. (2011). *Coders' Desk Reference 2012—Procedures.* Salt Lake City, UT: Ingenix.

OptumInsight. (2011). *Coders' Desk Reference 2012—Diagnoses.* Salt Lake City, UT: Ingenix.

Centers for Medicare & Medicaid Services. (2011). *National Correct Coding Initiative Policy Manual for Medicare Services,*

Chapter 10. Retrieved November 2, 2011, from Centers for Medicare & Medicaid Services website: www.cms.gov/ Medicare/Coding/National CorrectCodInitEd/

CHAPTER 20

Tables 20.1 and 20.2: Data from CPT 2013. © 2013 American Medical Association. All rights reserved.

American Medical Association. (2012). *Current Procedural Terminology 2013—Professional Edition.* Chicago, IL: AMA Press.

OptumInsight. (2011). *International Classification of Diseases, 9th Revision, Clinical Modification* (6th ed.). Salt Lake City, UT: Ingenix.

AAPC. (2012). *International Classification of Diseases, 10th Revision, Clinical Modification* (2012 draft). Salt Lake City, UT: Contexo Media.

OptumInsight. (2011). *Coders' Desk Reference 2012—Procedures.* Salt Lake City, UT: Ingenix.

OptumInsight. (2011). *Coders' Desk Reference 2012—Diagnoses.* Salt Lake City, UT: Ingenix.

Centers for Medicare & Medicaid Services. (2011). *National Correct Coding Initiative Policy Manual for Medicare Services,* Chapter 11. Retrieved November 2, 2011, from Centers for Medicare & Medicaid Services website: www.cms.gov/ Medicare/Coding/National CorrectCodInitEd/

CHAPTER 21

Tables 21.1–21.5: Data from HCPCS (Healthcare Common Procedure Coding System) Level II National Codes, Centers for Medicare & Medicaid Services.

American Medical Association. (2012). *Current Procedural Terminology 2013—Professional Edition.* Chicago, IL: AMA Press.

Centers for Medicare & Medicaid Services. (2011). *National Correct Coding Initiative Policy Manual for Medicare Services,* Chapter 12. Retrieved November 2, 2011, from Centers for Medicare & Medicaid Services website: www.cms.gov/ Medicare/Coding/National CorrectCodInitEd/

CHAPTER 22

Figure 22.1: CMS 1500 form from National Uniform Claim Committee.

Figure 22.2: ABN form from Centers for Medicare & Medicaid Services.

American Academy of Professional Coders. (2012). *AAPC Code of Ethics.* Retrieved June 26, 2012, from American Academy of Professional Coders website: www.aapc.com/aboutUs/ code-of-ethics.aspx

U.S. Department of Health and Human Services. (2009). *HITECH Breach Notification Interim Final Rule.* Retrieved June 20, 2012, from Health and Human Services website: www.hhs.gov/ocr/privacy/hipaa/understanding/ coveredentities/breachnotificationifr

Centers for Medicare & Medicaid Services. (2011). *Medicare Claims Processing Manual,* Chapter 30: "Financial Liability Protections." Retrieved June 20, 2012, from Centers for Medicare & Medicaid Services website: www.cms.gov/ Medicare/Medicare-General-Information/BNI/Downloads/ RevABNManualInstructions.pdf

Centers for Medicare & Medicaid Services. (2012). *Medicare Program—General Information.* Retrieved June 22, 2012, from Centers for Medicare & Medicaid Services website: www.cms.gov/Medicare/Medicare-General-Information/ MedicareGenInfo

Healthcare Economist. (2011). *The CMS HCC Model*. Retrieved June 3, 2012, from Healthcare Economist website: healthcare-economist.com/2011/05/17/cms-hcc-model

U.S. Department of Justice. (2010). *Office of Inspector General*. Retrieved June 6, 2012, from Department of Justice website: www.justice.gov/oig/

American Health Care Association. (2012). *Elements of an Effective Compliance Plan*. Retrieved June 3, 2012, from AHCA website: www.ahcancal.org/facility_operations/ComplianceProgram/Pages/BldgCompliancePrgm

Photo Credits

FRONTMATTER

p. v: (top left) Image Source/Getty Images; (middle left) Fuse/Getty Images; (bottom left) Ellen Pettengell; (top right) Ingram Publishing/AGE Fotostock; (bottom right) PIXTAL/PunchStock

p. vi: (top left) altrendo images/Getty Images; (middle left) Digital Vision; (bottom left) Ale Ventura/Photo Alto; (top right) Indeed/Digital Vision/Getty Images; (bottom right) MedicalRF.com

p. viii: (top left) © Jose Luis Pelaez Inc/Blend Images LLC; (bottom left) © Jim Wehtje/Getty Images RFl (right) Roy McMahon/Corbis

p. ix: (top left) Design Pics/Yuri Arcurs; (bottom left) Ingram Publishing; (top right) © PBNJ Productions/Blend Images LLC; (bottom right) © Blend Images/SuperStock

p. x: (top) © Cynthia Stewart; (bottom) © Cynthia Ward

CHAPTER 1

p. 1: (left) Image Source/Getty Images; (middle top left) Fuse/Getty Images; (middle top right) Ellen Pettengell; (middle bottom) Ingram Publishing/AGE Fotostock; (right) PIXTAL/PunchStock

pp. 2, 10–12: Image Source/Getty Images

CHAPTER 2

pp. 13, 26–28: Fuse/Getty Images

CHAPTER 3

pp. 29, 45–48: Ellen Pettengell

CHAPTER 4

pp. 49, 65–67: Ingram Publishing/AGE Fotostock

CHAPTER 5

pp. 68, 80–83: PIXTAL/PunchStock

CHAPTER 6

p. 87: (left) altrendo images/Getty Images; (middle) Digital Vision; (right) Indeed/Digital Vision/Getty Images

pp. 88, 110–113: altrendo images/Getty Images

CHAPTER 7

pp. 114, 122–128: Digital Vision

CHAPTER 8

pp. 129, 145–148: Indeed/Digital Vision/Getty Images

CHAPTER 9

p. 153: (left) Ale Ventura/Photo Alto; (middle left) MedicalRF.com

pp. 154, 180–184: Ale Ventura/Photo Alto

CHAPTER 10

pp. 185, 210–214: MedicalRF.com

p. 189: (top) The McGraw-Hill Companies, Inc.

CHAPTER 11

p. 221: Ryan McVay/Getty Images

CHAPTER 13

p. 285: (middle top right) © Jose Luis Pelaez Inc/Blend Images LLC; (right) Roy McMahon/Corbis

CHAPTER 15

pp. 351, 375–381: © Jose Luis Pelaez Inc/Blend Images LLC

CHAPTER 17

pp. 413, 435–441: Roy McMahon/Corbis

CHAPTER 18

p. 447: (left) © Jim Wehtje/Getty Images RF; (middle top left) Design Pics/Yuri Arcurs; (middle top right) Ingram Publishing; (middle bottom) © PBNJ Productions/Blend Images LLC; (right) © Blend Images/SuperStock

pp. 448, 464–468: © Jim Wehtje/Getty Images RF

p. 452: (top) © Dr. Kent M. Van De Graaff; (middle) © Walter Reiter/Phototake; (bottom) © SIU/Visuals Unlimited

p. 456: © Dr. P. Marazzi/Photo Researchers, Inc.

p. 461: © McGraw-Hill Higher Education, Inc./Eric Wise, photographer

p. 462: © The McGraw-Hill Companies, Inc./Timothy L. Vacula, photographer

CHAPTER 19

pp. 469, 481–486: Design Pics/Yuri Arcurs

p. 478: © JGI/Tom Grill/Blend Images LLC

CHAPTER 20

pp. 487, 505–512: Ingram Publishing

p. 491: Science Photo Library/Getty Images

p. 495: IMAGEMORE Co., Ltd./Getty Images

p. 497: © The McGraw-Hill Companies, Inc./Rick Brady, photographer

CHAPTER 21

pp. 513, 525–527: © PBNJ Productions/Blend Images LLC

p. 519: Ingram Publishing

p. 520: (top) © Ingram Publishing/AGE Fotostock; (bottom) Realistic Reflections

CHAPTER 22

pp. 528, 540–542: © Blend Images/SuperStock

INDEX

Page numbers followed by *f* or *t* indicate material in figures or tables, respectively.

Aorta, 246, 246*t*, 250–251, 250*f*
    atherosclerosis of, 260
    wounds of, CPT coding for, 264
Aortic aneurysm, 260
    repair of, CPT coding for, 267
Aortic dissection, 260
Aortic valve, 250, 250*t*
    CPT coding for, 264–265
    disorders of, ICD coding for
        not specified as rheumatic, 258
        rheumatic, 254
Aphakia, 493
Appendectomy, 124–125, 308
Appendicitis
    anesthesia in surgery for, 124–125
    ICD coding for, 292
Appendicular skeleton, 191, 191*t*–192*t*
Appendix
    CPT coding for, 308
    diseases of, ICD coding for, 292
Approach
    definition of, 131
    external, 226
    internal, 226
    surgical, 131–132, 132*t*
Arachnoid mater, 385*f*, 387*t*
ARDS; *see* Adult respiratory distress syndrome
Arms, bones of, 192*t*
ARRA; *see* American Recovery and
        Reinvestment Act
Arrhythmia, 259, 275, 275*t*
Arterial blood gas, 235*t*
Arteries
    CPT coding for, 262*t*, 268–271
    diseases of, ICD coding for, 253*t*, 260
    layers (tunics) of, 246*t*
    peripheral, 246*t*, 247*f*
    pulmonary, 246*t*
Arterioles, 246*t*, 250–251
    diseases of, ICD coding for, 253*t*, 260
Arteriovenous (AV) fistula, for hemodialysis
        access, 270
Arteriovenous malformation (AVM), 398
Arteritis, temporal, 275*t*
Arthrocentesis, 198
Arthrodesis, CPT coding for, 197, 203–204, 203*t*
Arthropathies, ICD coding for, 193*t*, 194–195
Arthroplasty, CPT coding for, 139–148
Arthroscopy, 132*t*, 147–148, 206
Artificial insemination, 367
AS; *see* Auris sinstra
ASA; *see* American Society of Anesthesiologists
Ascending colon, 288*t*
Ascites, 314*t*, 463*t*
ASD; *see* Atrial septal defect
Aspirate, 235*t*
Aspiration, 198
    spinal, 400
Asthma, 223–224, 236*t*
Ataxia, 405*t*
Atelectasis, 236*t*
Atherosclerosis
    of aorta and renal artery, ICD coding
        for, 260
    coronary, ICD coding for, 257–258
    of extremities, ICD coding for, 260
    of pulmonary artery, ICD coding for, 260
Atrial fibrillation, 279–280
    ICD coding for, 259
Atrial septal defect (ASD), 266
Atrioventricular block, 259
Atrioventricular (AV) node, 249–251, 249*f*, 249*t*
Atrophic conditions, of skin and subcutaneous
        tissue, 159

Atrophy, 208*t*
AU; *see* Auris unitas
Audiologic evaluation and therapeutic
        services, 493
Audiologic function tests, 493
Audiometry, 433, 433*t*
Auditory canal, external, 415*f*, 416*t*
Auditory system; *see also* Ear(s)
    CPT subsection on, 428–430, 428*t*
Auricle (pinna), 415*f*, 416*t*
    disorders of, ICD coding for, 423
Auris dextra (AD), 433, 433*t*
Auris sinstra (AS), 433, 433*t*
Auris unitas (AU), 433, 433*t*
Autograft, 161*t*, 170–171
Autonomic nervous system, 385, 386*t*
    CPT coding for, 402–403
    definition of, 402
Autopsy, 477
Avian influenza, 223
AVM; *see* Arteriovenous malformation
Axial plane, 461*f*, 461*t*, 463
Axial skeleton, 189*f*, 191, 191*t*

B codes, 517–518
Bacteriology, 476
Balance disorders, 423
Balance studies, 493
Balanitis, 333
Barman's operation, 426
Bartholin's glands, 352, 353, 353*t*
Base units, of anesthesia, 115
Basic life evaluation, CPT E/M coding for, 95
Basic life support (BLS), 515–516
Behavioral disorders, ICD chapter-specific
        guidelines for, 41*t*
Benign, definition of, 165
Benign hypertension, 255
Benign lesions
    destruction of, 161*t*, 173–174, 174*t*
    excision of, 165–166
Benign neoplasms, 59, 470
Benign prostatic hypertrophy (BPH),
        332, 342, 342*t*
Bethesda System, 477
Biliary tract
    anatomy of, 295*f*
    CPT coding for, 310
    diseases of, ICD coding for, 294–296
Billing language, 3
Biofeedback, 504, 504*t*
Biologic agent administration, 501
Biopsy, 137, 137*t*
    cervix, 366
    ear, 428–429
    integumentary, 160*t*, 164, 178*t*
    kidney, 335
    lip, 298
    liver, 309
    lymph node, 272
    musculoskeletal, 208*t*
    nasal, 228
    palate or uvula, 302
    pancreatic, 310
    prostate, 340
    rectal, 308
    respiratory system, 235*t*
    salivary glands or ducts, 302
    stomach, 305
    testes, 340
    thyroid gland, 430–431
    tongue or floor of mouth, 300–301
    uterus, 367
    vestibule of mouth, 299

Black lung disease, 224
Bladder; *see* Gallbladder; Urinary bladder
Bleeding; *see* Hemorrhage
Blepharoptosis, 433*t*
Blepharotomy, 427
Blindness, 420
Block (specimen), 480, 480*t*
Blood cells, 475, 475*f*
Blood disease, ICD chapter-specific guidelines
        for, 23*t*, 41*t*
Blood flow pathway, 250–251, 250*f*
Blood transfusion, 476
Blood vessels
    blood flow pathway through, 250–251, 250*f*
    great, 246*t*
    peripheral, 246*t*, 247*f*–248*f*
Blood-forming organs, diseases of, ICD coding
        for, 23*t*, 41*t*
BLS; *see* Basic life support
Body area, examination coding by, 102*t*, 104*t*
Body cavities, 462*f*
Body directions, 461, 462*t*
Body planes, 461, 461*f*, 461*t*
Bone(s), 190*t*
    of appendicular skeleton, 189*f*,
        191, 191*t*–192*t*
    of axial skeleton, 189*f*, 191, 191*t*
    compact, 190*t*
    CPT coding for, 185, 196–208, 208*t*
    flat, 189*f*
    ICD coding for, 193–196, 193*t*
    irregular, 190*f*
    long, 189*f*
    nuclear medicine studies of, 458, 459
    sesamoid, 190*f*
    short, 189*f*
    spongy, 190*t*
Bone density
    disorders of, ICD coding for, 195–196
    studies of, 456, 456*f*, 463, 463*t*
Bone marrow or stem cell services, CPT coding
        for, 271
Bone/joint studies, CPT subsection on, 456
BPH; *see* Benign prostatic hypertrophy
Brachytherapy
    clinical, CPT coding for, 457
    definition of, 457
Brackets, 19, 35–36
    slanted, 19
    square, 19, 35–36
Brain, 385, 386*t*
    anatomy of, 383*f*, 384*f*
    CPT coding for, 396–399
    other conditions of, ICD coding of, 393
Brainstem, 386*t*
Breast
    CPT coding for, 161*t*, 175–177
    infections or disorders of, related to
        childbirth and lactation, 362
    introduction of device to, 161*t*, 175–176
Breast cancer, case study of, 67
Breast mammography, CPT subsection on, 456
Breast repair/reconstruction, 161*t*, 176–177
Bronchi, 217*f*, 218, 218*t*
    CPT coding for, 231–233
Bronchiectasis, 223
Bronchiolitis, acute, 220
Bronchitis
    acute, 220
    chronic, 223–224
    not specified as acute or chronic, 223
Bronchoplasty, 233
Bronchoscopy, 132*t*, 232, 235*t*, 240–241
Bronchospasm, acute, 225

Critical illness, definition of, 92
Critical injury, definition of, 92
CRNA; *see* Certified Registered Nurse Anesthetist
Crohn's disease, 292, 314*t*
Cryptococcal meningitis, 389
Cryptococcosis, 389
Cryptorchidism, 342*t*
CT; *see* Computed tomography
CTA; *see* Computed tomography angiography
Cultures, 476
Current Procedural Terminology; *see* CPT
Cushing's syndrome, 434, 434*t*
Cutaneous papilloma, 159
Cutting or paring, 160*t*, 163
CVAD; *see* Central venous access device
Cyst(s), pilonidal, 158, 166
Cystectomy, 337
Cystitis, 332, 343*t*
Cystocele, 342*t*
Cystography, 342*t*
Cystometrogram (CMG), 337
Cystoscopy, 337
Cystourethrogram, voiding, 342*t*
Cystourethroscopy, 333, 337
Cytogenic studies, 480*t*
    CPT coding for, 477
    definition of, 477
Cytopathology, 480*t*
    CPT coding for, 477
    definition of, 477

Dacryoadenitis, 421
Data, in medical decision making, 103*t*, 105*t*
Deafness (hearing loss), 424
Debridement
    CPT coding for, 160*t*, 162–163, 178*t*, 502
    definition of, 162, 178*t*
    excisional versus nonexcisional, 163
    nonselective, 502
    selective, 502
Decision making; *See* Medical decision making
Decompressive spine procedures, 400–401, 401*t*
Decubitus ulcers, 159, 161*t*
Deductible, 532
Deep vein thrombosis (DVT), 260
Default codes, 37
Defibrillator
    CPT coding for, 263–264
    definition of, 263
Definitive identification, 476
Deformations, ICD chapter-specific guidelines for, 41*t*
Deforming dorsopathies, 195
Deformities, musculoskeletal, acquired, ICD coding for, 193*t*, 195–196
Degenerative diseases, of nervous system, ICD coding for, 390–391
Degenerative joint disease
    CPT coding for, 139–148
    ICD coding for, 194
Delivery
    case study of, 378–379
    complications occurring mainly in the course of, 361–362
    complications of, 361–362
    CPT modifiers for, 372–373, 372*t*
    CPT subsection on, 364, 369–371, 369*t*
    encounter for, 360–361
    exam questions on coding, 560–562
    global package of, 370–371
    ICD coding for, 360–362
    normal, 360–361
Delivery/birthing room attendance, 96

Dementia, 390–391, 405*t*
Demyelinating disease, ICD coding for, 392–394
Dental caries, 290
Dentoalveolar structures, CPT coding for, 301
Dentofacial abnormalities, 290
Department of Health and Human Services (HHS), 533
Dermal grafts, 171
Dermal lesions, shaving of, 160*t*, 164–165, 179*t*
Dermatitis, 158–159
Dermis, 155*f*, 156*t*
Descending colon, 288*t*
Destruction, 137, 137*t*
    benign, premalignant, and malignant lesions, 161*t*, 173–174, 174*t*
    ear, 430
    integumentary, 178*t*
    musculoskeletal, 208*t*
    nasal, 228
    nerve, 403
    palate or uvula, 302
    pulmonary, 233
    rectal, 308
    vagina, 365
    vestibule of mouth, 299
Deviated septum, 221
Diabetes mellitus
    anesthesia for patient with, 125–126
    complicating pregnancy, 360
    gestational, 360
    ICD chapter-specific guidelines for, 51*t*, 62–64
    ICD-9-CM codes for, 64*t*
    ICD-10-CM codes for, 64*t*
    insulin pump malfunction in, 63
    secondary, 62
    type 1, 62
    type 2, 62
Diabetic retinopathy, 418–419
Diagnosis
    first-listed, 24, 42
    in medical decision making, 103*t*, 105*t*
    principal, 24, 42
    unconfirmed terms, 24, 43
Diagnosis coding; *see* ICD-9-CM; ICD-10-CM
Diagnostic imaging; *see also* Radiology
    anatomical sites of, 452
    CPT subsection on, 452–454
    number of views/type of view in, 452
Diagnostic injections and infusions, 501
Diagnostic nuclear medicine study, 458–459
Diagnostic outpatient guidelines
    ICD-9-CM, 24
    ICD-10-CM, 42–43
Dialysis
    access for, CPT coding for, 270–271
    CPT coding for, 490–491
    hemodialysis, 270–271, 490, 491*f*
    hemofiltration, 491
    peritoneal, 491
    types of, 490–491
Diaphragm, 217*f*, 218, 218*t*
Diaphragm disorders, 225
Diaphragmatic hernia, 293*t*
Diaphysis, 190
Diastolic heart failure, 259
Digestive system, 286–322
    accessory organs of, 287, 287*f*, 289*t*
    anatomy of, 287, 287*f*, 287*t*–288*t*
    CPT subsection on, 296–312
        general heading code ranges of, 297, 297*t*
        modifiers in, 312–313, 312*t*
        subheadings and guidelines of, 298

CPT terms for, 313, 313*t*–314*t*
    exam questions on coding, 559–560
    functional disorders, not classified elsewhere, 294
    functions of, 286
    ICD chapter-specific guidelines for, 23*t*, 41*t*, 289–296, 289*t*
    ICD terms for, 313, 314*t*
    nuclear medicine studies of, 458
    other diseases of, 294–296
Dilation and curettage (D&C), 373*t*
    nonobstetrical, 367
    obstetric, 369
Diphtheria, tetanus, and pertussis (DTP), 504*t*
Diphtheria and tetanus (DT), 504*t*
Diplopia, 420
Direct examination, 226, 230
Direct laryngoscopy, 231
Direct (open) repair, of aneurysm, 267
Directions, body, 461, 462*t*
Disability evaluation services, CPT E/M coding for, 95
Discharge services, CPT E/M coding for
    hospital, 90
    nursing facility, 93
Disease-oriented panels, 471–472
Disk herniation, 409–410
Dislocations
    casts and strappings for, 205–206, 205*t*
    CPT coding for, 197, 200–202, 200*t*
    definition of, 205
    ICD coding for, 196
Distal, 462*t*
Distinct procedural service, Modifier 59, 537
Diverticula
    intestinal, 294
    urinary bladder, 332
Diverticulitis, 294
Diverticulosis, 294
Divinities, 426
DME; *see* Durable medical equipment
DNA, 474–475, 475*f*
Doctor of osteopathy (DO), 530
Dorsiflexion, 462*f*
Dorsopathies, ICD coding for, 193*t*, 195
Drainage; *see also* Incision and drainage
    spinal, 400
Drug(s)
    administered other than oral method, 519–520
    investigational, HCPCS Level II codes for, 517
    prescription, Medicare coverage of, 530
    table of, HCPCS Level II, 514
Drug abuse treatment services, 519
Drug assays, 473, 480*t*
Drug testing, 472–473
DT (diphtheria and tetanus), 504*t*
DTP (diphtheria, tetanus, and pertussis), 504*t*
Dual-energy x-ray absorptiometry (DXA) scans, 456, 463, 463*t*
Duodenal ulcer, 291
Duodenitis, 292
Duodenostomy tube, 311
Duodenotomy, 306
Duodenum, 288, 288*t*
    diseases of, ICD coding for, 291–292
    motility studies of, 492
Duplex scans, 496
Dura mater, 385*f*, 387*t*
Durable medical equipment (DME), 518, 519*f*
DVT; *see* Deep vein thrombosis
DXA; *see* Dual-energy x-ray absorptiometry scans
Dysphagia, 314*t*

Dyspnea, 236t
Dysrhythmias, cardiac, ICD coding for, 259
Dystocia, 362, 374, 374t

E codes, 518
Ear(s)
    anatomy of, 414–416, 415f, 416t
    audiologic services, CPT coding for, 493
    CPT sections on, 413, 428–430
        general headings and code ranges
            of, 428, 428t
        modifiers in, 432, 432t
    CPT terms for, 433, 433t
    exam questions on coding, 562–564
    functions of, 415
    ICD chapter-specific guidelines for, 41t, 413,
        422–424, 422t
Early pregnancy, 357
EBUS; see Endobronchial ultrasound
ECCE; see Extracapsular cataract extraction
ECG; see Electrocardiogram
Echocardiography, 495
Echoencephalography, 405t
-ectomy, 137t
Ectopic pregnancy, 358–359, 369
Eczema, 158–159
Edema, in pregnancy, CPT coding for, 359–360
EEG; see Electroencephalography
EHRs; see Electronic Health Records
Ejaculatory duct, 324, 326, 326f, 327t
Electric system, of heart, 249–251, 249f, 249t
    disorders of, ICD coding for, 259
Electrocardiogram (ECG), 494, 519
Electroencephalography (EEG), 405t, 499
Electrolyte panel, 472
Electromyography (EMG), 337, 499
Electronic Health Records (EHRs), 539
Electronic Protected Health Information
    (EPHI), 538
Electrophysiologic operative procedures, CPT
    coding for, 264
E/M codes; see Evaluation and Management
    (E/M) section, of CPT
Embolism
    pulmonary
        ICD coding for, 258, 362
        related to pregnancy, childbirth, or
            puerperium, 362
    renal artery, 331
    venous, ICD coding for, 260
Embolus, definition of, 275, 275t
Emergency condition, 116
Emergency department, definition of, 92
Emergency department services, CPT E/M
    coding for, 92
EMG; see Electromyography
Emphysema, 223–224
Empyema, 225
Encephalitis
    definition of, 388
    ICD coding for, 388–389
Encephalomyelitis, 389
Endartectomy, 274t
Endobronchial ultrasound (EBUS), 232
Endocarditis, acute rheumatic, 254
Endocardium, 246, 246t
    diseases of, ICD coding for, 258
Endocervical canal, 353t
Endocrine system
    anatomy of, 416, 416t–417t
    CPT sections on, 413, 430–432
        general headings and code ranges of,
            430, 430t
        modifiers in, 432, 432t

CPT terms for, 433, 434t
diagnostic nuclear studies of, 458
exam questions on coding, 562–564
function of, 416
ICD chapter-specific guidelines for, 23t, 41t,
    51t, 413
Endometriosis, 354, 355, 374t
Endometrium, 352, 353, 353t
Endophthalmitis, 418
Endoscopic retrograde cholangiopancreatography
    (ERCP), 304, 313t
Endoscopy, 131–132, 132t, 137, 137t, 206, 269;
        see also specific types
    cervix, 366
    digestive system, 298
    esophageal, 304
    laryngeal, 230–231
    nasal/sinus, 230
    rectal, 308–309
    small intestine and stomal, 307–308
    tracheal and bronchial, 232
    urinary bladder, 337
    urinary system, 333–334
    vagina, 366
Endotracheal intubation, 230
Endovascular repair, of aneurysm, 267
Endovascular therapy, 398
End-stage renal disease (ESRD), 329,
    330–331
    services for, CPT coding for, 491–492
Enteral therapy, 517
Enteritis
    noninfectious, ICD coding for, 292–293
    regional, 292
Enterolysis, 306, 307
Enteroscopy, small bowel, 320–322
Enterostomy, 307
Enterotomy, 306
Enucleation, 425
EP procedures, CPT coding for, 264
EPHI; see Electronic Protected Health Information
Epicardium, 246, 246t
Epidermal grafts, 171
Epidermal lesions, shaving of, 160t, 164–165, 179t
Epidermis, 155f, 156t
Epididymis, 324, 326f, 327, 327t
Epiglottis, 217f, 218
Epilepsy, ICD coding for, 392, 393
Epiphysis, 190
Episiotomy, 370, 373t
Episodic and paroxysmal disorders, ICD
    coding for, 392–394
Epistaxis, 229, 237t
Eponym, 75
ERCP; see Endoscopic retrograde
    cholangiopancreatography
Erythema, 158–159
Erythematosquamous dermatosis, 158
Erythropoiesis, 325, 325t
Erythropoietin, 325, 325t
Escharotomy, 173
Esophageal acid reflux test, 492
Esophageal perforation, 291, 305
Esophageal stenosis, 291
Esophageal strictures, 291
Esophageal ulcer, 291
Esophageal varices, 305, 314t
Esophagectomies, 303–304
Esophagoplasty, 313t
Esophagus, 287, 287f, 288t
    CPT coding for, 303–305
    diseases of, ICD coding for, 291–292
    motility studies of, 492
Esotropia, 422

ESRD; see End-stage renal disease
Established patients
    in CPT E/M coding, 89
        defining, 98–99
            home services, 94
    in ophthalmology, 493
Ethics, AAPC code of, 528, 529
Ethmoid sinus, 218, 218t, 221f
    CPT coding for, 229–230
Ethmoidectomy, 229
Etiology, 19–20
Eustachian tubes, 416t
Evaluation and management, exam questions
    on coding, 576–580
Evaluation and Management (E/M) section, of
    CPT, 88–113
    arranging codes in, 106–108
    chief complaint in, 97
    components of service in, 99–101, 101t
    determining level of code in, 101–108
    determining range of codes in, 97–99
    examination in, 99–108, 101t
    format and guidelines of, 89–97
    history in, 99–108, 101t
    medical decision making in, 99–108, 101t
    modifiers commonly used with codes,
        108–109, 109t
    patient status in, 97–99
    place of service or setting in, 97–99
    time as factor in, 100
Evisceration of eye, 425
Evocative/suppression testing, 473
Examination
    arranging codes for, 107–108
    in CPT E/M coding, 99–108, 101t
    in CPT surgical package, 133
    direct, 226, 230
    elements and subelements of, 102t–103t, 104t
    indirect, 226, 230
Excision, 137, 137t
    anal, 309
    appendix, 308
    biliary tract, 310
    breast, 161t, 175
    cervix, 366
    dentoalveolar structures, 301
    ear, 428–429, 429–430
    esophageal, 303–304
    integumentary lesions, 160t, 165–166, 179t
    intestinal, 306–307
    kidney, 335
    laryngeal, 230
    lip, 298
    liver, 309
    lymph node, 272
    Mohs surgery for, 160t, 174–175
    musculoskeletal, 196, 198, 199–200, 199t, 208t
    nasal, 228
    ovary, 368–369
    oviduct (fallopian tube), 368
    palate or uvula, 302
    pancreatic, 310–311
    penis, 339
    prostate, 340
    pulmonary or pleural, 233
    rectal, 308
    salivary glands or ducts, 302
    sinus, 229
    spine or spinal cord, 402
    stomach, 305
    testes, 340
    thyroid gland, 430–431
    tongue or floor of mouth, 300–301
    tracheal or bronchial, 233

ICD-9-CM, 13–28
    abbreviations in, 14–15
    chapter-specific guidelines of, 22,
        23t, 50t–51t
    circulatory system in, 253–261
    conventions, guidelines and notes in, 14–18
    diagnostic outpatient guidelines in, 24
    digestive system in, 289–296, 313, 314t
    ear in, 413
    endocrine system in, 413
    exam on, 546–581
    eye in, 413, 418–422, 418t
    female reproductive system in, 354–364,
        354t, 373, 374t
    format of manual, 14
    hierarchy in, 24
    index (Volume 2) of, 14, 20–22
    integumentary system in, 157–160, 158t, 178,
        179t
    locating appropriate code in, steps in, 21–22
    main terms in, 20–22
    male reproductive system in, 328, 328t,
        332–333, 341, 342t–343t
    musculoskeletal system in, 193–196, 193t
    nervous system in, 388–395, 388t, 404, 405t
    pathology/laboratory in, 470
    pregnancy, childbirth, and puerperium in,
        354–364, 355t, 373, 374t
    punctuation in, 19–20
    radiology in, 449–450
    respiratory system in, 219–226, 219t–220t,
        235, 236t–237t
    surgical diagnoses in, 141–142
    symptoms and signs in, 18–19, 23t
    tabular portion (Volume 1) of, 14
    translating provider documentation to, 25
    urinary system in, 328–332, 328t, 341,
        342t–343t
ICD-10-CM, 29–48
    abbreviations in, 31
    chapter-specific guidelines of, 40–42,
        41t–42t, 50t–51t
    circulatory system in, 253–261
    conventions, guidelines and instructional
        notes in, 31–35
    default codes of, 37
    diagnostic outpatient guidelines in, 42–43
    digestive system in, 289–296, 313, 314t
    ear in, 413
    endocrine system in, 413
    extenders in, 38
    eye in, 413, 418–422, 418t
    female reproductive system in, 354–364,
        354t, 373, 374t
    format of, 30
    impending or threatening conditions in, 39
    index of, 30, 37–40
    integumentary system in, 157–160, 158t, 178,
        179t
    locating appropriate codes in, steps in, 39–40
    main terms of, 30, 37
    male reproductive system in, 328, 328t, 332–
        333, 341, 342t–343t
    musculoskeletal system in, 193–196, 193t
    nervous system in, 388–395, 388t, 404, 405t
    pathology/laboratory in, 470
    placeholder characters in, 38
    pregnancy, childbirth, and puerperium in,
        354–364, 355t, 373, 374t
    punctuation in, 35–36
    radiology in, 449–450
    respiratory system in, 219–226, 219t–220t,
        235, 236t–237t
    sequela in, 38–39

subterms of, 30, 37
surgical diagnoses in, 142–143
symptoms and signs in, 34–35, 42t, 43
translating provider documentation to, 43–44
urinary system in, 328–332, 328t, 341,
    342t–343t
ICD-10-PCS, 30
ICF; See Intermediate care facility
Identifiers, HIPAA, 538
Idiopathic normal pressure hydrocephalus, 390
Ileum, 288, 288t
Iliac aneurysm, 267
Imaging; see Radiology
Immunity disorders
    ICD chapter-specific guidelines for, 23t, 51t
    ICD-9-CM codes for, 23t, 51t
    ICD-10-CM codes for, 51t
Immunization administration, 489
Immunology
    CPT coding for, 475–476, 497–498
    definition of, 475
Immunotherapy
    allergen, 498
    CPT coding for, 498
Impacted cerumen, 429
Impending conditions, 39
Impingement syndrome, 208t
Implants
    breast, 176–177
    musculoskeletal, 199
Incision, 137t, 179t, 208t, 235t
    anal, 309
    appendix, 308
    breast, 161t, 175
    ear, 430
    esophageal, 303
    integumentary, 162
    intestinal, 306
    kidney, 334–335
    liver, 309
    lymph node, 272
    middle ear, 429
    musculoskeletal, 196, 198, 199–200, 199t
    nasal, 227–228
    ovary, 368
    oviduct (fallopian tube), 368
    palate or uvula, 301–302
    pancreatic, 310
    penis, 339
    prostate, 340
    pulmonary or pleural, 233
    rectal, 308
    salivary glands or ducts, 302
    sinus, 229
    spine or spinal cord, 402
    stomach, 305
    thyroid gland, 430–431
    tongue or floor of mouth, 299–300
    tracheal, 231
    ureter, 336
    urethra, 337
    urinary bladder, 337
    vagina, 365
    vestibule of mouth, 299
Incision and drainage (I&D); see also Incision
    CPT coding for, 160t, 162, 179t
    definition of, 162, 179t
    ovary, 368
    thyroglossal duct, 430
Incisional hernia, 293t
Includes (note)
    in ICD-9-CM, 17–18
    in ICD-10-CM, 34
Incomplete abortion, 371

Incontinence, urinary, 325t
Index
    CPT, 75–76
    HCPCS Level II, 514
    ICD-9-CM, 14, 20–22
    ICD-10-CM, 30, 37–40
Indicator tests, 471
Indirect examination, 226, 230
Indirect laryngoscopy, 230
Infarction
    myocardial, acute, 256–257
    pulmonary embolism with, 258
    renal, 331
Infection(s); see also specific types
    definition of, 157
    opportunistic, 52
    skin and subcutaneous tissue, 157–158
Infectious arthropathies, ICD coding for, 194–195
Infectious diseases, ICD chapter-specific
    guidelines for, 23t, 41t, 50t
Inferior, 462t
Inferior vena cava, 246t, 250–251, 250f
    wounds of, CPT coding for, 264
Inflammatory polyarthropathies, ICD coding
    for, 195
Influenza, ICD coding for, 219t, 222–223
Infusion and injection procedures, 500–501
Ingestion challenge testing, 498
Inguinal hernia, 293t
Inhalation, 216, 218, 518t
Initial hospital care, 90
Initial infusion, 501
Initial nursing facility care, 93
Initial observation care, 90
Injection, spinal, 400
Injury, ICD chapter-specific guidelines for, 23t, 42t
Inner ear, 415f, 416t
    CPT coding for, 430
    disorders of, ICD coding for, 423
Inpatient, definition of, 97
Inpatient consultations, CPT E/M coding
    for, 91–92
Inpatient services, hospital, CPT E/M coding
    for, 90–91
Insomnia, organic, ICD coding for, 389
Inspiration, 216, 218
Instructional notes
    ICD-9-CM, 14–18
    ICD-10-CM, 31–35
Insufficiency, of heart valves, 254
Insulin pump malfunction, 63
Integumentary, definition of, 154
Integumentary system, 154–184
    anatomy of, 155–157, 155f, 156f, 156t
    CPT subsection on, 160–178, 160t–161t
    CPT terms for, 178, 178t
    exam questions on coding, 549–551
    ICD coding for, 157–160, 158t
    ICD terms for, 178, 179t
    modifiers for, 177–178, 178t
Intensive care services
    initial and continuing, 97
    neonatal and pediatric, 96–97
Interactive complexity, 490
Intermediate care facility (ICF), 93
Intermediate repair, 160t, 167
Internal approach, 226
Internal fixation, 201
Internal mammary artery graft, 266
International Classification of Diseases; see ICD;
    ICD-9-CM; ICD-10-CM; ICD-10-PCS
Interstitium, respiratory diseases principally
    affecting, 220t, 225–226
Interventional radiology, 448

Lymphatic system
    anatomy of, 251–252, 251t–252t
    CPT subsection on, 271–272, 271t
    CPT terms for, 273, 274t
    diseases of, ICD coding for, 253t, 260–261
    fluid exchange with cardiovascular
        system, 252f
    function of, 244
    ICD terms for, 273, 275t
Lymphatic vessels, 251, 251t
    diseases of, ICD coding for, 253t, 260
Lymphedema
    ICD definition of, 275t
    postmastectomy, 261
Lymphoid tissue, 251

M codes, 59
MAC; *see* Monitored anesthesia care
MACs; *see* Medicare Administrative
    Contractors
Magnetic resonance angiography (MRA), 453–454
Magnetic resonance imaging (MRI), 448
    contrast material, 454
    CPT coding for, 453–454
    definition of, 453
    specific anatomical area of, 454
Main terms
    CPT, 75–76
    HCPCS Level II, 514
    ICD-9-CM, 20–22
    ICD-10-CM, 30, 37
Male genital organ disorders, ICD coding for,
    332–333
Male reproductive system
    anatomy of, 326–328, 326f
    components of, 324, 326, 327t
    CPT subsection on, 338–340
        general guidelines of, 338
        general headings and code ranges of,
            339, 339t
        modifiers in, 340–341, 341t
        subheadings of, 339
    CPT terms for, 341, 342t
    definition of, 324
    exam questions on coding, 560–562
    functions of, 324
    ICD chapter-specific guidelines for, 328,
        328t, 332–333
    ICD terms for, 341, 342t–343t
Malignant, definition of, 165
Malignant hypertension, 255
Malignant lesions
    destruction of, 161t, 173–174, 174t
    excision of, 165–166
Malignant neoplasms, 59, 470
Malocclusion, 290
Malunion, 208t, 209
Mammaplasty, reduction, 176
Mammography, CPT subsection on, 456
Managed care entities, 528, 532
Management; *see* Evaluation and management
Management options, in medical decision
    making, 103t
Manifestation, 18, 19–20, 35
Manipulation
    chiropractic, 488, 504t
    CPT coding for, 197, 202
    definition of, 202
    esophageal, 305
    osteopathic, 488
    vagina, 366
Mastectomy, 161t, 176
    lymphedema after, 261
    sentinel node biopsy in, 272

Mastoid process, ICD chapter-specific
    guidelines for, 41t, 422–424, 422t
Mastoidectomy
    complications of, ICD coding for, 423
    CPT coding for, 429–430
Mastopexy, 176
Maternal (maternity) care; *see also* Delivery;
    Pregnancy
    CPT modifiers for, 372–373, 372t
    CPT subsection on, 364, 369–371, 369t
    exam questions on coding, 560–562
Maternal complications, other, ICD coding
    of, 363
Maxillary sinus, 218t, 221, 221f
    CPT coding for, 229–230
Maxillectomy, 229
MDM; *See* Medical decision making
Measles, mumps, rubella, and varicella
    (MMRV) vaccine, 489
Medial meniscus, tear of, 147–148
Median plane, 461t
Mediastinitis, 225
Medicaid, 528, 532
Medical coding; *see also specific codes*
    definition of, 2
    differentiation of languages in, 3
Medical decision making (MDM)
    arranging codes for, 107–108
    in CPT E/M coding, 99–108, 101t
    definition of, 106
    elements and subelements of, 103t, 105t–106t
Medical direction, 119
Medical disability evaluation services, CPT
    E/M coding for, 95
Medical insurance (Medicare Part B), 530
Medical necessity, 4
    CPT–ICD linkage for, 69, 69f
    ensuring
        translating to ICD-9-CM for, 25
        translating to ICD-10-CM for, 43–44
Medical supplies, HCPCS Level II codes for,
    516–517
Medically managed, 4
Medically unlikely edits (MUEs), 537
Medicare, 528, 530–532
    Advance Beneficiary Notice, 534–537, 535f
    claim forms of, 4–6, 5f, 6f, 69, 69f, 530, 531f
    Local Coverage Determinations, 534
    Outpatient Prospective Payment System, 518
    participating providers, 531
    parts of program, 530
Medicare Administrative Contractors (MACs),
    530, 533, 534
Medicare Advantage (Medicare Part C), 530
Medicare provider fee schedule (MPFS), 531
Medicine
    CPT section on, 487–512
        allergy testing in, 497
        audiologic services in, 493
        cardiovascular services in, 494–496
        dialysis in, 490–491
        gastroenterology in, 492
        general headings and code ranges of, 488t
        immunization administration in, 489
        immunology in, 497–498
        immunotherapy in, 498
        infusion and injection procedures in, 500–501
        modifiers in, 502–503, 503t
        neurology and neuromuscular procedures
            in, 498–500
        ophthalmology in, 492–493
        physical medicine and rehabilitation in,
            501–502
        psychiatry in, 489–490

pulmonary services in, 496–497
    sleep medicine testing in, 498–499
    terms used in operative reports, 503–504, 504t
    vaccines and toxoids in, 489
    exam questions on coding, 571–574
Medulla, renal, 325t
Medulla oblongata, 387t
Medullary cavity, 190t
Meninges, 387t
    of brain, 384f
    CPT coding for, 396–399
    of spinal cord, 385f
Meningitis
    definition of, 388
    ICD coding for, 388–389
Meniscal tear, 147–148
Menopause, 355–356
Menstrual disorders, 354, 355
Mental disorders, ICD chapter-specific
    guidelines for, 23t, 41t
Metabolic diseases, ICD chapter-specific
    guidelines for, 23t, 41t, 51t
Metabolic panel, 472
Methicillin-resistant *Staphylococcus aureus*
    (MRSA), 57
Microbiology, 476
Microcuries, 458
Micturition, 343, 343t
Middle ear, 415f
    anatomy of, 429f
    CPT coding for, 429–430
    disorders of, ICD coding for, 423
Migraines, ICD coding for, 392, 393
Military personnel, healthcare coverage
    for, 532
Millicures, 458
Miner's asthma, 224
Minimally invasive procedures, 487–488
Miscarriage, 358
Miscellaneous services, HCPCS Level II codes
    for, 517
Missed abortion, 371
Mitral valve, 250, 250t
    CPT coding for, 264–265
    disorders of, ICD coding for
        not specified as rheumatic, 258
        rheumatic, 254
M-mode ultrasound, 455
MMRV; *see* Measles, mumps, rubella, and
    varicella vaccine
Modalities
    definition of, 501
    in physical medicine and rehabilitation,
        501–502
Moderate sedation, 120
Modifiers, in CPT, 76, 77t–78t
    in ambulance codes, 516, 516t
    in anesthesia codes, 115–118
    in cardiovascular codes, 272–273, 273t
    in digestive system codes, 312–313, 312t
    in distinct procedural service
        (Modifier 59), 537
    in ear codes, 432, 432t
    in E/M codes, 108–109, 109t
    in endocrine system codes, 432, 432t
    in eye codes, 432, 432t
    in integumentary system codes, 177–178, 178t
    in male reproductive system codes, 340–341,
        341t
    in medicine codes, 502–503, 503t
    in musculoskeletal system codes,
        206–207, 207t
    in nervous system codes, 404, 404t
    in pathology/laboratory codes, 479, 479t

Modifiers, in CPT—*Cont.*
 in radiology codes, 459–460, 460*t*
 in respiratory system codes, 234–235, 234*t*
 in Surgery section, 134–136, 135*t*–136*t*
 in surgical procedures, 138, 144
 in urinary system codes, 340–341, 341*t*
Modifiers, in HCPCS Level II codes, 522, 522*t*
Modifiers, nonessential, in ICD-9-CM, 20
Mohs surgery, 161*t*, 174–175
Molar pregnancy, 358–359, 374*t*
Molecular pathology
 CPT coding for, 474–475
 definition of, 474
Monitored anesthesia care (MAC), 120
Mononeuritis, 394
Monotony, 426
Morbidity, external causes of; *see* External causes
Morphology (M) codes, 59
Motor studies, 499
Mouth, 287, 287*f*, 287*t*
 diseases of, ICD coding for, 290
 floor of, CPT coding for, 299–301
 vestibule of, CPT coding for, 299
Movement disorders, ICD coding
 for, 390–391
MPFS; *see* Medicare provider fee schedule
MRA; *see* Magnetic resonance angiography
MRI; *see* Magnetic resonance imaging
MRSA; *see* Methicillin-resistant *Staphylococcus
 aureus*
MUEs; *see* Medically unlikely edits
MUGA (multigated acquisition) scans, 459
Multiple sclerosis, 392
Muscle disorders, ICD coding for, 195, 394–395
Muscle fibers, 187*t*
Muscular dystrophy, 395
Muscular system; *see also* Musculoskeletal system
 anatomy of, 186, 186*f*–187*f*, 187*t*–188*t*
Musculoskeletal system, 185–214
 anatomy of, 186–193
 CPT subsection on, 185, 196–208
  general format of, 196–197, 197*t*
  general procedures in, 198–199
  modifiers in, 206–207, 207*t*
  subheadings of, 198–206, 202*t*
 CPT terms for, 208, 208*t*
 exam questions on coding, 551–552
 ICD chapter-specific guidelines for, 23*t*, 41*t*
 ICD coding for, 23*t*, 41*t*, 193–196, 193*t*
 ICD terms for, 208, 209*t*
 nuclear medicine studies of, 459
Mutations, 480, 480*t*
Myalgia, 208*t*
Mycology, 476
Myelitis
 ICD coding for, 388–389
 transverse, 392
Myocardial infarction, acute
 episode of care for, 257
 ICD coding for, 256–257
 sections of heart involved in, 256–257
Myocardial muscle, 188*t*
Myocardial perfusion studies, 459
Myocarditis
 acute rheumatic, 254
 septic, 258
Myocardium, 246*t*, 258
 diseases of, ICD coding for, 258
Myolysis, 208*t*
Myomectomy, 367
Myometrium, 352, 353, 353*t*
Myoneural junction disorders, ICD coding
 for, 394–395
Myopia, 420

Myotonic disorders, 395
Myringotomy, 429

Nail(s)
 anatomy of, 155, 155*f*, 156*f*, 157*t*
 CPT coding for, 160*t*, 166
 ICD coding for, 159–160
Nares/nostrils, 217*f*, 217*t*
Nasal cavity, 217*f*, 217*t*
Nasal hemorrhage
 anterior control of, 229
 CPT coding for, 229
 definition of, 229
 posterior control of, 229
Nasal polyps
 excision of, 228
 ICD coding for, 221
Nasal septum, 217*t*
 deviated, 221
 prosthesis or button insertion in, 228
Nasal turbinates, 227*f*
 CPT coding for, 227–229
Nasal vestibular stenosis, 228
Nasogastric tubes, 306
Nasopharyngitis
 acute, 220
 chronic, 221
National codes, in HCPCS, 70, 513–527; *see also*
 Level II, of HCPCS
National Correct Coding Initiative (NCCI), 537
National Coverage Determinations
 (NCDs), 534
National Provider Identifier (NPI), 538
NCCI; *see* National Correct Coding Initiative
NCDs; *see* National Coverage Determinations
Nearsightedness, 420
NEC (not elsewhere classified), 15, 31
Necropsy, 477, 480*t*
Neonatal critical care services, CPT E/M
 coding for, 96–97
Neonatal intensive care services, CPT E/M
 coding for, 96
Neoplasm(s), 59
 benign, 59, 470
 complications of treatment, 60
 encounters for treatment, 60–61
 ICD coding for, 23*t*, 41*t*, 51*t*, 59–62, 62*t*, 470
 lesions versus, 165
 malignant, 59, 470
 morphology (M) codes for, 59
 personal history of, 60
 primary, 59–60, 470
 secondary, 59–60, 470
 uncertain behavior of, 166, 470
 unspecified behavior of, 166, 470
Nephrorrhaphy, 336
Nephrectomy, 335–336
Nephritis, ICD coding for, 329–330
Nephrolithiasis, 343*t*
Nephrolithotomy, 335, 342*t*
Nephrons, 325, 325*t*
Nephroptosis, 343*t*
Nephrosis, 329–330
Nephrostomy, 335
Nephrotic syndrome, ICD coding for, 329–330
Nerve(s), CPT coding for, 402–403
Nerve block, 402
Nerve cells, of eye, 415*t*
Nerve conduction studies
 CPT coding for, 499–500
 definition of, 499
 motor, 499
 sensory, 499
Nerve disorders, ICD coding for, 394–395

Nerve plexus
 definition of, 394
 disorders of, ICD coding for, 394–395
Nerve roots, 387*t*
 disorders of, ICD coding for, 394–395
Nervous system, 382–412
 anatomy of, 383*f*–385*f*, 385–387, 386*t*–387*t*
 CPT subsection on, 395–404
  general headings and code ranges of,
  396, 396*t*
  modifiers in, 404, 404*t*
 CPT terms for, 404, 405*t*
 exam questions on coding, 562–564
 flow of information in, 385
 functions of, 382
 ICD chapter-specific guidelines for, 23*t*, 41*t*,
  388–395, 388*t*
 ICD terms for, 404, 405*t*
 other disorders of, ICD coding for, 391
Neuroendoscopy, 399
Neurology and neuromuscular procedures,
 498–500
Neurolytic agent, 403
Neuropathy, ICD coding for, 394–395
Neuroplasty, 403
Neurorrhaphy, 403, 405*t*
Neurostimulator(s), 399
 analysis-programming of, 500
 peripheral nerve, 402–403
Neurostimulator electrode implantation, 402
New patients
 in CPT E/M coding, 89
  defining, 98–99
  home services, 94
 in ophthalmology, 493
Newborn(s)
 ICD coding for, 23*t*
 sepsis in, 57
Newborn services
 CPT E/M coding for, 95–97
 normal, 96
Nines, rule of, 172
Nonautologous graft, 171
Nonessential modifiers, 20
Noninvasive procedures, 487–488
Noninvasive vascular diagnostic studies, 496
Nonparticipating (non-PAR) providers, 532
Nonsegmental instrumentation, 205
Nonselective debridement, 502
Nonunion, 208*t*, 209
NOS (not otherwise specified), 15, 31
Nose, 217*f*, 217*t*
 CPT coding for, 227–229
Not elsewhere classified (NEC), 15, 31
Not otherwise specified (NOS), 15, 31
Notes, instructional
 ICD-9-CM, 14–18
 ICD-10-CM, 31–35
Notes, parenthetical, in CPT, 72
NPI; *see* National Provider Identifier
Nuclear medicine
 CPT subsection on, 458–459
 definition of, 458
 diagnostic studies in, 458–459
 endocrine studies in, 458
 gastrointestinal studies in, 458
 therapeutic studies in, 459
Null zero, in CPT, 73, 73*t*
Nurse anesthetist, 117–118, 118*t*
Nurse practitioner (NP), 530
Nursing facility services, CPT E/M coding
 for, 93
Nutritional disease, ICD chapter-specific
 guidelines for, 23*t*, 41*t*

Obesity, complicating pregnancy, 357
Objective tinnitus, 424
Observation care discharge services, 90
Observation services, CPT E/M coding for, 89–90
Obstetric conditions; *see also* Delivery; Pregnancy
  other, not elsewhere specified, 363
Obstetric trauma, other, ICD coding for, 361
Obstetrical ultrasound, 455
Obstructive hydrocephalus, 390
Occipital lobe, 386*t*
OCR; *see* Office of Civil Rights
Ocular adnexa
  CPT sections on, 424, 424*t*, 427
  disorders of, ICD coding for, 41*t*,
    418–422, 418*t*
Ocular implant, secondary, 425
Oculus dexter (OD), 433, 433*t*
Oculus sinister (OS), 433, 433*t*
Oculus uterque (OU), 433, 433*t*
OD; *see* Oculus dexter
Office consultations, CPT E/M coding for, 91
Office of Civil Rights (OCR), 537–538
Office of Inspector General (OIG), 533–534
Office services, CPT E/M coding for, 89
OIG; *see* Office of Inspector General
OIs; *see* Opportunistic infections
Omentum, CPT coding for, 311–312
OMT; *see* Osteopathic manipulation treatment
Oncology, radiation; *see* Radiation oncology
Onychomycosis, 159–160
Open code-book exam, 8
Open fracture, 208*t*, 209
Open procedure, 132, 132*t*
Open treatment, of fractures, 201
Open-angle glaucoma, 419
Operating microscope, 430
Operative reports, terms used in, 136–138, 137*t*
  cardiovascular and lymphatic, 273, 274*t*–275*t*
  digestive, 313, 313*t*–314*t*
  ear, 433, 433*t*
  endocrine system, 433, 434*t*
  eye, 433, 433*t*
  female reproductive system, 373, 373*t*, 374*t*
  HCPCS Level II codes, 523, 523*t*
  integumentary, 178–179, 178*t*–179*t*
  male reproductive, 341, 342*t*–343*t*
  medicine, 503–504, 504*t*
  musculoskeletal, 208, 208*t*–209*t*
  nervous system, 404, 405*t*
  pathology/laboratory, 479–480, 480*t*
  radiology, 461–463, 461*t*, 462*t*, 463*t*
  respiratory, 235, 235*t*–236*t*
  urinary, 341, 342*t*–343*t*
Ophthalmology
  CPT coding for, 492–493
  general services in, 492–493
  new and established patients in, 493
  special services in, 493
  spectacle services in, 493
Opportunistic infections (OIs), 52
OPPS; *see* Outpatient Prospective Payment
    System
Optic disc, 415*t*
Optic nerve, 414*f*
  disorders affecting, ICD coding for, 421
Optic nerve head, 415*t*
Oral cavity
  diseases of, ICD coding for, 290
  vestibule of, CPT coding for, 299
Oral two-thirds, 301
Orbit
  CPT coding for, 427
  disorders of, ICD coding for, 421
Orchiopexy, 342*t*

Organ failure, in sepsis, 55–56
Organ panels, 471–472
Organ system; *see also specific systems*
  examination coding by, 103*t*, 104*t*
Orogastric tubes, 306
Orthoroentgenograms, 456
Orthotic procedures and devices, 520, 520*f*
OS; *see* Oculus sinister
-oscopy, 137*t*
Ossicles, 415*f*, 416*t*
Osteoarthritis
  definition of, 208*t*, 209
  ICD coding for, 194–195, 208*t*
Osteomyelitis, ICD coding for, 195–196
Osteopathic manipulation treatment
    (OMT), 488
Osteopathies, ICD coding for, 193*t*,
    195–196
Osteopathy, doctor of (DO), 530
Osteoporosis, 208*t*, 209, 456, 456*f*
-ostomy, 137*t*
Otalgia (ear pain), 423
Otitis externa, 423, 433*t*
Otitis media, 423, 438–439
-otomy, 137*t*
Otorhinolaryngologic services, 493
OU; *see* Oculus uterque
Outer ear; *see* External ear
Outpatient, definition of, 98
Outpatient consultations, CPT E/M coding
    for, 91
Outpatient guidelines
  ICD-9-CM, 24
  ICD-10-CM, 42–43
Outpatient Prospective Payment System
    (OPPS), 518
Outpatient services, CPT E/M coding for, 89
Oval window, 416*t*
Ovarian malignancy, 368–369
Ovary(ies), 352, 352*f*, 353, 353*t*
  CPT coding for, 368–369
  disorders of, ICD coding for, 355–356
  endocrine function of, 416
  pathology/laboratory studies of, 485–486
Overactive bladder, 332
Oviducts (fallopian tubes), 352, 352*f*, 353, 353*t*
  CPT coding for, 368
  disorders of, ICD coding for, 355–356
  pathology/laboratory studies of, 485–486
Oximetry, 235*t*
Oxygen, transport in blood, 250–251

Pacemaker
  CPT coding for, 263–264
  placement of, case study of, 279–280
Pacing cardioverter-defibrillator, CPT coding
    for, 263–264
PACU; *see* Postanesthesia care unit
Pain
  ear, 423
  ICD coding for, 391
Palate, CPT coding for, 301–302
Pancreas, 287, 287*f*, 289*t*
  anatomy of, 295*f*
  CPT coding for, 310–311, 431–432
  diseases of, ICD coding for, 294–296
  endocrine function of, 416
Pancreatotomy, 311
Pap smears, 477
Papilloma, cutaneous, 159
Paracentesis, abdominal, 311
Paralytic ileus, 294
Paralytic syndromes, ICD coding for, 392–394
Paranasal sinuses, 217*f*, 218*t*, 221, 221*f*

Parasitic disease, ICD chapter-specific
    guidelines for, 23*t*, 41*t*, 50*t*
Parasitology, 476
Parasomnia, 390
Parasympathetic nervous system, 386*t*
Parathyroid gland, 417*t*, 431*f*
  CPT coding for, 431–432
Paravaginal defect repair, 366
Parenteral therapy, 517
Parentheses, 20, 36
Parenthetical notes, 72
Parietal lobe, 386*t*
Paring
  CPT coding for, 160*t*, 163
  definition of, 163
Parkinson's disease, 390–391
Paronychia, 159–160
Paroxysmal disorders, ICD coding for, 392–394
Partial-thickness burns, 172*f*
Participating (PAR) providers, 531
Past, family, and social history (PFSH), 102*t*,
    104*t*, 107
Pathologic fracture, 208*t*, 209, 450
Pathology/laboratory, 469–486
  CPT section on, 470–480, 470*t*
    anatomic pathology in, 477
    chemistry in, 475
    consultations (clinical pathology) in, 473
    cytogenic studies in, 477
    cytopathology in, 477
    drug testing in, 472–473
    evocative/suppression testing in, 473
    guidelines in, 471
    hematology and coagulation in, 475
    immunology in, 475–476
    microbiology in, 476
    modifiers in, 479, 479*t*
    molecular pathology in, 474–475
    organ or disease-oriented panels in,
      471–472
    surgical pathology in, 477–478
    therapeutic drug assays in, 473
    transfusion medicine in, 476
    urinalysis in, 473–474
  CPT terms for, 479–480, 480*t*
  exam questions on coding, 567–571
  ICD guidelines for, 470
  ICD neoplasm table in, 470
Patient status, in CPT E/M coding, 97–99
Patients
  established; *See* Established patients
  new; *See* New patients
Payer(s), 528, 530–533
Payer language, 3
PDT; *see* Photodynamic therapy
Pediatric critical care services, CPT E/M
    coding for, 96–97
Pediatric intensive care services, CPT E/M
    coding for, 96
Pelvic bones, 192*t*
Pelvic organs, female
  inflammatory disease of, ICD coding
    for, 355
  noninflammatory disease of, ICD coding for,
    355–356
  ultrasound of, 455
Pelvis, ultrasound of, 455
Penis, 324, 326, 326*f*, 327*t*
  CPT coding for, 339–340
  disorders of, ICD coding for, 333
Peptic ulcer, 291
Percutaneous balloon valvuloplasty, 494
Percutaneous procedure, 132, 132*t*
Percutaneous skeletal fixation treatment, 201

ICD-9-CM codes for, 23*t*
ICD-10-CM codes for, 41*t*
Pulmonary arteries, 246*t*
 atherosclerosis of, 260
 wounds of, CPT coding for, 264
Pulmonary artery balloon angioplasty, 494
Pulmonary circulation, 245
 diseases of, ICD coding for, 253*t*, 258
Pulmonary collapse, 225
Pulmonary congestion and hypostasis, 225
Pulmonary diagnostic testing and therapies, 497
Pulmonary edema, 225
Pulmonary embolism
 with infarction, ICD coding for, 258
 related to pregnancy, childbirth, or
  puerperium, 362
Pulmonary fibrosis, 225
Pulmonary function tests, 497
Pulmonary heart disease, ICD coding for, 258
Pulmonary infiltrates, 242–243
Pulmonary insufficiency, 225
Pulmonary services, CPT coding for, 496–497
Pulmonary valve, 250*t*
 CPT coding for, 264–265
 disorders of, ICD coding for
  not specified as rheumatic, 258
  rheumatic, 254
Pulmonary veins, 246*t*
Pulp, tooth, disorders of, 290
Pump implantation, spinal, 400
Punctuation
 in ICD-9-CM, 19–20
 in ICD-10-CM, 35–36
Pupil, 414*f*, 415*t*
Purkinje fibers, 249–251, 249*f*, 249*t*
Pyelonephritis, 343*t*
 acute, 331
 chronic, 331
Pyeloplasty, 336
Pyloromyotomy, 305
Pyogenic arthritis, 194

Q codes, 521
Qualifying-circumstance modifiers, 116–117, 116*t*
Qualitative analysis, 472
Quantitative analysis, 473

Radial artery graft, 268
Radiation oncology
 clinical brachytherapy in, 457
 clinical treatment planning in, 457
 CPT subsection on, 456–457
 simulation-aided field setting in, 457
 treatment delivery in, 457
 treatment management in, 457
Radiation treatment delivery, 457
Radiation treatment management, 457
Radiation-related disorders, of skin and
  subcutaneous tissue, 158–159
Radiology, 448–468
 CPT section on, 70, 71*t*, 449–463
  bone/joint studies subsection in, 456
  breast mammography subsection in, 456
  component coding in, 451
  contrast material in, 450
  diagnostic imaging subsection in, 452–454
  diagnostic ultrasound subsection in, 454–456
  fluoroscopy in, 451
  format of, 449, 449*t*
  guidelines in, 450–451
  modifiers in, 459–460, 460*t*
  nuclear medicine subsection in, 458–459
  number of views in, 451
  radiation oncology subsection in, 456–457

CPT terms for, 461–463, 461*t*, 462*t*, 463*t*
exam questions on coding, 564–567
ICD guidelines for, 449–450
 abnormal findings in, 449
 aftercare in, 450
 encounter for therapy in, 449–450
 history of (personal or family) in, 450
 screening in, 450
 signs and symptoms in, 449
Radionuclide, 458
Radiopharmaceutical, 458, 463, 463*t*, 517
Radiosurgery, stereotactic, 399
Rales, 237*t*
Reconstruction
 breast, 161*t*, 176–177
 musculoskeletal, 202
Rectum, CPT coding for, 308–309
Red blood cell count, 475
Reduction mammaplasty, 176
Referral, 91
Refraction disorders, 420
Regional enteritis, 292
Regional nerve block, 402
Regulations
 American Recovery and Reinvestment Act
  and, 539
 Centers for Medicare and Medicaid Services
  and, 534–537
 compliance with, 3–6, 528, 533–539
 HIPAA and, 537–538
 National Correct Coding Initiative and, 537
 Office of Civil Rights and, 537–538
 Office of Inspector General and, 533–534
Regurgitation, cardiac valve, 265
Reimbursement, 3–6, 528, 530–533
Relative Value Guide (RVG), for anesthesia, 115
Removal
 from abdomen, peritoneum or omentum, 311
 from ear, 429
 from eye, 425
 of eye, 424–425
 from lung, 233
 of lung, 233
 from musculoskeletal system, 196, 198
 urinary bladder, 337
Renal artery atherosclerosis, 260
Renal artery embolism, 331
Renal failure, 343*t*
 acute, 330, 343*t*
 dialysis for, 490–491
 unspecified, 331
Renal infarction, 331
Renal pelvis, 325*t*
 catheter introduction to, 336
 surgical repair of, 336
Renal tubules, 325*t*
Renal tubulointerstitial diseases, 329
Repair, 137, 137*t*
 abdominal, peritoneal or omental, 311
 breast, 161*t*, 176–177
 ear, 429, 430
 esophageal, 304–305
 integumentary (closure), 160*t*,
  166–168, 179*t*
  complex, 160*t*, 167
  intermediate, 160*t*, 167
  simple, 160*t*, 167
 kidney, 336
 laryngeal, 231
 lip, 298–299
 liver, 310
 musculoskeletal, 197, 202, 208*t*
 nasal, 228
 nerve, 403

oviduct (fallopian tube), 368
palate or uvula, 302
penis, 340
respiratory system, 236*t*
salivary glands or ducts, 302
skull base, 397
spine or spinal cord, 402
tongue or floor of mouth, 301
tracheal or bronchial, 233
ureter, 336
urethra, 337–338
uterus, 367
vagina, 366
vestibule of mouth, 299
Replantation, musculoskeletal, 199
Resection, pulmonary, 233
Reservoir/pump implantation, spinal, 400
Respiratory failure
 acute, 225
 chronic, 225
Respiratory infections, acute, ICD coding for,
  219*t*, 220–221
Respiratory system, 215–243
 anatomy of, 216–219, 217*f*, 217*t*–218*t*
 CPT subsection on, 226–235
  general heading code ranges of, 227
  modifiers in, 234–235, 234*t*
  subheadings and guidelines of, 227
 CPT terms for, 235, 235*t*–236*t*
 exam questions on coding, 553–559
 function of, 215
 gas exchange in, 215, 216*f*
 ICD chapter-specific guidelines for, 23*t*, 41*t*,
  219–226
 ICD subheadings for, 219*t*–220*t*
 ICD terms for, 235, 236*t*–237*t*
 intraoperative and postprocedural
  complications and disorders of, 220*t*
 nuclear medicine studies of, 459
 other diseases of, 220*t*, 225–226
Restless legs syndrome, 391
Resuscitation, cardiopulmonary, 494
Resuscitation services, newborn, 96
Retina, 414*f*, 415*t*
 CPT coding for, 426
 disorders of, ICD coding for, 418–419
 other disorders of, 418–419
Retinal defects, 418
Retinal detachment, 418, 426
Retinopathy, 418–419
Retroperitoneum
 diseases of, ICD coding for, 294
 ultrasound of, 455
Revascularization, percutaneous
  transluminal, 494
Revenue cycle, 4
Reversible ischemia, 265
Review of systems (ROS), 104*t*, 106
Revision
 abdominal, peritoneal or omental, 311
 musculoskeletal, 202
Rheumatic chorea, 254, 275*t*
Rheumatic endocarditis, acute, 254
Rheumatic fever, acute
 ICD coding for, 253–254, 253*t*
  with mention of heart involvement, 253
  without mention of heart involvement, 253
Rheumatic heart disease, chronic
 ICD coding for, 253*t*, 254
 includes note on, 254
Rheumatic myocarditis, acute, 254
Rheumatic pericarditis, acute, 253
Rheumatism, ICD coding for, 193*t*, 195
Rheumatoid arthritis, ICD coding for, 194

Rhinitis, chronic or allergic, 222
Rhinoplasty, 228
Right heart failure, 259
Rinne test, 433*t*
Risk, table of, 103*t*, 105*t*
ROS; *See* Review of systems
Route of administration, 517–518, 518*t*
Rule of nines, 172
RVG; *see* Relative Value Guide

Sagittal plane, 461*f*, 461*t*
Salivary ducts, CPT coding for, 302
Salivary glands, 287, 287*f*, 289*t*
    CPT coding for, 302
    diseases of, ICD coding for, 290
Salpingitis, 355, 374*t*
Salpingostomy, 368
Saphenous vein graft, 266
SARS; *see* Severe acute respiratory syndrome
Scan grams, 456
Schilling tests, 458
Sclera, 414, 414*f*, 414*t*
    anterior, CPT coding for, 426
Screening, in radiology, 450
Scrotum, 326, 327*t*
Secondary cataracts, 419, 426
Secondary diabetes mellitus, 62
Secondary neoplasms, 59–60, 470
Secondary ocular implant, 425
Second-degree burns, 171–173, 172*f*
Security, HIPAA and, 538
Sedation, conscious or moderate, 120
Segmental instrumentation, 205
Selective debridement, 502
Semicolon, in CPT, 73–74
Seminal vesicles, 324, 326, 326*f*, 327, 327*t*
Seminiferous tubules, 327, 327*t*
Senile cataracts, 419, 440–441
Sense organs; *see also specific organs*
    diseases of, ICD chapter-specific guidelines
        for, 23*t*, 41*t*
Sensorineural hearing loss, 424
Sensory nerve studies, 499
Sentinel lymph node, 272
Separate procedure, in CPT, 74
Sepsis
    abortion and pregnancy complicated by, 57
    code selection flowchart for, 56*f*
    definition of, 55
    due to postprocedural infection, 57
    ICD chapter-specific guidelines for, 50*t*, 55–58
    ICD-9-CM codes for, 58*t*
    ICD-10-CM codes for, 58*t*
    in newborns, 57
    organ failure in, 55–56
    puerperal, 362–363
Septal graft, CPT coding for, 266
Septic myocarditis, 258
Septic shock, 50*t*, 55–58, 58*t*
Septicemia, 55–58
Septum, 246, 246*t*, 266
Sequela, 38–39
Sequential infusion, 501
Sesamoid bone, 190*f*
Setting, in CPT E/M coding, 97–99
Seventh-character extenders, 38
Severe acute respiratory syndrome (SARS), 237*t*
Severe sepsis, 50*t*, 55–58, 56*f*, 58*t*
Shaving
    definition of, 164, 179*t*
    of epidermal or dermal lesions, 160*t*,
        164–165, 179*t*
Shin splint, 209*t*
Shock, septic, 50*t*, 55–58, 56*f*, 58*t*

Short bones, 189*f*
Shoulder bones, 191*t*
Shunt, 274*t*
Shunt, CSF, 399, 402
Sick sinus syndrome (SSS), 275*t*
Sigmoid colon, 288*t*
Sigmoidoscopy, 308–309, 314*t*
Signs, 18
    in ICD-9-CM, 18–19, 23*t*
    in ICD-10-CM, 34–35, 42*t*, 43
    in radiology report, 449
Simple repair, 160*t*, 167
Simulation-aided field setting, 457
Single-layer (simple) repair, 160*t*, 167
Single-photon emission computed
        tomography (SPECT), 458, 459, 463*t*
Sinoatrial (SA) node, 249–251, 249*f*, 249*t*
Sinuses
    accessory, 229–230
    paranasal, 217*f*, 218*t*, 221, 221*f*, 229–230
Sinusitis
    acute, 220
    chronic, 221
SIRS; *see* Systemic inflammatory response
        syndrome
Sixth-degree burns, 172
Skeletal muscles, 188*t*
Skeletal system; *see also* Musculoskeletal
        system
    anatomy of, 189*f*, 190*t*–192*t*
Skeletal traction, 202
Skilled nursing facility (SNF), 93
Skin
    CPT coding for, 160–177, 160*t*–161*t*
    exam questions on coding, 549–551
    ICD coding for, 23*t*, 41*t*, 157–160, 158*t*
Skin, anatomy of, 155–157, 155*f*, 156*t*
Skin appendages, disorders of, 159–160
Skin grafts, 161*t*, 170–171
Skin infections, ICD coding for, 157–158
Skin replacement, 161*t*, 170–171
Skin tags, 159
    removal of, 160*t*, 164
Skin traction, 202
Skull
    bones of, 191*t*, 200, 201*f*
    CPT coding for, 396–399
Skull base surgery, 397
Slanted brackets, 19
Sleep apnea, organic, 389
Sleep disorders, organic, ICD coding
        for, 389–390
Sleep medicine testing, 498–499
Small bowel enteroscopy, 320–322
Small intestine, 287, 287*f*, 288*t*
    anatomy of, 293*f*
    CPT coding for, 306–308
    disorders of, ICD coding for, 291–294
Smooth muscles, 188*t*
SNF; *See* Skilled nursing facility
Soft tissue disorders, ICD coding for, 195
Somatic nervous system, 385, 386*t*
Somatics, definition of, 480*t*
Somnolence, excessive, ICD coding for, 389
Sonography; *see* Ultrasound
Sonohysterography, 367
Specificity, coding to highest level of, 20, 24, 43
Specimen, 480, 480*t*
SPECT; *see* Single-photon emission computed
        tomography
Spectacle services, 493
Spermatic cord, 327, 327*t*
    disorders of, ICD coding for, 333
Spermatogenesis, 327*t*

Sphenoid sinus, 217*f*, 218, 218*t*, 221*f*
    CPT coding for, 229–230
Spina bifida, 361
Spinal arthrodesis, 203–204, 203*t*
Spinal column, 204*f*
Spinal cord, 385, 387*t*
    anatomy of, 384*f*, 385*f*
    CPT coding for, 400–402
Spinal decompressive procedures, 400–401, 401*t*
Spinal instrumentation, 204–205
    nonsegmental, 205
    segmental, 205
Spine, CPT coding for, 400–402
Spinocerebellar diseases, 391
Spirometry, 236*t*, 497, 497*f*
Spleen, 251, 252*t*
    CPT coding for, 271, 271*t*
Splenectomy, 271
Split-thickness grafts, 171
Spondylopathies, ICD coding for, 195
Spongy bone, 190*t*
Spontaneous abortion, 358
Sports injuries, 209*t*
Sprain, 209, 209*t*
Square brackets, 19, 35–36
SSS; *see* Sick sinus syndrome
Staphylococcus aureus, methicillin-resistant, 57
Status migrainosus, 393
Stem cell services, CPT coding for, 271
Stenosis
    of esophagus, 291
    of heart valves, 254, 265
    nasal vestibular, 228
    of trachea, 240–241
Stent, 274*t*
Stent, intracoronary, 494
Stereotactic, definition of, 398, 405*t*
Stereotactic radiosurgery, 399
Stereotaxis, CPT coding for, 398–399
Stomach, 287, 287*f*, 288*t*
    anatomy of, 291*f*
    CPT coding for, 305–306
    diseases of, ICD coding for, 291–292
    motility studies of, 492
    x-ray of, 452*f*
Strabismus, 421–422, 427
Strain, 209*t*
Strapping application, 205–206, 205*t*
Strictures, esophageal, 291
Subarachnoid hemorrhage, 259
Subcutaneous administration, 518*t*
Subcutaneous infections, ICD coding
        for, 157–158
Subcutaneous tissue, 155*f*, 156*t*
Subcutaneous tissue disease(s)
    CPT coding for, 160–177, 160*t*–161*t*
    ICD chapter-specific guidelines for, 23*t*, 41*t*
    ICD coding for, 157–160, 158*t*
Subdural hematoma, 411–412
Subjective tinnitus, 424
Subsequent hospital care, 91
Subsequent nursing facility care, 93
Subsequent observation care, 90
Subterms, ICD-10-CM, 30, 37
Superficial veins, 246*t*
Superior, 462*t*
Superior vena cava, 246*t*, 250–251, 250*f*
    wounds of, CPT coding for, 264
Supination, 462*f*, 463, 463*t*
Suppression testing, 473
Surgery section, of CPT, 70, 71*t*, 129–138;
        see also specific systems and procedures
    approach in, 131–132, 132*t*
    global surgical package in, 133–134

global surgical period in, 133–134
guidelines and format of, 72, 130–133
modifiers in, 134–136, 135t–136t
subsections of, 130–131, 130t
Surgical package, global, 133–134
Surgical pathology, 477–478, 478f, 480t
Surgical period, global, 133–134
Surgical procedures; *see also specific procedures*
  CPT coding for, 129–138, 140
  diagnostic coding for, 138, 140–143
  ICD-9-CM coding for, 141–142
  ICD-10-CM coding for, 142–143
  indexing, 138–144
  modifiers for, adding, 138, 144
  procedural coding for, 138–140
  terms used in operative reports, 136–138, 137t
Surgical supplies, HCPCS Level II codes for, 516–517
Suture joint, 190t
Symbols, CPT, 73, 73t
Sympathetic nervous system, 386t
Symptoms, 18
  in ICD-9-CM, 18–19, 23t
  in ICD-10-CM, 34–35, 42t, 43
  in radiology report, 449
Syncope, 405t
Synovial disorders, ICD coding for, 195
Synovial joint, 191t
Syringobulbia, 391
Syringomyelia, 391
Systemic circulation, 245
Systemic connective tissue disorders, ICD coding for, 194–195
Systemic inflammatory response syndrome (SIRS), 55–58, 56f
Systemic lupus erythematosus, 194
Systolic heart failure, 259

T codes, 524
Table of neoplasms, 470
Table of risk, 103t, 105t
Tabular List of ICD-10-CM, 30
Tabular portion of ICD-9-CM, 14
TAVI; *see* Transcatheter aortic valve implantation
TAVR; *see* Transcatheter aortic valve replacement
TBSA; *See* Total body surface area
TEE; *see* Transesophageal echocardiography
Teeth
  CPT coding for, 301
  disorders of, ICD coding for, 290
Temporal arteritis, 275t
Temporal lobe, 386t
Temporary (category III) codes, 524
Temporary miscellaneous services, 521
Temporary national codes (non-Medicare), 521
Temporary procedures/professional services, 519
Tendon, 188, 188f, 188t
Tendon disorders, ICD coding for, 195
Tension headaches, 392
Tentorium, 386t
Terminology
  exam questions on, 575–576
  operative report; *see* Operative reports, terms used in
Testes, 324, 326, 326f, 327, 327t
  CPT coding for, 340
  disorders of, ICD coding for, 333
  endocrine function of, 416
Testicular torsion, 333
Test-taking skills, 8–9
Thalamus, 387t
Therapeutic injections and infusions, 501

Therapeutic nuclear medicine studies, 459
Third-degree burns, 171–173, 172f
Third-party payers, 528, 530–533
Thoracentesis, 233
Thoracic aortic aneurysm, 267
Thoracoscopy, 132t, 233
Thoracostomy, tube, 233
Thoracotomy, 233
Threatening conditions, 39
Thrombolysis, 494
Thrombophlebitis, ICD coding for, 260
Thrombosis, portal vein, 275t
Thrombus, definition of, 275, 275t
Thymus, 251, 252t, 417, 417t
Thyroid gland, 417, 417t, 431f
  CPT coding for, 430–431
  diagnostic nuclear studies of, 458
Thyroid storm, 434, 434t
Thyroid uptake studies, 458
Thyroidectomy, 431
Thyroid-stimulating hormone (TSH), 434t
Time
  in anesthesia care, 115
  in evaluation and management, 100
Tinnitus, 423–424
Tissue transfer, adjacent, 161t, 169–170, 178t
Toes, bones of, 192t
Tongue, CPT coding for, 299–301
Tonsil(s)
  chronic diseases of, 221
  CPT coding for, 303
Tonsillectomy, 303, 319–320
Tonsillitis
  acute, 220
  chronic, 319–320
  peritonsillar abscess with, 221
Torsion dystonia, 391
Total body surface area (TBSA), 172
Total hysterectomy, 367, 379–381
Toxoids, CPT coding for, 489
Trabeculoplasty, 426
Trabeculotomy ab externo, 426
Trachea, 217f, 218, 218t
  CPT coding for, 231–233
Tracheal puncture, 231
Tracheal stenosis, 240–241
Tracheitis, acute, 220
Trachelectomy, 366
Tracheobronchitis, diffuse, 242–243
Tracheoplasty, 233
Tracheostoma revision, 231
Tracheostomy, 231
Tracheostomy complications, 225
Traction, 202
  skeletal, 202
  skin, 202
TRALI; *see* Transfusion-related acute lung injury
Transactions and code sets, HIPAA, 538
Transcatheter aortic valve implantation (TAVI), 265
Transcatheter aortic valve replacement (TAVR), 265
Transesophageal echocardiography (TEE), 495
Transfer of care, 91
Transfusion medicine, 476
Transfusion-related acute lung injury (TRALI), 225
Transitional care management services, 97
Transplantation
  cornea, 425
  heart/lung, 267
  intestinal, 306–307
  islet cell, 311
  kidney, 335–336

liver, 310
lung, 233–234
Transportation services
  advanced life support in, 515–516
  basic life support in, 515–516
  HCPCS Level II codes for, 515–516
  HCPCS modifiers for, 516, 516t
Transurethral resection of the prostate (TURP), 342t
Transvaginal ultrasound, 455
Transverse colon, 288t
Transverse myelitis, 392
Transverse plane, 461f, 461t
Traumatic cataracts, 419
Traumatic fracture, 196, 450
Triangle, in CPT, 73, 73t
TRICARE, 528, 532
Tricuspid valve, 250, 250t
  CPT coding for, 264–265
  disorders of, ICD coding for
    not specified as rheumatic, 258
    rheumatic, 254
Trigeminal nerve disorders, 394
Trimesters of pregnancy, 357
TSH; *see* Thyroid-stimulating hormone
Tube thoracostomy, 233
Tunica externa, 246t
Tunica intima, 246t
Tunica media, 246t
TURP; *see* Transurethral resection of the prostate
Tympanic membrane, 415f, 416, 416t
  CPT coding for, 429–430
  disorders of, ICD coding for, 423
Tympanoplasty, 430
Tympanostomy, 429, 429f, 438–439

UB-04 claim form, 530
UFR; *see* Uroflowmetry
Ulcer(s)
  duodenal, 291
  esophageal, 291
  gastric, 291
  gastrojejunal, 292
  peptic, 291
  pressure, 159, 161t
Ulcerative colitis, 292
Ulnar artery graft, 268
Ultrasound, 448
  abdomen, 455
  A-mode, M-mode, and B-scan, 455
  cardiac, 495
  definition of, 454
  diagnostic, CPT coding for, 454–456
  endobronchial, 232
  extremities, 455
  gallbladder, 467–468
  head and neck, 455
  obstetrical versus nonobstetrical, 455
  pelvis, 455
  retroperitoneum, 455
Ultrasound guidance, 456
Umbilical hernia, 293t
Uncertain behavior, neoplasms of, 166, 470
Unconfirmed diagnosis term, 24, 43
Unspecified behavior, of neoplasms, 166, 470
UPP; *see* Ureteral pressure profile
Upper respiratory tract, 216
  acute infections of, 219t, 220–221
  other diseases of, 219t, 221–222
Ureter(s), 323, 324f, 325, 325t
  CPT coding for, 336
  other disorders of, ICD coding for, 331
Ureter stones (calculi), 331
Ureteral pressure profile (UPP), 337

Ureterocalycostomy, 336
Ureterolysis, 336
Ureteroplasty, 336
Ureteropyelostomy, 336
Ureterostomy, 336
Ureterotomy, 336
Urethra, 323, 324f, 325, 325t
    CPT coding for, 337–338
    male, 324, 326, 326f, 327t
Urethroplasty, 337–338, 340, 342t
Urethrotomy, 337
Urinalysis, 473–474
Urinary bladder, 323, 324, 324f, 325t
    anatomy of, 324f
    CPT coding for, 337
    diverticulum of, 332
    neck obstruction, 332
    other disorders of, ICD coding for, 332
    overactive, 332
    spontaneous rupture of, 347–348
Urinary system
    anatomy of, 324–326, 324f
    components of, 323, 325t
    CPT subsection on, 333–338
        general guidelines of, 333–334
        general headings and code ranges of,
            334, 334t
        modifiers in, 340–341, 341t
        subheadings of, 334
    CPT terms for, 341, 342t
    definition of, 324
    exam questions on coding, 560–562
    functions of, 323
    ICD chapter-specific guidelines for, 23t, 41t,
        328–332, 328t
    ICD terms for, 341, 342t–343t
    other diseases of, ICD coding for, 331–332
    symptoms and signs involving, 331
    symptoms involving, 331
Urinary tract, lower, calculus of, 332
Urinary tract infection (UTI), 332, 343t
Urodynamics, CPT coding for, 337
Uroflowmetry (UFR), 337
Urteroenterostomy, 336
Urticaria, 158–159
Use additional code, 18–19, 35
Uterine fibroids, 374t, 379–381
Uterine prolapse, 354, 374t
Uterus, 352, 352f, 353t
    body of (corpus uteri), 352f, 353, 353t, 367
    CPT coding for, 367

disorders of, ICD coding for, 355–356
full-term fetus in, 352f
neck of; see Cervix uteri
rupture of, 362, 370
ultrasound of, 455
UTI; see Urinary tract infection
Uvula, CPT coding for, 301–302
Uvulectomy, 302

V codes, 521
Vaccines, CPT coding for, 489
VAD; see Ventricular assist device
Vagina, 352, 352f, 353, 353t
    CPT coding for, 365–366
    disorders of, ICD coding for, 355–356
Vaginal delivery
    CPT coding for, 370–371
    ICD coding for, 360–361
Vaginectomy, 365
Vagotomy, 305
Valves, cardiac, 249–250, 250t
    CPT coding for, 264–265
    disorders of, ICD coding for
        not specified as rheumatic, 258
        rheumatic, 254
    insufficiency of, 254
    stenosis of, 254, 265
Valvuloplasty, 494
VAP; see Ventilator associated pneumonia
Varicose veins of extremities, 261
Vas deferens, 324, 326, 326f, 327, 327t
Vascular diagnostic studies, noninvasive, 496
Vascular disease, CPT coding for, 398
Vascular injection procedures
    CPT coding for, 268–269
    first, second and third order in, 269
    nonselective versus selective placement in,
        268–269
Vascular insufficiency, of intestine, 293
Vasectomy, 340, 342t, 349–350
VATS; see Video-assisted thoracic surgery
VCUG; see Voiding cystourethrogram
Vein(s)
    CPT coding for, 262t, 268–271
    deep, 246t
    diseases of, ICD coding for, 253t, 260–261
    peripheral, 246t, 248f
    pulmonary, 246t
    superficial, 246t
Vein transposition, for hemodialysis
        access, 270

Vena cavae, 246t, 250–251, 250f
    wounds of, CPT coding for, 264
Venous embolism, ICD coding for, 260
Ventilation/perfusion scan, 236t, 459
Ventilator associated pneumonia (VAP), 223
Ventilator management, 496–497
Ventral hernia, 293t
Ventricles, cerebral, 383f, 387t
Ventricular assist device (VAD), 267
Ventricular fibrillation, 259
Ventricular septal defect (VSD), 266
Ventriculogram, 509–510
Venules, 250–251
Vertebrae, 191t
Vertebral interspace, 401
Vertebral segment, 401
Vestibular function tests, 493
Vestibule of ear, 415f, 416t
Vestibule of mouth, CPT coding for, 299
Vestibuloplasty, 299
Video-assisted thoracic surgery (VATS), 233
Virology, 476
Vision services; see also Ophthalmology
    HCPCS Level II codes for, 521
Visual acuity, 420
Visual field examinations, 493
Visual impairment, 420, 420t
Vitamin B$_{12}$ absorption studies, 458
Vitreous fluid conditions, 426
Voiding cystourethrogram (VCUG), 342t
Volvulus, 294
VSD; see Ventricular septal defect
Vulva, 352, 353, 353t
    CPT coding for, 365
    disorders of, ICD coding for, 355–356
    trauma, in delivery, 361

Waiver of liability statement on file, 537
Weber test, 433t
White blood cell count, 475
With, in ICD-10-CM, 32–33
Without, in ICD-10-CM, 32–33
Work-related evaluation services, 95
Wound care management, active, 502
Wound exploration–trauma, 198
Wrist bones, 192t

Xenografts, 171, 179t
X-rays, 448, 452f